A wellness way of life

fifth edition

GWEN ROBBINS · DEBBIE POWERS · SHARON BURGESS

Ball State University

Mc
Graw
Hill

Boston   Burr Ridge, IL   Dubuque, IA   Madison, WI   New York   San Francisco   St. Louis
Bangkok   Bogotá   Caracas   Kuala Lumpur   Lisbon   London   Madrid   Mexico City
Milan   Montreal   New Delhi   Santiago   Seoul   Singapore   Sydney   Taipei   Toronto

McGraw-Hill Higher Education

A Division of The McGraw-Hill Companies

A WELLNESS WAY OF LIFE, FIFTH EDITION

Published by McGraw-Hill, a business unit of The McGraw-Hill Companies, Inc., 1221 Avenue of the Americas, New York, NY 10020. Copyright © 2002, 1999, 1997, 1994, 1991 by The McGraw-Hill Companies, Inc. All rights reserved. No part of this publication may be reproduced or distributed in any form or by any means, or stored in a database or retrieval system, without the prior written consent of The McGraw-Hill Companies, Inc., including, but not limited to, in any network or other electronic storage or tranmission, or broadcast or distance learning.

Some ancillaries, including electronic and print components, may not be available to customers outside the United States.

 This book is printed on recycled, acid-free paper containing 10% postconsumer waste.

1 2 3 4 5 6 7 8 9 0 QPD/QPD 0 9 8 7 6 5 4 3 2 1

ISBN 0-07-235328-7

Vice president and editor-in-chief: *Thalia Dorwick*
Executive editor: *Vicki Malinee*
Developmental editor: *Lynda Huenefeld*
Senior marketing manager: *Pamela S. Cooper*
Senior project manager: *Susan J. Brusch*
Production supervisor: *Sherry L. Kane*
Coordinator of freelance design: *Michelle D. Whitaker*
Freelance cover/interior designer: *Kaye Farmer*
Cover image: *The Stock Market*
Photo research coordinator: *John C. Leland*
Supplement producer: *Jodi K. Banowetz*
Media technology producer: *Judi David*
Compositor: *Carlisle Communications, Ltd.*
Typeface: *10/12 Goudy*
Printer: *Quebecor World Dubuque, IA*

Any photos not listed below are courtesy of: Gwen Robbins, Debra Powers, Sharon Burgess

Photo Credit
Pg. 3 © Corbis/Vol. 154; p. 8: © Photodisc/Vol. 58; p. 10 top © Corbis/Vol. 85; p. 10 bottom: © Photodisc/Vol. 40; p. 13 © Photodisc/Vol 9; p. 30: © Photodisc/Vol. 51; p. 32: © Photodisc/Vol. 41; p. 36: © Photodisc/Vol. 32; p. 39: © Photodisc/Vol. 67; p. 113: © Photodisc/Vol. 46: p. 116: © Photodisc/Vol. 63; p.121: © Photodisc/Vol. 10: p. 124 © Photodisc/Vol. 46; p. 134: © Photodisc/Vol. 67; p. 138: © Corbis/Vol. 103; p. 207: © Corbis/Vol. 103; p. 207: © Photodisc/Vol. 18; p. 208: © Photodisc/Vol. 67; p. 212: © Photodisc/Vol. 51; p. 235: © Photodisc/Vol. 54; p. 243: © Photodisc/Vol. 25; p. 245: © Corbis/Vol. 124; p. 246: © Photodisc/Vol. 58; p. 247: © Photodisc/Vol. 40; p. 251: © Photodisc/Vol. 18; p. 271: © Photodisc/Vol. 41; p. 278; © Photodisc/Website; p. 284: © Photodisc/Vol. 67; p. 284: © Photodisc/Vol. 67; p. 323: © Photodisc/Vol. 58; p. 336: © Corbis/Vol. 115; p. 339: © Photodisc/Vol. 48; p. 344: © Photodisc/Vol. 48; p. 345: © Photodisc/Vol. 67; p. 376: © Photodisc/Vol. 67; p. 377: © Photodisc/Vol. 45; p. 380 © Photodisc/Website; p. 387: © Photodisc/Vol. 20; p. 390: © Photodisc/Vol. 51; p. 395: © Corbis/Vol. 32; p. 417: © Photodisc/Vol. 18; p. 419: © Photodisc/Vol. 67; p. 420: © Photodisc/Vol. 67; p. 426: © Corbis/Vol. 94; p. 427: © Photodisc/Vol. 67; p. 459: © Photodisc/Vol. 18; p. 466: © Photodisc/Website; p. 469: © Photodisc/Vol. 25; p. 476: © Photodisc/Website; p. 501: © Corbis/Vol. 94; p. 506: © Photodisc/Vol. 25; p. 522: © Photodisc/Vol. 35; p. 524: © Photodisc/Vol. 63; p. 527: © Photodisc/Vol. 35; p. 529: © Photodisc/Vol. 40; p. 531: © Photodisc/Vol. 51

The Internet addresses listed in the text were accurate at the time of publication. The inclusion of a website does not indicate an endorsement by the authors or McGraw-Hill, and McGraw-Hill does not guarantee the accuracy of the information presented at these sites.

www.mhhe.com

brief contents

contents

chapter 4

Pursuing Lifetime Exercise Activities   111

chapter 8

Coping with Stress   267

chapter 9

Preventing Common Injuries and Caring for the Lower Back   311

chapter 10

Eating for Wellness   335

chapter 11

Aiming for a Healthy Weight   375

chapter 12

Preventing Cancer   413

chapter 13

Understanding Substance Abuse and Addictive Behavior   445

chapter 14

Preventing Sexually Transmitted Disease   495

chapter 15

Planning Wellness for a Lifetime   519

preface

This book is about enjoying life—living it to your fullest potential. The purpose of *A Wellness Way of Life* is to help you pursue a wellness lifestyle. Everyone has a wellness goal—lose a couple of pounds, quit smoking, start exercising, learn how to eat right, manage stress. But how do you make that goal a reality? *A Wellness Way of Life* can motivate and guide you toward making positive, healthy lifestyle changes that last.

We wanted to provide a book that would present a body of knowledge that goes beyond fitness. This knowledge helps you make informed, responsible decisions affecting your wellness. However, we know it takes much more than knowledge. It takes personal commitment, self-management skills, and coping strategies to live a healthy lifestyle. Therefore, a primary focus of this book is identifying behavior changes that you can easily incorporate into your life. Our goal is not only to deliver fitness and health information, but also to motivate and guide you toward making positive choices.

Abraham Lincoln said, "We are about as happy as we make up our minds to be." We believe that one secret to happiness is having the competence and confidence to make informed decisions that affect your daily well-being. Self-responsibility and self-empowerment are means of increasing the quality and quantity of life. There is no better feeling than to know that you are doing something good for yourself! As you read each chapter, you will learn strategies for taking control of your life and discover the joy in traveling the wellness journey. This book will help you wade through the myriad of health and wellness information and ultimately make you an informed wellness consumer. The result will be the indescribable joy in knowing you are attaining your highest potential for well-being.

Audience

This text is designed to meet the needs of a course that goes beyond the basics of physical fitness to encompass the broader scope of wellness. The content—covering all aspects of fitness, heart health, stress management, nutrition, weight management, and substance use and abuse—easily accommodates a variety of fitness, wellness, and health courses. It is a flexible book that fits nicely into a lecture/fitness activity format. The text has been classroom-tested since the late 1980s in one of the first fitness/wellness programs that started the trend sweeping the nation.

New Features in This Edition

Based on the idea of self-responsibility, *A Wellness Way of Life* gives students practical information about how to make good decisions that will positively affect their well-being throughout their lives. It's an open, accessible resource that minimizes technical jargon and presents health as a positive, dynamic process. New features for this fifth edition include:

- New four-color design brings the book to life and helps to easily identify important information.
- Updated information on national objectives for physical activity from *Healthy People 2010*.
- Expanded information on the spiritual dimension of wellness.
- Updated facts, figures, and statistics included in every chapter.
- Prochaska's Transtheoretical Model of Behavior Change has been thoroughly explained and expanded.
- Exciting and practical learning activity labs that include HealthQuest activities are located in each chapter.
- Expanded information broadens students' understanding of eating disorders, heart health, weight management, prevention of date rape, STDs, and stress management.

- Two additional principles of fitness development have been added—The Principle of Reversibility and The Principle of Individual Differences.
- New chapter, "Pursuing Lifetime Exercise Activities," includes information on a number of fitness activities and how to pursue them properly.
- New *2000 Dietary Guidelines* are included.
- New information included on fiber, trans fats, calcium (osteoporosis), antioxidants, phytochemicals, and phytoestrogens.
- Cancer chapter expanded to include new information on the contribution of diet to cancer risk and top cancer-fighting foods and a section on coping with cancer.
- Top Ten lists that give important information on various topics are now included in each chapter.
- Interesting tidbits of fitness and wellness trivia included in each chapter as a Wellness Flash.
- Boxes featuring information about Diversity Issues included in each chapter.
- Appendix includes Nutrition Values of Popular Fast Foods.

Why the Prochaska Transtheoretical Model of Behavior Change?

The Prochaska transtheoretical model of behavior change is included in this text because of its proven effectiveness in changing behavior. This revolutionary new model presents concrete strategies rather than vague resolutions to help people make permanent lifestyle changes. Psychologists James Prochaska, John Norcross, and Carlo DiClemente studied individuals who had successfully changed health-related behaviors on their own. What these researchers discovered during their years of studying behavior change is that individuals progress through distinct stages of change on their way to improved well-being. Their initial research was done on people who quit smoking but has expanded to cover other health behaviors. The stages of change are as follows:

1. *Precontemplation.* People at this stage see no problem with their behavior and have no intention of changing it.
2. *Contemplation.* In this stage, people come to understand their problem and its causes, and they start to think about taking action to solve it.
3. *Preparation.* In the preparation stage, people are planning to take action within the next month and are putting together a plan of action.
4. *Action.* A person in the action stage has taken the leap and is actively making behavior changes.

5. *Maintenance.* Even after action has been taken successfully, it must be maintained to prevent relapse.

Prochaska and his colleagues noted that certain behavioral change techniques work better than others in some stages of change. This model has received a great deal of attention in the popular press and among health educators. Prochaska, et al. published a successful trade book called *Changing for Good* on how to use their model to change behavior successfully. We hope this method assists you in your wellness journey.

Pedagogical Highlights

A Wellness Way of Life includes a number of built-in resources that make learning easy:

Chapter Objectives

Found at the beginning of each chapter, the objectives provide a starting point and focus for readers.

Key Terms

Important terms are highlighted in boldface to catch students' attention, increase retention, and indicate glossary terms.

Top 10 Lists

Located throughout each chapter, the Top 10 boxes give additional insight to topics discussed. Includes such topics as "Top 10 Ways to Protect Your Heart" and "Top 10 Immune System Boosters."

Wellness Flash

These boxes are located throughout each chapter and highlight interesting facts such as how many people are diagnosed with diabetes every day.

Diversity Issues

Located throughout the text, this feature discusses fitness and wellness issues for various cultures and ethnic backgrounds. Important topics such as the nutritional value of foods from different countries and the occurrence of heart disease among different genders and races appear throughout the chapters.

Using HealthQuest

Each chapter contains a new lab to complement the HealthQuest CD-ROM that accompanies the text. These activities allow students to assess their health behavior in nine areas.

Chapter Summary

The key points from each chapter are summarized at the end to increase student comprehension and retention of vital information.

Internet Addresses

Selected Internet sites are included to help students explore wellness topics outside of the classroom.

Resources

A listing of additional current resources is provided to encourage further exploration.

Activity Labs

Located at the end of each chapter, these labs help students apply chapter information into everyday action.

Appendices

These include a nutritional value table on fast food restaurants, as well as additional worksheets for classroom use.

Supplements

Course Integrator Guide

This manual includes all the features of a useful instructor's manual, including learning objectives, suggested lecture outlines, suggested activities, media resources, and web links. It also integrates the text with all the health resources McGraw-Hill offers, such as the HealthQuest CD, the Online Learning Center, the Visual Resource Library, the AIDS booklet, the video clips CD, and the Health and Human Performance Discipline Page. The guide also includes references to relevant print and broadcast media. (0-07-244466-5)

HealthQuest 3.0 by Bob Gold and Nancy Atkinson

HealthQuest 3.0 comes free with new texts and helps students explore the behavioral aspects of wellness through a state-of-the-art interactive CD-ROM. Your students will be able to assess their current health and wellness status, determine their health risks, and explore options to improve the behaviors that will impact their health.

Online Learning Center

This website offers resources to students and instructors. It includes downloadable ancillaries, web links, student quizzing, additional information on topics of interest and much, much more.

Resources for the instructor include:

- Downloadable PowerPoint Presentation
- Lecture outlines
- Discussion questions
- Concept summaries

Resources for the student include:

- Flashcards
- Online chapter reviews
- Interactive quizzes

Micro Test III Computerized Test Bank

Available on Hybrid CD for Windows and Macintosh, the latest version of our computerized testing software is available. This allows you to custom design your own tests, use the expanded test bank, and to add your own testing questions. (0-07-235332-5)

Test Bank

This printed manual includes multiple choice, true/false, and fill in the blank questions for each chapter. All questions have been entered into the computerized test bank. (0-07-235330-9)

PageOut: The Course Website Development Center

PageOut enables you to develop a website for your course. The site includes:

- A course home page
- An instructor home page
- A syllabus (interactive, customizable, and includes quizzing, instructor notes, and links to the Online Learning Center)
- Web links
- Discussions (multiple discussion areas per class)
- An online grade book
- Student web pages
- Design templates

This program is now available to registered adopters of McGraw-Hill textbooks.

Visual Resource Library

The Visual Resource Library is a bank of images for use in the classroom and in the accompanying PowerPoint presentation.

A slide editor tool allows the user to create customized slide shows. (0-07-244469-X)

Fitsolve II Software

This enhances learning of health-related fitness concepts by personalizing information and by explaining the meaning of the results rather than just merely "grading students" as other programs do. It begins with a coronary heart disease risk questionnaire, followed by input of fitness test scores. Features include score summary, heart attack risk categorization, and health-related fitness status. (Windows 0-697-33950-5)

The AIDS Booklet 6/e, by Frank Cox

This booklet provides current facts about AIDS and HIV: what it is, how the virus is transmitted, its prevalence among various population groups, symptoms of HIV infection, strategies for prevention, etc. It also covers the legal, social, medical, and ethical issues related to AIDS and HIV. After publication, additional updates are posted to the website at http://www.mhhe.com/catalogs/sem/hhp/student. It is available for $1.00 when combined with any McGraw-Hill product to create a package. (0-697-29428-5)

Testwell by the National Wellness Institute

This is a self-scoring, pencil-and-paper wellness assessment developed by the National Wellness Institute in Stevens Point, Wisconsin, and distributed exclusively by McGraw-Hill Publishers. It adds flexibility to any personal health or wellness course by allowing adopters to offer pre- and post-assessments at the beginning, end, or at anytime during the course. (0-697-21131-2)

Diet and Fitness Log by McGraw-Hill

This logbook helps students track their diet and exercise programs. It serves as a diary to help students log their behaviors. It may be packaged with Corbin for an additional $1.00. (0-8151-2524-0)

FoodWise College Edition 2.0

Based on the widely tested professional version of Food-Works, this dietary analysis software has been developed for use in college courses. It offers a variety of functions based on the latest release of the USDA database. FoodWise College Edition 2.0 features a novice-friendly interface and contains approximately 7,500 foods. It generates a wide variety of standard, easy-to-grade reports and allows the user to add their own foods to the database. (0-07-243775-8)

Health & Human Performance Discipline Page

http://www.mhhe.com/hhp
McGraw-Hill's Health and Human Performance Discipline Page provides a wide variety of information for instructors and students—including monthly articles about current issues, monthly articles that celebrate our diversity, text ancillaries, a "how to" guide to technology, study tips, and athletic training exam preparation materials. It includes professional organization, convention, and career information, and includes information on how to become a McGraw-Hill author. Additional features of the Discipline Page include:

- *This Just In*—This feature provides information on the latest hot topics, the best web resources, and more—all updated monthly!
- *Faculty Support*—Access online course supplements such as lecture outlines and PowerPoint presentations, and create your own course website with PageOut!
- *Student Success Center*—Find online study guides and other resources to improve your academic performance. Explore scholarship opportunities, and learn how to launch your career!
- *Author Arena*—Interested in writing a textbook or supplement for the college market? Read the McGraw-Hill proposal guidelines and links to the Editorial and Marketing teams, and meet and converse with our current authors!

Acknowledgements

We would like to thank the reviewers of our earlier four editions of this text: Christopher A. Ayres (East Tennessee State University), Bonnie Marrs (East Tennessee State University), Thomas Battinelli (Fitchburg State College), Lisa Farley (Butler University), Ergun Yurdadon (Butler University), Debra Felice (Jefferson Community College), Jeffrey Wiley (Jefferson Community College), Edna Gillis (Valdosta State University), Richard Wilkinson (Cochise College), Ben Davidson (Southern Utah University), Brian F. Geiger (University of Alabama at Birmingham), Detty Moore (Lamar University), Mary P. Schleirmacher (Keuka College), Carl Stockton (Radford University), Kathy Noe (University of Iowa).

Don Bergey (Wake Forest University), Robert Case (Sam Houston State University), Sally Hokanson (Gustavus Adolphus University), Cameron Howes (Northern Michigan University), Nancy Meyer (Calvin College), Max Oldham (Missouri Southern State College), Jim Scott (Jackson Community College), James A. Streater (Armstrong State College), Larry Thouin (L. A. Pierce College), Cheryl Tucker (Northeast Missouri State University),

Roberta Verley (Northern Michigan University), and Earl Watson (University of West Florida).

John S. Carter (The Citadel), Denyce Stokes (Ford-Howard University), Jean Martin Frazier (East Tennessee State University), Warren Hammer (University of Richmond), Cindy L. Hanawalt (University of Iowa), Patsy Livingston (Point Loma Nazarene College), Jeryl J. Neff (University of Wisconsin–Superior), Cynthia J. Petri (University of Alabama–Birmingham), Jacquie Rainey, Michael L. Teague (University of Iowa), and Donna J. Terbizan (North Dakota State University).

Thomas L. Dezelsky (Arizona State University), Robert Koslow (James Madison University), Rebecca R. Leas (Clarion University), Patsy Livingston (Point Loma Nazarene College), Jacqueline T. Poythress (Dekalb College), and Timothy Voss (Trinity College).

We would especially like to thank the reviewers of this edition for their time and assistance:

Kitty Baird
Centre College

Martha E. Beagle
Berea College

Todd Bowden
John Brown University

John Burgess
Suffolk Community College

Lisa Farley,
Eugenia Scott
Butler University

Debra Felice
Jefferson Community College, Watertown, NY

David Harackiewicz
Central Connecticut State University

Diane Lowry
Kennesaw State University

Sharon G. Rifkin
Broward Community College

Barbara Saperstone
Northern Virginia Community College

Mary P. Schleiermacher
Keuka College

Amy Jo Sutterlwety
Baldwin Wallace College

Judith D. Walton
University of Texas–Brownsville

Tillman (Chuck) Williams
Southwest Missouri State University

Ben Zhou
California State University at Dominquez Hills

We wish to express our gratitude to the following individuals for their assistance in the development of this book:

Sam Minor II, Department of Art, College of Fine Arts, Ball State University for artwork

Edgar Self and John Huffer for photography

Margaret Phillips, Boung Jin Kang, Chris Powers, Melissa Smith, Kelley Jarvis, Erika Hogan, Karlyn Rent, Jamie Troxell and Lowell Faison for modeling for photographs.

A very generous thank you goes to the dedicated Physical Education Fitness/Wellness (PEFWL) faculty for their vigorous commitment to quality teaching.

Special recognition is extended to Dr. John Reno, Chair, School of Physical Education, Dr. Donald F. Smith, Dean of the College of Applied Sciences and Technology, and Dr. C. Warren Vander Hill, Provost and Vice President for Academic Affairs for their continuing support of the fitness/wellness program at Ball State University. We are fortunate to have administrators who have the vision to recognize that participating in a fitness/wellness program will have a positive impact on students' lives now and in the future.

We dedicate this fifth edition to our families for their love and continuing support.

Gwen Robbins
Debbie Powers
Sharon Burgess

Life is not merely to be alive, but to be well.
Martial

1

Understanding Wellness

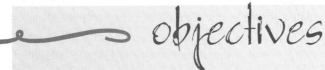 **objectives**

After reading this chapter, you will be able to:
1. Explain the relationship between lifestyle and health/longevity.
2. Explain the focus of the publication *Healthy People 2010.*
3. List ten health habits that, when practiced, can reduce the risk of health problems.
4. Distinguish between health and wellness.
5. Define *wellness*.
6. Identify the seven dimensions of wellness, and give three examples within each dimension.
7. List and describe the six factors that influence growth in wellness, as shown on the wellness wheel.
8. Give four examples of ways society supports wellness and four examples of ways society detracts from wellness.

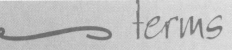 **terms**

- Emotional dimension
- Environmental dimension
- Extrinsic motivation
- Health
- Health promotion
- Intellectual dimension
- Intrinsic motivation
- Occupational dimension
- Physical dimension
- Social dimension
- Societal norm
- Spiritual dimension
- Wellness

As Rob lay in the coronary care unit, his eyes surveyed various tubes and wires connected to his tired body. The nightmare of the last 24 hours was over, but the pain and confusion lingered.

"How can this be? I'm only 49 years old. How could I have had a heart attack? What if I die? What about my wife? My son? My daughter? I've just become a grandpa. I was given a big promotion at work. Why now?" Rob's mind drifted.

"But I'm an athlete! Well, I *was* an athlete, back in high school. Once I started college there was no time for sports or exercise. Started smoking, too. Figured I'd stop when the pressure was off, but the pressure never stopped. Drank too much, too; partied a lot. Still like several drinks to end the day. I always thought I'd lose those extra 30 pounds—always next year, always a New Year's resolution. Diet? Too busy. Vending machines, hot dog stands, snacks in front of the TV, fast food. No time. Too much to do. Money to make. A lot of stress. Can't stop now. There'll be time later."

Rob's mind drifted back to his room. He could hear his doctor's voice—"stop smoking. Change in lifestyle. Low-fat diet. Start exercising. Cholesterol is 280. Break old habits." Rob thought, "How I wish I could turn back the clock!"

This scenario is too common in the United States. More than half of all deaths in this country are attributed to coronary heart disease and stroke. Although most heart attacks occur after middle age, many are a result of years of lifestyle abuse. Table 1-1 lists the leading causes of death in the United States. One hundred years ago the leading causes of death were infectious diseases such as tuberculosis, polio, diphtheria, pneumonia, and influenza and various diseases of infancy. Advances in medicine, the discovery of antibiotics, and improved sanitation diminished these ravaging diseases and in-

creased the average life span. Through scientific discovery, technology, industrial growth, and automation, the entire American lifestyle has changed. We use remote controls to change television channels and to open garage doors. Appliances wash our clothes, dishes, and teeth. We ride vehicles to work, school, and even while playing golf. "Surfing the 'Net" is much more popular than surfing the ocean. We allow ourselves to be bused and trucked, elevated and escalated, and then wonder why we grow fat and are out of shape. This so-called "good life" has created sedentary living, changes in eating habits (fast foods, increased fats and sweets, processed foods), stress, alcohol and drug abuse, and obesity. Although social scientists predicted in the 1960s that technology would create a future of abundant leisure time, most of us face an unrelenting pace of increased expectations and demands. Chronic hurrying has created chronic stress. Life feels out of balance. As Mahatma Gandhi once said, "There is more to life than increasing its speed."

Statistics released by the American Heart Association are startling. In a single year, diseases of the heart and blood vessels kill far more Americans than were killed in World Wars I and II, the Korean War, and the Vietnam War, combined. Those who survive a coronary incident are often faced with a restricted, less fulfilling life that causes an unnecessary, costly drain on the resources available for health care. Such horrendous figures should outrage the public and should cause a de-

table 1-1   Leading Causes of Death in the United States

All Ages	Ages 15–24	Ages 25–44
1 Heart disease 726,974	1. Accidents	1. Accidents
2. Cancer 539,577	2. Homicide	2. Cancer
3. Stroke 226,136	3. Suicide	3. Heart disease
4. Chronic obstructive lung disease 109,029	4. Cancer	4. Suicide
5. Accidents 95,644	5. Heart disease	5. HIV
6. Pneumonia and influenza 86,449	6. Congenital anomalies	6. Homicide
7. Diabetes mellitus 64,574	7. HIV	7. Chronic liver disease and cirrhosis

Source: Centers for Disease Control and Prevention, National Center of Health Statistics, National Vital Statistics Systems, 1999.

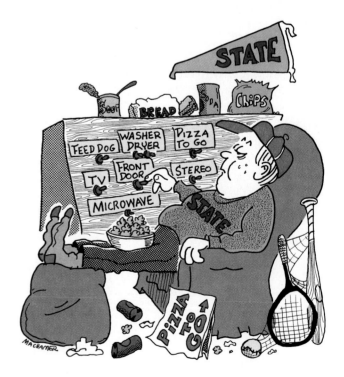

The "good life"?

mand for reform, because carnage is normally the basis for alarm and legislation. Instead, apathy is the general response of many. Good health is often taken for granted until it is lost.

The harsh truth is that a high percentage of disease and disability affecting the American people is preventable, a consequence of unwise behavior and lifestyle choices. The decision to smoke, for instance, is responsible for one of every six deaths in the United States each year. Twenty-one percent of heart disease deaths, 87 percent of lung cancer deaths, and 30 percent of cancer deaths are linked to smoking. Smoking costs our society over $100 billion annually in health care costs and lost productivity. Also, in 2000, cardiovascular disease cost the nation an estimated $326 billion in health care expenditure and lost productivity. This burden is growing as the population ages. Information from the Centers for Disease Control and Prevention states that as much as two-thirds of disability and death up to age 65 would be preventable in total or in part if we applied what we know about the effects of lifestyle on premature illness and death. Former U.S. Surgeon General C. Everett Koop states, "We are in an era of self-induced premature deaths." Figures 1-1 and 1-2 illustrate the extent to which our longevity is affected by a combination of our lifestyle decisions.

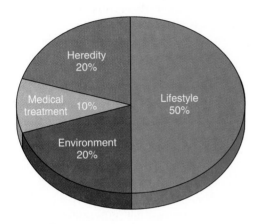

Figure 1-1   Factors affecting longevity.
Our longevity is affected by a combination of factors—only heredity is beyond our power.

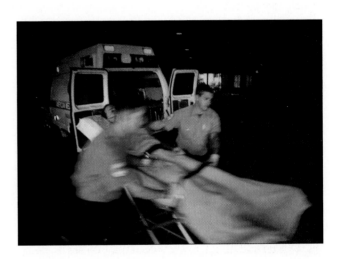

Heart disease, the number one killer of Americans, is considered a "lifestyle" disease.

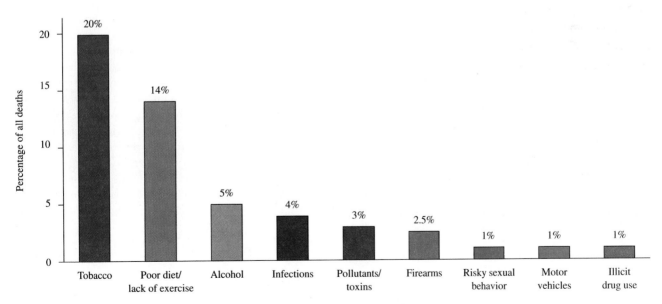

Figure 1-2   Contributors to premature deaths in the United States.
Source: National Center of Health Statistics, National Vital Statistics Systems, 1999

wellness flash

Sixty-three percent of adolescents possess two or more risk behaviors for heart disease and cancer. The five risk behaviors are:

*1. Consuming too few fruits and vegetables.
*2. Consuming too many high-fat foods.
 3. A sedentary lifestyle.
 4. Smoking.
 5. Binge drinking.

*The two most frequently occurring risk behaviors.

You may already possess some knowledge about these and other health topics. If you are like most, however, you underestimate your future risk of lifestyle diseases. Studies show that many adolescents already possess several risk factors that can lead to chronic diseases. Underestimation of your risk is of substantial concern because action should be an outcome of your health knowledge. After all, the truly educated individual understands cause and effect. Nevertheless, many young adults are much more interested in the present than the future. The evidence is clear—health and longevity are not solely a result of genetics and luck but an outcome of personal behavior. This personal behavior involves responsible choices, self-discipline, and a commitment to wellness.

This chapter introduces the basic concept of health, the impact of lifestyle on well-being, and the dynamics of high-level wellness. You will see that the news is exciting! Wellness living and healthy lifestyle interventions that begin early in life can shape your health destiny.

Concepts of Health

Traditionally **health** has been viewed as the "lack of disease." If you show no signs or symptoms of illness, you are healthy. Health is seen as a state of being. You are either ill or healthy. Some health-care facilities still reflect this simplistic view. Many insurance companies pay for treatments and hospitalization when sickness occurs but pay nothing for preventive checkups or procedures. Employers allow "sick days," yet personal days or vacation days must be used for pursuing health-promoting activities. Because of this curative focus, a majority of our health-care dollars are spent on procedures for patching people up after the damage has been done. Billions of dollars are spent to treat the results of bad eating and drinking habits, stress, sedentary living, and smoking. This is a "sickness-care" system rather than a "health-care" system. Because of the medical procedures, drugs, and technologies presently available, many people have become complacent about their health habits. They think they can be "bailed out" by medical science (at the cost of billions of dollars a year to society).

Expanding the focus of health to include many different aspects of life (social, psychological, spiritual, and so on) as well as empowering individual responsibility involves health promotion. **Health promotion** is the science and art of helping people change their lifestyles to move toward a state of optimal health. Health promotion involves systematic efforts by organizations to create healthy policies and supportive environments as well as the reorienting of health services to include more than clinical and curative care. Lifestyle change is motivated not by knowledge alone, but also by supportive social environments and the availability of facilitative services. Examples of health promotion programs are weight-loss workshops, smoking cessation clinics, and stress management seminars. Laws and policies such as those prohibiting drunk driving, those curtailing pollution, and those establishing smoke-free workplaces also assist in health promotion.

Another trend in health care is renewed emphasis on medical self-care. Medical self-care includes all actions taken by an individual with respect to a medical problem. It accounts for 85 percent to 95 percent of all medical care. Medical self-care promotes self-sufficiency in diagnosis and requires decision making about whether a physician's services are needed. It is usually used for minor illnesses or injuries such as colds, flu, cuts, and sprains. Individual decision making becomes the focus. Do I need a physician for this problem? What can I do for myself? What can I expect from the health-care profession? However, medical self-care goes beyond minor illness. Individuals with diabetes, asthma, and allergies have a major responsibility for their own care. Even emergency procedures such as cardiopulmonary resuscitation (CPR) and the Heimlich maneuver fall into the realm of medical self-care. No longer are thermometers the only diagnostic tool in home medicine cabinets. It is now common to find blood pressure kits, home pregnancy tests, colon-rectal cancer detection kits, and blood sugar and cholesterol self-tests. The purpose of self-care is not to replace the physician but to promote personal responsibility for health, rather than total dependence on physicians.

Lifestyle and Health

The preventive aspects of health have become increasingly clear, and research studies often become instant headlines (e.g., Which is better . . . butter or margarine? coffee or tea? protein or carbohydrate?). Sometimes the information is only partially reported, resulting in confusion, contradiction, even sensationalism. Bewildered and wary, many Americans reject or ignore many legitimate health pronouncements: *Cut fat to under 30 percent of calories. Exercise aerobically 30 minutes five times per week. Eat five or more fruits and vegetables daily.* Regardless of the messages, a majority of present-day Americans continue to be sedentary and overweight. Stress levels and blood cholesterol readings continue to soar. Though the relationship between lifestyle and health is clear, adopting healthy lifestyle habits has been difficult for many.

Healthy People 2010

Because of the concern for our nation's health and vitality, a vigorous national crusade for health promotion has been initiated. *Healthy People 2010: Understanding and Improving Health*, is a publication facilitated by the U.S. Department of Health and Human Services. *Healthy People 2010* is a statement of national opportunities and challenges communities to support health-promoting policies.

This document is a road map for improving the health of all people in the United States during the first decade of the twenty-first century. *Healthy People 2010* is committed to one overarching purpose: promoting health and preventing illness, disability, and premature death. The document identifies two broad goals as the means of bringing about fuller human potential:

1. Increase quality and years of healthy life
2. Eliminate health disparities

To achieve these goals, 467 objectives have been targeted for the year 2010 in areas including environmental health, violence, cancer prevention, and obesity reduction among others.

Table 1-2 lists a few of the objectives found in *Healthy People 2010*. Because of the diversity and varying needs of Americans, reaching these goals is a challenge. (See Diversity Issues.) Nevertheless, the federal government is playing a leadership role in cultivating a culture of healthier, life-enhancing habits for all Americans, regardless of income, race, sex, or other status. We must do our part to help. The current national health expenditure has more than tripled since 1980. More than $1 trillion is spent annually in the United States on treating disease—more than any other country in the world. Unfortunately, only 4 percent goes toward prevention. America is great at expensive, heroic care but very poor at low-cost preventive care.

Many of the proposals in *Healthy People 2010* to eliminate disease and create health are linked to everyday practices. Therefore, it is up to each of us to develop strategies for incorporating healthy habits into our daily lives. Look at the Top Ten Lifestyle Practices That Enhance Wellness. How many of these habits do you practice?

There is nothing extreme or magical in this list. It does shift the main responsibility for health to the individual, rather than relegating the individual to a position of passivity amidst excessive surgeries, medications, and medical

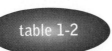

A Sample of Health Objectives from *Healthy People 2010*

table 1-2

- Increase moderate or vigorous daily physical activity to at least 60 percent of all ages/populations (currently 38 percent)
- Reduce cigarette smoking prevalence to no more than 12 percent of all adults (currently 25 percent)
- Reduce overall breast cancer deaths to 22.2 per 100,000 females (currently 27.7)
- Increase the use of seatbelts to 92 percent of the population (currently 69 percent)
- Reduce obesity to a prevalence of no more than 15 percent of adults (current 22.3 percent)
- Increase the daily consumption of vegetables to 3 or more servings per person for 50 percent of the population (currently 3 percent)
- Reduce overall colorectal cancer deaths to 13.9 per 100,000 people (currently 21.1)
- Reduce coronary heart disease deaths to no more than 166 per 100,000 people (currently 208)
- Increase to 75 percent the number of people who consume 30 percent or less of calories from fats (currently 33 percent)
- Increase the use of sun protection measures to 75 percent of the total population (currently 49 percent)

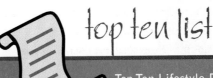

top ten list

Top Ten Lifestyle Practices That Enhance Wellness

1. Exercise aerobically at least four to five times per week.
2. Eliminate all tobacco products.
3. Limit animal fats, cholesterol, and saturated fats in the diet.
4. Eat at least five daily servings of fruits and vegetables, and include other high fiber foods and whole grains every day in the diet.
5. Assess personal stressors, and practice stress management techniques.
6. Limit the consumption of alcohol to no more than one drink (women) or two drinks (men) per day.
7. Pursue and maintain a healthy weight.
8. Fasten seat belts.
9. Practice safe sex habits.
10. Balance work; social; and personal time, including getting seven to nine hours of sleep every night.

tests. One physician has appropriately summarized the issue by stating, "One of my frustrations in medicine was having people come to me expecting way too much of me and not expecting anything of themselves."

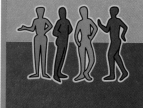

diversity issues

Although the diversity of the American population may be one of our nation's greatest assets, diversity also presents a range of health improvement challenges. *Healthy People 2010* identifies 93 areas in which the disparity between the general population and at least one select population is 25 percent or greater. A few examples of major disparities include:

- HIV/AIDS is the eighth leading cause of death for the total population, but the leading cause of death for African American men ages 25–44.
- Native Americans suffer from Type 2 diabetes 3 times the average rate.
- Lung cancer kills twice as many men as women.
- African American women die from breast cancer 1.3 times more than white women, 2 times more than Hispanic women, and almost 3 times more than Native Americans.
- Lower income persons consume fewer fruits and vegetables than those with higher income levels.

- African American men suffer from heart disease twice the rate of other men.
- Whites die from lung cancer 2 1/2 times more than Hispanics.
- Whites suffer 1 1/2 times more coronary heart disease deaths than Native Americans.
- African Americans and Hispanics are generally less active than whites.
- Major depression affects approximately twice as many women as men.
- Forty percent of white teens smoke, compared to 25 percent of white adults (over age 18)
- People from households with an annual income of at least $25,000 live an average of 3 to 7 years longer than people from households with annual incomes of less than $10,000.
- African American men die from prostate cancer more than twice the rate of other men.

"Lifestyle" consists of patterns of behavior in the *circumstances of one's life*. It is our responsibility, individually and collectively as a highly industrialized society, to create the circumstances of life and ways of living in those circumstances to live long and well. To evaluate your personal lifestyle habits, look to *Healthy Lifestyle: A Self-Assessment*, Lab Activity 1-1.

Understanding Risks

Often in this book we will talk about risks. In an effort to prevent disease and to promote health, it is important to identify the factors that cause disease and injury. From this, probabilities are determined as to the chances for occurrence. Like placing a bet at a race track, identifying risks is a way of quoting the odds. No one can honestly promise you that doing something or refraining from doing it will keep you safe or that doing one thing will positively kill you. You must draw your own conclusions from the evidence. There is no such thing as absolute safety, so you only can choose to widen or narrow your risk margins with your habits.

One ongoing study has resulted in much of the information we know about the risk factors associated with coronary heart disease. The people of Framingham, Massachusetts, a community 18 miles west of Boston, have been studied and charted since 1950. The Framingham Study, as it has become known, has resulted in information about how heredity, environment, medical care, and lifestyle factors affect heart disease and well-being. A comprehensive longitudinal study such as this, in contrast to a short-term, isolated study involving few people, results in reputable data. We hope you are thinking beyond mere "risk avoidance" to a life full of enrichment, self-fulfillment, and satisfaction. This dramatic shift in emphasis toward self-responsibility and an expanded quality of life has evolved into a concept called *wellness*.

High-Level Wellness

It is reassuring to know that we have a considerable amount of control over our health destiny. However, what are the upper limits of health? What is the ultimate in health? In the late 1950s, Dr. Halbert Dunn first used the term *wellness* in his writings about the pursuit of optimal well-being. He talked about "health" as a relatively passive state of existence—in contrast to "wellness," which he described as an everchanging process of growth toward an *elevated* state of superb well-being. Today, **wellness** is defined as *an integrated and dynamic level of functioning oriented toward maximizing potential, depend-*

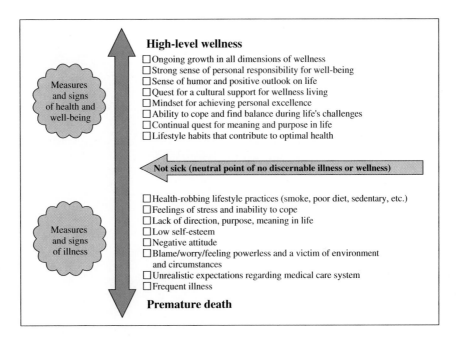

Figure 1-3   Wellness/illness continuum.
In the boxes to the left of the descriptors, check off how many fit you. In which direction are you traveling on the wellness continuum?

ent upon self-responsibility. Wellness involves not only preventive health behaviors, but a shift in *thinking* and *attitude*. Wellness is a mind-set of lifelong growth and achievement in the emotional, spiritual, physical, occupational, intellectual, environmental, and social dimensions. It means a lifetime of striving toward ever-higher levels of functioning.

High-level wellness is applicable to all ages (old and young), all socioeconomic groups (poor and wealthy), and all types of people (able-bodied and disabled). It means working toward becoming the best you can be without accepting "traditional" limitations (i.e., age, race, gender, genetics). Wellness is a way of living in which growth and improvement are sought in all areas. It involves a lifestyle of deliberate choices and self-responsibility, requiring conscientious management and planning. Living a wellness lifestyle does not come about by accident or luck. It also involves much more than curing sickness, counting fat grams, jogging, or measuring body fat. It is a *mind-set* of personal empowerment. It means approaching life with optimism, confidence, and energy. Unlike sickness-care, which involves treatment, wellness is a lifelong quest toward optimal functioning in which *you* take charge. It involves accepting the changes in life while seeking the positive payoffs of change. Individuals who strive for wellness have an exceptional openness to experience. Rather than fearing new experiences and life's changes, they welcome them as a way to grow. They do not allow prejudices or stereotypes to distort their perceptions. They take control of life and face it with creativity and freshness. Living a wellness lifestyle has good

potential for increasing longevity. However, this is not the sole purpose of wellness living. Wellness author and advocate Donald Ardell agrees. He states, "Wellness is not a goal to be attained but a process to be maintained."

Figure 1-3 shows a wellness/illness continuum. You do not attain a "state of wellness" and then stop. Your personal choices dictate whether you are moving upward toward high-level wellness or downward away from your wellness potential.

The Dimensions of Wellness

The wellness lifestyle is a coordinated and integrated living pattern involving seven dimensions: physical, intellectual, emotional, social, spiritual, environmental, and occupational. There is a strong interdependence between dimensions, though they function separately. For example, joining an exercise class in your community most notably enhances your physical well-being. But it can also be socially enriching and intellectually stimulating as you learn more about the functional capacity of the human body. It can also help relieve emotional stress. Attending the class with coworkers after work may improve your occupational wellness. In each dimension there is opportunity for personal growth, and, due to the dimensions' interrelationships, growth in one area often sparks interest in another. *Balancing* these dimensions, however, is important in pursuing wellness. For example, being an avid reader yet not being able to get along with anyone is not an example of balanced wellness.

Physical Dimension

The **physical dimension** deals with the functional operation of the body. Ask yourself if your body is the best machine possible. The physical dimension involves the health-related components of physical fitness—muscular strength, muscular endurance, cardiorespiratory endurance, flexibility, and body composition. Dietary habits have a significant effect on physical well-being. Your sexual, drinking, and drug behaviors also play a role in physical health. Do you smoke? Do you get an adequate amount of sleep? Are you overweight? Do you catch many colds? These questions deal with physical health.

The physical dimension also includes medical self-care—regular self-tests, checkups, proper use of medications, taking necessary steps when you are ill, and appropriate use of the medical system. Managing your environment also affects physical well-being. For example, do you try to minimize your exposure to tobacco smoke and harmful pollutants? Positive health habits are critical to physical well-being.

Intellectual Dimension

The **intellectual dimension** involves the use of your mind. Maintaining an active mind contributes to total well-being. Intellectual growth is not restricted to formal education— that is, school learning. It involves a continuous acquisition of knowledge throughout life, engaging your mind in creative and stimulating mental activities. Curiosity and learning should never stop. Reading, writing, and keeping abreast of current events are intellectual pursuits. Being able to think critically and analyze, evaluate, and apply knowledge are also associated with this dimension. Do you ever visit museums or attend cultural events? The link between intellectual stimulation and healthy living is undeniable.

Emotional Dimension

Having a positive mental state is directly linked to wellness. Emotional wellness includes three areas: awareness, acceptance, and management. Emotional awareness involves recognizing your feelings, as well as the feelings of others. Emotional acceptance means understanding the normality of human emotion, in addition to realistically assessing your personal abilities and limitations. Emotional management is the ability to control or cope with personal feelings and knowing how to seek interpersonal support when necessary. The ability to maintain emotional stability at some midrange between the highs and the lows is essential. The abilities to laugh, to enjoy life, to adjust to change, to cope with stress, and to maintain intimate relationships are examples of the **emotional dimension** of wellness.

Social Dimension

Everyone, with the possible exception of a hermit, must interact with people. Social wellness involves the ability to get

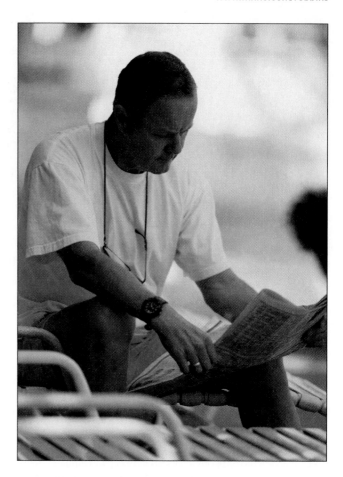

Learning should continue throughout life.

along with others and to appreciate the uniqueness of others. It means exhibiting concern for the welfare of your community and fairness and justice toward others. The **social dimension** of wellness also includes concern for humanity as a whole. You have achieved social wellness when you feel a genuine sense of belonging to a large social unit. Good friends, close family ties, volunteerism, community involvement, and trusting relationships go hand in hand with high-level wellness. Whereas feelings of isolation and loneliness are linked to ill health, feeling "connected" to a person, group, cause, or even a pet is a health strengthener.

Spiritual Dimension

Spiritual wellness is not always synonymous with religion. The **spiritual dimension** may or may not identify a creator, a god, or a specific religion. It involves the development of the inner self and one's soul. Spiritual wellness involves experiencing life and reflecting on that experience in order to discover a personal meaning and purpose in life. Why am I here? What path will lead to fulfillment in my life? What is life about? What are my values? These questions are most often answered within the context of a larger reality beyond the physical and material aspects of existence. Selflessness;

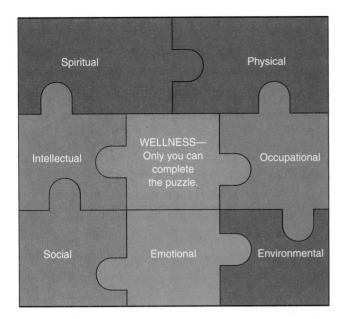

compassion; honesty; forgiveness; charity; and the development of a clear, comfortable sense of right and wrong are components of spiritual wellness. The Top Ten Components for Developing Spirituality will help you gain an understanding of the components of a spiritual life.

There is a strong connection between spirituality and self-esteem because of the internal feelings of self-worth that occur when a sense of hope, purpose, and morality are developed. Attempts to achieve long-term self-esteem by external constructs of power, socioeconomic status, or physical appearance fail. Like all dimensions of wellness, spirituality does not "happen." It is a process of growth requiring time and attention. Medicine has begun to recognize the strong influence of spirituality on health and illness.

Environmental Dimension

The **environmental dimension** of wellness deals with the preservation of natural resources, as well as the protection of plant and animal wildlife. We have basic biological needs that include adequate air, water, and food. Our dependence on the automobile, and the general industrialization of our world, have created worldwide pollution and changes in the atmosphere. Habits such as recycling, limiting the use of pesticides, carpooling, and conserving electricity show positive involvement in the environmental dimension of wellness. Demonstrating a commitment to the protection of wildlife and plants is also a component of environmental wellness. We must *all* take part in sustaining and improving the quality of the environment for current and future generations.

Occupational Dimension

The **occupational dimension** involves deriving personal satisfaction from your vocation. Much of your life will be spent

at work. Therefore, it is important that your chosen career provide the internal and external rewards you value. Do you want a job that allows for creativity, interaction with others, daily challenge, autonomy? Do you prefer opportunities for advancement, personal entrepreneurship, leadership, or helping others? How do you feel about mobility? Is salary your major motivation? Answering these questions may help you with career selection. Occupational wellness also involves maintaining a satisfying balance between work time and leisure time. It involves a work environment that minimizes stress and exposure to physical health hazards. A majority of your college life is spent analyzing and integrating your skills and interests with career choices. It is vital that your vocational choice be personally enriching and stimulating. If you are not happy with your occupation, you will find that your entire well-being suffers.

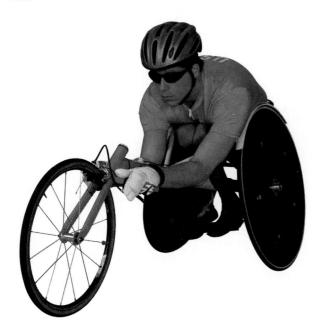

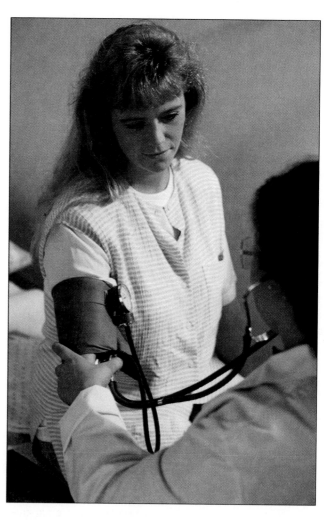

wellness is . . .

wellness is a continuous, active process—an ongoing, lifelong effort oriented toward maximizing one's potential.

wellness is commitment—a determined choice to move toward optimal well-being.

wellness is proactive—an approach to living, loving, working, playing based on your values.

wellness is a way of life—a lifestyle you design to achieve optimal health.

wellness is an integration—an appreciation that everything you do, think, feel, and believe has an impact on your well-being.

Wellness means striving to be the best you can be, regardless of life's situations or circumstances.

Wellness is a combination of all seven dimensions. It means striving for growth in each dimension, and appreciating the interconnectedness between all of them. Is there one dimension in which you are strongest? Which dimension is your weakest? Neglecting any dimension destroys the balance critical to high-level wellness. Certain dimensions may take on a greater importance at different times throughout your life. Nevertheless, striving for balance contributes to your wholeness. To evaluate your wellness in the seven dimensions, you are encouraged to do Lab Activity 1-2, *Assessing Your Wellness*. Taking this assessment will also help you understand the broad array of choices within each dimension.

Growth in Wellness

We have described wellness as a dynamic course of action based on self-responsibility. The goal is to assume greater responsibility for your quality of life by making positive lifestyle decisions. How do you begin making positive lifestyle choices? How do you know the options available to you? How do you grow in wellness? As Figure 1-4 shows, growth in wellness is influenced by many factors. Wellness living is an *active* process, so understanding how each of the factors contributes to your growth in each dimension is important.

Awareness

Before you can grow in wellness you must have an awareness of the wellness option. It is an exciting alternative! This chapter differentiates between the state of wellness and

Having your blood pressure checked is an example of a wellness assessment.

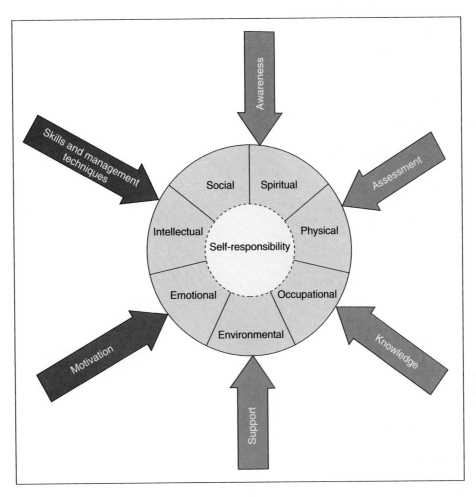

Figure 1-4   Factors affecting growth in wellness.

"treatment" health. You are now aware that your health, happiness, and quality of life are strongly affected by your willingness to make wellness choices. The increasing general interest in wellness has made it easier for an individual to adopt a wellness lifestyle, because wellness choices now are not only available, but valued.

Assessment

Once you are aware of the wellness option, you should assess your lifestyle. Assessment allows you to see how you are presently conducting your life and identify where changes should occur. An assessment can be anything from medical tests (blood lipid profile, blood pressure, etc.) to physical fitness tests. They can be stress inventories, health-risk appraisals, dietary logs, or even attitude questionnaires. Personality assessments can help you understand your social and professional relationships. Assessment offers an opportunity to begin the process of self-observation as you confront a wellness issue.

Knowledge

Having knowledge in the lifestyle areas helps you make decisions. For example, suppose from an assessment you learn your blood cholesterol level. What level constitutes a high blood cholesterol? What does this mean? How do you go about reducing your cholesterol? What dietary changes can make an impact? Will exercise help? Knowledge in lifestyle areas can help you to understand your risk and can guide you in accomplishing your goal.

Skills and Management Techniques

Skills and management techniques help you try some of the options. Skills in goal setting, behavior modification, and personal strategy building enable you to make the necessary lifestyle changes. How do I go about managing stress? Eating nutritiously in the residence hall or on a tight budget? Fitting regular exercise into my busy schedule? Skills and management techniques help you incorporate strategies of self-change into your life so that daily lifestyle choices are habitually "wellness choices." Realize that it takes time and practice to develop these skills into lifetime habits.

Motivation

Motivation is a powerful force in the wellness lifestyle. Motivation gets you started and keeps you going as you strive for continued wellness growth. Motivation is personal and complex. It changes throughout life and is specific to each person. At age 19 you may want to lose weight to look better. The 65-year-old may want to lose weight to help reduce high blood pressure.

Human behavior is purposeful and goal directed. **Extrinsic** (or external) **motivation,** including rewards such as certificates, trophies, recognition, and T-shirts, often stimulate one to action. However, **intrinsic** (or internal) **motivation** is more sustaining. One feels intrinsic motivation when the task is pleasant and satisfying without external rewards. Internal feelings of accomplishment are most likely to help you persist in the attainment of your goals. Three factors are essential for motivation:

1. Perceived autonomy (doing it because you want to, rather than being forced).
2. Perceived competence (believing in your ability to do it).
3. Perceived relatedness (feeling connected to others).

Therefore, by feeling choiceful, competent, and connected, a person can be energized by challenges, and persist when the going gets tough!

A powerful factor affecting motivation is how much you value what it is you wish to change. We usually value things we believe make life worth living or satisfying. Whether the goal is to lose weight, to manage stress, or to get along better with your parents, a variety of complex factors affect your ability to sustain motivation.

Support

Maintaining positive lifestyle choices is best achieved when there is support and encouragement from the organizations and environments surrounding you. For example, suppose you join a smoking cessation class and are trying to quit smoking. You are starting your climb toward permanent behavior change. If you face returning every day to a roommate who smokes or to a workplace where coworkers smoke, your chances of maintaining your new behavior are considerably lower. Your family, friends, and group affiliations have a strong influence on your behavior. It has been found that there are significant correlations among self-esteem, social support, and a healthy lifestyle. Choices are not made in a vacuum, so the aim should be to establish a health-promoting environment in which persons like you can easily make health-significant decisions. Choosing a living or working environment where others strive for wellness can assist you in wellness growth.

That is why it is important for schools, communities, and government agencies to provide wellness support to cultivate lifestyle changes. Do you feel your roommates, friends, and family are supportive of wellness? How about your campus? Why or why not?

Self-Responsibility

At the center of wellness growth is self-responsibility. The goal is to assume greater responsibility for your quality of life by making positive lifestyle decisions. Understandably, for every decision to be made, there are alternatives and consequences. Your challenge is to make thoughtful decisions that direct you toward high-level wellness. It is a satisfying feeling to work toward being your best. You know what you can and cannot control. Some circumstances are beyond your control. Part of self-responsibility is recognizing this and adjusting to continually strive toward full potential. Heredity is an example of something you cannot control. You had no voice in selecting your genetic tendencies. A physical disability is another uncontrollable life situation. Self-responsibility in wellness is making the best of the "hand you are dealt" regardless of your stage in life or your circumstances.

Self-responsibility in wellness means active involvement. Having realistic expectations, a sense of personal accountability, and a sense of humor will help you see wellness living as a joyful experience. Self-responsibility involves self-control as opposed to going along with the crowd or merely reacting to what seems to happen. Because everyone else is eating a triple order of french fries does not mean you must. When everyone else is grumbling about the weather, why not find something positive about it? Wellness is about personal empowerment—having a sense of ownership and control of the decision-making process. With that in mind, how do you make lifestyle changes? To make any permanent behavior change, you need a distinct, systematic plan of action.

As you travel this wellness path, you will probably become more aware of how society can help and hinder your trip. Societal or environmental support has the most powerful influence on promoting and maintaining a wellness lifestyle. A challenge we all face in attempting to pursue a wellness lifestyle is societal norms.

Societal Norms

We are constantly bombarded by subtle yet extremely powerful messages that are often obstacles to wellness. Our behavioral choices are strongly affected by unwritten codes that permeate our daily lives and can contradict and sabotage a wellness lifestyle. **Societal norms** are those behaviors or practices that are expected in a culture and that are accepted and supported by its members.

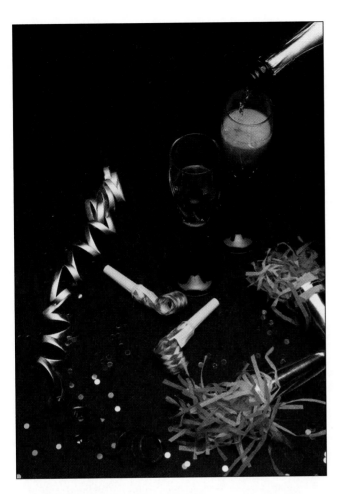

Occasions where alcohol abuse is accepted or even expected are examples of unhealthy societal norms.

table 1-3 Societal Norms that Promote "Unwellness"

- The idea that everyone must be extremely thin (especially women)
- The assumption that alcohol abuse is an acceptable rite of passage into college
- The media's portrayal of sex as being glamorous, without commitment or consequences
- Social events, parties, celebrations where alcohol and food abuse is expected (New Year's Eve, wedding receptions, Super Bowl parties, etc.)
- The number of high-sugar and high-fat gifts associated with holidays such as Valentine's Day, Easter, Halloween, and Christmas
- The habit of driving a car to go short distances
- Equating tanned skin with beauty, wealth, power, and sex appeal (thus, the emergence of thousands of tanning salons)
- Vending machines at offices and schools loaded with candy bars, chips, cookies, and doughnuts
- Fast-food restaurants that offer only burgers and fries (with no healthy alternatives)
- Miles and miles of roads built *without* sidewalks
- The elimination of daily physical education in the schools coupled with the parental push for private sports lessons and competitive Little League football, baseball, soccer, etc. (often servicing only the best athletes and emphasizing "winning" rather than lifetime participation)
- Access to television 24 hours a day, with a choice of 100 cable stations—all changed by remote control
- Meals built around a red meat entree
- The notion that as you grow older it is okay to be inactive and fat
- Consistently driving 5–15 mph over the speed limit.

These unwritten rules are carried on from generation to generation. Table 1-3 lists circumstances and norms you have probably grown up with. As you look at them, consider the messages they give. Do they promote wellness as you know it? You can probably think of more examples than those listed. For years it was considered rude or inappropriate for a woman to reapply her makeup after dinner at a restaurant table. Yet it was acceptable for her to pull a cigarette from her purse, light it, inhale, and then blow carcinogens into the air!

Many of our norms encourage a sedentary lifestyle. Somehow we've absorbed the notion that minimal exertion is better. Heaven forbid if, when operating your car, you have to roll down your own windows, walk around the car to unlock the doors, or keep constant pressure on the accelerator while driving on the interstate. You can go to the bank, a fast-food restaurant, a dry cleaners, and a milk store without ever leaving the comfort of your car. What kind of message is this sending?

The advertising industry is especially effective at mesmerizing us with messages. We are told, "It's doctor recommended." We see former athletes guzzling beer that is "less filling." Every Saturday morning high-sugar snacks that are fun to eat and that "your mother trusts" are displayed on television. If the thin, attractive models on billboards enjoy smoking, perhaps you will, too.

In traveling the road to optimum well-being, be aware of these pitfalls and obstacles present in our society. Remember, it is you who will make the daily choices as to how to live your life. You are the one who must assess the traps that may impede your pursuit of wellness. Self-responsibility is the key.

Changing Times: Making Wellness the Norm

Now that the wellness concept has begun to invade the health-care profession and society as a whole, we can see some norms already changing. Fifteen years ago the only people jogging were athletes in training or fitness "nuts." Now no one takes a second look even at senior citizens trudging along roads. Businesspeople pack their workout gear next to their business reports. Hotels hand out jogging maps to guests. Stress management, parenting, addictive behavior management, smoking cessation, and a multitude of other wellness topics are offered in community classes and workshops. As wellness permeates our society, there are more resources that support this lifestyle. There are positive choices available in grocery stores—more whole-wheat breads and cereals, low-sugar and low-salt products, low-fat dairy items, even take-out salad and fruit bars. Restaurants are also responding to the consumer demand for more nutritious food selections. These are a few of the positive changes that reflect wellness awareness. Only by drawing together all available resources (individual, community, media, school, corporate, government) will we fix current health problems. This multilevel approach is necessary to bring about changes in societal norms.

Beyond the physical, health-related factors of wellness, it is important to change people's attitudes. It should not be considered bizarre for people to arrive at work or at a class full of enthusiasm rather than full of complaints. It is also not weird to take a few moments to stretch or close your eyes to relax during the day, congratulate another person for doing well on an exam, adhere to the speed limit, have a fruit juice rather than a beer at a party, give someone a hug, or have fun in life. These are behaviors that reflect wellness and are brought about by awareness, education, and growth in wellness.

Not everyone has responded to this trend of positive lifestyle choices. It will take time. You can do your part by encouraging those around you to make wellness a lifetime pursuit. Pass these attitudes and behaviors on to your children. Help continue to make wellness and self-responsibility society's norm.

 frequently asked questions

Q. I am 20 years old. I realize I don't have the best health habits. Like many college students I eat a lot of fast foods at the food courts and am too busy to exercise. I smoke to relieve stress, and I drink alcohol. What's the point of adopting all these "healthy habits" at my age when I feel fine and have no symptoms of disease?

A. It is normal for young adults to feel healthy and invulnerable to future disease despite poor lifestyle choices. Nevertheless, these poor habits often become *lifetime habits!* Chronic diseases such as cancer, heart disease, Type 2 diabetes, and osteoporosis take years to develop. Damage accumulates over time. Look at older friends and relatives who have practiced these habits for 20 or 30 years. Do you like what you see? Knowing this, it may be easier to gradually make moderate lifestyle changes now rather than having to change "cold turkey" once a health scare has occurred. Those things you cannot feel (cells, artery walls, bones, organ tissues, etc.) will thank you in the long run. Also, there may be an immediate payoff. Do you feel as energized as you possibly could? If you begin now to change some of these habits, you'll reap the benefits immediately—and for years.

Q. My father had a heart attack at age 50, and my mom has cancer. What impact does genetics play in my future health and longevity?

A. For some, familial tendencies constitute a psychological trap. If your father has heart disease and your mother has cancer, your chances for following in their footsteps are greater than those of someone whose parents are healthy at age 75. However, this is only the case if your parents' health problems were a result of genetics rather than environment or lifestyle abuse. If you inherited a genetic liability, this knowledge should give you additional motivation to live in such a way as to fight it—controlling your blood pressure and cholesterol, exercising regularly, not smoking, eating healthy foods, and so on. Heredity is only one factor in the link to health and well-being. Although our biological inheritance predisposes us to certain illnesses and protects us from others, it is the interaction of genetics, culture, environment, and habits that counts. Your environment and personal health habits can either magnify or inhibit the tendencies with which you were born.

Q. Considering the health disparities and challenging diversity issues surrounding the health status of Americans, what can I do to make it better?

A. *Healthy People 2010* defines the nation's health agenda through broad reaching goals. By identifying specific objectives within these goals, national, state, and local organizations and agencies can work together to disseminate preventive health information. Through school programs, Internet and media communications, and community programming a lot can be accomplished. However, change occurs one person at a time. As you assimilate the knowledge and practices that surround a wellness lifestyle and attitude, you are setting an example for those around you. You can communicate to others the benefits and advantages of taking personal responsibility for one's health destiny. You can become an advocate for wellness alternatives in your school and workplace. It can start with you!

summary

Many adults in the United States die prematurely from diseases that are primarily a result of lifestyle abuse. Health promoters stress the importance of healthy behaviors in deterring the ravaging effects of these "diseases of choice." With the cost of health care increasing so rapidly, *Healthy People 2010* was published by the federal government in an effort to spark a national commitment to self-responsibility for well-being and acknowledge the need for support systems to help those pursuing wellness lifestyles. Whereas health is often viewed as a neutral state of nonsickness, high-level wellness is a dynamic level of functioning that is oriented toward maximizing potential. It is an integrated living pattern involving seven dimensions—physical, intellectual, emotional, social, spiritual, environmental, and occupational. It is a lifelong journey that involves a conscientious effort to reach full potential. The cornerstone of wellness living is self-responsibility. Wellness growth involves a multi-faceted approach of awareness, assessment, motivation, knowledge, support, and self-management skills. It includes intelligent deciphering of societal norms, recognizing your power, making choices, interpreting risks, and understanding personal limitations.

The objective of wellness is a richer, more satisfying life. Wellness is an attitude, not an end. Our time on this earth is too short to be drawn toward complacency and futility. We should consider and absorb the wisdom of W. Mitchell, former mayor of Crested Butte, Colorado, who, though paralyzed from an airplane crash, maintains an active schedule. He writes, "The way I look at it, before I was paralyzed, there were ten thousand things I could do; ten thousand things I was capable of doing. Now there are nine thousand. I can dwell on the one thousand, or concentrate on the nine thousand I have left. And, of course, the joke is that none of us in our lifetime is going to do more than two or three thousand of these things in any event."

additional information resources

American Council on Science and Health
www.acsh.org

American Medical Association
www.ama-assn.org

Center for Science in the Public Interest
www.cspinet.org

CNN's Health Report
www.cnn.com/HEALTH

Mayo Clinic Health Information
www.mayo.ivi.com

National Institutes of Health
www.nih.gov

U.S. Centers for Disease Control and Prevention
www.cdc.gov

U.S. Department of Health and Human Services
www.os.dhhs.gov

National Health Information Center
www.healthfinder.gov

www.discoveryhealth.com
www.drkoop.com
www.health.gov/healthypeople/
www.healthy.net
www.healthyideas.com
www.intelihealth.com
www.onhealth.com
www.realage.com
www.thriveonline.com
www.vitality.com
www.wellnessjunction.com

lab activity
1–1

Healthy Lifestyle:
A Self-Assessment

Everyone wants good health. However, many people do not have habits that contribute to health, well-being, and vitality. Health professionals now describe *lifestyle* as one of the most important factors affecting health. It is estimated that as many as *seven of the ten* leading causes of death could be reduced through simple, common-sense changes in lifestyle. This lifestyle assessment will help you see how well you are doing at managing the factors that strongly affect your present and future health.

1. I exercise aerobically (continuous, vigorous exercise producing a sweat for a minimum of 30 minutes) _____ times per week.
   a. 5 or more
   b. 3 to 4
   c. 2
   d. less than 2

2. Whenever possible, I try to increase my activity level by walking or biking rather than driving, participating in leisure sports, taking the stairs rather than the elevator, and so on.
   a. almost always
   b. frequently
   c. occasionally
   d. almost never

3. I make sure my diet is varied and well-balanced each day (fruits, vegetables, lean meats, dairy products, and whole grains).
   a. almost always
   b. frequently
   c. occasionally
   d. almost never

4. I intentionally include fiber in my diet on a daily basis.
   a. almost always
   b. frequently
   c. occasionally
   d. almost never

5. I limit the amount of fat, saturated fat, and cholesterol I eat (including animal fats, eggs, butter, oils, shortenings, and fast foods).
   a. almost always
   b. frequently
   c. occasionally
   d. almost never

lab activity @ chapter one

6. I smoke _____ packs of cigarettes per day.
   a. 0
   b. less than 1
   c. 1 to 2
   d. more than 2

7. I use other forms of tobacco products (smokeless, snuff, cigars, pipe) _____ times per day.
   a. 0
   b. 1 to 2
   c. 3 to 4
   d. 4 or more

8. I wear a seat belt while riding in a car.
   a. almost always
   b. frequently
   c. occasionally
   d. almost never

9. I obey traffic rules and the speed limit when driving.
   a. almost always
   b. frequently
   c. occasionally
   d. almost never

10. I examine my breasts (females) or testicles (males) on a monthly basis.
    a. almost always
    b. frequently
    c. occasionally
    d. almost never

11. I use healthy coping skills for the stress in my life.
    a. almost always
    b. frequently
    c. occasionally
    d. almost never

12. I include relaxation or "me" time as part of my daily routine.
    a. almost always
    b. frequently
    c. occasionally
    d. almost never

13. My consumption of alcoholic beverages can be approximated to be _____ drinks per month.
    a. 0
    b. 1 to 7
    c. 8 to 12
    d. 13 or more

14. I schedule health/medical screenings on a regular basis, including blood pressure and cholesterol checks, Pap tests (female), physical examinations, dental checkups, and so on.
    a. almost always
    b. frequently
    c. occasionally
    d. almost never

15. I would characterize my weight/body fat to be:
    a. within 5 pounds of ideal
    b. 6 to 15 pounds overweight/underweight
    c. 16 to 25 pounds overweight/underweight
    d. more than 25 pounds overweight/underweight

16. I am able to develop and maintain close personal relationships.
    a. almost always
    b. frequently
    c. occasionally
    d. almost never

17. I practice safe sex habits.
    a. almost always
    b. frequently
    c. occasionally
    d. almost never

18. I get 7–9 hours of restful sleep every night.
    a. almost always
    b. frequently
    c. occasionally
    d. almost never

19. I feel enthusiastic and happy about my life.
    a. almost always
    b. frequently
    c. occasionally
    d. almost never

20. I feel that my life has purpose and meaning.
    a. almost always
    b. frequently
    c. occasionally
    d. almost never

Scoring

Give yourself 3 points for every a; 2 points for every b; 1 point for every c; 0 points for every d.
Total Points = _____

Scores of 44 and Above
Excellent! You are aware of the importance of healthy lifestyle habits. More important, you are putting your knowledge to work by practicing good health habits. Most likely you are setting a good example for your family and friends. Keep up the good work!

Scores of 36 to 43
Good, but there is some room for improvement. Look again at the items you answered with a b, c, or d. What changes can you make to improve your score? Even a small change can make a difference!

Scores of 27 to 35
Your health risks are showing. You need to look over this assessment and identify some lifestyle habits that you can begin changing NOW. Plan your strategies for making this change. Write them out in contract form. Remember: habits (good and bad) are *learned* behaviors.

Scores of 26 and Below
You need to take a critical look at your lifestyle. Your present habits could seriously jeopardize your future health. Change is within your grasp. Your well-being is worth it!

Evaluation

Finish the following statements:

After completing "Healthy Lifestyle: A Self-Assessment,"

1. I discovered I am strong in _____

_____

_____

_____

_____

_____

_____

_____

2. I discovered I am weak in _____

_____

_____

_____

_____

_____

_____

_____

_____

3. I feel I can change _____

_____

_____

_____

_____

_____

_____

_____

_____

lab activity
1-2

Assessing Your Wellness

Read each statement carefully and respond honestly by using the following scoring:

    Almost always = **2** points

    Sometimes/occasionally = **1** point

    Very seldom = **0** points

Physical Dimension

_____ 1. I exercise aerobically (vigorous, continuous exercise producing a sweat) for a minimum of 30 minutes at least four times per week.

_____ 2. I eat fruits, vegetables, and whole grains every day.

_____ 3. I avoid tobacco products.

_____ 4. I wear a seat belt while riding in and driving a car.

_____ 5. I deliberately minimize my intake of cholesterol, dietary fats, and oils.

_____ 6. I avoid drinking alcoholic beverages *or* I consume no more than one drink per day.

_____ 7. I get 7–9 hours of sleep most nights.

_____ 8. I have adequate coping mechanisms for dealing with stress.

_____ 9. I maintain a regular schedule of immunizations, physical and dental checkups (including Pap smears and blood pressure and cholesterol checks), and monthly self-exams of breasts or testicles.

_____ 10. I maintain a reasonable weight, avoiding extremes of overweight and underweight.

_____ **Physical total**

Intellectual Dimension

_____ 1. I seek opportunities to learn new things.

_____ 2. I try to keep abreast of current affairs—locally, nationally, and internationally.

_____ 3. I enjoy attending special lectures, plays, musical performances, museums, galleries, and/or libraries.

_____ 4. I enjoy watching educational programs on TV.

_____ 5. I enjoy creative and stimulating mental activities/games.

_____ 6. I am happy with the amount and variety that I read.

_____ 7. I make an effort to improve my verbal, writing, and expression skills.

_____ 8. A continuing education program is/will be important to me in my career.

_____ 9. I am able to analyze, synthesize, and see more than one side of an issue.

_____ 10. I enjoy engaging in intellectual discussions.

_____ **Intellectual total**

Emotional Dimension

_____ 1. I am able to develop and maintain close relationships.

_____ 2. I accept responsibility for my actions.

_____ 3. I see challenges and change as opportunities for growth.

_____ 4. I feel I have considerable control over my life.

_____ 5. I am able to laugh at life and myself.

_____ 6. I feel good about myself.

_____ 7. I am able to appropriately cope with stress and tension and make time for leisure pursuits.

_____ 8. I am able to recognize my personal shortcomings and learn from my mistakes.

_____ 9. I am able to recognize and express my feelings.

_____ 10. I relax and enjoy life without the use of alcohol or drugs.

_____ **Emotional total**

Social Dimension

_____ 1. I contribute time and/or money to social and community projects.

_____ 2. I am committed to a lifetime of volunteerism.

_____ 3. I exhibit fairness and justice in dealing with people.

_____ 4. I have a network of close friends and/or family.

_____ 5. I am interested in others, including those from different backgrounds than my own.

_____ 6. I am able to balance my needs with the needs of others.

_____ 7. I am able to communicate with and get along with a wide variety of people.

_____ 8. I obey the laws and rules of our society.

_____ 9. I am a compassionate person and try to help others when I can.

_____ 10. I support and help with family, neighborhood, and work social gatherings.

_____ **Social total**

Spiritual Dimension

_____ 1. I feel comfortable and at ease with my spiritual life.

_____ 2. There is a direct relationship between my personal values and daily actions.

_____ 3. When I get depressed or frustrated by problems, my spiritual beliefs and values give me direction.

_____ 4. Prayer, meditation, and/or quiet personal reflection is/are important in my life.

_____ 5. Life is meaningful for me, and I feel a purpose in life.

_____ 6. I am able to speak comfortably about my personal values and beliefs.

_____ 7. I am consistently striving to grow spiritually and I see it as a lifelong process.

_____ 8. I am tolerant of and try to learn about others' beliefs and values.

_____ 9. I have a strong sense of hope and optimism in my life and use my thoughts and attitudes in life-affirming ways.

_____ 10. I appreciate the natural forces that exist in the universe.

_____ **Spiritual total**

Environmental Dimension

_____ 1. I consciously conserve energy (electricity, heat, light, water, etc.) in my place of residence.

_____ 2. I practice recycling (glass, paper, plastic, etc.).

_____ 3. I am committed to cleaning up the environment (air, soil, water, etc.).

_____ 4. I consciously carpool, ride a bicycle, walk, and so on to conserve fuel energy and to lessen the pollution in the atmosphere.

_____ 5. I limit the use of fertilizers and chemicals when managing my yard/lawn/outdoor living space.

_____ 6. I do not use aerosol sprays.

_____ 7. I do not litter.

_____ 8. I volunteer my time for environmental conservation projects.

_____ 9. I purchase recycled items when possible, even if they cost more.

_____ 10. I feel strongly about doing *my* part to preserve the environment.

_____ **Environmental total**

Occupational Dimension

_____ 1. I am happy with my career choice.

_____ 2. I look forward to working in my career area.

_____ 3. The job responsibilities/duties of my career choice are consistent with my values.

_____ 4. The payoffs/advantages in my career choice are consistent with my values.

_____ 5. I am happy with the balance between my work time and leisure time.

_____ 6. I am happy with the amount of control I have in my work.

_____ 7. My work gives me personal satisfaction and stimulation.

_____ 8. I am happy with the professional/personal growth provided by my job.

_____ 9. I feel my job allows me to make a difference in the world.

_____ 10. My job contributes positively to my overall well-being.

_____ **Occupational total**

Figure A.1   Wellness wheel.

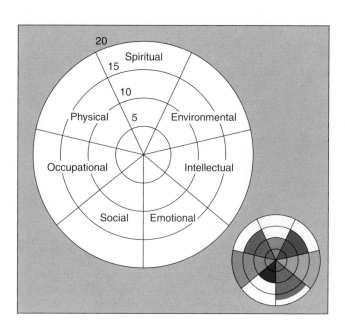

Scoring

Add your total score for each dimension of wellness.

Total Points = _____

Scores of 15 to 20 Points
Excellent strength in this dimension.

Scores of 9 to 14 Points
There is room for improvement. Look again at the items in which you scored 1 or 0. What changes can you make to improve your score?

Scores of 0 to 8 Points
This dimension needs a lot of work. Look again at this dimension and challenge yourself to begin making small steps toward growth. Remember: The goal is balanced wellness.

Take your score in each dimension of wellness and shade it in on Figure A.1. How smoothly will your wellness wheel roll? A smooth ride indicates *balanced* wellness, and the LARGER the wheel, the better!

Evaluation

Finish the following statements:
After completing "Assessing Your Wellness,"

1. I discovered I am strong in _____

_____

_____

2. I discovered I am weak in _____

_____

_____

3. I feel I can change _____

_____

_____

_____

lab activity

1-4

Is Your Campus/ Community Supportive of Wellness?

List ways your campus and/or community supports or promotes wellness living in each dimension of wellness. List as many resources as you can.

Can you think of *improvements* that could be made?

Physical Dimension

Intellectual Dimension

Emotional Dimension

lab activity @ chapter one

Social Dimension

Spiritual Dimension

Environmental Dimension

Occupational Dimension

There are three kinds of people in this world:
-those who make things happen;
-those who see things happen;
-and far too many who say— "what happened?"
—Anonymous

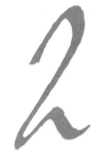

Changing Behavior

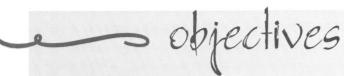

After reading this chapter, you will be able to:

1. Explain why willpower alone is not enough to permanently change a behavior.
2. Identify and describe the five stages of change in the transtheoretical model of behavior change.
3. Describe the nine processes of change and relate them to the stages of change in the transtheoretical model.
4. Describe the elements of a well-designed behavior change plan, and write a personal behavior change contract using the transtheoretical model.
5. Explain ways to prevent relapses during behavior change.

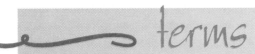

- action stage
- contemplation stage
- maintenance stage
- precontemplation stage
- preparation stage
- processes of change
- transtheoretical model of behavior change

T hough there is evidence linking lifestyle abuse and lack of well-being, many still smoke cigarettes, drink excessive amounts of alcohol and caffeine, never exercise, burn out due to stress, eat vast amounts of high-fat foods, and refuse to fasten their seat belts. It is perplexing that knowledge is not always linked to action. Knowledge is not power; rather, knowledge is only potential power! Information is necessary but not sufficient for creating meaningful change. Traditional educational messages devised to arouse fear (antismoking brochures showing blackened lungs, seat belt campaigns exhibiting crumpled cars, "this is your brain on drugs") have eliminated high-risk behaviors in some people, but not in the majority of the population. Fear of a heart attack or cancer has not kept many Americans involved in ongoing programs of exercise and dietary change. Even when the information is positive or inspirational, many still have difficulty making lifestyle behavior changes. Our everyday behaviors are learned responses. We were not born craving cigarettes, needing alcohol to have a good time, liking fruits and vegetables, or even automatically fastening our seat belts when we get into a car. These are learned behaviors. These behaviors occur as we respond to a variety of societal influences—parents, friends, role models, advertising, and so on. Called habits, these learned behaviors can also be unlearned. What is missing in the link between knowledge and action is a systematic strategy or plan.

More Than Willpower

Change is difficult. All of us who have tried to give up old habits or start new ones know how hard it is. Attempts to change can leave us feeling overwhelmed and demoralized. We may feel like giving up, feeling it's easier to hang on to old habits. Change can be especially difficult when someone else tells us to do—our physician, friend, parent, or spouse. For many of us who face imposed change, our first reaction is to get angry and defensive. We do not like feeling forced to do something, even when the change may appear to be in our best interest. ("I'll change when I'm ready, thank you very much!") When *we* initiate change, we feel free. When someone else initiates change, we may feel pressured or manipulated.

Changing a behavior or breaking an unhealthy habit involves *learning new behavior*. Just as in learning anything else, you must understand and practice the basic skills and techniques of behavior change. Some people are already excellent managers of their lives. They can study when they need to, exercise regularly, turn down an offer of chocolate creme pie, and refuse a beer at a party. These are powerful

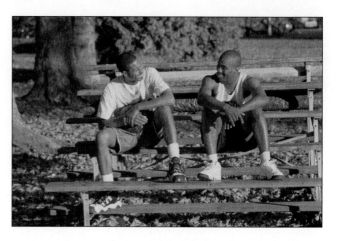

It's never too early to begin making sound wellness decisions. Your choices today will be reflected in your vitality and quality of life tomorrow.

choices; choices that are linked to wellness. Do these people have a lot of good old willpower? Is that what it takes? Willpower is an ambiguous entity. Others believe that merely *wanting* to change is enough. Isn't it as simple as making a New Year's resolution? No! Certainly desire for change is important, but it has no strategy to follow through. Most of us can relate to the top ten list, "Top Ten Excuses for Not Changing a Behavior."

The key to permanent change is having a plan. Successful behavior change involves choosing goals and designing strategies to meet them. It is a learned skill that involves conscious decisions, including how to deal with setbacks. Successful change occurs when *knowledge* and *action* are linked for the purpose of controlling behavior.

The Transtheoretical Model of Behavior Change

Changing a behavior is a complex process. It has puzzled behavioral scientists for years how some people can successfully self-initiate and maintain major lifestyle changes (stop smoking, lose weight, stick with exercise, cut fat in their diet, etc.), while others fail to even make moderate changes, even after participating in professional group programs (exercise groups, smoking cessation classes, low-fat cooking seminars, etc.). After spending years studying individuals who had successfully changed health-related behaviors by themselves, James Prochaska, John Norcross, and Carlo DiClemente revolutionized behavior-change theory. They concluded that individuals engaging in a new behavior move through five distinct stages of change. This is called the **transtheoretical model of behavior change.** Rather than viewing behavior change as a single *event*, such as quit-

top ten list

Top Ten Excuses for Not Changing a Behavior

Whether it involves our activity level, diet, anger control, or drinking habits, we seem to have a natural resistance to change. Here are the top ten common excuses for not changing.

1. "It can't happen to me."
   Denial is the first psychological barrier. Denial prevents us from seeing things the way they are. A wellness lifestyle requires an honest assessment of things as they are and a willingness to change.

2. "I'll do it later."
   Change is achieved in little steps, and the time to start is now. The rest of your life starts *today*, not "after Christmas" or "when it gets warm."

3. "I'll have to give up and lose the things I love."
   Instead of focusing on the benefits of change, most people have a tendency to focus on what they're losing. Instead of mourning the loss of your chocolate cake, alcohol, or cigarettes, focus instead on the gains: money saved, a better figure, more self-respect, and so on.

4. "It's someone else's fault that I am the way I am."
   Wellness and lifestyle changes begin with self-responsibility and taking ownership of your problem. Blaming others is a trap, a way of avoiding self-responsibility.

5. "The task is too overwhelming."
   When you were a 1-year-old, the task of running around the block was also overwhelming! You started with baby steps (and some falls along the way).

6. "It's too late to change."
   Nonsense! Whether it's because of your age or length of time, you will benefit from any positive lifestyle change.

7. "If I fail, I'll look silly."
   There is no such thing as failure; there are only learning experiences. Thomas Edison, for example, learned hundreds of way *not* to make a light bulb. All of us have setbacks from time to time.

8. "I don't deserve to succeed."
   One way of breaking through the barrier of negative self-dialog is by affirming the positive. An affirmation is a conscious, positive statement or image that channels your energy into action. When you catch yourself feeling "that you don't deserve success," try visualizing that positive image or repeating positive self-talk statements like: "I deserve success" or "I've worked hard for success."

9. "My family/friends aren't particularly supportive."
   This is a tough one. Have you discussed your plan with them? You may be surprised at how supportive (and proud) of you they are once you tell them how important it is to you.

10. "I don't know how to begin."
    Behavior change is a complex process that doesn't happen overnight. As you study the transtheoretical model in this chapter, you'll identify your current stage and the behavior processes that will help you move along. Formulate your plan and act on it.

---

ting overeating or smoking, the transtheoretical model identifies the change as a *progression* through five stages. These stages are identified as precontemplation, contemplation, preparation, action, and maintenance. This is a self-help approach in which the person is fully involved in the process of change. The old "just do it," "cold turkey" approach often decreases involvement and leads to stress, disappointment, and resistance.

The following is a brief description of each stage, followed by typical statements spoken by people in each stage:

Stage 1—**Precontemplation** ("I don't have a problem!")
Precomtemplation is the stage in which people are not intending to take action in the foreseeable future. People may be in this stage because they are uninformed or underinformed about the consequences of their behavior. Or they may have tried to change a

number of times and became demoralized about their abilities to change. Precontemplators are often viewed as unmotivated, uncooperative, and defensive. They tend to avoid reading, talking, or thinking about their behavior. Denial is common.

Typical statements made by precontemplators: "I think my diet is fine." "Smoking doesn't cause heart disease." "Individual recycling won't really make a difference." "My weight is not a problem."

Stage 2—**Contemplation** ("Is change worth it?")
Contemplators have a sense of awareness about their problem behavior. In this stage, they are intending to take action or are seriously thinking about it, but have not yet made a commitment to take action. They have to be convinced that the trip is worth the effort. People may remain stuck in this stage for years as they contemplate the pros and cons of changing.

wellness flash

The maintenance stage in the transtheoretical model is estimated to last 6 months to 5 years. To lend research support to this time frame, of smokers who quit for 12 months, 43 percent return to regular smoking; after 5 years of continuous abstinence the risk for relapse drops to 7 percent.

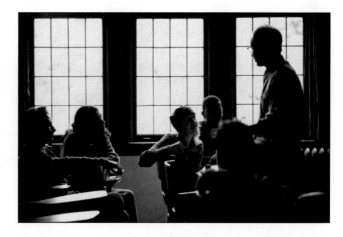

Joining a support group is especially helpful to someone in the action stage of change.

Typical statements made by contemplators: "I really should eat more fruits and vegetables, but I'm not ready." "I know drinking is bad, and maybe someday I'll quit." "Exercise would be good for me, but I don't want to do it." "I really get stressed out, but I don't have the time to work on stress management skills."

Stage 3—**Preparation** ("Count me in!")

In this stage people are intending to take action in the immediate future, usually within the next month. These individuals are putting together a plan of action, having resolved that the pros of changing outweigh the cons. They are making a commitment to the change effort and taking small steps to change.

Typical statements made by someone in the preparation stage: "Monday I start my diet." "I signed up for a Bible study class." "I purchased a treadmill and am going to start a walking program." "I bought a low-fat cookbook to help cut the fat from my diet."

Stage 4—**Action** ("I'm doing it!")

In this stage the individual overtly takes action, requiring considerable commitment of time and energy. This stage is most visible to others who see the new behaviors taking place. This is a busy stage of change where the person uses strategies to resist temptations, cope with everyday challenges, and prevent a relapse. Having a strong belief and confidence in the ability to change is a key element in this stage. That's why working toward small, attainable goals is important during the action stage. Most experts agree that one must be in the action stage for 6 months before moving to the maintenance stage.

Typical statements made by someone in the action stage: "My roommate and I now go to the library to study three nights a week from 8:00 to 10:00 P.M." "I've switched from donuts to a wholegrain cereal for breakfast and have a lot more energy throughout the morning as a result." "When I feel the urge to smoke, a sugar-free mint satisfies my urge."

Stage 5—**Maintenance** ("It's hard to imagine how it used to be.")

Maintenance is the stage in which a person is sustaining their new behavior, usually for 6 months to 5 years. Patterns are becoming more automatic. Maintainers are experiencing the benefits of their change and are increasingly confident in their ability to sustain this new lifestyle. The main goal in maintenance is relapse prevention. For this reason, maintenance is a long, ongoing process.

Typical statements made by maintainers: "I do my breast self-exam on the same day every month." "I haven't had a cigarette for 2 years and really don't miss them." "I prefer skim milk over 2% milk." "My day isn't complete without my evening workout."

Take a look at the algorithm in Figure 2-1. By answering each question you can identify your current stage of change.

The transtheoretical model acknowledges that each stage is equally important in the change process. To apply this model, you should understand the following principles:

- Movement through the five stages does not always occur in a distinct, linear manner. Some people cycle back and forth between stages, and may be stuck in one stage for many years before the goal is reached (e.g., relapse from the "action" stage back to the "contemplation" stage).
- Successful behavior change is a process that unfolds over time; it doesn't happen all at once. There is no "magic moment."
- You may be at different stages of change for different behaviors (e.g., be in maintenance as far as an exercise program, but in contemplation as far as consumption of fruits and vegetables).
- The majority of at-risk populations are not prepared for action and will not be served by traditional action-oriented prevention programs.
- Specific processes must be applied at the specific stages if progress through the stages is to occur.

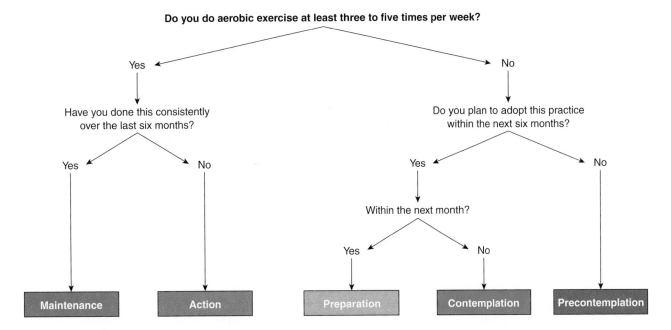

Do you do aerobic exercise at least three to five times per week?

You can substitute a variety of lifestyle questions for the initial question in this algorithm.
Try substituting: Do you recycle used newspapers, glass bottles, and aluminum cans?
                     Do you wear sunscreen when you know you'll be out in the sun for an hour or more?
                     Do you consistently limit the fat in your diet?
                     Do you get seven to nine hours of sleep most nights of the week?

Can you think of other questions?
Lab Activity 2-1 (found at the end of the chapter) allows you to insert any lifestyle question you choose on a blank algorithm.

figure 2-1   An algorithm for determining your stage of change.

- The key to successful behavior change is *identifying what stage of change you are in, and then applying the processes of change that fit that particular stage* to move on to the next stage.

The Processes of Change

Prochaska and his colleagues discovered that to help people progress through the stages toward maintenance, distinct behavior strategies known as **processes of change** need to be practiced at different stages. These processes are covert and overt activities and experiences that individuals engage in when they attempt to modify problem behaviors. These nine processes and the behavior change strategies that they incorporate have been shown to be the *best* predictors of permanent lifestyle change because they incorporate personal decision-making, feelings of self-involvement, and individual confidence. The degree of confidence individuals have that they can practice healthful behaviors across a broad range of daily situations has been shown to be critically important in progressing through behavior change. Table 2-1 explains the nine processes of change that Prochaska, Norcross, and DiClemente have

identified. Examples of behavioral strategies are listed for each process.

After looking over these strategies you may say, "But I tried many of these techniques and *still* went back to my old habits!" The most dramatic implication of this behavior change research is that efficient self-change depends on doing the right behavior strategies (processes) at the right time (stages). In this way, the key to successful change is *identifying* what stage you are in and matching the change processes to maximize the problem-solving efforts. Figure 2-2 identifies the five stages of change and the nine processes that work best within each stage.

To use an example, suppose Rick uses chewing tobacco. He doesn't believe that it will harm him, and he has no immediate intention to quit. He is in the precontemplation stage. The best chance of him moving into the contemplation stage would be to experience the *consciousness-raising*, *social liberation*, and *emotional arousal* processes.

Examples of consciousness-raising: In his wellness class, Rick learns the long-term effects of chewing tobacco; a week later he sees a news story about a major league baseball player who is diagnosed with mouth cancer—the result of regular use of chewing tobacco; a few days later he picks

table 2-1   The Processes of Change

Process	Definition	Example Behavior Strategies
Consciousness-raising	Providing information regarding the nature and risk of unsafe behaviors; efforts by the individual to gain awareness and feedback about a problem behavior.	• Assessing, "What foods in my diet are high in fat?" • Asking, "How many calories will I burn when I jog?" • Investigating, "What actually triggers my angry outbursts?" • Investigating, "What do I spend too much money on?" • Thinking, "What would be the benefits of losing weight?" • Using lifestyle and health assessments
Social liberation	Understanding and changing the contingencies that control or maintain the problem behavior; accepting and using new alternatives provided by the external environment; social opportunities that support change.	• Creating alternative atmospheres (community-sponsored postprom parties; smoke-free buildings, school lunch salad bars, etc.) • Identifying self-help groups and support groups • Identifying advocacy groups, minority health promotions • Using low-fat menu choices in restaurants and supporting designated driver programs • Empowering policy changes (quiet hours, recycling requirements, etc.)
Emotional arousal	Experiencing emotions related to the problem behavior.	• Watching a dramatic movie pertaining to the situation or problem • Using mental imagery to construct a scene (for example, imagining everyone alienated you because of your temper or obnoxiousness when you're drinking) • Blowing cigarette smoke into a handkerchief to see the yellow stain • Grieving over the illness or death of someone with heart disease, lung cancer, in a DWI accident, and so on
Self-reevaluation	Combines emotional and cognitive assessment of one's self-image with and without a particular habit; reevaluating values; weighing pros and cons.	• Listing pros and cons of changing • Asking, "Do I really want this beer?" • Reflecting, "Is tanning that important to me?" • Analyzing, "Will being more assertive be threatening to my boyfriend?" • Considering, "Will my parents respect me more if I stop smoking?" • Asking, "Will going to the library three nights per week diminish my social life?"
Self-liberation	Accepting personal responsibility for changing, especially the belief that it *can* be done; committing and recommitting to act on that belief.	• Publicly announcing your intentions; making New Year's resolutions • Creating a plan of action and taking small steps • Setting a specific date • Posting motivational signs, pictures, affirmations • Keeping a log, chart, diary
Reward	Rewarding one's self or receiving rewards and reinforcement from others for positive changes.	• Using self-talk ("way to go," "it feels good to be in control," "I like the compliments I'm receiving") • Making bets, pacts; using money, gifts • Incorporating a step-by-step approach with reinforcements at each step
Countering	Substituting alternative behaviors for problem behaviors.	• Walking with your spouse rather than watching TV • Practicing relaxation rather than arguing/retaliating • Thinking positive, self-supporting thoughts • Drinking soda instead of beer • Chewing gum rather than smoking

table 2-1   The Processes of Change (Continued)

Process	Definition	Example Behavior Strategies
Environment control	Restructuring the environment to reduce temptations; avoiding or controlling the situations that trigger the problem behavior.	• Removing ashtrays from the house • Never shopping at the grocery store when hungry • Not buying high-fat foods • Posting signs and reminders • Planning ahead by visualizing your action when confronted with a temptation/trigger • Having exercise clothes/gym locker conveniently ready
Helping relationships	Trusting, accepting, and using the support of others during attempts to change the problem behavior.	• Discussing your plans with others • Writing a contract with goals, countering techniques, and helpers' commitments • Enlisting someone else to "buddy up" and change with you; having someone to talk to • Using support groups; being with others who are doing the same things

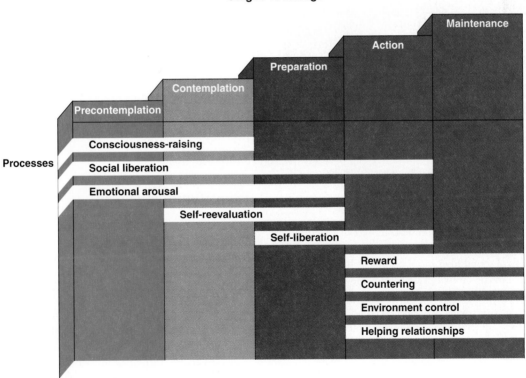

figure 2-2   Stages of change and the processes found to be most useful per stage.

Source: James O. Prochaska, Cancer Prevention Research Center, University of Rhode Island

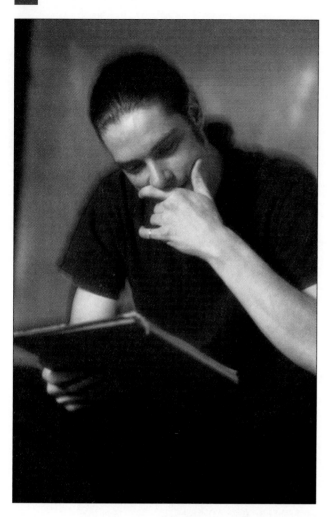

Reading and learning about a risky behavior is an example of the *"consciousness-raising"* process of change. This can help someone in the precontemplation or contemplation stage of change.

up and reads a pamphlet on gum and mouth disease while sitting in the dentist's waiting room.

Examples of social liberation: Now that he's in college and without a car, the closest place to buy chewing tobacco is 5 miles away; Rick's roommate (a former tobacco user) asks Rick not to use tobacco in the room or around him; Rick hopes to try out for the baseball team and learns of the team policy disallowing the use of chewing tobacco during practices or games.

Examples of emotional arousal: Rick learns that his favorite uncle (the one who used to take him fishing *and* the one who introduced Rick to chewing tobacco) has been diagnosed with cancer of the tongue and will soon have surgery to remove half of his tongue.

With these influences, Rick begins considering quitting the habit. Rick has transitioned from the precontemplation to the contemplation stage. To start Rick out with forced attendance in a tobacco addiction class or buying him

nicotine gums would have been futile. Rick was not initially ready for "action." Unfortunately, many health promotion programs in society address the needs of those select persons in the "action" stage of change (e.g., aerobics classes, low-fat cooking classes, stress management seminars). Yet a large proportion of individuals are precontemplators and contemplators who need other strategies. For these individuals to join an action-oriented program often results in failure, guilt, or blame for the lack of willpower or motivation. Prochaska's stages-of-change model can be a self-directed model as you begin applying the correct *processes* according to the stage of change you are in. Understanding this transtheoretical model should help you reach your behavior-change goals more effectively.

Making a Plan

One specific way to initiate a lifestyle change is to write a personal behavior-change contract or plan incorporating the processes for the change. Writing it out makes you think through your plan in its entirety, rather than letting things happen as they may. It specifies the *details* for carrying out your plan. Figure 2-3 shows a sample behavior-change contract. The changes you choose to make can pertain to any dimension of wellness—anything from improving study skills to losing weight to reducing stress to controlling anger. The most important outcomes of writing a contract are the self-evaluating and planning involved. Having a *plan* is what differentiates between successful change and a fleeting New Year's resolution. A blank contract and a behavior-change log are provided in the lab activities at the end of the chapter for your use.

Identifying Your Goal

Being able to identify your goal is an important first step. Some make the mistake of selecting too broad a goal or trying to change too many things at once. There are a few key points to remember in goal identification:

1. *Prioritize your goals.* Do not attempt to change everything at once. You may fail if you try all at once to lose weight, stop smoking, get along better with your mother-in-law, and make the dean's list every semester. Start with only one goal.
2. *Make your goal realistic and achievable.* For example, if your goal is to lose 30 pounds in three weeks, study every Friday night, go to church every Sunday, jog 4 miles every day, never lose your temper, or make straight A's every semester, your plan is probably doomed!
3. *Specify the situation.* Goal identification is easier if you can specify the situation in which the behavior occurs. For example, instead of saying, "I eat too

Behavior-Change Contract (using the transtheoretical model)

Name Kate Christopher

Date February 10

Goal: To keep my dietary fat grams under 50 per day

Pros: Better for my arteries/overall health; lose weight; reduce future cancer and heart disease risk; feel less sluggish; relatively easy to do with substitutes

Cons: I love high-fat foods; many of the people I eat with eat high-fat foods; high-fat foods are readily available

Identify stage of change currently in:

_____ Precontemplation _____ Contemplation _____ Preparation

___X___ Action _____ Maintenance

Processes (with accompanying behavior strategies)

1. Consciousness-raising
   — record the foods I typically eat and calculate the fat grams consumed
   — make a list of foods high in fat/low in fat
   — research the long-term health benefits of low-fat eating
   — read about people who have had success in cutting fat from their diets

2. Social liberation
   — take a low-fat cooking class
   — read the brochures provided in restaurants to see what foods are low in fat
   — investigate low-fat/no-fat alternative products at the grocery store
   — campaign for fat-free alternatives in the cafeteria

3. Emotional arousal
   — visualize my coronary arteries clogging
   — visit the hospital coronary care unit
   — watch a "beach movie"—all those thin people in bikinis!
   — think about my overweight uncle with a 320 cholesterol

4. Self-reevaluation
   — reflect on how eating fatty foods is not that important to me—only a moment's pleasure!
   — I really want to be healthier and know this is what I need to do.
   — review my list of pros of eating low-fat
   — reassess that being happy and content with myself includes changing my diet

5. Self-liberation
   — keep a daily log of fat grams eaten
   — write out possible menus for a day
   — keep a chart of healthy food substitutes
   — post motivational signs/pictures in the kitchen

6. Reward
   — $1.00 per day in a jar . . . eventually a new outfit
   — use self-talk ("I have gone eight days in a row and don't want to blow it now"; "I am doing great", etc.)

7. Countering
   — use low-fat substitutes (nonfat sour cream, salsa on potatoes, no-fat salad dressings)
   — eat bagels rather than donuts, pretzels instead of chips, etc.
   — have veggie burgers rather than hamburgers
   — switch to skim milk rather than 2%

8. Environment control
   — don't buy junk food
   — take my lunch to school
   — have veggies and low-fat foods ready in the refrigerator
   — post a sign in the kitchen with fat grams in a donut, cheese, potato chips, etc.

9. Helping relationships
   — discuss with nutrition professor
   — ask roommate to do this with me
   — tell Mom about my plan (prepare her for my summer eating)

figure 2-3

Behavior-change contract (Note: This sample contract gives suggested strategies for each process though Kate, having identified herself as being in the "action" stage, is best addressed by only six of the processes. Can you identify those six? (see below)

[Social liberation, self-liberation, reward, countering, environment control, helping relationships]

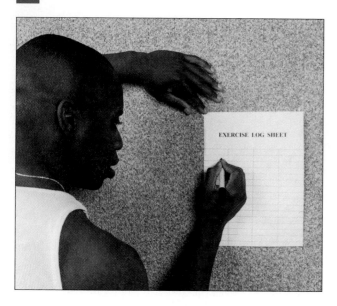

Keeping a log, diary, or chart allows you to see your progress and can be a great motivator

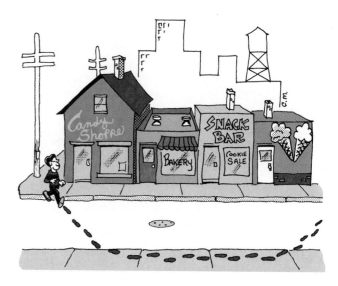

There are many ways to avoid temptations.

much," you might say, "I can't resist desserts." Or, instead of saying, "I'm self-centered," you might pinpoint, "I talk about myself too much." When you are identifying a goal, be truthful with yourself. It is not a time for denial: "But I'm not a big eater!" (spoken as you devour an entire sausage pizza!).

4. *Make your goal specific and measurable.* Not "lose some weight," but "lose 10 pounds in 16 weeks." Not "eat more nutritiously," but "eat four fruits/vegetables daily." Not "smoke less," but "cut down to three cigarettes per day." Not "get along with my roommate better," but "sincerely compliment my roommate in some way every day." Not "study more," but "study every Monday, Tuesday, and Wednesday, from 7:00 to 10:00 P.M. for the remainder of the semester." Self-change strategies are more effective when goals are stated in behavioral terms and quantified. Also, try to express your goals in positive terms. If a goal is to start doing something that you are not presently doing (for example, fastening your seat belt), state the goal in terms of what you want to do and in what situation you will do it.

Listing Pros and Cons

A lot of the decision to move from one stage to the next is based on the weight given to the pros and cons of changing behavior. The pros represent positive aspects of changing, including facilitators of change. The cons represent negative aspects of changing behavior and may be thought of as barriers to change. It's helpful to make a list of the pros and cons as you contemplate a change. Seriously ask yourself how your life will be affected by your changed behavior. Realize

that changing behavior brings consequences to yourself and, most likely, others. (By quitting drinking I will have better health and less likelihood of suffering from an alcohol-related accident. However, I will lose some social friends and my "mood medication.")

In the precontemplation stage of the transtheoretical model, the cons of changing outweigh the pros. In the contemplation stage, the pros may begin to match the cons. However, because they are so close to being equal, the resulting indecision and lack of commitment causes many individuals to become stuck in the contemplation stage. These individuals substitute *thinking* for *action* while continually weighing the costs and benefits of changing. As individuals move into preparation and through the final two stages, the positive aspects (pros) of changing progressively outweigh the negative aspects (cons).

Honestly assessing the costs of changing will help you face yourself and your true motivations. This will help you anticipate the obstacles asked of you. To increase your motivation, you might talk to acquaintances who have successfully made the change you are attempting.

Preventing Relapse

In the first line of his best-selling book *The Road Less Traveled*, Dr. M. Scott Peck writes, "Life is difficult." He further adds, "life is always difficult and is full of pain as well as joy." Changing a habit takes *effort*; but the joy in the growth and self-empowerment is the wellness journey. In our society we have become accustomed to the quick fix: instant cash at the ATM machine, fast food, 24-hour shopping, FAX machines. Setbacks may occur when you are trying to change a behavior. It is common to float back and forth between stages of change. Instead of throwing in the towel, try to learn from these experiences. Maintaining

top ten list

Top Ten Keys for Success in Changing Behavior

1. Divide large tasks into a number of small steps.
2. Use positive attitudes and affirmations when working on a change.
3. Find someone who will actively support you.
4. Spend time with people who already do what you are trying to do. ("It's hard to soar like an eagle if you hang around with turkeys.")
5. Practice stress management strategies daily.
6. Make a list each day of three things you *can* and *will* do to reach your goal.
7. Take action to change your immediate surroundings. (For example, get tempting snacks out of the house.)
8. Break up routines that reinforce the things you want to change.
9. Expect occasional setbacks; they are part of change. Plan ahead what you'll do if things don't work out as expected.
10. Don't let the change be an obsession; try to maintain a sense of humor, and don't take yourself too seriously.

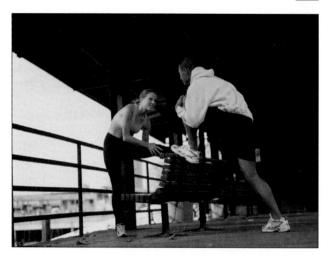

It is much easier to stick with a program when you have someone doing it with you (an example of the helping relationships process of change).

your plan will require flexibility, particularly if the plan is not working properly, if unexpected obstacles arise, or if a support system is failing. Reevaluation is a necessary component in making a permanent lifestyle change. Often the first line of defense against relapse is *planning*. If chocolate chip cookies are your downfall, don't buy any. (They'll keep calling your name from the cupboard.) If you've tried and can't get up 45 minutes earlier in the mornings to exercise, what about using your lunch hour to exercise? Take your walking shoes to work with you and invite a colleague to exercise with you. Plan so you'll *succeed*. Check out the top ten list, "Top Ten Keys for Success in Changing Behavior." Keep these in mind as you use the behavior strategies that correspond with your stage of change.

As you become the *cause* rather than the *effect* of actions, your confidence and self-esteem are enhanced. Emphasize the positive. Value your successes and your worth as

frequently asked questions

Q. One of the processes of change in the transtheoretical model is called "countering." What are some specific countering strategies?

A. Countering behaviors replace the problem behavior. This strategy is useful when one faces a craving or a social pressure. Try reading a magazine article; abdominal breathing; calling a friend; surfing the Internet; playing a musical instrument; putting on a CD and dancing or singing; going for a walk; watching a television program; playing a game of solitaire; practicing positive self-talk; doing sit-ups/pushups; cross-stitching; watching a movie; reading scriptures; chewing gum; closing your eyes and practicing imagery; shooting baskets; practicing a new skill; drinking a diet soda; e-mailing a friend/family member. There are many more. The intent is to divert your attention for 10–15 minutes while you refocus on your goals.

Q. My behavior change needs involve time management—specifically making myself go to the library four nights per week from 7:00 to 10:00 P.M. to do homework. I wrote a contract and did well for 4 weeks; then I missed several nights. Now I feel like a failure and am having a hard time getting back on track. Help!

A. The problem of relapse is an important challenge in changing behavior. When individuals experience a *lapse* (a few days of not complying with a new behavior) they need to avoid the feeling that they are doomed. For dieters, it is the belief that one cookie terminates a diet. For exercisers, it is the belief that one missed exercise class means that they are no longer "exercisers." Remember a lapse is a slip, a *relapse* is a string of lapses, and a *collapse* is when the person gives up and returns to past behaviors. Everyone has lapses. Analyze what influenced your lapse. Did you have some other commitments? An invitation to go shopping? A birthday party to attend? Maybe you'd be better off scheduling your three hours at the library from 2:00 to 5:00 P.M. Readjust, refocus, recommit and don't let a mere lapse turn into a major relapse or collapse.

a human being. Most of us do not realize that the majority of our supportive messages come from our internal thought processes rather than from external sources. We carry on continual dialogue with ourselves each day. Called *self-talk*, our inner voice can be a positive source of motivation. Self-talk that encourages us and reminds us of our achievements helps increase our self-esteem. Self-talk can also be negative, and, as a result, a source of discouragement.

The top three factors that contribute to relapses are:

1. Stress (Remedy: develop and maintain stress management skills—see Chapter 8)
2. Social situations (Remedy: plan ahead and be prepared for societal challenges)

3. Cravings (Remedy: practice self-talk, imagery, and countering strategies)

If a relapse or setback does occur, analyze what happened. Rather than throwing in the towel, learn what you could do better in the next similar situation.

Remember that high-level wellness is a process involving growth and pursuit of a fuller life. The process of self-managing behavior means reassessing goals, monitoring behavior, reviewing strategies, learning from setbacks, and acknowledging the joy in the effort to be the best you can be.

summary

It takes more than willpower to successfully change a behavior. Permanent behavior change involves passing through five distinct transitional stages, while using the corresponding problem-solving processes and strategies within each stage. Making a plan, goal setting, listing pros and cons, and understanding relapses are important skills. Writing a contract helps to construct a plan in its entirety, and keeping a behavior-change log helps monitor daily activity. Though setbacks may occur, a mind-set of commitment and self-empowerment can help continue the wellness journey.

Think about a business that places a sign in its window: "UNDER NEW MANAGEMENT." Imagine that your body/life is your "business" and you're the new manager who's been brought in to turn this business around. It's going to be challenging, and you're going to have to make some tough decisions. It'll take effort and commitment, but it is your job! And think of the benefits! So, declare it now . . . "MY LIFE IS UNDER NEW MANAGEMENT!"

additional information resources

University of Rhode Island Cancer Prevention Research Center
(Home of the Transtheoretical Model)
2 Chafee Road
Kingston, Rhode Island 02881
www.uri.edu/research/cprc

lab activity

2-1

Identify Your Current Stage of Change

On the line, write a lifestyle question (see Fig. 2-1). Then, using a highlighter, trace a path on the algorithm as you answer each question. Highlight your stage of change. On the back of this sheet, write another lifestyle question and highlight your stage of change for that particular habit.

Do you _____?

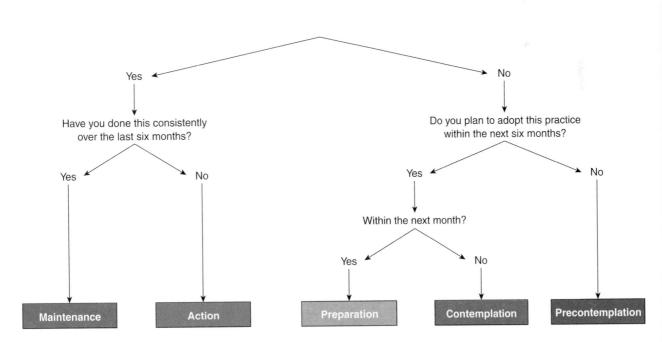

lab activity @ chapter two

Do you _____ ?

Yes ← → No

Have you done this consistently
over the last six months?

Yes ← → No

Do you plan to adopt this practice
within the next six months?

Yes ← → No

Within the next month?

Yes ← → No

| Maintenance | Action | Preparation | Contemplation | Precontemplation |

Behavior-Change Contract

Goal:

Pros:

Cons:

Identify stage of change currently in:

_____ Precontemplation   _____ Preparation   _____ Maintenance

_____ Contemplation   _____ Action

Processes:

Identify and circle the *processes* that correspond to the stage of change you are in (refer to fig. 2-2). Then, list three specific behavioral strategies you will use for each process.

1. Consciousness-raising

    a.

    b.

    c.

2. Social liberation

    a.

    b.

    c.

3. Emotional arousal

   a.

   b.

   c.

4. Self-reevaluation

   a.

   b.

   c.

5. Self-liberation

   a.

   b.

   c.

6. Reward

   a.

   b.

   c.

7. Countering

   a.

   b.

   c.

8. Environment control

   a.

   b.

   c.

9. Helping relationships

   a.

   b.

   c.

lab activity

2-3

Behavior-Change Log

Keeping a regular log can help you monitor your behavior, identify stumbling blocks, incorporate coping behavior strategies, and readjust your plan as circumstances dictate. (Make copies of this log as needed.)

Goal (long-term):

Goal (short-term):

Potential obstacles/challenges/triggers:

Behavioral/coping strategies to overcome obstacles:

Day/Date	Today's Challenges/Obstacles	Today's Behavioral/ Coping Strategies	Comments (student and/ or instructor)

lab activity @ chapter two

Day/Date	Today's Challenges/Obstacles	Today's Behavioral/ Coping Strategies	Comments (student and/ or instructor)

Name _____

Class/Activity Section _____

Date _____

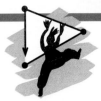

Using HealthQuest

1. Insert HealthQuest CD into your computer.

2. From the table of contents click on one of the nine lifestyle areas ("Fitness," "Nutrition & Weight Control," "Communicable Diseases," etc.)—NOT "Wellboard." Select a lifestyle area that interests you as a personal behavior change.

   LIFESTYLE AREA SELECTED _____

3. Click on "Introduction"; click on "Wellness Activities"; click on "Stages of Change Module." Click on "Overview" and read it.

4. Click on "Back," then click on "Assess Yourself." Go through the assessment. In what stage of change did the assessment show for you?

   STAGE OF CHANGE _____

   Click on the step icon and read about your stage. What are the suggestions/feedback for you?

5. Go "Back" and click on "Explore the Stages." Click on the various stages and read about each stage. Select one particular stage (one you're not in).

   STAGE _____

   What are the behavior tips for this stage?

6. Go "Back" and click on "Contract for Change." Go through the contract steps and print them.

Developing and Assessing Physical Fitness

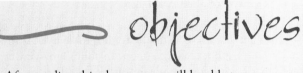

After reading this chapter, you will be able to:

1. Define the chapter terms.
2. Identify the five health-related fitness components.
3. Identify benefits of cardiorespiratory fitness.
4. Define and apply the FITT prescription factors for developing physical fitness.
5. Calculate training heart rate using the Karvonen formula and explain how to use the Rate of Perceived Exertion Scale to measure workout intensity.
6. Describe the purpose, content, and time of the three parts of a workout.
7. Identify one or more tests for each component of health-related fitness.
8. Complete the personal fitness assessment at the end of this chapter.
9. Use textbook norms to identify fitness levels in four fitness components, based on the results of fitness assessments.
10. Determine an appropriate fitness program using workout charts for specific aerobic activities in the appendix and the results of a cardiorespiratory fitness assessment.

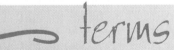

terms

- Aerobic
- Anaerobic
- Ballistic stretching
- Body composition
- Cardiorespiratory endurance (CRE)
- Conditioning bout
- Cool-down
- Cross training
- Exercise tolerance test
- Fat-free tissue
- FITT prescription factors

- Flexibility
- Heart rate reserve (HRR)
- Hypokinetic disease
- Karvonen equation
- Lean body mass
- Maximal heart rate (Max.HR)
- Maximal oxygen uptake (max VO₂)
- Muscular endurance
- Muscular strength
- Physical fitness
- Principle of individual differences

- Principle of reversibility
- Principle of specificity
- Progressive overload
- Rate of perceived exertion (RPE)
- Skinfold calipers
- Static stretching
- Subcutaneous fat
- Target heart rate (THR)
- Task specific activity
- Training effect
- Warm-up

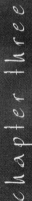

If there was a pill that you could take to increase your energy; help you manage weight; decrease stress, feel better, and decrease your risk of heart disease, cancer, and diabetes, would you be interested? The benefits of regular physical activity include these and many more. It is perhaps our cheapest preventive medicine. To live a wellness lifestyle, you must be physically active. While moderate levels of activity produce improvements in health, physical fitness requires higher intensity activity and produces greater benefits. Physical fitness is possibly the most important component of wellness, because what affects the body ultimately affects the mind. Physical fitness enables you to function at the peak of your capacity physically and mentally—to enjoy life more fully—to be all that you can be.

So, you want to become more physically fit. How do you begin? This chapter discusses the benefits of physical activity and how much activity is needed to maintain health. It reviews basic principles of developing physical fitness, gives a prescription for physical fitness, and details methods of assessing the health-related physical fitness components. This enables you to measure your current fitness levels, set goals, and develop a plan for working toward those goals. It will provide you the information you need to begin a fitness program so that you can reap the benefits for life!

Importance of Exercise

The natural peak of fitness occurs at physiological maturity, in the late teens to early twenties. After this, life becomes a slide down the aging curve for sedentary individuals, who gradually lose 1–3 percent per year of their cardiorespiratory endurance, muscle mass, flexibility, and so on. If you have observed friends who are older, late twenties to thirties, you see that many of them are beginning to show physical deterioration due to lack of exercise: decreasing energy levels, increasing body fat, loss of muscle tone. Our bodies were designed for physical activity, but few occupations provide enough to maintain health or fitness. The homemaker, office worker, attorney, and student have busy, stressful lives and may feel tired at the end of the day, but they lack the physical activity vital to tone muscles, stimulate the heart and lungs, or produce a training effect. This has resulted in an epidemic of **hypokinetic diseases** related to an inactive lifestyle such as obesity, coronary heart disease, cancer, osteoporosis, and diabetes. Unfortunately, too many people feel that they don't have time for exercise and are satisfied with minimal exertion in their lives. Approximately 250,000 premature deaths per year in the United States can be attributed to lack of exercise. According to Dr. Steven Blair, epidemiologist for the Cooper Institute for Aerobics Research, a sedentary lifestyle is as much a risk factor for disease as smoking, obesity, and high blood pressure, but inactivity is more prevalent.

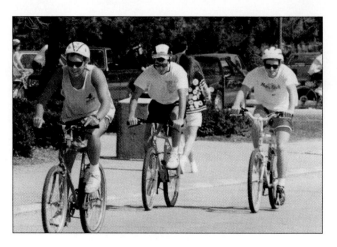

It is more fun to be a participant than a spectator.

Inactivity also contributes to the problem of obesity in our country. About half of American adults are overweight and nearly a quarter are obese. In the last 10 years, adults have shown an average weight gain of nearly eight pounds per person. Our nation's children are fatter, too, and about half are not physically active enough for aerobic benefit, which increases their risk of heart disease. Too many calories consumed and not enough exercise are to blame. The problem is compounded by the abundance of labor-saving devices, in other words, remote controls, computers, and riding lawn mowers. Children's playtime often consists of watching television; surfing the Internet; or sports lessons where sitting, standing, or watching consumes a major portion of the time. To make matters worse, although childhood is the best time to develop a lifelong habit of physical activity, many physical education programs face elimination because they are considered a frill when educational budgets are crunched. While we do not need a high level of physical fitness to get along in a world dominated by labor-saving technology, our bodies need physical activity throughout our lives for optimal health and well-being.

For young people, levels of physical activity decline sharply through adolescence. Many college students show early signs of hypokinetic disease. If you are concerned about slowly gaining weight from pizza, shakes, and fries, a good fitness program can reverse the trend. If normal daily activities leave you feeling worn out, you can boost your energy with regular exercise three to five days a week. Because routine activities such as sitting in class, watching TV, or walking across campus seldom require adequate physical effort needed to develop fitness, we must plan for daily vigorous exercise. The old saying "Use it or lose it" has never been more true.

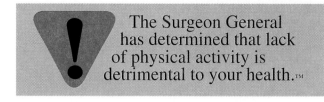

The Surgeon General has determined that lack of physical activity is detrimental to your health.™

Physical Activity and Health: A Report of the Surgeon General

We know that many people can improve their health and the quality of their lives with lifelong physical activity, yet about 60 percent of Americans are not regularly active, and worse, 25 percent are not active at all. Nearly 85 percent need more physical activity to improve their health. Almost half of our young people are not vigorously active. To encourage Americans to get moving and to reverse the increasing toll of health care costs related to chronic diseases, the office of the surgeon general produced a report, *Physical Activity and Health*. This report summarized the literature on the role of physical activity in preventing disease and came to these conclusions:

1. People of all ages can benefit from regular physical activity.

2. People can gain significant health benefits by including a moderate amount of physical activity on most, if not all, days of the week. This is equal to physical activity that uses 150 calories of energy per day, about 1,000 calories per week (Table 3-1). With a modest increase in physical activity, Americans can improve their health and quality of life.

3. Because amount of activity is related to frequency, intensity, and duration, the same amount of activity can be obtained in longer sessions of moderately intense activities (such as brisk walking) and shorter sessions of more vigorous activities (such as running).

4. Cardiorespiratory endurance activity should be supplemented with strength developing exercises at least twice per week.

5. Greater amounts of physical activity (longer duration or greater intensity) can provide additional health benefits.

table 3-1   Light, Moderate, and Vigorous Levels of Activity

Daily moderate activity improves the health and quality of life.
Activity in the moderate-intensity range that uses approximately 150 calories (kcal) of energy per day (3–6 METS),* is recommended for enhancing health benefits. CRE fitness gains and lower mortality rates occur when exercise is in the vigorous-intensity range (6+METS)*.

Light (<3 METS)	Moderate (3–6 METS) (as intensity increases, time decreases)	Vigorous (6+ METS)
• strolling <3 mph	• washing and waxing car 45–60 min.	• fast walking (>4 mph)
• archery	• washing windows or floors for 45–60 min.	• fitness activities that follow the FITT
• bowling	• playing volleyball for 45 min.	prescription
• golf (with a foursome)	• playing touch football for 30–45 min.	• racket sports (singles)
• conditioning exercises	• heavy gardening, raking leaves, jobs	• hill climbing
• light stretching	around the house for 30–45 min.	• rope skipping (>15 min.)
• hatha yoga	• wheeling self in wheelchair for 30–40	• snow shoveling (>15 min.)
• fishing	min.	• mowing lawn with hand mower
• mowing lawn (riding mower)	• walking 1¾ miles in 35 min. (20	• splitting wood
	min./mile)	• vigorous calisthenics
	• cycling 5 miles in 30 min.	• mountain biking
	• dancing fast (social) for 30 min.	• canoeing (>4 mph)
	• pushing stroller 1½ miles in 30 min.	
	• walking 2 miles in 30 min. (15 min./mile)	
	• water aerobics for 30 min.	
	• low impact aerobics for 20–30 min.	
	• swimming laps for 20 min.	
	• wheelchair basketball for 20 min.	
	• basketball (playing a game) for 15–20 min.	
	• cycling 4 miles in 15 min.	
	• jumping rope for 15 min.	
	• running 1½ miles in 15 min. (10 min./mile)	
	• shoveling snow for 15 min.	
	• stair walking for 15 min.	

*METS (metabolic equivalents) is a measure of calorie intensity and a method of classifying various activities and exercises. It represents the rate of energy (calories) expended at rest and is used to rate activities in multiples above rest. One MET represents the energy expended at rest (approximately 1.25 calories per minute or 3.5 ml of oxygen per kg [2.2 pounds] of body weight per minute). Six METS, for instance, means that the activity requires six times more energy than required at rest (about 8 calories per minute).

6. Physical activity provides the following benefits:
   - Reduces risk of premature death
   - Reduces risk of dying from coronary heart disease and of developing high blood pressure, cancer, and diabetes (see Fig. 3-1).
   - Helps reduce body fat and control weight
   - Helps reduce blood pressure in some people who already have high blood pressure
   - Helps build and maintain healthy bones, muscles, and joints
   - Reduces anxiety and depression, improves mood
   - Promotes psychological well-being

An important study conducted at the Institute for Aerobics Research in Dallas by Steven Blair, et al., provides evidence that physical fitness is associated with longevity (Fig. 3-2). In this eight-year study, physical fitness was quantified using an exercise tolerance test on a treadmill. The subjects were categorized into five levels of physical fitness based on the treadmill test. The greatest reduction in risk of death occurred between the two lowest levels of fitness. Therefore, a modest improvement in fitness among the most unfit can bring about substantial health benefits.

Healthy People 2010 (see Chap. 1) also contains exercise objectives, which include:

- To reduce to 20 percent the proportion of adults who engage in no leisure-time physical activity.

- To increase to 30 percent the proportion of adults who engage regularly in moderate physical activity at least 30 minutes or more.

Accomplishing these objectives would greatly reduce mortality rates. Then, perhaps, these individuals will enjoy a new active lifestyle and begin to see and feel the benefits of exercise. Eventually, they may invest additional time and energy increasing the potential to acquire greater benefits from increased levels of activity.

Moderate Physical Activity for Health Promotion

There are differences in the intensity and duration of physical activity needed for health; for physical fitness, and for performance, such as in athletics. What is involved in adopting a moderately active lifestyle?

First, realize physical activity does not have to be punishing to be beneficial. The emphasis should be on exercise of *moderate* intensity. This would be equivalent to walking

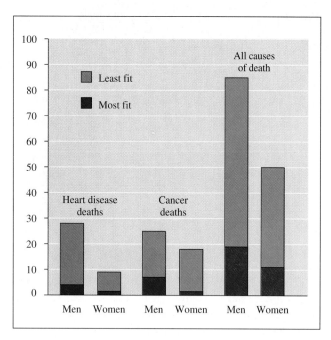

figure 3-1   Exercise and health. An 8-year study of 13,344 people (10,224 men, 3,120 women) shows that physical activity reduces the risk of death from most causes. Charts compare death rates.

Source: Institute for Aerobics Research, "Physical Fitness and All-Cause Mortality." *Journal of the American Medical Association* 262, no. 17 (Nov. 3, 1989).

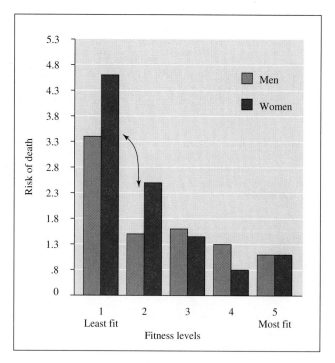

figure 3-2   Comparison of fitness levels and risk of death. The death rates for the least fit men (level 1) were 3.4 times higher than for the most fit men (level 5). Death rates for the least fit women (level 1) were 4.6 times higher than for the most fit women (level 5). The most dramatic drop in risk of death occurs between levels 1 and 2 (from 3.4 to 1.4 for men; from 4.6 to 2.4 for women).

Source: Blair, Steven, et al. "Physical Fitness and All-Cause Mortality: A Prospective Study of Healthy Men and Women." *Journal of the American Medical Association* 262 (Nov. 3, 1989): 2395-401.

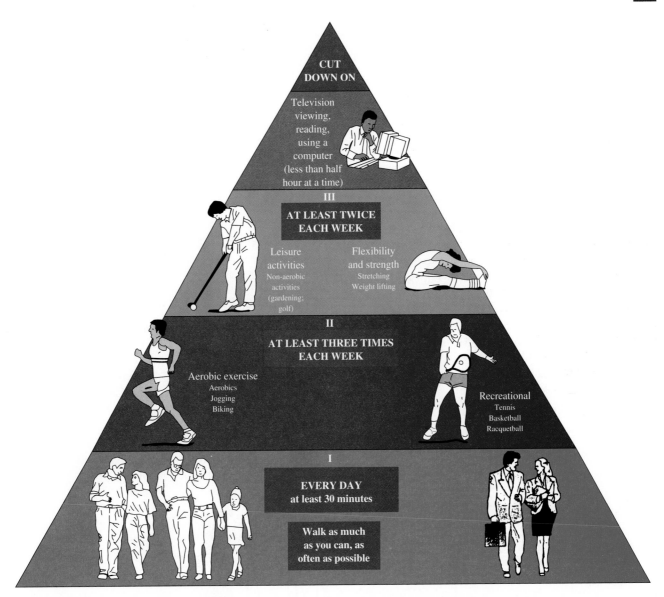

CUT DOWN ON

Television viewing, reading, using a computer (less than half hour at a time)

III

AT LEAST TWICE EACH WEEK

Leisure activities
Non-aerobic activities (gardening; golf)

Flexibility and strength
Stretching
Weight lifting

II

AT LEAST THREE TIMES EACH WEEK

Aerobic exercise
Aerobics
Jogging
Biking

Recreational
Tennis
Basketball
Racquetball

I

EVERY DAY
at least 30 minutes

Walk as much as you can, as often as possible

figure 3-3   The activity pyramid.

approximately 2 miles at a 15-minute-per-mile pace. You don't have to be soaked with sweat for improvements in health to occur.

Second, exercise does not have to be all at one time. We know that 20–30 minutes of vigorous exercise is recommended for high-level fitness (full cardiorespiratory benefit), but all activity is beneficial to our health. Something is better than nothing. Incorporate bits of activity into every day whenever and wherever you can. For example: Ride your bike to mail a letter; play racquetball, walk, swim, or run at noon; take a walk after dinner; walk to the grocery when you need only a few items. *Look* for opportunities to add daily activity—get up earlier, use TV commercial time, when working out a problem, when visiting a friend, and so on.

The Activity Pyramid

The Activity Pyramid (Fig. 3-3), like the Food Guide Pyramid, is a guide to help you choose activities to improve your health and fitness level. The activities at the base of the pyramid, such as walking the dog or using the stairs more often, can be built into your everyday life. If you are currently sedentary, this is the place to start. If you are already moderately active, begin a formal exercise program (the second level of the pyramid) at least three times per week. Aerobic exercise is the most beneficial in promoting health benefits and cardiorespiratory fitness. Recreational sports also promote cardiorespiratory fitness if the FITT (Frequency, Intensity, Time, Type) prescription is followed. Extra healthful benefits can be achieved at the third level, which recommends flexibility and strength exercises at least twice per week to build balanced fitness, especially if you already do aerobic exercise regularly. The top of the pyramid suggests what to do *least,* including sitting and watching TV.

You are faced with a tremendous challenge. As our nation's future homemakers, parents, and leaders, the responsibility for the health and well-being of the next generation rests in your hands. You can make an enormous impact on the activity patterns of your children, family, friends, and neighbors by setting a good example. So go to it . . . get up off the sofa, turn off the TV, and accept the challenge to enjoy exercise daily.

Encourage your friends and neighbors to get out and work in the garden, walk around the block, mow the lawn, walk the dog, participate in recreational sports (bowling, tennis, golf, softball), and go dancing. Anyone can begin the journey toward wellness with a single step and begin reaping health benefits immediately.

While moderate activity can improve health, physical fitness requires more vigorous exercise to cause long-term beneficial physiological changes. Next, we will look at the components of physical fitness, basic principles of fitness development, benefits of cardiorespiratory fitness, and a prescription for developing cardiorespiratory fitness.

What Is Physical Fitness?

Physical fitness is the ability of the body to function at optimal efficiency. The fit individual is able to complete the normal routine for the day and still have ample reserve energy to meet the other demands of daily life—recreational sports and other leisure activities, and energy to handle life's emergency situations. Physical fitness involves skill-related and health-related components. The *skill-related* components of fitness include speed, power, agility, balance, reaction time, and coordination. These are important to athletic success and are not crucial for health. The five *health-related components* of fitness include: cardiorespiratory endurance, muscular strength, muscular endurance, flexibility, and body composition.

Cardiorespiratory Endurance

Probably the most important fitness component is **cardiorespiratory endurance (CRE),** the ability of the heart, blood vessels, and lungs to deliver oxygen and essential nutrients to the working muscles and to remove waste products during vigorous physical activity. Cardiorespiratory endurance is often expressed in terms of your **maximal oxygen**

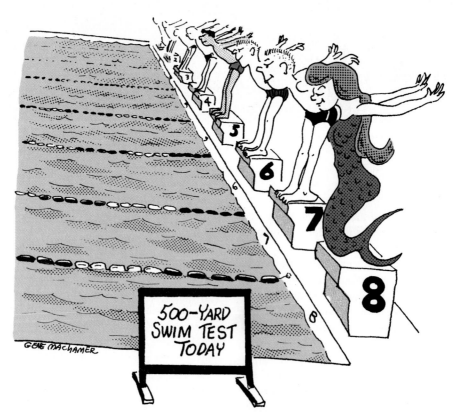

Cardiorespiratory potential varies among individuals.

uptake (max VO_2), the greatest amount of oxygen that can be used by the body during intense exercise. This is one of the best overall indicators of physiological well-being. You can go several days without water, several weeks without food, but only minutes without oxygen. Your life depends on the efficient functioning of your cardiorespiratory system. Research shows that vigorous exercise is needed to keep your heart healthy and to prevent heart disease. Good CRE is also needed if you want to enjoy running, swimming, cycling, and other vigorous activities to live at the peak of health and enjoy a full life.

Muscular Strength

Muscular strength is the ability of a muscle to exert one maximal force against resistance. Short-duration, high-intensity efforts such as moving furniture, lifting a heavy suitcase, or lifting a 100-pound weight one time are examples. Strength is important in sports, whether you are hitting a tennis ball, running, jumping, or throwing. Weight training (Chap. 5) is the best way to enhance strength.

Muscular Endurance

Muscular endurance is the ability of the muscle to exert repeated force against resistance or to sustain muscular contraction. It is characterized by activities of long duration but low intensity such as doing repetitions of push-ups or sit-ups. Muscular endurance is essential in everyday activities such as housework, yard work, and recreational sports. Muscular strength and endurance tend to decline with age along with activity levels. This loss can be delayed and muscular fitness maintained by participating in a resistance training program.

Flexibility

Flexibility is movement of a joint through a full range of motion. Flexibility is essential to smooth, efficient movement and may help prevent muscle strains. Can you sit and touch your toes without bending your knees? This requires hamstring flexibility. You need arm and shoulder flexibility to scratch your back. Women usually have more joint flexibility than men because men have bulkier skeletal muscles. Older adults may have trouble performing routine tasks such as getting in and out of an automobile, turning to watch traffic while driving, and dressing when clothes fasten at the back because flexibility diminishes with age. This loss can be countered if stretching is part of your lifetime exercise program. Chapter 5 has more information about flexibility.

Body Composition

Body composition is the amount of body fat in proportion to fat-free weight. The ratio between body fat and fat-free weight is a better gauge of fatness than body weight alone.

There are various ways to measure body composition and all are superior to the height/weight chart method. For instance, a height/weight chart may label a 6-foot, 210-pound football player as overweight, when in reality he has only 10 percent body fat, as measured with skinfold calipers. On the other hand, a sedentary person may look okay, but when body composition is analyzed, it is calculated to be 30 percent body fat. Have your body composition analyzed by a professional. Obesity is not only unhealthy and uncomfortable, it is associated with increased risk for heart disease, diabetes, high blood pressure, and joint and lower back problems.

Physical Fitness and Wellness

Becoming physically fit is a positive health habit that has a major impact on all dimensions of wellness (Table 3-2). It is one area where you can assume control of your lifestyle.

table 3-2 **Benefits of Physical Fitness on Wellness Dimensions**

Physical	Slows the aging process; increases energy; improves posture and physical appearance; helps control weight; improves flexibility; improves muscular strength and endurance; strengthens bones, reduces osteoporosis; reduces risk for coronary heart disease.
Emotional	Relieves tension; aids in stress management; improves self-image; evens emotional swings; provides time for adult play; promotes psychological well-being.
Social	Enhances relationships with family and friends; increases opportunity for social contacts.
Intellectual	Develops concepts of mind and body oneness; increases alertness; enhances concentration; motivates toward improved personal habits (smoking cessation, reducing drug and alcohol use, better nutrition); stimulates creative thoughts.
Occupational	Decreases absenteeism; increases productivity; decreases disability days; lowers medical care costs; lowers job turnover rate; increases networking possibilities.
Spiritual	Develops appreciation of body/mind connection; enhances appreciation for healthy environment; builds compassion for those less able.
Environmental	Develops appreciation for healthy air and water; increases concern for recycling and preservation of our natural resources; increases interest in eliminating toxins and chemicals from food chain.

Benefits of Aerobic Exercise

The number one reason people begin exercising is they want to improve their physical appearance—to decrease body fat and develop firm, well-toned muscles. These are not the only benefits. There are a number of physiological (cardiorespiratory, body composition, and metabolic) and psychological (mental and emotional) health benefits. Exercise has short- and long-term effects. The immediate effects of vigorous exercise, regardless of fitness level, are an increase in the respiration rate, an increase in the heart rate, and some sweating. After a few weeks of regular, vigorous exercise, the body begins to adapt to meeting the demands. These physiological adaptations (the total beneficial changes) are called the **training effect** and are detailed in the following lists. Benefits of flexibility and muscular fitness will be discussed in Chapter 5.

Cardiorespiratory Benefits:
1. lower resting heart rate
2. increased stroke volume (the amount of blood pumped out of the heart with each beat), improving heart efficiency
3. increased rest for the heart between beats due to slower resting heart rate and increased stroke volume
4. increased oxygen-carrying capacity of the blood, due to the greater supply of red blood cells and hemoglobin; greater endurance in exercising muscles due to increased energy and improved elimination of waste products
5. improved exercise performance on timed tests (due to more efficient use of oxygen)
6. possible reduction in blood pressure
7. improved blood lipid profile by increasing the number of protective high-density lipoproteins
8. quicker recovery to resting heart rate after vigorous exercise due to improved cardiac efficiency
9. possible regression of atherosclerosis
10. fewer illnesses and deaths due to coronary heart disease

Body Composition/Physical Appearance Benefits:
1. reduced body fat percentage
2. increased lean body mass
3. firmer, more toned muscles

Psychological Benefits:
1. enhanced sense of well-being and self-esteem, resulting in increased energy, alertness, and vitality
2. increased sense of self-discipline due to the determination needed to stick to an exercise program
3. reduced state of anxiety and mental tension, thereby increasing stress coping ability
4. improved quality of sleep, resulting in the ability to fall asleep faster and with less tossing and turning during sleeping time
5. decreased level of mild to moderate depression
6. improved mental acuity, learning, and memory
7. feeling of relaxation

The psychological benefits are the most rewarding and are often the main reason people keep exercising. Fitness produces other important benefits. You burn extra calories while exercising, which helps to promote weight loss and reverse obesity. Exercise and weight management help prevent and manage diabetes and reduce risk of certain cancers. Fit people can exercise longer at the same level of intensity, and their perception of how hard they are working decreases.

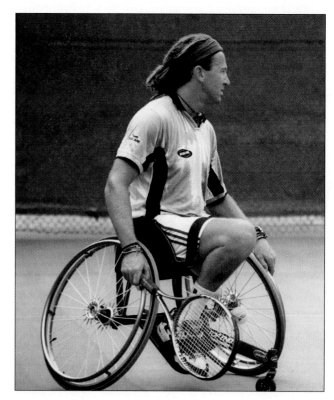

Everybody benefits from physical activity.

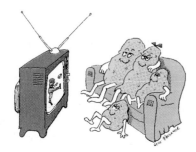

"We have become a nation of spectators"

This is due to increased muscular strength and endurance. Tendons, ligaments, and joints are strengthened through exercise. Also, exercise stimulates bone strengthening and may help counteract and reverse osteoporosis. Vigorous exercise improves the functioning of the cardiorespiratory system and is directly related to reduced coronary risk. CRE alone, however is not a panacea and does not guarantee immunity from heart disease. It cannot "cancel" other risk factors. If you smoke cigarettes, eat a high-fat diet or have coronary risk factors, you may still be at risk.

The FITT Prescription for Cardiorespiratory Fitness

Cardiorespiratory fitness development involves the four **FITT prescription factors:** Frequency, Intensity, and Time and Type of exercise (see Fig. 3-4). This prescription is recommended for high-level physical fitness. It is not the recommended training program for athletes or for the person who wishes to run a marathon. However, many athletes use the FITT prescription to maintain their fitness in the off-season.

"F" Equals Frequency

How often should you exercise? Exercise three to five times per week with no more than 48 hours between workouts. After 48 hours, the body starts to decondition and lose some of the benefits gained in the last workout. It is not necessary to exercise every day of the week to develop fitness, although five-day-a-week programs produce greater improvements than do three-day-a-week programs. If your goal is to lose weight or reduce stress, five days of exercise a week are recommended. However, time for recovery is important, especially if you are just beginning a fitness program. The body needs time to adapt, so start slowly, working out every other day, gradually increasing the frequency as your fitness improves.

"I" Equals Intensity

How hard should you exercise? In athletics, a coach may ask you to give 100 percent, but this intensity is not needed to develop health-related fitness. A little over half to over three-quarters effort allows adequate stimulation of the cardiorespiratory system to produce training effect benefits. The American College of Sports Medicine (ACSM) recommends a workout intensity of 60 to 80 percent of your heart rate reserve. Intensity of effort is directly reflected by exercise pulse rate and is perhaps the most important factor in gaining training effect benefits from your exercise program.

FITT=

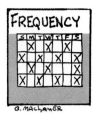

3–5 times/wk.

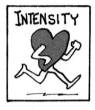

60–80% HRR*

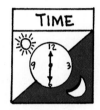

20–30 min.

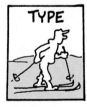

Continuous and rhythmic

*HRR = Heart rate reserve

figure 3-4   The FITT formula is the prescription for cardiorespiratory fitness.

You must put in enough effort to force the body to adapt and produce fitness improvements. If intensity is too low, there will still be health benefits, but no increase in physical fitness. There are two ways to judge intensity: target heart rate and rate of perceived exertion.

Target Heart Rate: Karvonen Equation

To determine your **target heart rate (THR)** range for exercise, we will use the **Karvonen equation,** which takes into account your fitness level based on your resting heart rate (RHR). Karvonen, a Finnish researcher, discovered that the heart rate during exercise must be raised by at least 60 percent of the difference between resting and maximal heart rates (called the **heart rate reserve, HRR**) to gain cardiorespiratory fitness. An adequate upper intensity is 80 percent of HRR.

It is necessary to know your **maximal heart rate (Max.HR)** to calculate your target heart rate range. The Max.HR is your highest possible heart rate. It can be directly determined during a treadmill exercise tolerance test in a laboratory or can be estimated. The maximal heart rate ranges from 180 to 200 beats per minute (bpm) in young people and decreases with age. Most people can estimate their Max.HR by subtracting their age from 220. For example, if you are 20 years old, your estimated Max.HR is 220 − 20 = 200.

Next, you will need to know your RHR for one minute. Check it using a stopwatch or a watch with a second hand. You can find the pulse with your finger tips (not the thumb) at the carotid artery in the neck or on the thumb side of the wrist (Figs. 3-5 and 3-6). Count the number of beats for 30 seconds and multiply by two to calculate your one-minute pulse. By using your age and your RHR, you can calculate your target heart rate range (Table 3-3). There is also a target heart rate worksheet in Lab Activity 3-4.

Now that you know your target heart rate range, you will be able to measure the intensity of every workout. Count your pulse during exercise and immediately after conditioning. Because your pulse drops rapidly when you stop exercising, rather than counting your pulse for a full minute, you may find it easier to count for 6 or 10 seconds (i.e., if you count 15 beats in 10 seconds, your pulse is 150). It will take some practice, but in time you will become accurate at checking your heart rate.

Exercise heart rates differ by age (Fig. 3-7). For most young adults, a THR is in the range of 150 to 170 beats per minute, but for older adults, a rate of 120 to 140 beats per minute may be adequate. Exercising at a heart rate above your THR is not necessary for fitness, but is fine as long as you are comfortable. Keep in mind that because the maximal heart rate is estimated, any error in that estimate is carried over into the THR calculation. Actual THR can vary plus or minus 10 beats. Rating of perceived exertion can be helpful in adjusting intensity when you begin an exercise program. A general rule is to apply the *talk test*. You should be able to comfortably carry on a conversation with a companion while exercising. If you are too breathless to talk, you are exercising too hard.

THR During Nonweight-bearing Activities. When you swim, bike, or water run, an adequate target pulse rate is lower than when running. Weight-bearing activities, such as running and walking, use more oxygen and make your heart

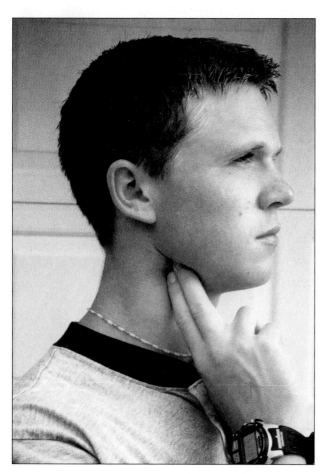

figure 3-5   Pulse at carotid artery.

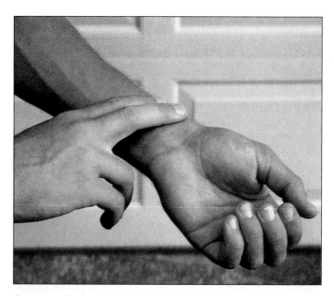

figure 3-6   Pulse at the thumb side of wrist

table 3-3

Calculating the Target Heart Rate Range Using the Karvonen Formula

$$THR = \left[\begin{array}{c} \text{(maximal} \\ \text{heart} \\ \text{rate} \end{array} - \begin{array}{c} \text{resting} \\ \text{heart} \\ \text{rate)} \end{array} \right] \times \begin{array}{c} \text{intensity} \\ \text{factor} \end{array} + \begin{array}{c} \text{resting} \\ \text{heart} \\ \text{rate} \end{array}$$

This example shows a 20-year-old with a resting rate of 70 bpm:
- Estimation of maximal heart rate = 220 minus age 20
- Resting heart rate = pulse at complete rest for 1 minute
- Intensity = range of 60% to 80%

$$
\begin{aligned}
\text{THR at 60\%} &= [(220 - 20) - 70] \times 0.60 + 70 \\
&= [200 - 70] \times 0.60 + 70 \\
&= 130 \times 0.60 + 70 \\
&= 78 + 70 \\
&= 148 \\
\text{THR at 80\%} &= [(200 - 20) - 70] \times 0.80 + 70 \\
&= [200 - 70] \times 0.80 + 70 \\
&= 130 \times 0.80 + 70 \\
&= 104 + 70 \\
&= 174
\end{aligned}
$$

Target heart rate range = 148 to 174.

beat faster than when you work out by cycling or swimming—at the same perceived level of effort. As a general rule, reduce cycling THR by 5 percent and swimming THR by 10 percent. In any case, you should be able to pass the talk test. For example, if your THR for running/walking is 150–170 bpm, your swimming THR would be:

1. 150 × .10 = 15; 170 × .10 = 17
2. 150 − 15 = 135; 170 − 17 = 153
3. THR = 135 − 153 bpm

Also remember to set different goals for cross training. A good way to achieve an effective workout is to monitor your rate of perceived exertion (RPE).

Target Heart Rate: Percentage of Maximal Heart Rate

An old method of determining the target heart rate used a straight percentage of the maximal heart rate. Early researchers used 70 to 85 percent of an individual's maximal heart rate to set exercise intensity. For example, if a person's estimated maximal pulse was 200, the target heart rate range would be 140 (200 × .7) to 170 (200 × .85) beats per minute. Its advantage is it is simple to compute. The drawback of this method is that it does not take different fitness levels, as measured by resting pulse, into account.

Rate of Perceived Exertion (RPE)

Many people do not check their heart rate during exercise and judge intensity of exercise by **rate of perceived exertion (RPE),** paying attention to how hard or easy your workout feels. This method uses a scale developed by Gunnar Borg (see Table 3-4). Borg discovered that exercisers are able to "sense" their exercise intensity levels. He found that the RPE scale correlated with heart rate. Borg found that the descriptive words in the right column closely paralleled the heart rate of the exerciser, which is illustrated by the numbers in the left column. To develop fitness, exercisers should feel the effort is "Somewhat hard" to "Hard." It is helpful to cross-check your heart rate with your perceived rating when first beginning to use this method. After several workouts, you should be able to predict your exercise heart rate by your perceived exertion of the exercise session. When exercising ask "How do I feel?" Describe how you feel using the descriptors on the Borg scale. Adjust the intensity of your

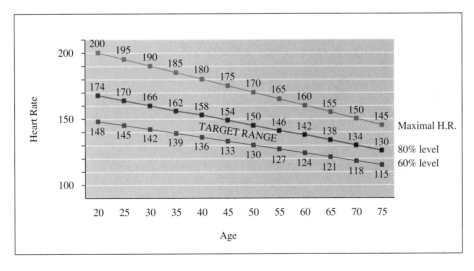

figure 3-7   Estimated target heart rate range (based on RHR of 70 bpm).

table 3-4   Borg's Rate of Perceived Exertion (RPE)

(RPE) Chart

6		
7	Very, very light	Warm-up/cool-down zone
8		
9	Very light	
10		
11	Fairly light	
12		
13	Somewhat hard	Target zone
14		
15	Hard	
16		
17	Very hard	
18		Working too hard zone
19	Very, very hard	
20		

Source: G. Borg, "Psychophysical Bases of Physical Exertion—Perceived Rate of Exertion," *Medicine and Science in Sports & Exercise*, 14, 344-86, 1982, © by The American College of Sports Medicine.

workout accordingly. This is a safe and accurate way to monitor exercise intensity anywhere, anytime without using a stopwatch.

"T" Equals Time

How long should each workout be? The ACSM recommends a conditioning bout of 20 to 30 minutes at an intensity of 60 to 80 percent not including warm-up and cool-down. Intensity and time of a workout interact to produce a caloric expenditure necessary to achieve health and fitness goals. A similar workout may be obtained at a low intensity and longer time (60 percent intensity, 30 minutes) or a higher intensity and shorter time (80 percent intensity, 20 minutes). However, risk of injury does increase at higher intensities. If time permits and the exercise session is enjoyable, or if you are training for a long distance event (i.e., minimarathon), exercising for longer than 30 minutes is fine, but it is not necessary for basic fitness. A typical workout would be as follows:

Warm-up		Conditioning bout		Cool down
5–15 min.	+	20–30 min.	+	5–15 min.

When beginning a fitness program, it is best to limit your conditioning periods to 20 minutes or less (i.e., 4, 5-minute bouts with a rest in between if needed), then progress slowly until you can comfortably work out for 20 to 30 minutes in your target heart rate range. While many people feel that

they don't have time to exercise, if you do the minimum 20 minutes, 3 days per week, it takes one hour out of 168 hours in your week—a small investment that pays big dividends.

"T" Equals Type

What type of exercise promotes aerobic fitness? The term **aerobic** means "with oxygen." Aerobic activities are those that demand large amounts of oxygen and improve cardiorespiratory endurance, which produces many physiological and psychological benefits. They are vigorous, continuous, and rhythmic. This includes activities that accelerate respiration and maintain a heart rate in the target range. Aerobic dancing, swimming, cycling, and jogging are all good, as are other vigorous activities that sustain a target heart rate (see Chap. 4). However, riding a bike a short distance across campus is not adequate in intensity or time to develop fitness. Ask, "Did I keep my heart rate in the target heart range for 20 to 30 minutes or more?" On the other hand, rope jumping or even stair climbing can be an aerobic activity, providing the FITT prescription factors are met. Bowling, golf, and softball, although enjoyable recreational activities, are not aerobic. What other activities meet the FITT prescription?

Anaerobic exercise means "without oxygen." Anaerobic activities are high intensity and short duration, such as sprinting. This type of activity demands more oxygen than the body can supply while exercising, causing an oxygen debt. Anaerobic exercise causes waste products (lactic acid) to accumulate in muscles, which, along with the depletion of stored energy, leads to exhaustion. Many activities—tennis, volleyball, and weight training—are anaerobic. They aid in the development of agility, eye-hand coordination, and muscular strength and endurance, as well as flexibility, but they are not aerobic and do not produce a cardiorespiratory training effect.

How Long Before Results Become Apparent?

It varies with the individual. Within the first few exercise sessions, many people report that they feel better. Measurable differences such as decreased heart rate or improved aerobic fitness can occur within 8 to 12 weeks. The key is staying with the exercise program. Studies indicate over 50 percent of adults who start an exercise program quit within the first 3 to 6 months. Regular exercisers focus on the positive benefits of exercise, reminding themselves how good they feel after a workout and pat themselves on the back for progress. So how do you stay with an exercise program long enough to experience the benefits of the training effect? First, review in Chapter 2 the stages of change that people go through who want to make a change in their lives. See the top ten list, "Top Ten Ways

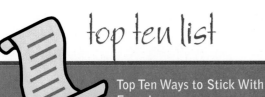

Top Ten Ways to Stick With Exercise

1. *Pick an activity you enjoy.* Exercise should be fun, not only work. Try different activities until you find one or two you like.
2. *Make exercise social.* Exercising with a partner or group of friends is more fun than working out alone. Friends rely on each other for moral support and help each other stay committed to their fitness program. An "exercise date" once or twice a week can keep you going.
3. *Take lessons.* Join an aerobic dance class or a health club. Start slowly and progress gradually to avoid injuries. If exercise is too difficult or too intense, you are not likely to want to stay on your program.
4. *Make it convenient.* Develop a home gym or purchase a couple exercise videos. Keep your exercise gear available so that you can squeeze in a quick workout.
5. *Treat exercise like an appointment.* Schedule a time that works best for you, whether that be morning, noon, or evening.
6. *Keep a chart to monitor your progress.* It's rewarding to see how much you have progressed.
7. *Add variety.* To keep your program fresh, walk or jog different routes, exercise in a park or around a golf course. Alternate swimming, walking, and bicycling. While pedaling a stationary bike, read, listen to music, or watch TV. (But don't wear headphones when exercising outside near traffic.)
8. *Have a backup plan in case of bad weather or conflicts.*
9. *Be patient with yourself.* Expect ups and downs. Some days you will be more energetic, some days less. If you're not feeling like a workout, tell yourself you will do a little and you may find that after a few minutes you perk up. On the other hand, if you have been doing too much, a rest may do you more good than another workout.
10. *Finally, don't stop!* It's difficult to get going again. Remember to plan for changes in your schedule (for example, pack your exercise equipment when you travel). However, don't feel guilty if you miss an exercise session. A few days off due to illness or injury aren't a disaster. Consider this a lifetime commitment, and resume exercising as soon as possible.

to Stick with Exercise," for examples of how to apply the processes to your current stage of change.

Three-Part Workout

A workout includes three parts: A warm-up, a conditioning bout, and a cool-down.

Warm-Up

The **warm-up** is an important beginning to a workout session. Two important physiological changes occur during the warm-up. The internal temperature of the muscles increases, enhancing their elasticity. Heart rate and respiration increase, thus providing greater blood flow to the exercising muscles. The warm-up prepares the body physically and mentally for the conditioning bout and may reduce the chance of injury while exercising. There is no set length of time for the warm-up, although 5 to 15 minutes is adequate. On cold days, or times when you feel sluggish, the warm-up may take longer. When you're feeling energetic or when the temperature is warm, the warm-up period may be shorter. A good method of gauging whether you have had an adequate warm-up is to pay attention to how you feel. Do you feel ready to exercise vigorously? If you still feel stiff and sluggish, you need a longer warm-up. A slight sweat is a good indication of an adequate warm-up.

Three activities may be included in the warm-up: calisthenics (such as jumping jacks), mild stretching exercises, and a short period of task specific activity. Stretching during warm-up is mainly preparation for the activity, not for flexibility. Gentle **static stretching,** in which a stretch is held for 10 to 30 seconds, is best. **Ballistic stretching,** with jerking and bouncing movements, should not be used because it can strain cold muscles. Most experts agree that the best time to stretch for flexibility is during the cool-down phase because the muscles are warmer and more elastic.

The **task specific activity** is an exercise using the same muscles that will be used in the conditioning bout but at a lowered intensity level (lower heart rate). For example, joggers should include a short period of walking or slow jogging before increasing to a normal workout intensity. See Chapter 5 for exercises that can be used for warm-up and cool-down.

Conditioning Bout

The **conditioning bout** contains vigorous aerobic exercise that stimulates the cardiorespiratory system. It should follow the FITT formula. Progress slowly and listen to your body. Gradually increase the frequency and time of your workouts until you reach a maintenance level. Your goal is a lifetime of exercise. Select an aerobic activity you will enjoy. Depending on your age, current fitness level, and physical abilities, enjoy walking, cycling, or any other vigorous activity you prefer.

Cool-Down

The **cool-down** is the final segment of the workout. The purpose of the cool-down is to ease your body back to its resting state. It will usually take 5 to 15 minutes to gradually reduce the intensity of exercise. It should begin with the same activity performed in the conditioning bout, but at a lowered intensity. For example, if you jog, reduce the pace and end with a period of walking. Failure to cool-down may allow the muscles to further tighten, potentially causing soreness and stiffness. Another problem with inadequate cool-down is the possibility of venous blood pooling in the lower extremities, resulting in faintness and dizziness. Cool-down should continue until the heart rate is approximately 100 to 110 beats per minute or less. In the cool-down, spend a few minutes stretching while the muscles are thoroughly warm and elastic. Use the stretching exercises illustrated in Chapter 5. Greater flexibility is achieved when stretching occurs in the cool-down segment of the workout.

Principles of Fitness Development

When a person begins an exercise program, over time the body adapts to the demands placed upon it. The beneficial long-term changes that occur with regular exercise depend on several factors. To put together an effective exercise program, it is important to understand several principles of fitness development, including overload, specificity, reversibility, and individual differences.

Progressive Overload

Progressive overload is a gradual increase in physical activity, working a muscle group or body system beyond accustomed levels. Overload is perhaps the most important factor in developing physical fitness. When the amount of exercise is gradually increased, the muscle group or system, such as the cardiorespiratory system, gradually adapts, resulting in improved physiological functioning. In addition, a decrease in the severity and a delay in the onset of fatigue occur. If there is insufficient overload, there is no fitness improvement, but too much overload can cause injury. The key to gradual overload is to adapt the FITT formula to FTI (i.e., Frequency, Time, Intensity).

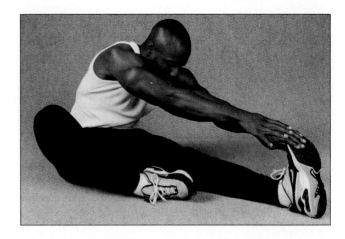

Flexibility gains are greatest during cool-down stretching.

First, there should be a gradual increase in the *frequency* of workouts, starting with 3 and progressing to 5 workouts per week, adding 1 more workout each week. Second, increase *time*. Start with workouts of 20 minutes (or less, if you are in poor condition) and gradually lengthen the workouts to 30 minutes by no more than 10 percent per week. For example, if the conditioning bout is 20 minutes, the next week's workouts can be 22 minutes. Third, increase the workout *intensity*. Begin at 60 percent intensity and progress to the 80 percent range by no more than 10 percent a week.

The old saying, "No pain, no gain!" is inappropriate advice for fitness exercisers. To increase your workout and minimize risk of overuse injury, follow the prescription factors in the correct order and listen to your body. Don't rush to get into shape in a couple weeks. Exercise is for a lifetime.

Specificity

The **principle of specificity** means that only the muscles or body systems being exercised will show beneficial changes. To improve the cardiorespiratory system, exercise the heart and lungs through aerobic activities; to improve flexibility, do stretching exercises; and to improve muscular strength, lift weights. You cannot strengthen the muscles of the arms by jogging, nor can you increase cardiorespiratory fitness by doing yoga. This principle also helps to explain why you are "wiped out" after swimming 10 minutes, even though you can run for 30 minutes.

Reversibility

The **principle of reversibility** states that changes occurring with exercise are reversible and if a person stops exercising, the body will decondition and adapt to the decreased activity level. Rate of fitness loss varies, but if a person stops exercising, a gradual loss of fitness begins within 48 hours. All fitness improvements can be lost within 2 to 4 months. If a person must decrease activity, greatest benefits can be retained by maintaining intensity while decreasing frequency or time of exercise. For example, if a person is traveling for two weeks and doesn't have time for the regular 30-minute run, 5 days a week, dropping to 20 minutes or 3 days a week at the usual THR will help maintain training effect benefits.

Individual Differences

The **principle of individual differences** states that people vary in their ability to develop fitness components. Some people find that it is relatively easy for them to build strength, but they have to work hard to maintain their desired body composition. Others find that it is easier for them to increase their cardiorespiratory endurance than their flexibility. We differ in our genetic endowment, and there are limits on our ability to improve any particular fitness component. Some have estimated that maximal oxygen uptake can be improved by only about 15 to 30 percent with aerobic exercise. Still, that amount of increase can make a tremendous difference in a person's quality of life. Within our genetic endowment, we have potential for improvement. You don't have to be an Olympic athlete to gain the health benefits of physical activity.

Cross Training

Cross training involves developing all five health-related components of fitness. Traditionally, cardiorespiratory endurance has been the most emphasized fitness component because it is essential to high-level health, but the other four health-related components are also important. Cross training develops balanced fitness by emphasizing comprehensive conditioning in the major muscle groups. Advantages of cross training are given in Table 3-5.

Originally, cross training referred to a conditioning regimen used by triathletes to train in three events—running, biking, and swimming. In the strictest sense, training for a triathlon is not cross training because all three events emphasize cardiorespiratory endurance. An example of cross training would be to add one swimming session and two weight-training workouts to a three-time-per-week jogging program. Add some stretching exercises after each workout and you have a balanced fitness program. (See Table 3-6 for other cross-training activities.) Expand your fitness program to include cross-training activities. The time and energy you invest will give big payoffs.

Assessing Physical Fitness

Physical fitness tests are often divided into two categories: health related and skill related. Skill-related tests, such as a vertical jump or shuttle run, are performance based and are related to athletic ability. Health-related tests are related to functional well-being in the areas of cardiorespiratory endurance, muscular strength and endurance, flexibility, and body composition. These areas of physiological functioning

table 3-5 Advantages of Cross Training

1. Cross training builds overall fitness because all five fitness components are emphasized. It entices the exerciser to apply the overload principle in workouts, thus improving fitness gains in every component.
2. Cross training develops high levels of fitness. By participating in a variety of activities, new muscle fibers are recruited and neuromuscular pathways, formerly left untapped, are developed. Higher levels of cardiorespiratory endurance can result.
3. Cross training reduces risk of overtraining and injury. When a person uses one activity to develop CRE, the same body parts are continually stressed, especially in weight-bearing activities such as running. Repetitive impact injuries (i.e., shin splints) can result. Because the stress imposed by cross training is spread to different muscle groups, a high volume of training can be performed without overtraining and injury.
4. Cross training develops muscle symmetry, a balance of strength and flexibility in opposing muscle groups. Using only one activity, some muscles become strong and their opposing muscles disproportionately weak. Well-balanced muscle pairs working in concert allow for more effective and efficient movement and minimize risk of injury.
5. Cross training reduces boredom and provides motivation. Cross training, with its variety of activities, stimulates interest in exercise, thereby improving adherence.

table 3-6 Activities for Cross Training

Exercise Goal	Activity
Cardiorespiratory Endurance	Running, fitness walking, aerobic dance, bench and stair stepping, rope jumping, cross-country skiing, swimming, cycling, water exercise, in-line skating, ice skating, full-court basketball, ultimate frisbee, soccer
Flexibility	Stretching, yoga
Muscular Strength	Resistance training with weight machines, free weights, elastic bands, gymnastics
Muscular Endurance	Calisthenics (push-ups, pull-ups, abdominal curls) weight training with light weights and high repetitions
Body Composition	Cardiorespiratory endurance exercises burn calories at the highest rate per minute. Resistance training builds muscle, which increases metabolic rate for a greater calorie burn 24 hours a day

can be improved or maintained through regular exercise and offer protection from the negative effects of a sedentary lifestyle.

Do you know how fit you are? We seem to have a natural curiosity about how we compare to others. The purpose of fitness testing is to help you identify your current fitness levels in several health-related categories. Such an evaluation should tell you whether your current lifestyle is effective in developing and maintaining a level of fitness conductive to optimal wellness. Your results can be used as a basis for setting personal fitness goals; for developing an appropriate individualized exercise prescription; and finally, for measuring the effectiveness of your fitness program in reaching your goals.

The remainder of this chapter gives norms that enable you to compare your fitness levels with those of other students. Norms reflect achievements of people who have completed a 12- to 15-week fitness course. When evaluating your fitness and setting goals, keep in mind that scoring in the "low" category does not reflect negatively on you. While "excellent" is an attainable goal for some, relatively few people achieve this level in one or more areas of fitness. Bodies are different. Your current fitness level does not indicate your potential. Physical capacity to achieve any particular level of fitness is partially genetically determined. You may find that you gain strength easily but must constantly work on flexibility or vice versa. Health-related fitness benefits can be experienced at the "average" fitness level. Also keep in mind that all tests are subject to some measurement variability. Use these norms as guidelines. Finally, testing should not dominate your program but help you measure its effectiveness. You may wish to measure at the beginning of your program and remeasure 8 to 12 weeks into the program to see how you are progressing.

A *Personal Fitness Profile* is located in Lab Activity 3-5. When completed, it will indicate areas of fitness you can maintain and areas needing improvement. It will help you decide where to begin in your fitness program.

Guidelines for Medical Clearance

According to American College of Sports Medicine guidelines, it is generally safe to begin a vigorous exercise program if you are under 40 years of age for men and under 50 for women, are healthy, and have had a satisfactory medical checkup in the past 2 years. Also, if you have been exercising regularly, it is probably safe to continue progressing gradually from your current activity level. Prior to participation, you should complete the *Health/Exercise Assessment Form* found in Lab Activity 3-1 to identify any potential health concerns.

If you are over these age guidelines or if, regardless of age, you have had health concerns noted on the *Health/Exercise Assessment Form*, it is important to check with your physician before taking a cardiorespiratory fitness test or participating in vigorous exercise. The *Exercise Clearance Form* in Lab Activity 3-2 is designed for individuals with special health concerns to assist your instructor in individualizing your fitness program according to your physician's recommendations. You may need to have a medical checkup and diagnostic exercise test. If you smoke cigarettes, have been sedentary over the past several months, are pregnant, have diabetes, are 20 or more pounds overweight, or have family members who have positive risk factors for heart disease, it is particularly important that you see your physician and ask him or her to fill out the *Exercise Clearance Form*. Also, check with your physician if you are unsure or have concerns about your health.

Cardiorespiratory Endurance Tests

A person with a high level of cardiorespiratory fitness can do more work with less fatigue than can a person with low cardiorespiratory fitness. Increased cardiorespiratory fitness can enhance quality of life by increasing the rate of energy production during physical activity. Low levels of cardiorespiratory fitness may result in a limited lifestyle due to low energy reserves, quick exhaustion with moderate exertion, and resulting inability to participate in vigorous, oxygen-demanding activities. High-level wellness is inextricably tied to a physically active lifestyle. If you want to be an active participant in life—not just a spectator—cardiorespiratory fitness is essential. The ability of your heart and lungs to supply oxygen during activity is one of the best indicators of overall physical fitness. There are several ways to measure your body's ability to use oxygen. The most accurate method is an **exercise tolerance test** on a treadmill or on a bicycle ergometer in a laboratory (see Fig. 3-8). In an exercise tolerance test, a person exercises strenuously while heart rate and oxygen consumption are measured. This, however, is complex, expensive, and time consuming and requires elaborate equipment and trained personnel. It is impractical for testing large numbers of people.

Cardiorespiratory fitness can also be measured in field tests conducted out of the laboratory setting. What they lose in accuracy they make up in the practicality of self-testing or testing many people at the same time. Field tests of cardiorespiratory endurance are generally based on physiological performance (distance or time tests) or a parameter such as pulse rate (step test).

A field test used to estimate oxygen consumption measures the time it takes you to jog 1.5 miles. Studies have

piratory endurance are the *1-Mile Walk Test*, the *3-Mile Bicycling Test*, the *500-Yard Swim Test*, the *500-Yard Water Run Test*, and the *3-Minute Step Test*. You can choose the test most appropriate for your chosen physical conditioning activity.

Pretest Instructions

For any of the cardiorespiratory endurance tests, you will need comfortable clothes appropriate for the activity and a stopwatch or a watch with a second hand.

- If possible, avoid taking the test under conditions of extreme heat or cold, particularly if you are not accustomed to exercising under those conditions.
- Do not eat a heavy meal, consume alcohol, caffeine, or smoke for up to 3 hours prior to the test.
- Drink plenty of fluids the day before testing.
- Rest from vigorous exercise at least 1 day prior to taking the test.
- Get adequate sleep (7 to 9 hours) the night before testing.
- Warm up and stretch before taking the test and then cool down and restretch afterward.
- If at any point during the test you begin to feel ill, dizzy, faint, or extremely short of breath, stop! Your body is telling you that you are not ready for this level of exertion.

Do not be ashamed of stopping before completing the test, especially if you are unfit. Test performance may be limited by local muscular endurance or by aerobic capacity. You may record the amount of time in the test you were able to complete and work toward a fitness level that will enable you to complete the test.

1.5-Mile Run Test

The *1.5-Mile Run Test* requires six laps around a standard quarter-mile track, or it can be done on a measured section of road. Consider taking this test only if you have been exercising previously. The *1-Mile Walk Test* may be more appropriate for you if you are over 35 years of age or 20 or more pounds overweight or if you have been out of shape for some time but are otherwise in good health.

    Goal: To run 1.5 miles as quickly as you can.
    Directions:

1. Locate a standard quarter-mile track or measure a section of road that has few stoplights.
2. Have a stopwatch or a watch with a second hand.
3. Warm up before taking the test.
4. This is a test of your maximum capacity, so do the best you can. Push yourself to cover the distance as fast as possible without overdoing. Try to maintain a continuous, even pace. Run as long as you can and

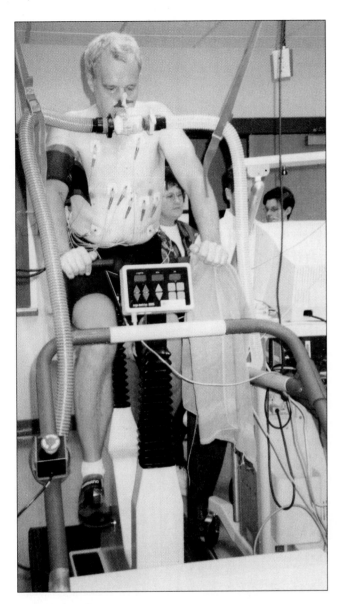

figure 3-8   Exercise tolerance test on a bicycle ergometer.

shown that time on the 1.5-mile run correlates well with maximal oxygen uptake. The faster you cover the distance, the more efficient your heart and lungs are at their job of supplying oxygenated blood and nutrients to the working muscles and in carrying away waste products. Field tests make it easy for you to measure your fitness and to detect progress as you train. Keep in mind that if you retest within a few weeks, early improvements may be due to a "learning effect" rather than true cardiovascular changes. That is, you will learn to pace yourself better throughout the distance. It will take 8 to 12 weeks for significant cardiovascular improvement to occur. You should only take the *1.5-Mile Run Test* if you are conditioned for it. It is best if you have been building up to the distance gradually for several weeks prior to taking the test. Other field tests that measure cardiores-

then walk when necessary. In a group of runners, it is helpful for runners to be given the right-of-way on the inner lanes and people who need to walk to move to the outer lanes.

5. When you complete the 1.5-mile distance, record your time and cool down with walking and stretching.
6. Check Table 3-7 for your fitness level.

1-Mile Walk Test

For those starting a walking program or for whom the *1.5 Mile Run Test* may be too vigorous, the *1-Mile Walk Test* is an option. You will need a 1-mile measured course (four laps of a quarter-mile track), your walking shoes, and a watch with a second hand.

Goal: To walk 1 mile as quickly as you can.
Directions:

1. Warm up and stretch before beginning.
2. Walk 1 mile as quickly as you can.
3. Record your time to the nearest second.
4. Cool down and stretch.
5. Locate your fitness level in Table 3-8.

3-Mile Bicycling Test

If your main fitness activity is bicycling, you can test your cardiorespiratory fitness with a timed 3-mile bicycle ride.

table 3-7   1.5-Mile Run Norms

	Men				
Age	18–29	30–39	40–49	50–59	60+
Excellent	<8:26	<9:10	<9:55	<10:40	<11:25
Good	8:26–10:24	9:10–11:10	9:55–12:00	10:40–12:50	11:25–13:40
Average	10:25–12:31	11:11–13:45	12:01–14:55	12:51–16:05	13:41–17:15
Low	12:32–14:39	13:46–16:00	14:56–17:15	16:06–18:30	17:16–19:45
Very Low	>14:39	>16:00	>17:15	>18:30	>19:45
	Women				
Age	18–29	30–39	40–49	50–59	60+
Excellent	<12:34	<13:34	<14:34	<15:34	<16:34
Good	12:34–13:40	13:34–14:40	14:34–15:40	15:34–16:40	16:34–17:40
Average	13:41–14:45	14:41–15:45	15:41–16:45	16:41–17:45	17:41–18:45
Low	14:46–16:00	15:46–17:00	16:45–18:00	17:46–19:00	18:46–20:00
Very Low	>16:00	>17:00	>18:00	>19:00	>20:00

table 3-8   1-Mile Walk Norms

	Men				
Age	18–29	30–39	40–49	50–59	60+
Excellent	<11:39	<12:40	<13:40	<14:10	<15:10
Good	11:39–12:59	12:40–14:00	13:40–14:40	14:10–15:20	15:10–16:10
Average	13:00–14:21	14:01–15:20	14:41–15:55	15:21–16:25	16:11–17:05
Low	14:22–15:43	15:21–16:15	15:56–16:45	16:26–17:25	17:06–18:05
Very Low	>15:43	>16:15	>16:45	>17:25	>18:05
	Women				
Age	18–29	30–39	40–49	50–59	60+
Excellent	<12:34	<13:34	<14:34	<15:34	<16:34
Good	12:34–13:40	13:34–14:40	14:34–15:40	15:34–16:40	16:34–17:40
Average	13:41–14:45	14:41–15:45	15:41–16:45	16:41–17:45	17:41–18:45
Low	14:46–16:00	15:46–17:00	16:46–18:00	17:46–19:00	18:46–20:00
Very Low	>16:00	>17:00	>18:00	>19:00	>20:00

This test can be done on a bike track or on a measured section of road with few stoplights or stop signs.

Goal: To bicycle 3 miles as quickly as possible.
Directions:

1. Warm up by riding for a few minutes and stretching.
2. Cycle 3 miles as quickly as you can. If you are doing this on the road, be careful to obey traffic rules.
3. Try to pace evenly. Time the ride with a stopwatch or a watch with a second hand. Record the time.
4. Cool down and stretch.
5. Check your results in Table 3-9.

500-Yard Swim Test

If your fitness program primarily involves swimming, you will find a swimming endurance test useful. A regulation 25-yard pool is recommended, and you will need a friend to time you. You may swim any stroke, although best results will be obtained with the front crawl.

Goal: To swim 500 yards as quickly as you can.
Directions:

1. Warm up.
2. Have a friend time you and count lengths. In a 25-yard pool, 500 yards is 20 lengths.
3. Record your time, cool down, and stretch.
4. Check Table 3-10 for your fitness level.

500-Yard Water Run Test

The *500-Yard Water Run Test* (Fig. 3-9) was designed for those involved in aerobic water exercise programs in which swimming skills are not required. It can be done lengthwise in a pool of constant depth or widthwise across the shallow

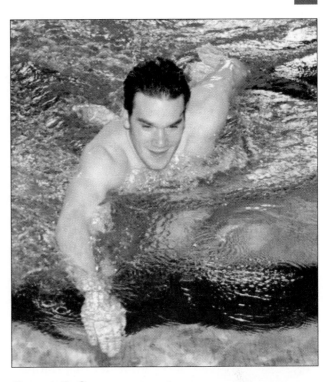

figure 3-9   500-yard water run test. This is a valid field test for nonswimmers. (Note: The water level should be midpoint between navel and nipple.)

end of a pool of variable depth. It helps to work in pairs, with one partner on deck counting completed laps for the other. For most accurate results, runners should carve their own paths through the water and avoid drafting in the wake of other runners. Runners should use their arms to pull as they run but must maintain a vertical body position. No swimming is allowed.

table 3-9   3-Mile Bicycling Norms

Men					
Age	18–29	30–39	40–49	50–59	60+
Excellent	<8:24	<9:00	<9:36	<10:12	<10:48
Good	8:24–9:12	9:00–9:42	9:36–10:12	10:12–10:42	10:48–11:12
Average	9:13–10:12	9:43–10:48	10:13–11:24	10:43–12:00	11:13–12:36
Low	10:13–11:06	10:49–11:35	11:25–12:06	12:01–12:48	12:37–13:12
Very Low	>11:06	>11:35	>12:06	>12:48	>13:12
Women					
Age	18–29	30–39	40–49	50–59	60+
Excellent	<9:18	<9:54	<10:30	<11:06	<11:42
Good	9:18–10:06	9:54–10:42	10:30–11:06	11:06–11:36	11:42–12:06
Average	10:07–11:06	10:43–11:42	11:07–12:18	11:37–12:54	12:07–13:30
Low	11:07–12:00	11:43–12:30	12:19–13:00	12:55–13:30	13:31–14:00
Very Low	>12:00	>12:30	>13:00	>13:30	>14:00

table 3-10   500-Yard Swim Norms

Men					
Age	18–29	30–39	40–49	50–59	60+
Excellent	<6:12	<6:30	<7:00	<7:30	<8:00
Good	6:12–7:44	6:30–8:14	7:00–8:44	7:30–9:14	8:00–9:44
Average	7:45–9:19	8:15–9:49	8:45–10:19	9:15–10:49	9:45–11:19
Low	9:20–10:51	9:50–11:22	10:20–11:52	10:50–11:22	11:20–12:52
Very Low	>10:52	>11:22	>11:52	>11:22	>12:52
Women					
Age	18–29	30–39	40–49	50–59	60+
Excellent	<7:05	<7:35	<8:05	<8:35	<9:05
Good	7:05–8:49	7:35–9:19	8:05–9:49	8:35–10:19	9:05–10:49
Average	8:50–10:34	9:20–11:04	9:50–11:34	10:20–12:04	10:50–12:34
Low	10:35–12:19	11:05–12:49	11:35–13:19	12:05–13:49	12:35–14:49
Very Low	>12:19	>12:49	>13:19	>13:49	>14:49

table 3-11   500-Yard Water Run Norms

Men					
Age	18–29	30–39	40–49	50–59	60+
Excellent	<6:53	<7:20	<7:50	<8:20	<9:50
Good	6:43–7:44	7:20–8:15	7:50–8:45	8:20–9:15	9:50–10:45
Average	7:45–8:38	8:16–9:05	8:46–9:35	9:16–10:05	10:46–11:05
Low	8:39–9:32	9:06–10:00	9:36–10:30	10:06–11:00	11:06–11:30
Very Low	>9:32	>10:00	>10:30	>11:00	>11:30
Women					
Age	18–29	30–39	40–49	50–59	60+
Excellent	<7:59	<8:30	<9:00	<9:30	<10:00
Good	7:59–8:38	8:30–9:08	9:00–9:38	9:30–10:08	10:00–10:38
Average	8:39–9:18	9:09–9:48	9:39–10:18	10:09–10:48	10:39–11:18
Low	9:19–9:58	9:49–10:28	10:19–10:58	10:49–11:28	11:19–11:58
Very Low	>9:58	>10:28	>10:58	>11:28	>11:58

Goal: To run 500 yards in the water as quickly as possible.

Directions:

1. Measure pool width and calculate the number of lengths required to cover 500 yards.
2. Have a partner on deck count laps and keep the time.
3. Warm up with a couple minutes of easy jogging in the water.
4. To give runners of different heights a similar level of water resistance in a variable depth pool, select a starting point along the pool wall where the water level is at a midpoint between the runner's navel and nipple. Shorter runners will start in shallower water, taller runners in deeper water.
5. Take a position in the water, note your starting time, and run the necessary number of widths. Record your time to the nearest second.
6. Cool down and stretch.
7. Check Table 3-11 for your fitness level.

3-Minute Step Test

There are a variety of step tests useful for testing cardiorespiratory fitness indoors. They involve stepping on and off a bench for a 3- to 5-minute period and measuring the heart

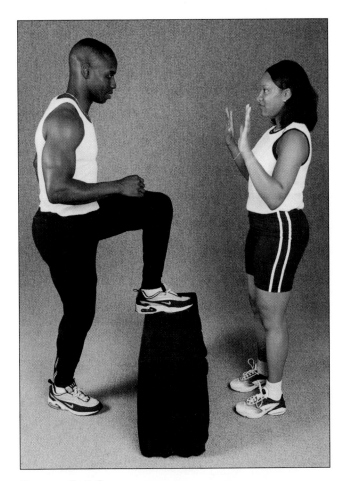

figure 3-10   Step test.

table 3-12	3-Minute Step Test Norms	
	Men	Women
Excellent	<31	<37
Good	31–37	37–41
Average	38–41	42–44
Low	42–45	45–49
Very Low	>45	>49

your right and then your left. Continue for 3 minutes. Straighten your knees as you step up on the bench. To prevent leg soreness, you may want to switch lead legs about halfway through the test.

5. Stop at the end of 3 minutes and sit down. Five seconds after completing the test, the tester should count the partner's pulse for 15 seconds. The tester can check the partner's carotid pulse by lightly pressing against the neck under the jawbone. The partner being tested can double-check his or her own pulse at the radial artery, located on the thumb side of the wrist. The partners' pulse counts should not vary more than one or two beats if counting is accurate.

6. Record the pulse.

7. Cool down and stretch.

8. Compare your pulse with the norms given in Table 3-12 to assess your cardiorespiratory fitness. If you are unable to keep the cadence for the full 3 minutes, consider yourself to have low cardiorespiratory endurance.

rate recovery. The step test is based on the fact that the heart rate of a person who is physically fit is lower at any work load and recovers faster than does the heart rate of a person who is unfit. Although it is not the best measure of cardiorespiratory fitness, it is a quick and simple way to evaluate the heart's response to exercise. It is easy to administer to an individual or to large groups, requires no special skill to perform, and requires little equipment (Fig. 3-10).

Goal: To step on and off a bench for 3 minutes.
Directions:

1. Locate a 15-inch bench or a 16-inch roll-out bleacher step.

2. Warm up.

3. Work with a partner. While your partner is stepping on and off the bench, stand in front of him or her to prevent falling. Then switch.

4. You will need to step up and down at 96 counts per minute. A metronome or recorded music at a tempo of 96 beats per minute will help you keep cadence, or your instructor will call the cadence: "Up-up-down-down." At the signal "Begin," step up with your right foot and then your left foot and then step down with

Muscular Strength and Endurance Tests

Muscular strength and endurance are assets in the ability to perform daily activities—lifting, carrying, pushing, pulling—without strain or undue fatigue. Strength and endurance of the abdominal muscles are particularly important for good posture and lower back health. Muscular fitness activities add shape and firmness to muscles, resulting in a trim, well-toned appearance.

Muscular strength and muscular endurance tests have been used as a measure of physical fitness for years. Physical conditioning activities require and can develop both components. Strength is best developed by weight training and is often measured by one maximal lift with weights (see Chap. 5). Muscular endurance can be measured without special equipment, using tests provided here. Abdominal curls are perhaps the best way to assess the endurance of the abdominal muscles. The traditional *Bent-Knee Sit-Up Test* requires use of the thighs and hip flexors as well as abdominals and may put the back at risk. Abdominal curls isolate and test only abdominal muscles, decreasing risk to the lower back. Directions and norms for abdominal curls are given. To test the muscular endurance of the arms and upper body muscles, norms are also given for push-ups.

Abdominal Curls

Goal: To complete as many abdominal curls as possible in 1 minute.
Directions:

1. Tape a 3-inch wide strip on the floor, and lie on your back on the floor with your fingertips at the edge of the strip. Bend your knees, and bring your heels as close as possible toward your buttocks.
2. Curl forward until your fingertips have moved forward across the 3-inch strip and then curl back until your shoulder blades touch the floor. Your shoulders should lift from the floor with each curl,

but the lower back should stay on the ground (Fig. 3-11). If you are working with a partner who is counting your curls, your partner should not hold your feet down, nor should your feet lift off the ground—if they do, you are curling too high.
3. Complete as many curls as possible in 1 minute; then check the results in Table 3-13.

Push-Ups

Goal: To complete as many push-ups as possible in 1 minute.
Directions:

1. Start in an "up" position with your weight on your toes (men) or knees (women) and hands (Figs. 3-12 and 3-13).
2. Lower yourself until your elbows form a right angle and your upper arm is parallel to the floor.
3. Complete as many full push-ups as you can in 1 minute. Be sure to keep your abdominals tight, hips slightly

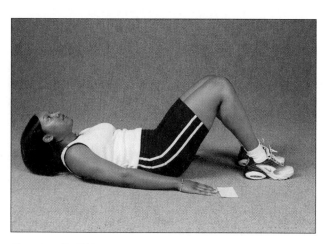

figure 3-11   Abdominal curls (fingertips move forward 3 inches).

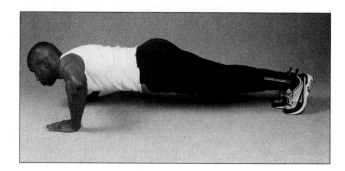

figure 3-12   Push-up—standard position. (Note the 90 degree elbow angle.)

table 3-13   1-Minute Abdominal Curl Norms

Men					
Age	18–29	30–39	40–49	50–59	60+
Excellent	>93	>78	>65	>49	>44
Good	79–93	62–78	53–65	42–49	33–44
Average	64–78	51–61	45–52	35–41	27–32
Low	50–63	40–50	36–44	28–34	22–26
Very Low	<50	<40	<36	<28	<22
Women					
Age	18–29	30–39	40–49	50–59	60+
Excellent	>88	>70	>56	>45	>36
Good	75–88	60–70	48–56	38–45	30–36
Average	60–74	47–59	37–47	29–37	22–30
Low	45–59	35–46	27–36	21–28	16–21
Very Low	<45	<35	<27	<21	<16

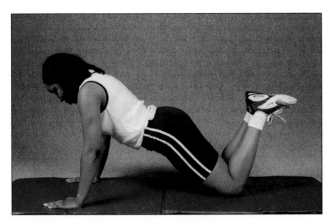

figure 3-13   Push-up—modified position.

piked, and your back straight to protect your lower back. Record, and check your score in Table 3-14.

Flexibility Tests

Flexibility is a valuable asset in daily activities or in any type of vigorous exercise program. The ability to move joints through a full range of motion without stiffness or tightness makes exercise more comfortable and may decrease risk of injury. The tests included in this section will indicate whether you have a normal range of motion in the lower back and other important areas.

Quick Checks for Flexibility

The quick checks for flexibility shown in Figures 3-14 to 3-19 are easy ways of measuring flexibility of major muscle groups often shortened and tightened in daily activities.

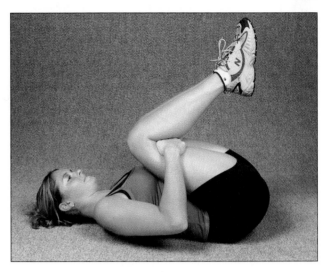

figure 3-14   Lower back flexibility test.
Muscle: Erector spinae (lower back)
Test: Lying on your back, pull thighs to chest.
Passing: Thighs should touch chest.

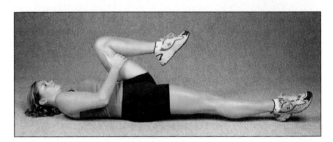

figure 3-15   Hip flexor flexibility test.
Muscle: Iliopsoas (hip flexor)
Test: Lying on your back, pull one knee to chest, keeping other leg fully extended on the floor.
Passing: Calf of extended leg must remain on the floor; knee must not bend.

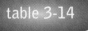
table 3-14   1-Minute Push-Up Norms

Standard Position				
Age	18–29	30–39	40–49	50–59	60+
Excellent	>64	>54	>43	>33	>23
Good	51–64	41–54	32–43	26–33	18–23
Average	37–50	27–40	22–31	17–25	11–17
Low	23–36	18–26	13–21	8–16	6–10
Very Low	<23	<18	<13	<8	<6
Modified Position				
Age	18–29	30–39	40–49	50–59	60+
Excellent	>54	>43	>33	>23	>17
Good	44–54	32–43	26–33	18–23	15–17
Average	32–43	22–31	17–25	11–17	10–14
Low	20–31	13–21	8–16	6–10	4–9
Very Low	<20	<13	<8	<6	<4

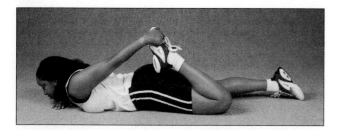

figure 3-16   Quadriceps flexibility test. Caution: Avoid if you have or experience knee problems.

Muscle: Quadriceps (front of thigh)
Test: Lying face down with knees together, pull heel toward buttocks.
Passing: Heel should comfortably touch buttocks.

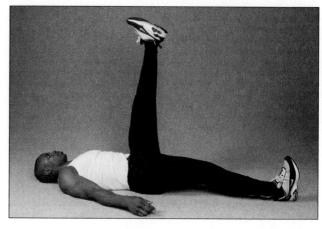

figure 3-17   Hamstring flexibility test.

Muscle: Hamstrings (back of thigh)
Test: Lying on your back, lift one leg, keeping other leg flat on floor without bending either knee.
Passing: The raised leg must reach vertical (90 degrees).

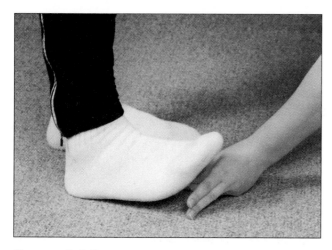

figure 3-18   Calf flexibility test.

Muscle: Gastrocnemius (calf)
Test: Standing without shoes, raise one forefoot off floor, keeping knees relaxed and heels down.
Passing: Ball of foot should clear floor by height equal to width of two fingers.

Each quick check is also a stretch, so if your range of motion is limited or if you feel excessive tightness in a joint or muscle group, use the same position to improve flexibility in that area (see Chap. 5 for basic fitness flexibility guidelines).

Sit and Reach Test

The *Sit and Reach Test*, which measures hamstring flexibility, can be done with a flex box. If you do not have a flex box, the test can be performed with a ruler on a bench or on the ground with feet flexed (Fig. 3-20). Norms are given using the soles of the feet as the 0 inches mark.

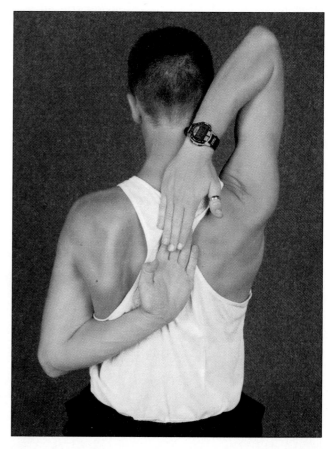

figure 3-19   Shoulder girdle flexibility test.

Muscle: Shoulder girdle
Test: Try to touch fingertips behind back both ways.
Passing: Fingertips touch.

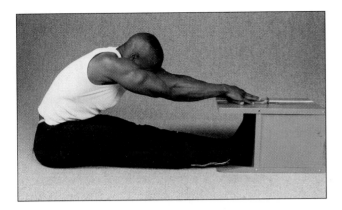

figure 3-20   Sit and reach test.

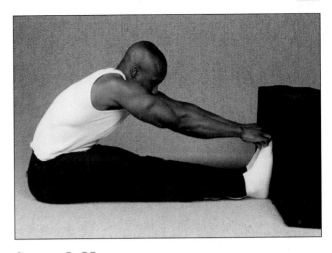

figure 3-21   Sit and reach wall test.

Goal: To measure flexibility of the hamstrings.
Directions:

1. Warm up.
2. Sit with your feet flat against the flex box about 5 inches apart. Keep your legs straight.
3. Place your hands together. Without bending your knees, reach as far forward as possible, extending fingertips along the box. Hold the position for 3 seconds.
4. Find your flexibility in Table 3-15.

Sit and Reach Wall Test

The *Sit and Reach Wall Test* is a self-check for flexibility and can quickly be performed by a large number of people. All you need is a wall! (Fig. 3-21).

Goal: To measure flexibility of the hamstrings.
Directions:

1. Warm up by walking and static stretching.
2. Remove shoes, sit facing a wall, and keep your feet flat against the wall and your knees straight.
3. Reach forward as far as possible to touch your fingertips, knuckles, or palms to the wall and hold the position for 3 seconds.
4. Check your flexibility evaluation in Table 3-16.

Body Composition Tests

A certain amount of body fat is essential to good health. Fat acts as an insulator, conserving body heat. It pads bones and cushions internal organs, and it stores and supplies energy for later use.

table 3-15   Sit and Reach Norms

Men					
Age	18–29	30–39	40–49	50–59	60+
Excellent	>7.0	>6	>5	>4	>3
Good	4.0–7.0	3–6	2–5	1–4	0–3
Average	1.0–3.9	0–2.9	−1–1.9	−3–0	−1.–0.1
Low	−2.0–0.9	−3.–0.1	−4.–1.1	−5.–3.1	−7.–4.1
Very Low	<−2.0	<−3	<−4	<−5	<−7
Women					
Age	18–29	30–39	40–49	50–59	60+
Excellent	>8.5	>8	>7	>6	>5
Good	6.5–8.5	5–8	4–7	3–6	2–5
Average	4.0–6.4	3–4.9	2–3.9	0–2.9	−1–1.9
Low	1.0–3.9	0–2.9	−1–1.9	−2–0.1	−3–1.1
Very Low	<1.0	<0	<−1	<−2	<−3

table 3-16 — Sit and Reach Wall Test Scores

Result	Flexibility
Cannot touch wall	Low
Fingertips touch wall	Average
Knuckles touch wall	Good
Palms touch wall	Excellent

In a diet-obsessed society in which both obesity and eating disorders abound, few people realize that excessive leanness can be as unhealthy as excessive fatness. For young adults, an average range of body fat for women is 21 to 24 percent and for men it is 14 to 17 percent (Table 3-17). Keep in mind that each of us has inherited a certain body build and fat distribution; it is natural for some bodies to carry more fat than others. It is also natural to increase body fat slightly as we age.

While weight scales can tell you how much you weigh, they cannot tell you how much of your body is composed of fat or lean tissue. A sedentary individual may maintain a normal weight for height but increase fat and lose **lean body mass** (muscle tissue) over time. A body builder may be "overweight" according to height-weight charts, but this is due to development of muscle and bone rather than fat. Being overweight due to having a substantial amount of lean muscle tissue is not the same as being overweight due to excess fat tissue. A person who has a muscular build may think she is too heavy when the weight is mainly lean tissue. She could jeopardize her health trying to lose weight unneces-

sarily. On the other hand, a sedentary person who is satisfied with her weight may be shocked to discover her body fat percentage is over 30 percent, high enough to pose a health risk. In the early stages of a fitness program, excess fat will often be lost and lean muscle weight will increase as fitness improves. Even if no significant weight change occurs, the exerciser is leaner and appears trimmer because a pound of muscle is denser than a pound of fat.

Body fat is most accurately measured by underwater weighing in a laboratory. Because fat is more buoyant than muscle tissue, underwater weighing can estimate body composition within plus or minus 2 to 3 percent. However, this requires elaborate equipment, trained personnel, and considerable time to test each individual. Other laboratory tests of body composition being researched include bioelectrical impedance, near-infrared spectrophotometry, ultrasound, and photon absorptiometry.

Bioelectrical impedance is based on the fact that an electrical current travels through **fat-free tissue** (all parts of the body except fat) with its high water and electrolyte content more readily than it does through fat. The current is not harmful because it is too mild to be felt. Results vary with differences in hydration, placement of electrodes, skin temperature, and type of machine used. The validity of this technique has not been determined, and studies have found both over- and underestimation of body fat by 2 to 5 percent when compared to other criterion measures.

Infrared technology traditionally has been used to determine the moisture, protein, and fat composition of food. When used to measure body composition, it tends to underestimate body fat, though some feel it is more accurate than other methods for lean or obese individuals.

table 3-17 — Body Fat Norm Percentages

Men			
Ages	18–29	30–39	40–49	50+
Very low fat	<10	<11	<13	<15
Low fat (trim)	10–13	11–16	13–18	15–19
Average	14–17	17–19	19–21	20–22
Above average (fat)	18–20	20–22	22–23	23–24
High fat	21–25	23–25	24–25	25–26
Obese	>25	>25	>25	>26
Women			
Ages	18–29	30–39	40–49	50+
Very low fat	<17	<18	<19	<20
Low fat (trim)	17–20	18–20	19–21	20–22
Average	21–24	21–24	22–24	23–25
Above average (fat)	25–27	25–27	25–27	26–28
High fat	28–30	28–30	28–30	29–31
Obese	>30	>30	>30	>31

Ultrasound devices measure the variation in diffusion rates of ultrasound waves through fat and lean tissue. Accuracy varies with the pressure exerted on the skin, body fluid balance, and the number of sites measured.

Photon absorptiometry is based on the variations in the rate of photon emissions from bone, lean, and fat tissue after the body is exposed to low-dose radiation. It is not commonly used due to its limited availability, expense, and complexity and due to concern over radiation exposure.

A practical technique for measuring body composition involves the use of **skinfold calipers.** A caliper is a device that compresses the skin at a pressure determined by a spring. Skinfold measurements can be used to assess your proportion of fat to lean tissue because about 50 percent of your fat is **subcutaneous fat**—located directly under the skin. The amount of subcutaneous fat you have correlates highly with total body fat. An experienced measurer can assess body fat with skinfold calipers to within a range of plus or minus 2 to 5 percent. Two or more body sites may be measured, and accuracy increases with the number of sites sampled. Accuracy diminishes at the ends of the scale—for the very obese and the very lean—but for the average individual, skinfolds are reliable.

Self-tests of body composition, though considerably less accurate than skinfold caliper measurements, involve body girth measures of body fat and the pinch test. Keep in mind that greater fitness is not guaranteed by low body fat, and what constitutes a healthy fat percentage for you is an individual matter.

Body Composition Assessment Using Skinfold Calipers

Goal: To accurately measure subcutaneous body fat.
Directions: Have a person trained in the use of skinfold calipers perform the following steps.

1. Measure skinfolds on the right side of the body using a skinfold caliper.
2. Grasp a fold of skin between thumb and forefinger, pulling it away from the underlying muscle.
3. Apply the calipers about 0.25 inch below the fingers holding the skinfold (Fig. 3-22).
4. Take triceps and thigh measurements on a vertical skinfold. Take subscapular and suprailiac measures on a slight lateral slant along the natural fold of the skin.
5. Measure twice. Take readings to the nearest half millimeter. If the readings do not match, take a third measurement and average the closest two measurements.
6. Skinfold sites for women are the following:
   a. Triceps. Measure a vertical skinfold on the back of the arm midway between the shoulder and the elbow (Fig. 3-23).

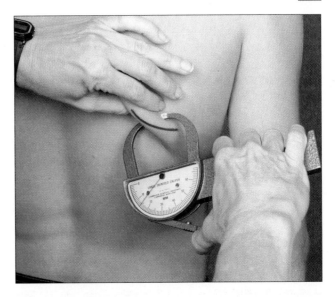

figure 3-22   Skinfold measuring technique.

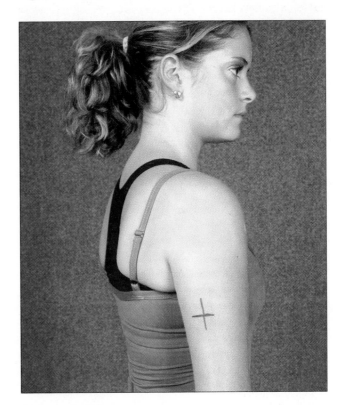

figure 3-23   Triceps.

   b. Suprailiac. Measure a slightly lateral fold at the middle of the side of the body just above the hip bone (iliac crest) (Fig. 3-24).
7. Skinfold sites for men are the following:
   a. Thigh. Measure a vertical fold on the front of the thigh midway between the inguinal fold (where the hip bends in front) and the top of the patella (knee cap) (Fig. 3-25).

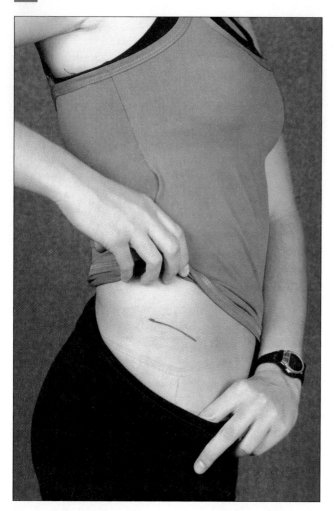

figure 3-24   Suprailiac.

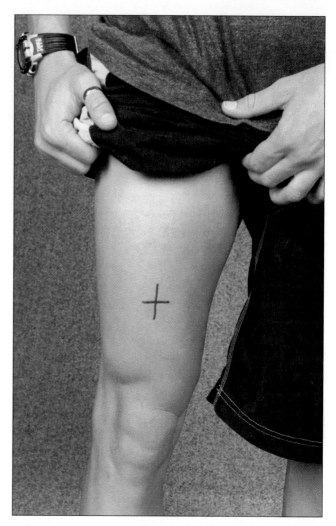

figure 3-25   Thigh.

b. Subscapular. Measure a diagonal fold just under the right shoulder blade (scapula) (Fig. 3-26).

8. Mark your two skinfold measurements on the *Percent Body Fat Nomogram* (Fig. 3-27) and connect the marks with a straight line. Read your percent of fat on the centers scale. See Table 3-17, Body Fat Norm Percentages, for your body composition evaluation. If your body fat is not on the nomogram, use the following formula:

Female (percent body fat formula)

% Body fat [Sloan-Weir] = [4.57/[1.0764 − (0.00081 × suprailiac skinfold, mm) − (0.00088 × triceps skinfold, mm)] − 4.142] × 100

Male (percent body fat formula)

Percent body fat = [4.57/[1.1043 − (0.00133 × thigh skinfold, mm) − (0.00131 × subscapula skinfold, mm)] − 4.142] × 100

How to Determine Desirable Weight

Once you have measured your body fat percentage, it is useful to determine your desirable weight based on your present fat-free mass. For young adults, a reasonable body fat level in the trim range for women is 17 percent to 20 percent fat, and for men it is 10 percent to 13 percent fat (Table 3-17). The following steps use an example of a person who has 26 percent body fat and weighs 140 pounds to illustrate how to determine desirable weight at 18 percent body fat for females and 12 percent fat for males.

Goal: To calculate desirable weight at 18 percent fat for women and 12 percent fat for men.
Directions: Perform the calculations that follow using your measurements:

- Body fat percentage = 26 percent.
- Weight = 140 lbs.

1. Body fat percentage × body weight = fat 0.26 × 140 lbs. = 36.4 lbs.
2. Body weight − fat = fat-free mass 140 lbs. − 36.4 lbs. = 103.6 lbs.
3. Fat-free mass ÷ 0.82 = desired weight for women at 18 percent fat.
   103.6 lbs. ÷ 0.82 = 126 lbs.
   Fat-free mass ÷ 0.88 = desired weight for men at 12 percent fat.
   103.6 lbs. ÷ 0.88 = 117 lbs.

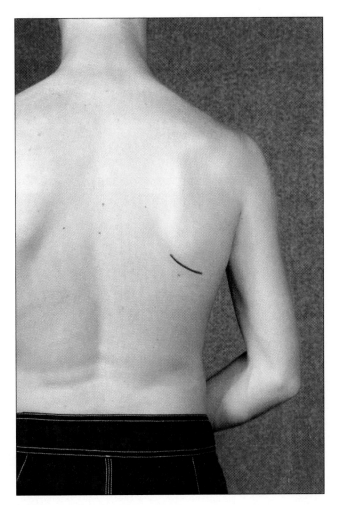

figure 3-26 Subscapular.

Body Girth Measures

One reason many people begin a fitness program is that they are concerned about their physical appearance. Basic body build is an inherited characteristic, and only about 5 percent of the population can aspire to the current cultural "ideal" of model-like proportions. Take a look at your parents and grandparents to get an idea of your genetic endowment and what is realistic for you. While your basic structure cannot be altered, as fitness improves, fat may be lost from deposit areas and muscles will become firmer, enhancing body contours. You may notice a loss of unwanted inches from the waist, hips, or thighs or a desirable reshaping of body contours before noticing any weight change. Body girth measures will help you set goals to work for a trim, healthy body shape.

Goal: To measure body girths.
Directions: Recruit a partner to measure you. You will need a measuring tape. For each measurement, pull the tape snugly, but do not indent the flesh. Take the measurements at the following sites (Fig. 3-28):

- *Chest:* across the nipple line at the midpoint of a normal breath
- *Abdominal 1:* across the floating ribs, halfway between the chest and waist, at the midpoint of a normal breath
- *Waist:* the narrowest point, across the navel
- *Abdominal 2:* across the iliac crest (hip bones), midway between waist and hips
- *Hips:* with feet together, across the pubic bone in front and across the widest part in back
- *Thigh:* right side, widest part, 1 inch below the crotch
- *Calf:* widest part
- *Wrist:* narrow part, above the bone, with palm up

Body Girth Measures of Body Fat

Body girth measures of fatness are considerably less accurate than other measures of body fat such as skinfolds. However, their advantage is that they do not require special equipment nor training, and they can be done with a measuring tape at home.

Directions:

1. Men should measure waist girth at the navel and women should measure hips at the widest point. Pull the tape so it is snug but does not indent the skin (Fig. 3-28).
2. Remove shoes. Men should measure their weight without clothing. Women should measure their height.
3. Mark the measurements on the appropriate circumference chart and connect them with a straight line (Fig. 3-29).

Waist-to-Hip Ratio

Investigations have begun pointing to the location of excess fat as a risk factor for heart disease and certain cancers. Fat

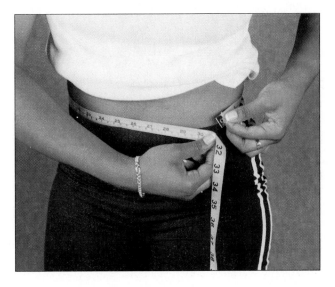

Waist-to-hip ratio identifies health risk.

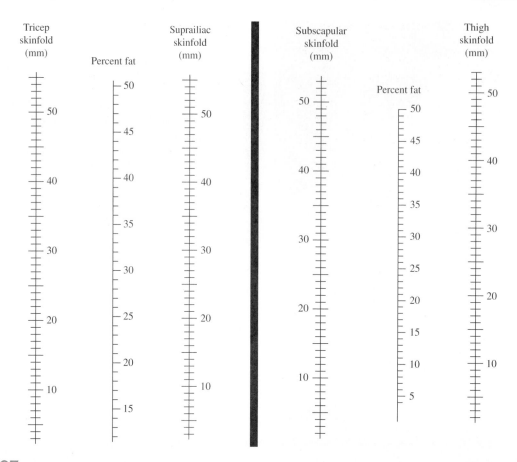

figure 3-27   Percent body fat nomogram.

Source: A. W. Sloan and J. Weir. "Nomograms for Prediction of Body Density and Total Body Fat from Skinfold Measurements." *Journal of Applied Physiology* 28:2 (1970): 221–22. Reprinted by permission of the American Physiological Society.

distributed in the abdominal area is linked to increased health risks; hip/thigh fat is not as risky. As a result, the waist-to-hip ratio has become a common assessment for health-risk identification. To compute this ratio, divide the waist measurement by the hip measurement.

$$\frac{29 \text{ in. waist}}{38 \text{ in. hip}} = 0.76 \qquad \frac{42 \text{ in. waist}}{36 \text{ in. hip}} = 1.17$$

Studies indicate that health problems are increased for women whose ratio is 0.80 or higher and for men whose ratio is 0.95 or higher. (See Chap. 11 for more information on waist-to-hip ratio as a health-risk factor.)

Pinch Test

Another simple measure of body fatness is the pinch test. Grasp a skinfold at the mid-point of your side, just above your hip bone (iliac crest). More than a 1-inch skinfold thickness may indicate excessive body fat.

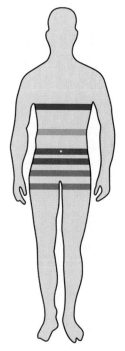

figure 3-28   Body girth measurement sites.

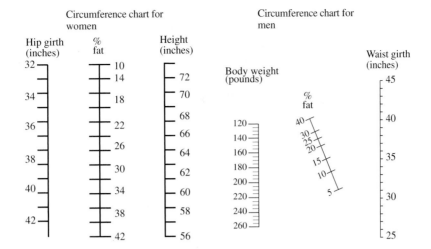

figure 3-29 Circumference charts.

Source: Nomograms developed by Jack Wilmore, University of Texas. Used by permission.

 frequently asked questions

Q. How many calories do I burn while walking or jogging a mile?

A. Caloric expenditure is based on body weight. You burn about 62 calories per 100 pounds per mile whether walking or jogging. It's a principle of physics. It takes a certain amount of energy to move weight a certain distance. If you weigh 150 pounds, you burn $62 \times 1.50 = 93$ calories per mile.

Q. I've seen a lot of ads for electrical muscle stimulators (EMS). Do they really make you lose weight, firm thighs, tone up?

A. There is no shortcut to fitness. EMS machines use an electric current to cause muscles to contract. They are often used in physical therapy to help heal weak or injured tissues. Research has shown them to be ineffective in strengthening healthy muscles. To get a strong enough contraction to be effective, you would have to turn up the current to painful levels. Also, the machines are expensive. If you want to lose weight and tone up, your time and money are better spent in the gym.

Q. I want to lose weight. Is it better to exercise for a longer time at a lower intensity or less time at a higher intensity?

A. If your main goal is weight control, the most important factor, besides a low-fat, nutritious diet, is to be consistent about working aerobic exercise—of any length and intensity—into your daily schedule. Work out at least 5 days per week. Total calories expended is more important than intensity of activity in maximizing weight loss. One or

two weight-training sessions per week also benefit weight control. Moderate intensity exercise is recommended because it allows you to exercise longer, accumulate more total work, thus burn more calories, and it is less likely to cause discomfort or injury. Moderate-intensity activity can also help you keep off lost weight. If your goal is high-level fitness, then exercise at a higher intensity is necessary.

Q. I swim/cycle regularly and feel like I'm in pretty good shape. Why did I only score "average" on the 1.5 mile walk/run?

A. It's the rule of specificity. Your aerobic fitness will show best if you use the test specific to your activity. Swimmers should use the 500 yard swim, cyclists the 3-mile ride for results, which are a better reflection of their aerobic fitness level. Likewise, someone who usually runs for exercise would find a cycling or swimming test more difficult.

Q. I had my body fat tested by skinfold calipers and bioelectrical impedance. They gave different results. Which is more accurate?

A. Both are reasonably accurate when used by an experienced tester, with average errors of 2 to 5 percent. Skinfold calipers are more accurate if multiple sites are measured to get a better picture of total fat distribution. Bioelectrical impedance can overestimate fat percentage if you are dehydrated, and results vary depending on where the electrodes are placed and the type of machine used.

summary

The sedentary lifestyle of most Americans is seriously undermining the health and welfare of our nation. We are fast becoming overfat and underfit, resulting in reduced levels of well-being. From the information you have acquired in this chapter, you now have the necessary tools to confidently develop a personalized physical fitness program, based on sound scientific principles and using your age, resting heart rate, interests, and abilities. You also have gained a better understanding of the health benefits that can be achieved by incorporating moderate levels of physical activity into your daily life. By applying the FITT prescription factors, the concept of a three-segment workout, and finding ways to increase daily activity, you can be on your way to a lifetime of improved health, fitness, and wellness.

Assessment is a critical tool in developing any dimension of wellness. It helps you to understand your strengths and weaknesses and to decide whether your current levels of cardiorespiratory endurance, muscular endurance, flexibility, and body fat are conducive to optimal wellness. With this knowledge, you can set reasonable fitness goals, establish a starting point for a fitness program, and develop a plan of action. Specific workout programs for different aerobic activities can be found in Chapter 4. A *Health/Exercise Assessment Form* and a *Personal Fitness Profile* are also available in the Lab Activities section of this chapter.

As you progress in your fitness program, it may be useful to retest occasionally. While testing should not dominate your program, it will allow you to monitor your progress and can give additional motivation to continue regular exercise.

additional information resources

Centers for Disease Control and Prevention
    www.cdc.gov

American College of Sports Medicine (ACSM)
    www.acsm.org
Indianapolis, IN
317–637–9200

Name _____

Class/Activity Section _____

Date _____

lab activity 3–2

Exercise Clearance Form

This form is designed for individuals with special health concerns to assist your instructor in individualizing your fitness program according to your physician's recommendations. If you have concerns about your health noted in Lab 3–1, are sedentary, diabetic, pregnant, 20 or more pounds overweight, smoke cigarettes or have a family history of heart disease, it is important to check with your physician before starting an exercise program.

This form must be taken to the health center or to your personal physician for a signature. It must be returned to your instructor by _____.

_____ is presently enrolled in _____. He/she has identified the following health problems that may affect participation in the activities of the course:

_____

_____

_____

_____

_____

_____

_____

The class will include the following activities:

After examining _____, I recommend the following level of participation in the course described.

____ Full participation

____ No participation*

____ Modified participation as indicated.

The student may participate in the class with the following modifications to activity: _____

_____

_____

_____

*If the student may not participate in this class, list activities in which the student may participate: _____

_____

_____

_____

_____

_____   _____   _____
Signature of physician   Phone #   Date

Health-Related Fitness Analysis Chart

After completing your *Personal Fitness Profile*, use norms in Chapter 3 to determine your fitness level on each of the tests. Use Figure A.2 to graph the results. Match fitness levels on the left with the norm ratings for each of the following tests: cardiorespiratory endurance, abdominal curls, push-ups, and sit and reach. Use the descriptors on the right for body fat norms. Place a dot in the center of the space that indicates your rating on each of the health-related fitness norms. Use straight lines to connect the dots.

Fitness level						Body fat descriptors
						Very low fat
Excellent						Low fat
Good						Average fat
Average						Above average fat
Low						High fat
Very low						Obese
	CR endur.	Curls	Push-ups	Sit & reach	Body fat	

Source: From Assmann, N. Muncie, Ind.: Ball State University. Used by permission.

1. In which fitness components did you score average or higher? Why?

lab activity @ chapter three

2. In which fitness components did you score below average? Why?

3. What are your fitness goals for the next 8–12 weeks, 6 months–1 year, 5 years or more?

8–12 weeks:

6 months–1 year:

5 years or more:

Name _____

Class/Activity Section _____

Date _____

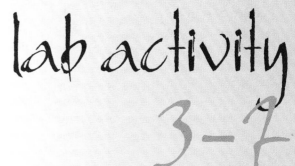

Understanding Health-Related Fitness Assessments

This exercise allows you to check your understanding of which assessments correspond to which fitness components and of how to interpret fitness test results based on age-adjusted norms. It also gives you practice in applying fitness test results to an appropriate workout in Chapter 4.

Jenny, age 23, completed her fitness assessments and the results follow. Using norms given in Chapter 3, evaluate her fitness levels and, for each assessment, determine what fitness component was being tested.

Assessment	Results	Fitness Level	Fitness Component Tested
1.5-mile run	16:30	_____	_____
Abdominal curls	45	_____	_____
Push-ups	45	_____	_____
Skinfolds:			
Tricep	20 mm	Percent fat _____	_____
Iliac	10 mm		
Sit and reach	3 inches	_____	_____

1. Using the *Run/Walk Program* chart in Chapter 4, what is her starting workout level?

2. From this *Run/Walk Program* chart, what is prescribed for her initial workout?

Cardiorespiratory Fitness Assessment

Equipment Needed:

1.5-Mile Run or 1-Mile Walk Test:	Track or premeasured course and stopwatch
3-Mile Bicycling Test:	Premeasured course and stopwatch
500-Yard Swim or Water Run Test:	Swimming pool and stopwatch
3-Minute Step Test:	15–16 inch bench or bleacher step, metronome or music at 96 beats per minute, and stopwatch

Purpose:

1. To evaluate your cardiorespiratory fitness.

2. To become familiar with different ways to measure cardiorespiratory fitness.

Procedure:

Read the "Pretest Instructions" through the "3-Minute Step Test" in the chapter. Perform one or more of the six cardiorespiratory fitness test described in Chapter 3. For best results, no more than two tests should be done in one day, and 15 to 20 minutes recovery should be allowed between tests.

Results:

Determine your fitness categories on the tests using norms given in Chapter 3.

1.5-Mile Run Test

Time: _____
Fitness Category _____

1-Mile Walk Test

Time: _____
Fitness Category _____

3-Mile Bicycling Test

Time: _____
Fitness Category _____

500-Yard Swim Test

Time: _____
Fitness Category _____

500-Yard Water Run Test

Time: _____
Fitness Category _____

3-Minute Step Test

Pulse: _____
Fitness Category _____

Conclusions:

1. If you took more than one test, how did your fitness categories compare? Was one test a better measure of your cardiorespiratory fitness? Why?

2. Were the results what you expected? Why or why not?

3. Are you satisfied with your current level of cardiovascular fitness? Explain.

lab activity
3-9

Muscular Endurance Assessment

Equipment needed: A ruler, tape, and stopwatch

Purpose:

1. To evaluate your muscular endurance.

2. To become familiar with ways to measure muscular endurance for different muscle groups.

Procedure:

Read "Muscular Strength and Endurance Tests" in the chapter. Follow the instructions to complete the tests and record your results.

Results:

Determine your fitness category on the tests using norms given in Chapter 3.

Abdominal Curls (1 min):

Number: _____

Fitness Category: _____

Push-Ups (1 min):

Number: _____

Fitness Category: _____

lab activity @ chapter three

Conclusions:

1. What did you learn from these tests about your muscular endurance?

2. Were the results what you expected? Why or why not?

3. Are you satisfied with your current level of muscular endurance? Explain.

Flexibility Assessment

Equipment needed: *Flex box or ruler*

Purpose:

1. To evaluate your flexibility.
2. To become familiar with ways to assess flexibility of different muscle groups.

Procedure:

Read "Flexibility Tests" in the chapter. Follow the instructions to complete the tests and record your results.

Results:

	Pass	Fail
Lower back flexibility test	___	___
Hip flexor flexibility test	___	___
Quadriceps flexibility test	___	___
Hamstrings flexibility test	___	___
Calf flexibility test	___	___
Shoulder girdle flexibility test	___	___

Sit and reach test   **Sit and reach wall test**

Inches   _____   Result   _____

Fitness category   _____   Fitness category   _____

Conclusions:

1. How did your flexibility results compare for different body areas?

2. Were the results what you expected? Why or why not?

3. Are you satisfied with your current flexibility levels? Explain.

4. What area(s) do you need to work on most?

Body Composition Assessment

Equipment needed: *Skinfold calipers, measuring tape*

Purpose:

1. To evaluate your body composition
2. To compare different ways of assessing body composition

Procedure:

Read "Body Composition Tests" through "Body Girth Measurement" in the chapter. Follow the instructions to estimate body fat using skinfold calipers, if available, and/or body girth measurements.

Results:

Men		**Women**	
Subscapular skinfold	___	Triceps skinfold	___
Thigh skinfold	___	Suprailiac skinfold	___
Percent fat	___	Percent fat	___
Fitness category	___	Fitness category	___

Body Girth Measurement

Men		**Women**	
Waist girth	___	Hip girth	___
Weight	___	Height	___
Percent fat	___	Percent fat	___
Fitness category	___	Fitness category	___

Conclusions:

1. If you took more than one test, how did the categories compare? Was one category a better measure of your body composition? Why?

2. Were the results what you expected? Why or why not?

3. Are you satisfied with your current body composition? Explain.

lab activity 3-12

Body Mass, Waist-To-Hip Ratio, and Health Risk

Equipment needed: *Measuring tape*

Purpose:

1. To evaluate your health risk as indicated by waist-to-hip ratio and body mass index.

2. To compare different ways of assessing health risk factors.

Waist-to-Hip Ratio

Investigations have begun pointing to the location of excess fat as a risk factor for heart disease and certain cancers. Fat distributed in the abdominal area is linked to increased health risks; hip/thigh fat is not as risky. As a result, the waist-to-hip ratio has become a common assessment used for health-risk identification. To compute this ratio, divide the waist measurement by the hip measurement. Some experts feel that weight-related health problems are increased for women whose ratio is 0.80 or higher and for men whose ratio is 0.95 or higher.

Beth's waist is 29 inches and her hips are 38 inches.

$$\frac{29 \text{ in. (waist)}}{38 \text{ in. (hip)}} = 0.76 \text{ Waist-to-hip ratio does not indicate increased risk.}$$

Steve's waist is 42 inches and his hips measure 36 inches.

$$\frac{42 \text{ in. (waist)}}{36 \text{ in. (hip)}} = 1.17 \text{ Waist-to-hip ratio indicates increased risk.}$$

Calculate your waist-to-hip ratio:

Your waist measurement: ___ in.

Your hip measurement: ___ in.

Waist-to-hip ratio: ___

(Check one):

Increased risk ___

No risk ___

lab activity @ chapter three

Body Mass Index (BMI)

Read "Understanding Body Composition" in Chapter 11. Follow the instructions to calculate your body mass index.
Calculate your body mass index using the following formula:

1. Your body weight in pounds $\times$ 705 = A
2. A $\div$ your height in inches = B
3. B $\div$ your height in inches = BMI

Results:

Your BMI using the chart in Table 11.1 is _____

Your BMI using the formula is _____

Category _____

Conclusions:

1. How did the categories compare using different tests?

2. What do each of the measures indicate about your health risk level?

3. Were the results what you expected? Why or why not?

Cardiorespiratory Exercise Plan

Equipment needed: *None*

Purpose: *To design your cardiorespiratory exercise program.*

Type of Exercise: _____

Cardiorespiratory Fitness Rating: _____

(See Chapter 4 for suggested workouts based on your current fitness rating.)

Frequency	Day	M	T	W	Th	F	Sa	Su
Time:	Week 1	___	___	___	___	___	___	___
	Week 2	___	___	___	___	___	___	___
	Week 3	___	___	___	___	___	___	___

Warm-up activities: _____

_____

Cool-down activities: _____

_____

Intensity: Target Heart Rate Range (from Lab 3.4): ___ to ___ beats per minute.
10 sec pulse count for 60 percent = ___ 80 percent = ___

lab activity

3-14

Cross-Training Workout Plan

Using the following chart and a sample fitness program given in Chapters 4 and 5, develop a two-week individualized cross-training workout plan based on results of your cardiorespiratory fitness and muscular endurance assessments. Include frequency, intensity, time, and type of activities.

Type of activities:

CR fitness category: _____

Program starting level: _____

Frequency: _____

Target heart rate: _____

Sunday	Monday	Tuesday	Wednesday	Thursday	Friday	Saturday

Describe your warm-up activities:

Describe your cool-down activities:

lab activity @ chapter three

lab activity
3–15

Exercise/Activity Log Sheet

(Make extra copies of this form as needed.)

	S	M	T	W	Th	F	Sa
Week 1							
Week 2							
Week 3							
Week 4							

Goals:_____
_____
_____
_____
_____
_____
_____
_____

Comments: _____
_____
_____
_____
_____
_____
_____
_____
_____

lab activity @ chapter three

Exercise/Activity Log Sheet

(Make extra copies of this form as needed.)

	S	M	T	W	Th	F	Sa
Week 1							
Week 2							
Week 3							
Week 4							

Goals:_____
_____
_____
_____
_____
_____
_____

Comments: _____
_____
_____
_____
_____
_____
_____

A journey of a thousand miles starts with a single step.
— Lao Tse

4

Pursuing Lifetime Exercise Activities

objectives

After reading this chapter, you will be able to:
1. Have a greater understanding for the eight aerobic exercise activities found in this chapter. You will discover each to be an excellent method for developing cardiorespiratory endurance (CRE). The eight activities include: aerobic dance, bicycling, fitness swimming, fitness walking, indoor exercise equipment, in-line skating, jogging, water exercise/aqua aerobics.
2. Pursue a lifetime of aerobic activity by selecting one of the eight exercise activities and by following the guidelines established for that specific activity.

This chapter contains eight exercise activities, any of which will assist you in your quest for attaining high level fitness. The activities included are: aerobic dance, bicycling, fitness swimming, fitness walking, indoor exercise equipment, in-line skating, jogging, and water exercise/aqua aerobics. Any one of these activities is an excellent choice for improving cardiorespiratory endurance (CRE). Keep in mind, this is a "how-to" chapter. Select the activity you wish to pursue to reach your fitness goals, then follow the FITT prescription factors established in Chapter 3. Next, thoroughly read the activity unit of your choice. This will provide you with the helpful guidelines necessary to assist you in reaching these goals. Each activity unit contains these sections: Advantages/Disadvantages, What to Wear, Techniques and Safety Tips, How to Begin and Progress, Variety, Common Discomforts, and Resources.

At the end of this chapter you will find several Lab Activities. The "Exercise Across the U.S.A." Lab Activity is a fun and interesting way to stay motivated to exercise. A variety of exercise logs can also be found in the Lab Activity section. These are helpful tools that can be used for any of the activities in this chapter and are especially beneficial for recording the half-marathon and marathon mileage.

Healthy People 2010 states that only 15 percent of our nation's adults (18 years and older) perform the recommended amount of physical activity and an alarming 40 percent of our nation's adults engage in no leisure-time activity. We now recognize that a high level of physical activity is a primary indicator of optimal health, so the low level of activity depicted in *Healthy People 2010* illustrates that our nation's health is on the decline. You can do your part to help improve the health of our nation by selecting and participating in one of the eight exercise activities in this chapter. Don't delay. Get started today.

Though regular exercise may be the most important habit you can adopt to safeguard your health, exercise can also have negative consequences if you don't take proper precautions. Follow the guidelines established in Chapter 3 before assessing your fitness level or beginning the exercise activities in this chapter.

As a reminder, always:

- Attain medical clearance to exercise (follow guidelines outlined in Chap. 3).
- Warm-up and cool-down.
- Scale back your workouts, for outdoor activities, during extremely hot or cold weather. (See Chap. 6.)
- Progress slowly and always listen to your body.

As you begin your exercise program, let the thoughtful words of the Reverend Jesse Jackson inspire you. "Both tears and sweat are salty, but they render a different result. Tears will get you sympathy, sweat will get you change."

chapter four

Do it! Move it! Make it happen! No one ever sat their way to success.

—H. Jackson Brown, Jr., *Dad, a Father's Book of Wisdom*

Aerobic Dance

(Including Step Aerobics, Slide Training, Tae Bo, and Spinning)

Advantages/Disadvantages

Aerobic dancing is a popular fitness activity. Usually performed under the leadership of an instructor, it combines the cardiovascular benefits of jogging with the joy of dancing. The variety of movements not only strengthens the cardiorespiratory system but also increases flexibility, tones muscles, and enhances body composition. It is a total body workout. The upbeat music tempo creates an atmosphere of excitement; exercising in a group is fun and emotionally stimulating. The popular music and group comaraderie help prevent boredom and can keep you motivated. Aerobic dancing can be so much fun, you often forget you are exercising. Because the participants focus on the instructor, aerobic dance classes are good for the beginning or self-conscious exerciser. Aerobic dance allows for individualization of a workout. The same movement sequence or exercise can be done by a well-conditioned participant and a beginning exerciser with variation in the intensity or number of repetitions. Because aerobic dance is done indoors, the environment provides security and comfort.

Aerobic dance has excellent potential for developing all components of physical fitness, but it can have some drawbacks. Although participants are urged by instructors to work at their own pace, some exercisers overdo it. These exercisers try to keep up with the group or work as hard as the instructor, even though they may not be ready for this intensity. Many times the result is excessive soreness or fatigue. Performing aerobic dance on a hard, unyielding surface (like cement) or while wearing inappropriate shoes also increases the risk of injury. Some overzealous aerobics participants attend classes one or more times a day, leading to overuse. Excessive impact may cause leg and foot problems. Also, not all aerobic dance instructors have had training in exercise instruction and safety and may teach improper technique. Unless good body mechanics and reasonable progressions are emphasized in a class, the result can be discomfort rather than exhilaration and a desire to continue exercising. Having to join or travel to a fitness facility to take an aerobics class may be viewed as a disadvantage to some exercisers. Others find it motivating to have a set time, to have made a financial in-

vestment, and to have a group of friends to exercise with. Aerobic dance videotapes are available for the home exerciser. They allow exercising in private but lack the spontaneity, instruction, and enthusiasm available in a live class.

What to Wear

Although some aerobic dancers have color-coordinated leotards and fancy exercise apparel, any loose-fitting and comfortable clothing will do. A T-shirt and shorts are fine. More important than the clothing are supportive shoes. Shoes specially designed for the impact and movement of aerobic dance are recommended. A good aerobic shoe has a well-cushioned, resilient midsole to aid in shock dispersion and a sturdy heel counter to hold the foot in place. The shoe should allow for lateral movement and, as a result, not have a wide heel flair that is often seen in a jogging shoe. Like the jogger, the aerobic participant should replace old shoes when their cushioning ability has decreased.

Techniques and Safety Tips

Many injuries and discomforts can be avoided in aerobic dance with proper shoes, gradual progression, and exercising on a resilient surface. Chapter 9 gives several general suggestions for preventing injury in fitness activities. In aerobic dance, careful attention to technique and body mechanics further eliminates chance for injury and heightens the enjoyment of the activity.

1. *Always warm up with low-intensity, whole body movements.* Your warm-up should include slow, full range-of-motion joint movements. Static stretching should also be included in the warm-up.
2. *Keep abdominals pulled in and buttocks tucked under.*
3. *Avoid twisting the spinal column excessively* (windmill toe touches, elbow-to-knee lunges, etc.).
4. *Limit the hopping on one foot* to a maximum of four consecutive times.
5. *Soften your jumps and bounces by maintaining a slightly bent-knee landing position.*
6. *Try to make your heels go all the way to the floor when landing from jumps.*
7. *Never fling or throw your arms or legs.* Maintain control of limbs throughout movements.
8. *Avoid hyperextending your elbows, knees, or lower back.*
9. *Listen to your body.* If a stretch, exercise, or position causes pain or a burning sensation, do not do it.

The amount of concern for technique and safety in the class depends on your instructor. A wise wellness consumer chooses a knowledgeable, trained instructor. The popularity of aerobic dance has skyrocketed, and the number of qualified instructors has not kept pace. While standards and certification programs have been established, it is up to you to select a class. Do not be shy. Check the instructor's qualifications. Is she or he certified by a national fitness organization? Does the instructor have knowledge in anatomy, exercise physiology, kinesiology, and first aid? Is she or he currently certified in CPR (cardiopulmonary resuscitation)? Does the instructor do some health screening or fitness assessment of students? Is the class supervised effectively? Does the instructor monitor the intensity of the workout with periodic heart-rate checks? Does the class begin with a good warm-up and end with a cool-down period? Does the instructor give corrective cues and technique suggestions throughout the workout? Does she or he consider the variances in fitness levels in the class by showing how to modify the intensity of the workout? Is she or he easy to follow? Does he or she educate the participants on injury prevention and signs of fatigue? Looking good in a leotard and being a fluid dancer are not requirements for being a quality aerobic dance instructor. Most important is the ability to conduct a safe, yet invigorating, workout from which all participants can benefit.

How to Begin and Progress

As with any other fitness activity, begin slowly. Attend no more than three classes per week for several weeks. Start with 5 to 10 minutes of the aerobic phase and progress gradually. If the aerobic portion of the class is 30 minutes, do low-impact moves or walk in place while the experienced exercisers continue. Monitor your pulse and stay within your target heart-rate range. You should be able to talk or sing with the music throughout the entire workout. Gradually add a few minutes weekly to the aerobic phase until you can exercise aerobically for 20 to 30 minutes.

Some exercisers prefer low-impact aerobics to high-impact aerobics. Low-impact aerobics reduces the strain on knees and ankles by minimizing jumping and bouncing movements. In low-impact aerobics, one foot is in contact with the ground at all times. *Low impact* does not necessarily mean *low intensity.* To maintain a training heart rate, move your arms vigorously and travel along the floor by wide-stride walking, sliding, and sidestepping. Beginners and well-trained exercisers with joint problems can benefit from low-impact aerobics. You may want to combine low-impact and high-impact moves. Most jumps and steps can be modified to become low-impact steps.

Most aerobic dance classes incorporate in the workout a body toning segment. Once again, use common sense. Do not try to do as many repetitions as the teacher, unless you are equally fit. Stop and stretch if you feel pain or a burning sensation in the muscle. Aerobic dance participants often tend to compare themselves or compete with others in the class. Avoid falling into this trap. Work to be the best you can be without shame or guilt.

Variety

It is easy to add variety to aerobic dance. Vary the music. Use pop, jazz, country, or classical music. Try some holiday or

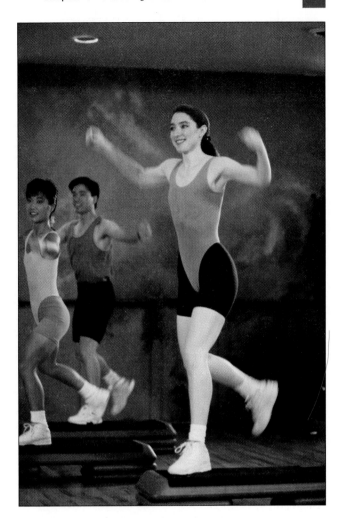

Working out in a class setting is social and fun.

theme music when appropriate. Vary the routines or steps. Aerobics can be taught by using set routines (repetitive movements in a programmed format) or in a freestyle format (participants mimic the instructor and change accordingly). Varying between learned routines and a freestyle approach helps keep interest high. Try circuit aerobic dance. Set up exercise stations around the room. Do different aerobic movements for 1 to 2 minutes per station and then jog to the next station to sustain your training heart rate. There are many other ways to add variety to aerobic dance. One-to 2-pound hand weights can be used during aerobic routines to increase upper body endurance and to maintain a training heart rate. Heavier hand weights are often used during stationary power moves to tone arms and legs. To prevent knee injuries, do not wear ankle weights while doing aerobic dance steps. Weights are, however, an effective way to add resistance while doing floor toning. Thick rubber bands and elastic tubing can also be used to increase the efficiency of body toning exercises.

Step Aerobics

Also known as *bench/step training*, step aerobics is an innovative activity that involves stepping up and down on a 4- to 12-inch platform. Combining a variety of stepping patterns with kicks, turns, and upper body movements results in a brisk workout. Step aerobics appeals to a wide range of exercisers for several reasons: It can be a high-intensity workout with low-impact force; it is adaptable to different fitness levels by adjusting the bench height, adding jumps, varying arm gestures, and adding light hand weights; and it is easy to do. Step aerobics has become especially popular with men, who may be put off by "dance-like" aerobics classes. As with all aerobic exercise activities, proper form and technique are necessary to prevent injury.

To prevent injury while stepping:

1. *As much as possible, keep your shoulders aligned over your hips.*
2. *Step up lightly, making sure the whole foot lands on the platform.*
3. *Keep your knees aligned over your feet when they're pulling your body weight onto the platform.*
4. *At the top, straighten your legs, but don't lock your knees.*
5. *Do not pivot a bent, supporting knee.*
6. *As you step down, stay close to the platform.*

If you are a beginner to step aerobics, start with the lowest bench, and keep your eyes on the bench until you adjust to the activity. Once you learn the stepping patterns, you can add arm movements and light hand weights or challenge yourself by raising the height of the bench. (However, never use a height that flexes your knees to an angle less than 90 degrees.)

Step aerobics is a great workout for the lower body and, when combined with a variety of arm movements, is an exciting new variation in aerobic exercise.

Slide Training

Slide training is a safe, low-impact activity that has gained popularity. It is offered as a class at many fitness centers or can be performed easily at home. Slide training involves side-to-side sliding, similar to a speed skater's motion, on a slick board. Most boards are 5 to 6 feet in length with small raised ends for pushing off. The slide boards, available at most sports/fitness retail outlets, are lightweight and can be rolled up for easy storage and handling.

While wearing special slippers, the exerciser glides from end to end in a low, crouched position. This exercise improves balance and agility, conditions the lower body, and provides a great cardiovascular workout. Medical and athletic training professionals have used slide training for many years to rehabilitate injured knees, legs, and backs. Arm lifts and various leg lifts can be added to the basic slide motion

for a varied workout. To avoid injury and heighten the enjoyment of sliding observe the following guidelines:

1. *Warm up, cool down, and stretch off the slide.*
2. *Keep your weight centered over your feet and slightly bent knees aligned with your toes.*
3. *Contract the abdominals and keep your eyes on the board to start.*
4. *Keep your hips squared and aligned with your torso and shoulders.*
5. *Tuck your shoelaces into the slide socks.*
6. *Control your speed by dragging your trail leg.*
7. *Only add arm movement when you are proficient with the basic slide.*
8. *Maintain the music tempo at 120 to 130 beats per minute (averages to about 30 slides across).*

Tae-Bo

Tae-Bo, developed by martial arts expert, Billy Blanks, blends the elements of the ancient art of self-defense, aerobic dance, and boxing. The workout features upbeat, energizing music and claims to be rated as the highest calorie-burning exercise. Tae-Bo strengthens and tones the legs, arms, chest, and abdominals. It also provides an excellent cardiorespiratory endurance workout. Billy Blanks popularized Tae-Bo by teaching the workout program to many Hollywood celebrities and superstar athletes. The exercise program appeals to men and women of all ages.

His nationally best-selling system includes three videos: Tae-Bo Instructional, Basic Tae-Bo Workout, and Advanced Tae-Bo Workout. An 8-minute Tae-Bo workout is often included as a free bonus video. To avoid injury and increase your enjoyment of Tae-Bo observe the following guidelines:

1. View and practice the movements illustrated on the Tae-Bo Instructional Video. You will learn the proper technique for the guard position, basic punches (i.e., jab, cross, hook, and upper cut), kicks, knee raises, and foot work patterns.
2. Thoroughly warm-up.
3. Control the movements of the arms and legs. Don't fling them about wildly.
4. Don't fully extend the elbow on the punches.
5. Keep the abdominals contracted.
6. When in guard position (or other half-squat positions), keep the knees over the toes—do not let the knees extend past the toes.
7. Use a chair or other support for balance when first learning the various kicks.
8. Keep an eye on the instructor.
9. Cool-down thoroughly.
10. The "double-time" sequences are too fast for some exercisers. It's okay to stay with single-time during these vigorous sequences.

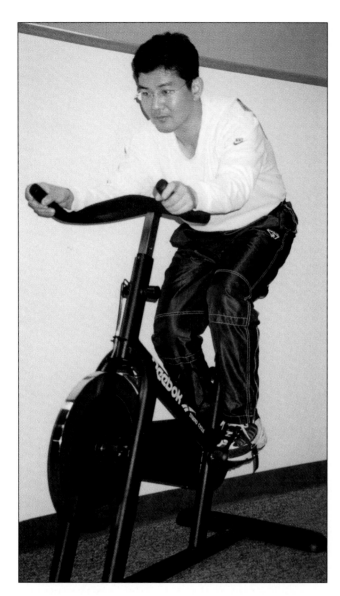

Spinning is a popular indoor fitness activity.

Spinning

The Spinning program, created by world-class cyclist Johnny G. (Goldberg) and managed by Mad Dogg Athletics, Inc. (MDA), is an indoor stationary cycling workout that uses general exercises, combined with heart-rate training and motivational techniques. Spinning and Spinner are registered trademarks of MDA.

This popular 40-minute workout, said to burn up to 500 calories per class, is taught by certified Spinning program instructors. The Spinning instructor leads a group of Spinners on a scenic stationary trail ride by using visualization techniques, motivational strategies, and video tapes and music. The Spinning program allows people of all ages

and fitness levels to take a stationary bike and transform it into a powerful workout. Participants vary their workout by making changes in the speed and resistance of their bike. Indoor cycling classes allow participants (about 15 to 30 per class) to experience road cycling without the associated dangers. The program is also a great choice for the cyclist who wants to take his/her outdoor program inside during inclement weather.

Drawbacks to this excellent aerobic exercise program is the necessity to join a class that provides the certified trained instructor and the Spinner bikes. Access to a health/fitness club or university fitness class is usually required for Spinning.

For added comfort and enjoyment while Spinning follow these guidelines:

1. Adjust the seat high enough so the leg fully extends at the bottom of each pedal stroke with a slight bend in the knee.
2. If possible, move the seat forward or back so the bent knee, at the top of the stroke, rests just above midfoot.
3. Attach toe clips to help prevent foot fatigue.
4. Tilt the seat slightly downward to avoid crotch numbness.
5. For added comfort, buy a cover to pad the seat (try Spinning Gel Seat, 1–888–988–3644) and invest in cycling shorts.
6. Adjust handlebar height to reduce hand/wrist pressure.
7. Add resistance when pedals (instead of your thigh muscles) are propelling your foot or the instructor advises you to do so.
8. Always warm-up and cool-down properly. Don't try to compete with class members, ride at your fitness level. Use your THR or PRE as a guide.
9. Listen to your body and stop before you feel fatigued.

Common Discomforts

As in most fitness activities, mild soreness can be anticipated by the beginning exerciser. Some discomforts may be avoided by emphasizing stretching and toning the first 3 to 4 weeks to condition muscles and connective tissue for the stress of impact and the new movements. Veteran exercisers can suffer pain or injury by increasing frequency, time, or intensity too rapidly. Most aerobic dance discomfort is found in the legs, so be sure to warm up and stretch this area. Exercise fatigue can also occur due to dehydration or lack of sleep/rest. Refer to Chapter 9 for further information about prevention and treatment of injuries. If you use hand weights, elbow and shoulder strain can be avoided by not flinging the weights. Always move the weights with control. Having a towel or exercise mat with you provides additional comfort and padding for floor exercises.

Potential just means you ain't done it yet.

—Darrell Royal, football coach

Bicycling

Advantages/Disadvantages

Cycling is a popular choice for people of all ages. You can fit in a cycling workout while running errands, while going to work, or while at home in front of the TV (on rollers or a stationary bike). You can cycle alone, with family, or with friends. If you have a small child, you can take him or her along in a bike seat instead of having to hire a sitter while you get a workout. It is nonimpact exercise, minimizing stress to the back, shins, and ankles.

There are a few drawbacks, though. You must have a bicycle, keep it in good working condition, and store it securely to prevent theft. Cycling in traffic requires alertness and use of defensive driving skills to prevent accidents. Cycling in rain, snow, or icy conditions is uncomfortable and hazardous. Also, bicycles are so efficient that they can do most of the work for you. Most people don't work hard enough to do themselves much good. Cycling to class or short distances is fine for transportation, but if you want to get in shape, you will need to put in more effort. Nevertheless, cycling produces cardiorespiratory benefits without impact, making it the third most popular activity in the United States. It can be enjoyed throughout a lifetime.

What to Wear

To be clearly visible to vehicles, wear bright-colored clothing during the day and light-colored clothing at night. Fancy bicycling gear is not necessary, although if you really get into cycling, you might find that a pair of bicycling shorts makes long rides more comfortable. Hard-soled, athletic, or bicycling shoes are fine.

Equipment

There are plenty of bike-pedestrian and bike-car accidents on campus, and usually it is the bicyclist who is at fault. Always wear a helmet, even if you're only going across campus. The sidewalk is as hard there as anywhere else. You may lose some skin in a slide or break some bones, but they will heal. Your brain won't. Head injuries account for over 75 percent of deaths and permanent disabilities in cycling crashes. If you hit something and go flying head first, wearing a good helmet is the best way to prevent serious injury.

When you are choosing a helmet, make sure that it has the following characteristics:

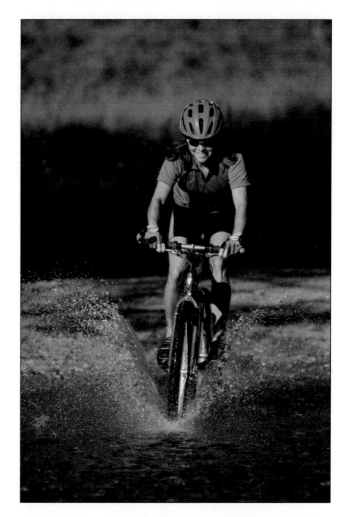

Bicycling is a great fitness activity across the lifespan.

Outer shell or cover that is brightly colored (i.e., yellow, white, or red) so that you are easily visible to drivers
Hard shell lined with polystyrene or polystyrene alone
Secure chin strap
Label indicating the helmet is ANSI or Snell approved

Helmets are single-use devices designed to crush and absorb shock upon impact. You should replace a helmet that has been in a significant crash.

A water bottle is essential for workouts, particularly in the heat. Because sweat evaporates so quickly while you are riding, you may not realize how quickly water is lost. Dehydration, leading to heat illness, can easily occur. Drinking regularly from a water bottle to maintain an adequate level of hydration during a workout is a necessity, not a luxury.

It doesn't matter what type of bike you ride—one speed, 10-speed, mountain—but it does matter that it be kept in good working order. If you are not mechanically inclined, your local bicycle shop can help. Most people ride with the bike seat too low, which is inefficient and can make the knees hurt. The bike seat should be high enough that when you sit centered on the seat with your heel on the pedal at its lowest point, your knee is straight. That way, when you move the ball of your foot to its proper position on the pedal, your knee will be almost fully extended at the bottom of the stroke. If the seat is too high, you'll tend to rock side to side with each footstroke and may develop a sore crotch. A sore crotch can also be caused by improper seat tilt. Start with the nose of the seat level. If it bothers you, tilt it down slightly. Pedals, wheels, and steering should turn or spin freely with no binding, catch, or click. The derailleur should shift smoothly. Brakes should close and release easily. Brake shoes should be ⅛ inch or less from and level with the rim of the bike. If they are badly worn, replace them. The air in the tires usually needs to be topped off weekly to keep them hard and rolling smoothly but use caution when filling them. The air pumps at service stations are designed for cars, and it's easy to explode a bicycle tire by overfilling it. If a bike wheel is badly out of true and wobbles, it may hit your brake shoe with each revolution. A bike shop can true a wheel; lubricate sticky brake cables; adjust the derailleur; and show you how to keep your machine running smoothly, which makes riding safe and enjoyable.

Technique and Safety Tips

Shifting

On 10-speeds, the gears overlap slightly and you have to shift by feel. To shift, continue pedaling but ease up on the pedal pressure. Shifting without pedaling can cause a bent or broken chain or gear teeth. As you shift, you should not hear a loud clunk nor a constant rubbing sound, if you are shifting smoothly and getting it into gear correctly.

Most beginners gear too high and pedal too slowly. They feel like they're not getting any exercise unless they're pushing against resistance. This is inefficient and can increase fatigue and cause knees to ache. It is better to pedal quickly against light resistance. An optimal pedal rate is 80 rpm, with a range of 60 to 100 rpm. Racers and experienced tourists often cycle at 90 to 110 rpm.

If your bike has several gears, practice using them. Gearing is a matter of maintaining an even cadence regardless of terrain, weather, or wind conditions. If you're going uphill, shift before you have to slow your cadence so that you can go up smoothly. Also practice downshifting before stop signs so that you don't have to stand on the pedals to get going again.

Pedaling

Ride with the ball of your foot on the pedal. If you have toe clips, you can try ankling—pulling up as well as pushing down on the pedal each stroke—which doubles your efficiency.

Braking

Use your brakes as little as possible. Look ahead, signal, slow down, and learn to anticipate problems instead of simply reacting to them. Be careful not to jam on your brakes too suddenly or you can pitch headfirst over the handlebars. The front brake is the most powerful because, as you decelerate, your weight shifts forward, lessening the weight over the back tire. For the most efficient stop, keep the body weight back, gradually increase pressure on the front brake, and hold pressure on the back brake just below the point where the wheel will skid. In wet conditions, brakes lose up to 90 percent of their braking ability. It is good to frequently apply the brakes lightly to wipe water off the rims and to allow extra stopping distance. When going downhill, pump the brakes to avoid overheating the wheel rims or brake shoes. When in doubt, favor the rear brake. It may skid the bike, but at least you won't land on your face.

Bumps

When you come up to bumps, holes, and railroad tracks, don't sit on the seat like a sack of potatoes. Shift your weight to pedals and handlebars to absorb the shock. Its better for you and for your bike.

Safety Tips

1. Wear brightly colored clothing, wear a helmet, and carry water.
2. Keep to the right side of the road and ride in a straight line. Always ride in single file with traffic.
3. Do not make sudden turns or swerves. Signal turns and stops.
4. Stay alert. Look out for cars pulling out into traffic or turning. Listen constantly for traffic approaching out of your line of vision.
5. Observe traffic regulations as if you were driving a car—red and green lights, one-way streets, stop signs. Slow down at all street intersections and look right and left before crossing.
6. Be sure your brakes are operating efficiently and keep your bicycle in perfect running condition. Keep your hands on or near the brakes at all times.
7. Keep speed under control, especially on long downhill runs. Speed should be low enough that you can stop quickly.

8. In rainy weather, allow much more distance for stopping and don't take corners too fast.

9. Watch for sudden door openings from parked cars. Ride at least 3 feet away from them.

10. Avoid sewer grates that parallel your direction.

11. If railroad tracks are rough, walk your bike across them (to prevent blowout or other damage to the bicycle). If you choose to ride over the tracks, cross them at a 90-degree angle.

12. Make sure you are at least 3 feet off the traveled portion of the road when you stop or park.

13. Hug the right-hand shoulder of the road on all curves.

14. Give pedestrians the right-of-way. Avoid sidewalks.

15. Watch out for child cyclists. Children on bicycles usually weave from side-to-side and turn unpredictably without signaling, and they can run into you when you are passing them.

16. Dogs are potential adversaries. If a dog is far enough away, you can probably outrun him. Water from your bottle or a bike pump may scare him off. If you stop, keep the bike between you and the dog. Walk slowly away. Usually, a dog will leave you alone, but watch him carefully before you get under way again. You can also buy a small can of "dog repellent," which will shoot a thin stream of chemical about 10 feet. Although the effects are potent, there is no permanent damage done to the animal. Don't try to run down or kick at a dog—this can cause a crash. If you are scared, you can yell, "Out" at the dog, mimicking a noise made by mother dogs when disciplining their puppies. This will usually startle a dog enough to give you a chance to escape.

17. Don't wear headphones—they block out street sounds that enable you to anticipate traffic.

18. Don't wear a heavy backpack. It can throw off your balance. Carry packages in baskets or bags attached to the cycle.

19. Learn to shift gears while keeping your eyes on the road.

How to Begin and Progress

First, measure your fitness level using the 5-mile timed ride test in Chapter 3. Remember that your *current* fitness level does not indicate your potential. Allow yourself several weeks to show significant improvement. Begin at the step indicated by your current fitness level. If you cannot complete the test, begin at level 1. Exercise 3 to 5 days a week at your training pulse. (An appropriate pulse for bicycling appears to be about 5 percent lower than for other exercise, so subtract 5 percent to adjust for this difference.) You may work at one level until you can comfortably handle the recommended distance and intensity; then move to the next step. To develop balanced fitness, add 25 to 30 push-ups, a minute of abdominal curls, and 5 to 15 minutes of stretching to each workout.

Bicycling Program

Fitness Category	Starting Level	
Very low	1 or 2	
Low	3	
Average	4	
Good	5	
Excellent	6	

Level	Cycling	Total Distance
1	20–30 min. (8-10 MPH)	3–5 miles
2	20–30 min. (10-12 MPH)	4–6 miles
3	30–45 min. (12 MPH)	4–8 miles
4	30–60 min. (15 MPH)	7–15 miles
5	40–75 min. (15 MPH)	10–18 miles
6	40–90 min. (15 MPH)	10–22 miles

Variety

Part of the appeal of bicycling is being able to explore an area and see things you wouldn't normally notice as you whizzed past in a car. Try cycling to a park, a lake, or a scenic spot or merely try exploring on a bicycle. Plan an outing with a picnic or refreshment break halfway. Ride to a nearby small town and back. Plan a bike rally, similar to a car rally with checkpoints, or a bike scavenger hunt in which you gather bits of information from certain locations (i.e., what is the name of the store at 21 Oak Street?). If you are interested in more, consult your local bicycle shop for bicycling organizations in your area and find out what rides and tours are planned.

Common Discomforts

Bicyclists beginning a conditioning program often experience a sore crotch the first week or two. As you and your saddle adjust to each other, the syndrome should disappear. Check to see that the seat is not too high. A too-high seat causes you to rock side-to-side with each pedal stroke, and the constant rubbing will prolong soreness. It may help to tilt the nose of the saddle down a bit (not so much you slide off!), to try a different saddle, one with padding under the "sit bones," or to consider padded cycling shorts.

Sore knees? A seat that is too low, so that your knees are excessively bent throughout the pedal stroke is one cause. Riding with excessive resistance at too low a cadence increases pressure on the knees and is another easily remedied cause. A relatively high cadence against light resistance reduces frequency of overuse injuries.

If your fingers feel numb after cycling, you need to change hand position more frequently and ride with elbows slightly bent, not locked. The ulnar nerve runs across the palm, and constant pressure on the hands can temporarily cut off sensation to the area. Wearing padded cycling gloves or cushioning your handlebars with foam grips may also help.

Neck or back soreness usually disappears in a week or so once you grow accustomed to riding. If they do not, try changing hand positions frequently, riding with elbows slightly bent, moving the seat forward a little, or perhaps switching to upright handlebars.

Do your toes tend to go numb on long rides? If you are using toe clips, it may be that pedaling tends to push your foot forward into your shoes until your toes touch the end, reducing blood flow to the area. Try lacing your shoes snugly enough so that they hold your foot back in the heel of the shoe but not so tightly that circulation is hindered. Also, try loosening your toe clips.

Basic Bicycle Tool Kit

If you wish to save money and time by doing much of your own maintenance, the following tools are recommended: tire patch kit, tire irons, adjustable wrench or set of crescent wrenches (best), third hand (for brakes), screwdriver, tire gauge, silicone lubricant, tire pump.

How to Fix a Flat Tire

1. *Remove wheel.* Caliper brakes may need to be loosened to permit wheel removal. Loosen axle nuts and remove the wheel from the forks. In the rear, you must also press the tension roller forward to wiggle the wheel out.

2. *Remove the tire.* Push the tire irons between the rim and bead. Pry up the tire carefully so as not to pinch and further damage the tube. Work around the tire.

3. *Push the valve stem into the rim and pull the tube out of the tire.* Locate the source of the puncture and remove it from the tire. Feel the inside of the tire to check for foreign objects. Also check the rim to make sure a spoke is not protruding. Mark the puncture on the tube. If the source of the leak is not readily apparent, slightly inflate the tire and listen for a hiss or put the tube in water and look for bubbles. Dry the tube and mark the hole with chalk. Deflate.

4. *Read and follow the patch kit directions.* Rough around the puncture with a roughing tool. Apply a thin layer of cement and let it dry thoroughly. Apply the patch, pressing out air bubbles.

5. *Replace the tube in the tire, valve first.*

6. *Replace the bead of the tire in the rim,* being careful to avoid pinching the tube between the bead and the tire. Use tire irons to replace the last few inches of the tire bead.

7. *Inflate the tire.* Replace it; center it between the forks; tighten the axle nuts and, if necessary, the brakes.

Bicycle Inspection Checklist

Name _____

Bicycle make & model _____ Serial no. _____

Note: Proper bicycle fit and maintenance are essential for comfort, safety, and riding efficiency. Any problems must be identified and corrected before the first ride.

	OK	FIX
Frame Size		
Can you straddle the frame with both feet flat on the ground? You need a 1- to 2-inch space between your crotch and the top bar for road bikes and 3 to 4 inches for all-terrain bikes.	_____	_____
Saddle		
Horizontal adjustment: The nose of the saddle should be 1 to 3 inches behind a vertical line drawn through the crank hanger. A cyclist 5 feet 6 inches tall would position the saddle 1 inch back (5 feet 10 inches: 2 inches back; 6 feet 3 inches: 3 inches back).	_____	_____
Vertical adjustment: Sit on the bike with your heel on the pedal at the lowest position. Your knee should be straight.	_____	_____
Tilt: Make sure it is horizontal or slightly downtilted.	_____	_____
Is the saddle tight and in good condition?	_____	_____
Handlebars		
Vertical adjustment: The top bar should be level with the nose of the saddle.	_____	_____
Horizontal adjustment: Place your elbow on the nose of the saddle. Your outstretched fingertips should just touch the center of the handlebars. The length of the stem may need to be changed.	_____	_____
The handlebars should be in line with the wheel and symmetrical.	_____	_____
The handlebars should be tight; there should be no horizontal or vertical movement.	_____	_____
The tubing ends should be plugged and the grips tight.	_____	_____
Tire Pressure		
The correct pressure (embossed on the side of the tire) for this bike is _____. Check the pressure once a week.	_____	_____

	OK	FIX
Bolts		
Check bolts for looseness monthly.	_____	_____
Hand Brakes		
Is there adequate space between the lever and the handlebar when the brakes are engaged? If not, tighten the cable.	_____	_____
The cable should be taut, with no kinks, rust, or frayed ends.	_____	_____
The brake shoes should be tight. The openings should face the rear of the bike.	_____	_____
Are the brake shoes level with and no more than $\frac{1}{8}$ inch from the rim?	_____	_____
Is there at least $\frac{3}{16}$ inch rubber remaining? Replace if needed.		
Test the operation of each brake separately. They must hold without catching.		
Front	_____	_____
Rear	_____	_____
Wheels		
Spin each wheel. They should run true, without wobbles.	_____	_____
They should have no bindings or looseness (bearings).	_____	_____
They should be centered between forks (and chain stays in the rear).	_____	_____
Rim: Is it dented or kinked?	_____	_____
Spokes: Are they intact and tight?	_____	_____
Tire: Is each tire properly seated? Is there at least $\frac{1}{8}$ inch of tread remaining?	_____	_____
Derailleurs		
Turn the bike upside down or have a partner lift the rear wheel while you crank the pedal and shift through first the front and then the rear gears. (Shift only while the pedal is turning!) The derailleur should shift the chain smoothly from one sprocket to the next without skipping a gear, catching, or throwing off the chain.	_____	_____
Chain and Sprocket		
Is the chain dirty? If so, clean it with silicone spray.	_____	_____
The sprocket teeth should be intact and not bent or broken.	_____	_____
Pedals		
The pedals should be intact and tight.	_____	_____
The tread should be intact and tight.	_____	_____
Press down on both pedals at once. Are they tight?	_____	_____

> *Don't let what you cannot do interface with what you can do.*
>
> —John Wooden

Fitness Swimming

Advantages/Disadvantages

Swimming is a superb form of exercise. It is a total body workout using major muscle groups of both the upper and lower body. Other forms of aerobic exercise, jogging for example, use mainly large muscles of the lower body. In addition, water exercise is a natural form of strength training. Resistance of the water against the body's movements enhances muscle strength. Swimmers are also subject to fewer injuries than are participants in many other activities. Joint and muscle injuries are not common among swimmers because of water buoyancy. Water supports the body, alleviating the jarring effects of weight-bearing exercise such as aerobics or jogging. Swimming is ideal for the overweight, the arthritic, the injured, the elderly, and those prone to joint problems.

Another advantage of swimming is the rare occurrence of heat exhaustion and heat stroke. This can be a concern when exercising in hot, humid weather. If you don't like to sweat, you will probably prefer to exercise in water.

Swimming does have its drawbacks. You must have some swimming ability and have access to a pool at a time convenient for you. That first plunge into the water may be difficult for some, but after a brief warm-up period, the cool water temperature will be invigorating. Warm water quickly becomes uncomfortable during a vigorous workout.

Although the injury rate is low, you may experience some minor annoyances as you train in water. Eye irritations and "swimmer's ear" are the most common.

The inconvenience of having to redo makeup and hair is minor when you measure the positive outcomes of aquatic exercise. After the workout, an efficient hair and makeup routine develops quickly.

What to Wear

Swimming is an inexpensive sport because the only equipment needed is a comfortable swimming suit. Many swimmers wear goggles to protect their eyes and, for added comfort, you may wish to use ear plugs and a swim cap. Swimmers can exercise indoors or outside, making it a year-round sport.

Technique and Safety Tips

Learn to swim the following five basic strokes efficiently: sidestroke, elementary backstroke, breaststroke, back crawl, and front crawl. Incorporate stroke mechanics sessions on these strokes into each workout. The butterfly stroke is too strenuous for most fitness swimmers.

Learn and practice the front crawl flip turn and the back crawl spin turn. These will make lap swimming more enjoyable. Construct your daily training program to include a water warm-up, conditioning bout, and water cool-down. Monitor your heart rate (or use the PRE), and do not allow it to exceed your swimming target zone. Use hand paddles, kickboards, pull buoys, and swim fins to increase muscular strength and stroke efficiency. Hyperextension of the lower back (arching) is natural in water exercise. It is important to strengthen the abdominal muscles and always stretch the lower back area to counteract this tendency.

Here are other safety tips:

1. *Never swim alone.* A lifeguard should be present. Safety equipment, such as a ring buoy and reaching pole, should also be available.
2. *Do not dive into the pool at the shallow end.* The risk is too great. Even experienced swimmers have misjudged the depth of the water and hit the bottom, resulting in serious injuries.
3. *Stay to the right of the lane and make your turns counterclockwise.*
4. *If resting at the pool edge, keep to one side of the lane to allow other swimmers to turn easily.*
5. *Be careful with electrical equipment around the pool* (radios, pace clocks, etc.). Make sure electrical outlets are grounded.
6. *Keep telephone and emergency rescue numbers in the pool area.*
7. *Keep all doors going into the pool area locked unless there is a lifeguard on duty.*

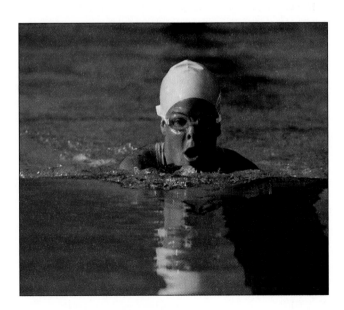

Swimming provides an excellent workout.

Heart Rate During Swimming

Do not use the same target heart rate range when you swim as when you perform land sports. Weight-bearing activities such as running, aerobic dance, and fitness walking cause the heart to beat faster. Thus, to avoid risk of overtraining and for more comfortable workouts, reduce your swimming THR by approximately *10 percent* (see Chapter 3).

For example, if your THR for land activities is 150 to 170 bpm, your swimming THR would be 135 to 153 bpm:

1. $150 \times 0.10 = 15$ $170 \times 0.10 = 17$
2. $150 - 15 = 135$ $170 - 17 = 153$
3. Swimming THR = 135–153 bpm

How to Begin and Progress

Assess your aerobic swimming fitness on the 500-yard swim test as described in Chapter 3. Based on your fitness category, begin at the appropriate starting level. Progress through each level, one step at a time. Do not skip steps and stay on each as long as necessary to adapt to that workload. Remember to monitor your pulse and do not exceed your swimming target heart rate range. When you have completed level M, you may want to swim continuously for distance or time or continue with the routine of four lengths and a brief rest for the measured distance or time. Keep in mind the FITT prescription factors covered in Chapter 3.

In this program, swim the number of lengths suggested, but if the workout feels too hard, rest a few seconds by climbing out of the pool and walking back to the starting point, or rest at the end of the pool for a few seconds before continuing the workout. Swim the front crawl, if possible, or any stroke that allows you to reach the prescribed swimming target heart rate. Consult the pool distance table.

Pool Distance

Most standard pools are 25 yards in length
One length = 25 yards
One lap = two lengths (50 yards)

18 lengths = 1/4 mile	(approx. 450 yds.)
35 lengths = 1/2 mile	(approx. 875 yds.)
53 lengths = 3/4 mile	(approx. 1325 yds.)
70 lengths = 1 mile	(approx. 1750 yds.)

25 Meter Pools

16 lengths	=	1/4 mile (approx. 402.25m)
32 lengths	=	1/2 mile (approx. 804.50 m)
48 lengths	=	3/4 mile (approx. 1206.75 m)
64 lengths	=	1 mile (approx. 1609 m)

Fitness Swim Program

Fitness Category	Starting Level
Very low	S
Low	S
Average	W
Good	I
Excellent	M

Swim Program

	Level S				Level W	
Lengths	Repeats	Distance	Lengths	Repeats	Distance	
1 ×	4	= 100 yds./m	2 ×	4	= 200 yds/m	
1 ×	6	= 150 yds./m	2 ×	5	= 250 yds/m	
1 ×	8	= 200 yds./m	2 ×	6	= 300 yds/m	
1 ×	10	= 250 yds./m	2 ×	7	= 350 yds/m	
			2 ×	8	= 400 yds/m	
			2 ×	9	= 450 yds/m	
			2 ×	10	= 500 yds/m	
			2 ×	11	= 550 yds/m	

	Level I				Level M	
Lengths	Repeats	Distance	Lengths	Repeats	Distance	
3 ×	7	= 525 yds./m	4 ×	7	= 700 yds./m	
3 ×	8	= 600 yds./m	4 ×	8	= 800 yds./m	
3 ×	9	= 675 yds./m	4 ×	9	= 900 yds./m	
3 ×	10	= 750 yds./m	4 ×	10	= 1000 yds./m	
3 ×	11	= 825 yds./m	4 ×	11	= 1100 yds./m	
3 ×	12	= 900 yds./m	4 ×	12	= 1200 yds./m	
3 ×	13	= 975 yds./m				
3 ×	14	= 1050 yds./m				

Variety

To add variety to your swimming workouts, practice stroke mechanics on the five basic strokes. This will allow you to use a variety of strokes in your workouts instead of being limited to one or two. Swim for time instead of distance for a change or vice versa. Use swim fins, pull buoys, swim trainers, hand paddles, kickboards, webbed gloves, or a tethering system to add interest to your workouts. These devices also improve strength and stroke efficiency. For a complete change of pace, try an aquacircuiting or water running session in shallow water or a deep water jogging workout using some type of flotation device. See Water Exercise/Aqua Aerobics.

Discomforts

While swimmers are less susceptible to injuries, they may experience a few minor discomforts. Eye irritations are caused by an imbalance in the pH of the water (balance of acidity and alkalinity) or excessive amounts of chlorine. Wear goggles and you will have no problem. Swimmer's ear refers to a rashlike inflammation of the ear canal that is caused by frequent exposure to moisture. Dry your ears thoroughly with a towel to prevent this nuisance. If you have frequent ear infections, it would be wise to purchase a pair of ear plugs. See a specialist to get a good fit; those purchased over the counter do not fit well enough to keep water out of the ear canal. A few swimmers complain of sore shoulders. A certain amount of soreness is normal during the first weeks of training. But if pain persists, you may be developing tendinitis. Shoulder tendinitis may be caused by an inherent structural shoulder problem, use of hand paddles, or improper stroke mechanics. See an orthopedic specialist if shoulder pain persists and use strokes with an underwater recovery (i.e., breaststroke, sidestroke, and elementary backstroke). Some swimmers experience knee pain, especially along the inner borders of the knees when swimming the breaststroke and elementary backstroke. This is caused by the kick used in these strokes. Do not swim the breaststroke or elementary backstroke until the pain subsides or avoid them. It is a common myth that you are more susceptible to colds if you participate in aquatic activities, especially during the winter. Colds and respiratory infections are caused by viruses and are spread by contact with infected individuals. You are more likely to catch a cold in a warm, dry, crowded room than in a swimming pool. Another myth is that swimming during menstruation is prohibited. Minor discomfort during this period may be alleviated by exercise. If cramps are severe, use your judgment.

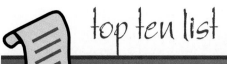

top ten list

Top Ten Reasons to Pursue Lifetime Exercise

In addition to helping maintain healthy weight, reducing unhealthy abdominal fat, and increasing energy, lifetime exercise:

1. Improves heart health by reducing heart disease.
2. Lowers blood pressure and risk of stroke.
3. Reduces risk of diabetes.
4. Increases bone density, reducing osteoporosis.
5. Lowers risk of some cancers, especially of the colon and breast.
6. Improves sleep.
7. Reduces joint pain in the arthritic.
8. Reduces likelihood of gallstone surgery.
9. Reduces stress, anxiety, and depression.
10. Increases HDL ("good") cholesterol and lowers triglycerides.

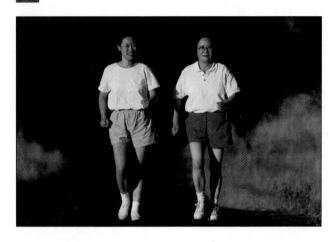

Fitness walking can be enjoyed inside or outside.

"Walking is man's best medicine."

—Hippocrates

Fitness Walking

Advantages/Disadvantages

Walking is simple, enjoyable, and probably the safest form of aerobic exercise known. It is inexpensive and can be done by almost anyone, any place, any time. There is no need to join a club or to find partners or opponents. It is a wise exercise choice for the overweight, the older adult, the very out-of-shape, the postsurgical patient, and the individual in a cardiac rehabilitation program. Appropriate shoes and comfortable clothes are the only equipment you need. Walking is excellent for weight control. You use as many calories walking a mile as you would jogging the same distance. The difference is that walking takes longer. Even though the injury rate is low, some walkers who try to increase distance and pace too quickly may experience sore muscles and knees or other discomforts. Another disadvantage to walking is that the already physically fit may not be able to elevate the heart rate into the target zone. In this case, try one of the advanced forms of fitness walking, such as power walking (with hand weights) or race walking. Dogs and inclement weather present other problems to the walker. Many shopping malls have opened their doors for early morning walking and also to provide a safe, weather-controlled environment year-round.

What to Wear

You don't have to buy special clothes; anything loose and comfortable will do. It is a good idea to have a pocket for carrying identification, keys, and a handkerchief. For sugges-

tions on dealing with weather, read the tips for hot and cold weather dressing provided in the section, Jogging.

Studies show that walking generates a downward force of about one and one-half times your body weight, so wearing appropriate shoes is important in helping you progress smoothly and injury free. You may save a few dollars on inexpensive shoes, but a good pair of shoes will help protect your feet, legs, and back. When purchasing new shoes, go to a reputable store and ask for a trained salesperson. Look for shoes with a cushioned heel, flexible sole, firm heel support, and arch supports that fit your feet. The toe box must provide room for the toes to work to prevent blisters. Several companies manufacture shoes designed for the sport of walking. Try one of these or one made for cross training or jogging but be sure it fits your foot. The shoe should never feel like it needs to be broken in. It should feel comfortable from day one.

Do you replace your worn-out shoes soon enough? A study at Tulane University found that all shoes, regardless of brand, price, or type of construction, lose most of their shock absorbency after 500 miles of use. This is a good reason for keeping records of your mileage. Take your old shoes with you when shopping for a new pair so that a knowledgeable salesperson can evaluate the wear pattern to help you choose a suitable shoe.

Technique and Safety Tips

Walking posture is erect but relaxed. To alleviate tension, the abdomen should be pulled in, the rib cage lifted, and the shoulders pulled down. This will help you keep relaxed and increase your endurance. Your arms should be bent at about a 90-degree angle, and your hands (loose fist) should swing slightly above your waist. Your arms counterbalance your leg motion. You may discover during your walk that your arms have dropped, resulting in a slower pace. Visualize that you are walking in a straight line. Hold your head up with eyes focused ahead, watching the ground but not your feet. Your foot contact should be a heel roll to the ball of the foot and toes for pushing off. Resist the tendency to lean forward at the waist.

While you are walking, keep in mind these tips for a safe workout:

1. *Always carry some form of identification* (include pertinent medical information).
2. *Choose a safe time and place to exercise.* Take keys with you and lock the car and/or house.
3. *Plan your route carefully.* Use well-populated, well-lighted areas. Avoid areas that are dark and have dense shrubs and alleys.
4. *Know where you can get help along your route.*
5. *Use sidewalks or walk facing oncoming traffic* and walk in single file.
6. *Obey traffic signals and signs.* Do not jaywalk.
7. *Keep alert at all times.* Give the right-of-way to cars. Don't assume the driver sees you.
8. *Wear bright, reflective clothing at dusk or night.*

Correct Walking Form

To check your form, have a friend watch you walk, or walk on a treadmill in front of a mirror. Here are the key points for good walking posture.

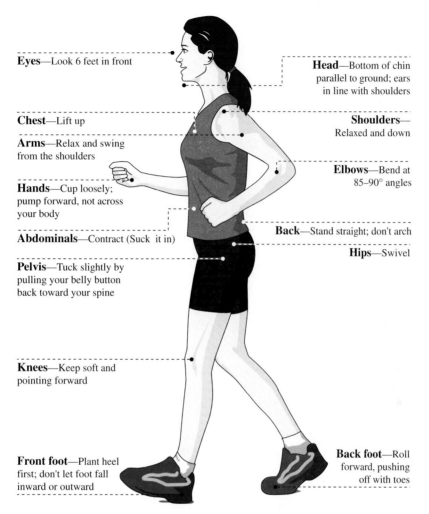

Eyes—Look 6 feet in front

Head—Bottom of chin parallel to ground; ears in line with shoulders

Chest—Lift up

Shoulders—Relaxed and down

Arms—Relax and swing from the shoulders

Elbows—Bend at 85–90° angles

Hands—Cup loosely; pump forward, not across your body

Back—Stand straight; don't arch

Abdominals—Contract (Suck it in)

Hips—Swivel

Pelvis—Tuck slightly by pulling your belly button back toward your spine

Knees—Keep soft and pointing forward

Front foot—Plant heel first; don't let foot fall inward or outward

Back foot—Roll forward, pushing off with toes

Feet—Point toes forward, keeping feet parallel

9. *Tell someone where you are going and when you think you will return.* Better yet, use the buddy system. It's more fun to walk with someone.

10. *Avoid dogs by selecting routes that are free of them.* The best advice is to ignore a barking dog, and never walk between a barking dog and its human, especially if the human is a child.

11. *For the cleanest air, walk in the morning.* The air is more polluted at midday, and pollution drops after rush hour in the evening.

12. *Don't wear a headset;* you would be losing one of your most valuable sensory aids. If you wear a headset, keep volume low so you can hear traffic or approaching strangers.

13. *Avoid walking on snow/ice-covered roads and walks.*

14. *Avoid peak traffic hours* unless you can use a jogging path or a sidewalk.

Tips for Increasing Walking Pace

What is your current walking pace? If you do not know, here is how you can measure your effort. Go to a quarter-mile track, or measure one mile on a road with your car odometer. Time yourself walking for one mile. If it takes you 20 minutes, you are walking at four mph; if it takes you about 13 minutes, you are walking at a 4.5 mph pace; if you do it in 12 minutes, you have reached a 5 mph pace.

If you would like to increase your fitness walking pace try The Top 10 Techniques for Increasing Walking Pace.

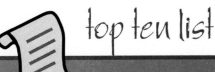

top ten list

Top 10 Techniques for Increasing Walking Pace

1. *Pump your arms.* When your arms drag, the tendency is to slow down. Resist this. Keep your arms pumping and your legs will be forced to keep pace. Bend the arms to a full 90-degree angle, keep the shoulders low and relaxed (not raised).

2. *Heel walks.* Walk on your heels, with your toes off the ground. This stretches and strengthens your calves and especially your shins, training that puts power in your stride by helping you develop a stronger push-off and prevents the development of shin splints.

3. *Crossovers.* On a track, road, or sidewalk, practice walking along an imaginary straight line. Engage your hips by crossing your foot across the line with each step. This forces you to adopt the signature race walking wiggle. Plus, extending your legs from your hips allows your pelvis to rotate forward so you can cover more ground with each step without overstriding.

4. *Use interval training.* Walk as fast as you can for 1 minute, then slow the pace for 4 minutes. Gradually increase the intervals by 1 minute every 2 weeks until you can do intense 4 minute intervals with only 1 minute at the slower pace.

5. *Simultaneously begin using the hard/easy system of training.* Go hard one day—either by taking a long walk or by doing intervals or hills—and easy the next. Practice at least two training days per week.

6. *Streamline your form.* Alter your strike to a straight-leg landing. When your heel touches the ground, the front leg should be straight. Your forefoot is flexed momentarily to land on the heel rather than the sole of the foot.

7. *Set "walk-to" targets.* Set a "walk-to" target a short distance in front of you (about 30 yards). Walk quickly to the target, reset the target, and walk fast to the new target. Keep resetting the walk-to targets throughout the route. Use mailboxes, driveways, road signs, and trees for targets. This technique helps to keep you mentally involved in your fitness walking workout and helps you resist the tendency to stroll.

8. *Add bends and straight-a-ways.* On a track, warm-up for 10 minutes then go your fastest on the straight-a-ways, using the curves for slow recovery walks. Start with six to eight laps, building to 15.

9. *Count steps.* Accelerate 100 steps 5 times in 30 minutes. This will teach your legs to move faster.

10. *Don't over do it.* Limit speed works to twice a week so sore muscles won't sideline you for the next day's walk.

How to Begin and Progress

Test your fitness using the 1-mile walk test described in Chapter 3. Then follow the appropriate level on the W.A.L.K.S. Program. After completing the "S" level, continue on the W.A.L.K.S. Maintenance Program for a lifetime of fitness.

Warm up for 5 to 10 minutes before starting the conditioning segment of your workout. The warm-up should be activity specific, so for fitness walking begin gradually increasing the pace to that at your conditioning level. During the conditioning bout, always check your heart rate to be sure it stays within the target zone. Listen to your body and progress slowly for optimal results.

Cool down for 5 to 10 minutes following the conditioning bout. As in the warm-up, the cool-down should be activity specific. Thus, reduce your pace, finishing with 5 to 10 minutes of slow walking.

For total fitness, stretch for flexibility. Improved flexibility is best achieved if it occurs at the end of the cool-down when the muscles and joints are thoroughly warmed and pliable. Use flexibility exercises for your stretching routine.

Take each step on the chart and don't skip ahead. If the increase is too difficult, go back to the preceding level for awhile. You should feel energized after your workout, not exhausted.

W.A.L.K.S. Program

Fitness Category	Starting Program
Very low	**W** Level
Low	**A** Level
Average	**L** Level
Good	**K** Level
Excellent	**S** Level

W Level

Week	1–2	3–4	5–6	7–8	9–10	11–12	13–14
Warm-up (min.)	5–10	5–10	5–10	5–10	5–10	5–10	5–10
Conditioning bout (mileage)	1.00	1.25	1.50	1.75	2.00	2.25	2.50
Intensity % (target heart rate)	60–75	60–75	60–75	60–75	60–75	60–75	60–75
Cool-down (min.)	5–10	5–10	5–10	5–10	5–10	5–10	5–10
Frequency	3	3	3	3	4	4	4

A Level

Week	1–2	3–4	5–6	7–8	9–10	11–12	13–14
Warm-up (min.)	5–10	5–10	5–10	5–10	5–10	5–10	5–10
Conditioning bout (mileage)	2.00	2.25	2.50	2.75	3.00	3.25	3.50
Intensity % (target heart rate)	60–75	60–75	60–75	60–75	60–75	60–75	60–75
Cool-down (min.)	5–10	5–10	5–10	5–10	5–10	5–10	5–10
Frequency	3	3	3	4	4	4	4

L Level

Week	1–2	3–4	5–6	7–8	9–10	11–12	13–14
Warm-up (min.)	5–10	5–10	5–10	5–10	5–10	5–10	5–10
Conditioning bout (mileage)	3.00	3.25	3.50	3.70	3.75	4.00	
Intensity % (target heart rate)	60–75	60–75	60–75	60–75	60–75	60–75	60–75
Cool-down (min.)	5–10	5–10	5–10	5–10	5–10	5–10	5–10
Frequency	3	3	4	4	4	4	4

K Level

Week	1–2	3–4	5–6	7–8	9–10	11–12	13–14
Warm-up (min.)	5–10	5–10	5–10	5–10	5–10	5–10	5–10
Conditioning bout (mileage)	3.50	3.75	3.75	4.00	4.00	4.00	4.00
Intensity % (target heart rate)	60–75	60–75	60–75	60–75	60–75	60–75	60–75
Cool-down (min.)	5–10	5–10	5–10	5–10	5–10	5–10	5–10
Frequency	4	4	4	4	5	5	5

S Level

Week	1–2	3–4	5–6	7–8	9–10	11–12	13–14
Warm-up (min.)	5–10	5–10	5–10	5–10	5–10	5–10	5–10
Conditioning bout (mileage)	4.00	4.00	4.00	4.25	4.25	4.50	4.50
Intensity % (target heart rate)	60–75	60–75	60–75	60–75	60–75	60–75	60–75
Cool-down (min.)	5–10	5–10	5–10	5–10	5–10	5–10	5–10
Frequency	5	5	5	5	5	5	5

W.A.L.K.S. Maintenance Program
(for a lifetime of fitness)

Warm-up:	5–10 min.
Conditioning bout:	3–5 miles per workout
Intensity %:	60–75
Cool-down:	5–10 min.
Frequency:	3–5 times per week
Weekly mileage:	9–25 miles

Variety

Adding variety to your walking workouts can keep you enthused about the sport for many years. Varying your walking routes gives you a change of scenery. Drive the car to a new area, park, and explore the surroundings during your workout. Mailing a letter, walking an errand, taking window shopping walks, and doing shopping mall workouts can be fun. Walk with a friend, in a group, or by yourself for a change. Get a dog; they make excellent walking companions. For a challenge, try an advanced exercise walking technique such as race walking, power walking, hill walking, or walking a fitness trail. Participate in a volksmarch, a competitive walking event, or join a Hashing Club (described in the Jogging section). Water walking (walking in waist-deep water) is popular in many areas; give it a try. Some people enjoy listening to music while exercising in a traffic-free area. Schedule walking meetings with coworkers. Train for a half-marathon (mini); see sample training program in the Jogging section. Try the "Exercise Across the U.S.A." Activity found later in this chapter for added incentives to keep walking. You won't become stale or bored with exercise if you vary your workouts.

Common Discomforts

As in running, most aches, pains, and injuries from walking occur from overuse. Listen to your body. Don't attempt to work through an injury. It will only aggravate the condition. The two most common walking complaints are shin splints and back-of-the-knee soreness. Refer to Chapter 9 for information about shin splints. Cut back on pace and distance until soreness subsides. Comfortable, well-fitting shoes will help prevent blisters. Consult a sports podiatrist if you suffer from foot problems such as calluses, bunions, heel spurs, ingrown toenails, high arches, flat feet, or an overly pronated foot. These conditions can be remedied but, if not corrected, may prevent you from fully enjoying your walking program.

Name _____

Date _____

W.A.L.K.S. Fitness Walking Log
(Make extra copies of this form as needed)

Week(s) _____　　　　　　　　　　　　　　　　　　　Level _____

Goals: _____

_____

_____

Date	Length of Walk (Time)	Distance of Walk	HR During Exercise	Location of Walk	Comments (How Felt, etc.)
Sun					
Mon					
Tues					
Wed					
Thurs					
Fri					
Sat					
Sun					
Mon					
Tues					
Wed					
Thurs					
Fri					
Sat					
Sun					
Mon					
Tues					
Wed					
Thurs					
Fri					
Sat					
Totals:	_____	_____			

Ninety-nine percent of the failures come from people who have the habit of making excuses.

—George Washington Carver

Indoor Exercise Equipment

(Including Stationary Bikes, Steppers, Treadmills, Ski Machines, Rowing Machines, and Elliptical Trainers)

Advantages/Disadvantages

When winter's plummeting temperatures, ice, snow, and chill winds make outdoor exercise difficult, indoor exercise equipment may be for you. If it is too rainy, too hot, too dark, or unsafe to exercise outside, you can work out in the relative comfort and safety of a health club or your home. Indoor exercise equipment allows you to alternate indoor and outdoor workouts according to weather, your schedule, and your mood.

Indoor workouts can be done either on your equipment at home or equipment in a health club. If you like working out with others, don't want to deal with equipment maintenance, and enjoy a variety of different types of exercise, a health club is a good place to start. At a club, you can try different types of equipment: bicycles, steppers, treadmills, skiers, rowers, and elliptical trainers and see what you like best. If, on the other hand, you can't seem to make time to get to the health club, with exercise equipment at home, you don't have to go anywhere. You can exercise before or after work, be with your family, and read or watch TV at the same time. If you have children, you can keep an eye on them and won't have to hire a baby-sitter while you work out. The main advantage to working out at home is the convenience.

Disadvantages of home exercise equipment are that you have to decide what type of equipment and features you want, purchase it, make room for it in your house, perform your own maintenance, find someone to repair it (or fix it yourself) if it breaks, will likely be working out alone, and may get bored with the same workout day after day. Also, if your enthusiasm wanes, the equipment may become a constant reminder of failed resolutions. However, working out in private is very appealing to many people. You know who used the equipment last, and, for what you pay for a 1-year club membership, you can have your own equipment at home.

Advantages of working out at a health club include that you can switch from one type of equipment to another to avoid boredom or work different muscle groups; you can meet a lot of people; professionals are readily available to answer your questions; you don't have to buy, maintain, and repair the equipment; and you don't have to make space at home for it year-round.

Disadvantages of working out at a health club include that you will have to pay membership fees, schedule it in your day, have transportation, and at popular workout times may have to wait to get on some equipment.

What to Wear

You are working out inside, so any comfortable workout gear will be fine; a T-shirt and shorts, supportive shoes, a water bottle, and a towel to wipe off sweat and you are ready to go.

Equipment

Equipment comes in two main types: aerobic and strength machines. Strength training information is covered in Chapter 5. This section will focus on aerobic equipment. Equipment ranges in price from a couple hundred to several thousand dollars, depending on quality and options desired, but indoor exercise equipment need not be expensive. A jump rope, an exercise mat, elastic resistance bands, a step or a slide mat, and an aerobics video are low budget. More costly exercise machines include steppers, cross-country ski simulators, climbers, treadmills, exercise bicycles, rowers, and elliptical trainers.

If you would like to work out at home and are not familiar with the variety of equipment available, join a health club for a 1- to 3-month trial period to try out and compare the different types. Then you will know what type of equipment you want to purchase and will be more familiar with features available. Do not, however, expect a $200 home unit to function like a $2,000 health club model. Shop informed. Ask friends and family about equipment and features they like.

Be choosy. Avoid cheap equipment, which may be flimsy, noisy, unstable, or jerky and can make the whole workout experience so unpleasant that you'll soon use the machine as a coat rack. Shop for well-designed exercise equipment from a specialty retailer rather than from a TV infomercial or chain department store. The quality and durability will be worth the cost in terms of ease of use and maintenance. Think compact. Unless you have a lot of space, you probably will not want equipment that takes up a whole room. Steppers and exercise bicycles have the smallest "footprint" and are easily moved to the side when not being used. Think simple. Not much can go wrong with a jump rope, but plenty can go wrong with a flimsy treadmill. The more complicated a piece of equipment is to use and adjust, the more maintenance it needs. Many devices have timers, heart rate monitors, and ergometers that calculate your work output in calories.

Before you invest in home exercise equipment, try out several models and ask these questions:

1. How much will I use this? Do I enjoy this type of exercise?
2. Does the sales staff ask about my needs and fitness goals before helping me select equipment rather than automatically recommending the most expensive machine?
3. Does it have the features I want?
4. Is it easy to assemble?
5. If it breaks, how will I get it repaired? Can it be fixed locally?
6. What kind of warranty comes with it? What is the store's return policy?
7. Is it well-constructed of steel or alloy to last 10 or more years?
8. What kind of maintenance is needed, according to the manual?
9. Are the seats and grips comfortable, durable, and easily adjustable?
10. Does it work smoothly? How stable is it? Is it relatively quiet? Is it safe?
11. Where will I put it? How much space does it require?
12. Does the manual show how to use the equipment correctly and how to reach my target heart rate?
13. Do I need all the fancy gadgets or will a more simple model do?
14. Can I get a workout with this machine that is intense enough for my current and future fitness levels?

Stationary Bikes

Advantages/Disadvantages

Most models work the lower body—primarily legs, hips, and buttocks—but some models have handlebars for exercising arms and shoulders. Some of the more expensive electronic models have programmed workouts such as interval training or hills to add variety. Upright models make efficient use of space, and you can read or watch TV as you exercise. They give you a good nonimpact workout, easier on the joints than treadmills. They are particularly good for overweight people who need to avoid extra stress on the back, knees, and ankles. Both upright and recumbent models are effective. Recumbent bikes, in which you sit back on a seat and pedal in front of the body tend to be more expensive and need at least 6 to 7 feet of space but are easier on the back. Bicycle trainers, which put your regular bicycle on a stand with resistance to the rear wheel, require balance but are less expensive than stationary bicycles. Another model, popularized by Health Rider, does not involve pedaling; rather, you push on both pedals simultaneously as you pull on handlebars, exercising both upper and lower body muscles.

How to Select

A good machine is easy to adjust, moves smoothly, and feels stable. The seat should be comfortable and should adjust to

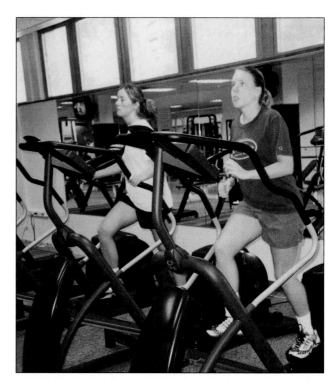

Add variety to your exercise program.

your height. In many models, handlebars are also adjustable. The controls should be within easy reach, and the workload should adjust smoothly and easily. Look for a smooth, quiet ride; a sturdy frame; a wide, comfortable, adjustable seat; and an easy-to-read instrument panel. Cheaper models are made of flimsier metal; the resistance mechanism may be grabby, the seat less comfortable, and the whole device more "tippy."

Technique and Safety Tips

Proper seat height and pedaling cadence are the keys to avoiding knee problems. Seat height should be adjusted so that when you sit on the seat, your knee is almost fully extended on the downstroke. Also, keep the resistance moderate so that you maintain a cadence of about 60 to 80 rpm.

Steppers

Advantages/Disadvantages

Steppers primarily work the legs, hips, and buttocks and do not work the upper body. They take relatively little space and allow you to read or watch TV as you exercise. They may aggravate some knee problems. They tend to work the calves more than other types of equipment do.

How to Select

Steppers come with either dependent or independent pedals. With dependent pedals, as one goes down, the other goes up. The machine does some of the work for you because you are exercising one foot at a time. Independent pedal models, in which both feet have to be working at the same time, take a little more work to get the rhythm and coordination but give a better workout. Hydraulic resistance mechanisms provide a fluid feel at an affordable price. High-end models have computerized interval resistance programs that can increase and decrease the workload through the exercise bout. Self-leveling pedals are a nice feature. Make sure pedals are big enough for you to balance on them comfortably. Some also come with poles for working the arms. Less expensive models are manually adjustable, so if you want to change resistance in the middle of a workout, you will have to get off and turn knobs or slide levers. They still give you a good workout, however, so the lower price may be worth some minor inconvenience.

Technique and Safety Tips

Rest your hands lightly on the handlebars or railings for balance and take small steps at first. Stand tall and gradually begin to take deeper steps after you warm up. Do not lean on the railings or you will decrease the effectiveness of the workout.

Treadmills

Advantages/Disadvantages

Treadmills are popular and easy to use, giving a good cardiovascular and lower body workout. They also tend to be used more than other types of equipment. However, they are noisy and more prone to breakdowns than other types of equipment. They also require a large space, about 6 by 4 feet, though you can purchase models that fold for storage.

How to Select

A motorized treadmill should have at least a 1.5 horsepower continuous-duty motor to be strong enough to maintain even speed. Walkers need a speed of at least 5 mph and joggers a speed faster than your normal pace. Ability to simulate at least a 10 percent incline is important for you to always be able to reach your target pulse. Look for a safety lock so a child cannot accidentally start the treadmill and an emergency shut-off button to cut power immediately. You need at least one handrail, preferably two for balance, and wide footrails. Also look for a wide 2-ply rubber belt for durability on the running surface, some flexibility so that it gives a little with each stride, and a belt long enough so that you can maintain a comfortable stride. Decide if you want a motorized or hand-crank incline and what other computerized features you desire, such as heart rate or calorie counting. Less expensive machines tend to have a shorter, narrower bed; lower horsepower; a faster starting speed; a lower top speed; a less durable 1-ply belt; and fewer computerized features. They are also noisier, wear out

faster, and may not keep the belt speed as consistent as the higher-end models do.

Nonmotorized treadmills are cheaper but move only with the pull of your feet on the belt, and they slow down if you do. They are better for walking than running and may be harder on the joints than motorized treadmills, which move continuously at a preset speed.

Technique and Safety Tips

Start the machine at a slow pace. Straddle the belt, step with one foot a few times to get a feel for the speed, and then begin. Increase to normal speed as you warm up. Keep near the front of the belt at all times.

Ski Machines

Advantages/Disadvantages

Ski simulators can work both upper and lower body muscles and give a smooth, nonimpact workout. They do require a lot of space, up to 9 by 3 feet, but some models fold for storage when not in use. They are not suitable for people with balance problems that lead to dizziness or difficulty coordinating movements when standing. You can listen to music or watch TV, but you cannot read while you ski. Ski machines do require practice to master the coordination, but they reward the effort with an excellent workout.

How to Select

Ski machines come in two basic types. One type, popularized by NordicTrack, has skilike rails onto which you place your feet. These glide back and forth on a track, and your hands alternately pull a cable. The other type has small platforms that slide back and forth on a track, and your hands usually pull on poles rather than cables. Cables are usually better than poles because they exercise your arms through a fuller range of motion, giving the muscles a better workout.

Like steppers, ski machines come in independent and dependent pedal models. Dependent pedal models are connected so that, as one foot slides backward, the other automatically comes forward, producing a stiff-legged gait. Independent pedal models require more learning, but the gait is more natural. The muscles in both legs have to work with each stride, and you get a fuller workout. Look for skis that move smoothly, have a base long enough for your stride, and offer adjustable leg and arm resistance.

Technique and Safety Tips

Be forewarned that with a skier it may take several weeks to master the coordination, and they are not for anyone who has balance problems.

Rowing Machines

Advantages/Disadvantages

Rowers provide an excellent upper as well as lower body workout, toning shoulders, back, arms, and legs. They do, however, require a lot of space, up to 8 feet by 3 feet. They can also be noisy, and you cannot read while working out.

How to Select

They come in piston and flywheel models. The piston models are cheaper and more compact, but flywheel models have smoother action. Some models give strokes per minute, total distance, time, and power output per stroke.

Technique and Safety Tips

Correct rowing technique takes practice to master and is important to avoid back injury. Do not lean into the pull, but keep upright throughout the range of motion. Your legs, arms, and shoulders, not your back, should do much of the work, and your arms should move forward before you bend your knees. With a flywheel model, pull the bar into your abdomen, not your chin. The workout can be intense.

Elliptical Trainers

Advantages/Disadvantages

This machine simulates a combination of walking, running, and stair climbing in one motion. The workout is weight-bearing, but there is none of the jarring impact caused when exercising on pavement, a track, or a treadmill. The motion is even smoother than step machines. Physical therapists and athletic trainers love these machines because they allow athletes to continue their training regime even while the athlete is rehabilitating an overuse injury, such as Achilles tendinitis, runner's knee, shin splints, even a stress fracture. Elliptical trainers offer the same cardiorespiratory endurance and muscular benefits of running as well as providing refuge from Mother Nature's wrath and the dangers of traffic dodging.

Like all exercise machines, elliptical trainers do have some drawbacks, though they are minimal. Because the muscles do not have to adjust for landing on the ground with each stride as they do with actual running, the overall mus-cle action (and thus, the overall workout), is not quite as intense on an elliptical trainer. The estimated overall workout benefit on an elliptical trainer is anywhere from 75 to 90 percent of a running workout. Ellipticals require minimal use of the arms and shoulders, so they do not offer a total body workout. Elliptical trainers with armpole attachments reduce this drawback.

Ellipticals tend to be rather large machines, so they do not offer the mobility and storability offered by some other indoor exercise machines. Cost may be a drawback unless you can comfortably afford the $300 to $3,000 (health club model) price tag. Keep in mind you get what you pay for.

How to Select

The elliptical trainer you select should have tension control that allows you to adjust and vary the resistance against the running ramps. The ramp elevation option on some machines is nice but not essential. You can get the same effect by running faster and/or adjusting the ramp resistance control to a higher tension setting. You may select a machine with arm poles—similar to those on cross-country ski machines. Thus, allowing you to use them for an upper body workout. These are nice but not essential.

Experts recommend selecting a machine that has a read-out screen that shows information such as calories burned, time and distance run, and strides per minute.

A final piece of advice if you plan on buying an elliptical trainer, try out a number of models before making a final decision.

Technique and Safety Tips

When you exercise on an elliptical trainer, you stand on two platforms, or ramps, "suspended" between wheel-gear and roller mechanisms. When you move your legs in a running motion, one ramp moves forward and slightly upward while the other ramp moves backward and slightly downward. You will leave your arms free (as in running) or hold on to the hand railing on the side of the machine.

Stand upright. Elliptical trainers can put pressure on the lower back if you lean forward or lean on the handrails while exercising. If you feel low back discomfort during or after the workout, check your posture. Feet that are too far apart can cause the hips to shift excessively, putting strain on the lumbar region. To stabilize, bring feet closer together on the pedals.

How to Begin and Progress

Consult the owner's manual for guidelines specific to your exercise equipment regarding how to begin and progress. In general, treadmills and stationary bikes have the quickest learning curves, steppers run third, with ski machines and rowers requiring more balance and skill. However, for the time invested in the latter two, you can get a better upper body workout along with aerobic fitness, so the time is well spent. Also, the rule of specificity applies, so if you are in great running shape but begin working out on a stepper or cycle, give yourself some time to build up to the same level of intensity and duration. If you are a beginner, start with 5 to 10 minutes, low intensity, 3 days the first week to get a feel for correct mechanics and how to use the equipment. Increase the workout by a couple of minutes each week. Pace your progress according to how you feel during and after the workout. If you feel tired and washed out, you are trying to progress too quickly and need to move back or maintain the same level until your endurance increases. If you feel good, then you can continue to add a couple of minutes a week to each workout until you reach 20 to 30 minutes of continuous activity. To increase frequency, add an additional day each month until you are exercising up to 5 days a week at your target pulse. A suggested workout schedule follows:

Sample Beginning Program

Week	1–2	3–4	5–6	7–8	9–10	11–15
Warm-up (min.)	5–10	5–10	5–10	5–10	5–10	5–10
Conditioning bout (min.)	5–10	8–14	12–18	17–22	21–26	25–30
Intensity (target heart rate)	50–60	60–75	60–75	60–75	60–75	60–75
Cool-down (min.)	5–10	5–10	5–10	5–10	5–10	5–10
Frequency	3	3	3	3–4	3–4	3–5

How to Select a Health Club

1. Ask friends and family about local clubs, equipment, and advantages and disadvantages.
2. Visit several clubs at times you would be going, such as after work, to see how crowded they are. Check out the bathrooms, locker room, pool, weight room. All should be clean and well-maintained. Equipment should be in good repair. Talk to the regulars to see how they judge it. See that it has the features and types of equipment you want to use.
3. Professionals should be available to show you how to use the equipment correctly for the most effective workout and to avoid injury. Ask about instructor qualifications. Certification by a professional group demonstrates a commitment to quality instruction. There are many national certifying organizations that certify instructors in different activities. Some of these are the American College of Sports Medicine, YMCA, YWCA, International Dance-Exercise Association, Aerobics and Fitness Association of America, and National Strength and Conditioning Association.
4. Look for a health club with at least 3 years of continuous operation. Call your local Better Business Bureau or your state or local consumer protection agency to check if any negative reports have been filed. Ask to see evidence of bonding from the club (this protects you if the club goes out of business).
5. Membership fees are negotiable, so no matter what is printed on the brochure, negotiate!
6. Start with a short-term membership. Only 10 percent of members are still working out after 3 months, so either pay on a monthly basis, or sign up for a 3-month trial membership.
7. Read the contract carefully before signing, making sure it covers everything you have discussed with the club employees. If you change your mind, most states have a 3-day cooling-off period during which you can void the contract and get a full refund.

The harder you work, the luckier you get.

—Gary Player

In-Line Skating

Advantages/Disadvantages

Modern skating has gone in-line. Instead of four wheels situated in box formation under the skate, the new skating gear consists of four urethane wheels positioned down the center of a supportive boot complete with brake pads. Skaters also need protective pads and a helmet to lower injury risk, which can be substantial.

Ice hockey players in Minnesota designed the first prototype for today's in-line skates. They enjoyed their dryland workouts so much that they began skating out of season for fun! The popularity of in-line skating exploded in the 1990s primarily because it is so easy to learn and convenient. People are no longer intimidated by the misconception that only the supercoordinated can skate on a single row of wheels.

In-line skating can be a competitive sport involving speed or fancy tricks, known as freestyle skating. Other sports such as basketball and hockey can be played on in-line skates, and skiers may cross train on in-line skates off-season. But the majority of in-line skaters do it primarily for fitness, recreational, social, or transportation purposes. Thirty-five percent of in-line skaters report using skates as a mode of transportation.

In-line skating has excellent potential for developing physical fitness, especially cardiorespiratory endurance and muscular endurance. Plus, it is invigoratingly fun. Vigorous and continuous striding can burn as many calories as jogging or cycling. Skating is one of the best activities for improving balance and ideal for cross training for any fitness activity. Serious skating increases muscular strength and endurance. It strengthens the musculature in the entire upper leg, including the hamstrings and quadriceps as well as the buttocks, hips, and lower back muscles. By swinging and pumping the arms vigorously during skating the biceps, triceps, and shoulder muscles can be strengthened and toned.

In-line skaters reap all the benefits of other forms of exercise: improved physical fitness; increased energy levels; lower blood pressure; weight control; relaxation; and a reduced risk of cancer, heart disease, and stroke. Physiological responses measured during in-line skating indicate that individuals with average fitness levels can achieve appropriate exercise training effect on flat terrain, although the highly fit may need to skate uphill or skate fast to achieve the same benefit.

In-line skating does have a few drawbacks. This fun, aerobic, low-impact sport can be dangerous to skaters who don't wear helmets and protective pads or who do not learn

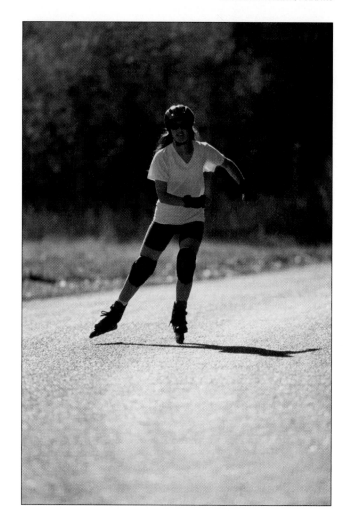

Enjoy exercise out-of-doors.

safe starting and stopping techniques. If you have a fear of falling, suffer from osteoporosis, or have balance problems, in-line skating is not a good exercise choice. Another disadvantage with in-line skating is cost. In-line skates and the necessary safety gear can be expensive.

What to Wear

You can in-line skate in almost any kind of weather if you dress appropriately. Dress in layers when it's cool (removing outer garments as you warm up) and as little as decently possible when it's hot. You will be most comfortable skating in stretchy or loose-fitting clothes. The lycra clothing worn by many runners is perfect. T-shirts are fine, and so are tights and bike shorts. Jeans are not usually comfortable and will bunch up under the knee pads or over the boot.

In-line skates are available in a spectrum of prices and styles. Before buying a pair, rent several types to see which suits you. Talk to knowledgeable salespeople; tell them about your skating activity and the type of skating you are planning to do. The cost of a good pair of skates ranges from $100 to $400 or more. Add another $50 to $200 for the protective gear. To try on skates, bring a pair of absorbent socks that you plan to wear while skating. A sock that helps "wick" sweat away from the foot and aids in preventing blisters is a good choice. When you rent or buy your first pair of in-line skates be sure to get a properly fitted helmet; knee and elbow pads; and wrist guards, specially designed gloves with extra padding at the palms. Treat protective gear like your seat belt; wear it everytime you skate.

Necessary Gear

- *Skates:* Good in-line skates are not cheap. Expect to pay between $100 to $400. The rule to follow is to buy the best possible skates you can afford. Originally, the skate boot was made from molded polyurethane, a lightweight but extremely sturdy material. But since 1994, the soft-boot in-line design skate boot has been the industry standard. The new boot fits like a hiking boot instead of a plastic ski boot. The fit of the boot should not be too tight or too loose. A snug fit, when the boot is laced, is good. It should allow some room for the toes (about one-fourth inch from the end of the longest toe to the end of the boot). In-line boots use laces, buckles, velcro straps, or a combination of laces and buckles to tighten and secure the boot. The most effective and popular style is a boot that laces on the lower part and buckles on the ankle for maximum support. Boots with vents, to allow liberal air circulation, are recommended. A foam liner, either built into the skate or an insert purchased separately, provides added comfort and helps to prevent blisters. Look for liners with vents to aid breathability.
- *Helmet:* Select a helmet that provides a snug, comfortable fit. Look for approval by the two national helmet testing bodies, SNELL and ANSI.
- *Wrist Guards:* This is a fingerless glove with a hard plastic splint running down the front. The plastic is curved slightly—not enough to hinder wrist and hand movement, but enough to act as shock absorber in the event of a fall.
- *Knee and Elbow Pads:* These are designed to prevent scrapes and bruises. Use only the style that has a hard plastic shield over the pad. Do not use cloth-covered pads from other sports such as volleyball.

Techniques and Safety Tips

Taking a few in-line skating lessons or studying an instructional video are the recommended methods for learning this sport. It is imperative to practice the following basic skills before you take to the street or trails: ready position, forward fall, forward stride and glide, basic turning, braking,

and making emergency stops. Find a conveniently located paved area where you can go often to practice. It must be smooth and level with enough room to move about unobstructed. Empty parking lots and unused ball courts are ideal, providing they are free of pedestrians, debris, and bike traffic. Avoid hills until your skills are proficient. While skating there are some safety guidelines you need to follow: see Table 4-1.

Skate Maintenance

In-line skates are relatively low maintenance, that is one of the inviting aspects of the sport. You can put on your skates and get a good workout without much set-up or clean-up time. However, your skates will need occasional attention.

Tools. It's a good idea to put together a skate repair kit that can be carried in your skate bag. Be sure to choose components and tools that fit your particular model of skate. Your local skate shop can help you with the selection of components and tools.

Wheel Rotation or Replacement. The most common maintenance activity is rotation of the wheels. Wheels wear down while skating; therefore, to get maximum mileage proper rotation is necessary. Rotation is changing the position of the wheels on the frame and turning the wheels over so the inside edges become the outside edges. To rotate your wheels, follow these directions:

Wheel in Position	Move to Position
1	3
2	4
3	1
4	2

table 4-1   Safety Guidelines for In-Line Skating

1. Always wear full protective gear.
2. Achieve a basic skating level before taking to the road. Practice basic skills on a smooth, flat surface away from traffic.
3. Stay alert and courteous at all times.
4. Always skate under control.
5. Skate on the right side of paths, trails, and sidewalks.
6. Overtake pedestrians, cyclists, and other skaters on the left. Announce your intentions by saying, "Passing on your left."
7. Avoid water, oil, or debris on the trail and uneven, broken pavement.
8. Obey all traffic regulations.
9. Avoid areas with heavy automotive traffic.
10. Always yield to pedestrians.
11. Keep your gear in proper working order.

Bearing Replacement. Bearings allow the wheels to spin smoothly and have the biggest effect on the performance of the skate. Buy the best bearings you can afford. Each skate has two sets of bearings, one on each side of the wheel. ABEC bearings range from 1 to 7, 1 creating the least amount of speed, 7 the greatest amount of speed. Fitness/recreation skaters usually use ABEC 3 bearings.

Brake Replacement. Brakes should be replaced when you have to lift your toe too high to be stable when stopping or when the bolt holding the brake in place begins to rub the ground. Loosen the bolt, remove the brake, and attach the new brake.

How to Begin and Progress. First, assess your fitness level using the 1.5-mile timed run test described in Chapter 3. Remember that your current fitness level does not indicate your potential. Based on your fitness category, begin at the appropriate starting level. Progress through each level, one step at a time. Do not skip steps and stay on each as long as necessary to adapt to that workload. Remember to monitor your pulse and do not exceed your target heart rate range. Or, if you prefer, use the PRE to monitor your intensity level during the workout. Keep in mind the FITT prescription factors covered in Chapter 3. Don't forget to warm-up and cool-down during each workout. To develop balanced fitness add 25 to 30 push-ups, 1 minute of abdominal curls, and 5 to 15 minutes of stretching per workout.

In-Line Skating Program

Fitness Category	Starting level
Very low	1 or 2
Low	3
Average	4
Good	5
Excellent	6

Level	Skating
1	10–15 min.
2	10–20 min.
3	15–25 min.
4	20–40 min.
5	30–45 min.
6	45–75 min.

Variety

Adding variety to your skating workouts can keep you enthused about the sport for many years. Varying your skating routes gives you a change of scenery. Drive the car to a new area, park, and explore the area. Find new trails, paths, sidewalks, and parking lots on which to skate. Use your skates for transportation to and from school or work several days a week. Keep your skates in the trunk of the car and strap them on for a spontaneous workout when you see an opportunity (i.e., at lunch time). Be sociable, skate with a friend or join a skating club. Pack a backpack with a water bottle and a snack for a longer than usual workout. Try speed skating, amateur racing, or freestyle or artistic skating, which is similar to ice figure skating. Extreme skating involves tricks, jumps, and ramps that might appeal to you. You won't become bored with exercise if you vary your workouts.

Common Discomforts

According to estimates by the Centers for Disease Control and Prevention about 1 in 225 in-line skaters sought emergency room treatment for skating injuries during a six-month study. Only 7 percent of the injured skaters had worn safety gear. Spontaneous loss of balance; falling due to debris or an irregularity on the skating surface; colliding with a fellow skater; or striking a stationary hazard, such as a tree, are the most common causes of falls by in-line skaters, studies show. Blisters, strains, sprains, and many other general complaints are addressed in Chapter 9.

Falling is the biggest concern when skating, so you won't be surprised to learn that the number one injury site is the wrist. The wrist can be strained, sprained, or even fractured during a fall. The U.S. Consumer Product Safety Commission (CPSC) and the International In-line Skating Association (IISA) recommend that a helmet, elbow and knee pads, and wrist guards with fingerless gloves be worn while skating to reduce the risk and severity of injuries, especially those involving the wrist.

In the games of life even the 50-yard line seats don't interest me. I came to play.

—H. Jackson Brown, Jr. *Dad, A Father's Book of Wisdom*

Jogging

Advantages/Disadvantages

Running is a simple way to develop cardiorespiratory endurance. You can do it alone, with a partner, or with a group. A good pair of running shoes is the only equipment you need. Finding a place to run is as simple as walking out your front door. Getting a full workout through running takes less time than many other aerobic activities. It can be done in most types of weather, on vacation, or during a lunch break. As a weight-bearing exercise, jogging provides stress to the long bones, which aids in maintenance of bone mineralization and decreases risk of osteoporosis. Like other aerobic activities, jogging has positive benefits in reducing obesity, stress, Type 2 diabetes, and several heart disease risk factors.

Drawbacks to running include traffic; uneven pavement; and, occasionally, an aggressive dog. Trying to progress too quickly may cause impact problems such as shin splints or sore knees. Jogging is not for everyone. For individuals prone to musculoskeletal problems, low- or nonimpact activities such as bicycling or water exercise are less likely to precipitate injury. If you are overweight or out of shape, it may be best to start with a less intense activity, such as walking. Nonetheless, a carefully planned program of progressive activity enables many people to enjoy running as part of their fitness program.

What to Wear

You can run in almost any kind of weather if you dress appropriately. On hot days, wear as little as decently possible—shoes, socks, shirt, and shorts. For cooler weather, add layers: a long-sleeved T-shirt and tights or long pants. In cold weather, add a jacket or a turtleneck sweater and, to protect ears and hands, a stocking cap and mittens. In wet weather, wear a cap with a brim to keep rain out of your eyes and rain-repellent clothing, if desired. Keep in mind that when you are running, you generate a great deal of body heat. When you are warmed up, it will feel about 20 degrees warmer than the actual temperature. A hot day would be 70 degrees or higher, a warm day 50 to 60 degrees, a cool day 30 to 40 degrees, and a cold day below freezing. High humidity on hot days and the windchill factor on cold days also should be considered (see Chap. 6).

A good pair of properly fitted running shoes is important in preventing injuries. When running, your foot strikes the ground with an impact of approximately three times your body weight. A well-made running shoe fitted by a trained salesperson can absorb shock and support the foot. A cheap pair of poor quality shoes is no bargain if it leaves you with blisters or shin splints.

Technique and Safety Tips

Good running form is relaxed and mechanically efficient. Your energy goes into moving you forward and is not dissipated in extraneous movements. Maintain a relaxed, erect posture, head up, eyes looking ahead. Keep your shoulders relaxed and level, arms swinging freely from the shoulder, hands unclenched, traveling between the hips and lower chest. Avoid hunching forward, your eyes watching your feet, your arms held stiffly or swinging across the midline of your body. Knees and feet should aim ahead, not to the center or side. Foot contact should be heel to ball or midfoot, not on the toes like a sprinter. Keep your stride length comfortable and effortless, with your foot landing under your center of gravity. Be careful not to overstride or bounce when you run. Stride length is a product of speed and leg strength. Unless you increase one of these elements, attempts to increase your stride length will waste energy. Breathe through your mouth and nose. It is hard to get enough air breathing through the nose alone.

While you are working on your running form, there are some safety guidelines you need to keep in mind:

1. *Before leaving home, let someone know your route* and when you expect to return. Carry identification.
2. *If you wear a headset, keep the volume low* enough so you can hear approaching traffic.
3. *Keep alert.*
4. *If there is a sidewalk, jog on it.*
5. *If there is no sidewalk, run facing traffic on the extreme left edge or shoulder of the road.*
6. *Respect private property.* Do not run across lawns.
7. *Obey traffic signs and signals.* When crossing a street at the light, cross with the green light only.
8. *Maintain eye contact with motorists* whenever you cross in front of them.
9. *Give the right-of-way to cars.* Don't antagonize drivers, even if they try your patience.
10. *If you run at night, wear light-colored clothing with reflective strips.*
11. *At night, do not run in unfamiliar areas.*
12. *Do not wear a vinyl sweat suit* while exercising, ever!

How to Begin and Progress

Begin at the level indicated by your cardiorespiratory fitness assessment (Chapter 3) and progress slowly. If you cannot complete a mile in 15 minutes, then begin with walking briskly 15 to 30 minutes until your heart rate stays within the target range. When you can comfortably handle 2 miles in

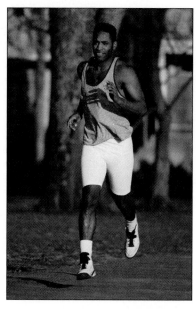

Vary your jogging workouts to avoid becoming bored and stale.

30 minutes, you may begin the jog/walk program. As in all activities, follow the FITT guidelines.

Run/Walk Program

Fitness Category	Starting Level
Very low	1, 2, or 3
Low	4
Average	5 or 6
Good	7 or 8
Excellent	9 or 10

Level	Run	Walk	Repeats
1	—	15–20 min.	1
2	—	20–30 min.	1
3	30 sec.	30 sec.	8–12 plus 10- to 15-min. walk
4	1 min.	30 sec.	6–10 plus 10-min. walk
5	2 min.	30 sec.	4–10 plus 5- to 10-min. walk
6	4 min.	1 min.	4–6
7	6 min.	1 min.	4–5
8	8 min.	1–2 min.	3–4
9	12 min.	2 min.	2
10	20–30 min.	5 min.	1

Start at the level appropriate for your fitness category. Remember that your starting level does not indicate your potential. For each run-walk interval, begin with the lowest number of repeats indicated and, each successive workout, add one repeat. When you can do the maximum number of intervals at one level, move to the next level. A 5-minute warm-up and 5-minute cool-down should accompany each workout. You may stay at one level as long as you need to or even move back a step if the beginning level is too difficult. If the workout has been appropriate, you should feel refreshed and relaxed, not exhausted, after exercise.

Variety

Much of the variety in running comes from running different routes and from observing the changing scenery and seasons. If you run alone, you may wish to occasionally run with a partner or a group. Instead of taking a long run at a continuous pace, you might try *fartlek*, a Swedish term for *speed-play*. Fartlek mixes fast-paced runs, brief all-out sprints, and slow-paced recovery intervals. It is best done on uneven or hilly terrain such as a park or golf course. Interval training done once or no more than twice a week can add a change of pace. This alternates a fast-paced run over a predetermined distance with walking or a slow recovery jog. An example might be running 220 yards, four to six times in 40 to 50 seconds with a 220-yard walk between each. With interval training, you may vary the distance run, recovery interval, number of repetitions, and time or pace of the run. These workouts are usually done on the track but can be done on the road by running and then walking a set amount of time, by running a certain number of telephone pole intervals, or by selecting a long hill on your route and running up it several times. A fitness trail, or parcour, with exercise stations linked by a running trail, may be available at a local park or university or you can make your own. To simulate a parcour on a regular running route, stop every 2 to 4 minutes to do a stretching or toning exercise (i.e., hamstring stretch, run 2 minutes, calf stretch, run 3 minutes, push-ups, run 3 minutes, abdominal curls, . . .).

Some activities are suitable for a small group. You can take a tennis or foam ball along to toss among some friends. You'll get quite a workout because it mixes sprinting and upper body exercise into the run. This is safer if your route has little traffic. Hashing is a popular club sport in the southern United States, Europe, and Russia. The idea is for a group to follow a marked course through an unfamiliar area. Elected group members meet at an earlier time to mark the route, usually with flour. Orienteering is popular in some areas. This is a cross-country type of activity in which participants navigate from point to point using a map and compass, covering distances from 2 to 10 miles. Local fun-runs give you a chance to run with and meet other runners in a noncompetitive atmosphere. If you like competition, you can get information on road races from your local running club or athletic shoe store.

Common Discomforts

Most aches and pains in running do not occur suddenly. They are often from overuse—a long steady erosion that wears down the body. Many general complaints are addressed in Chapter 9. Specific to running, two additional discomforts, easily avoided, occasionally occur. If you run with shoes that are too short or that don't fit well, in addition to developing blisters you could injure a toe. The toenail may turn black and possibly fall off. While painful, the condition is not permanent. The nail will grow back. If your thighs rub together when you run, you may suffer an abrasion. The solution is to apply vaseline to the area and to wear tights or shorts that cover your thighs.

Water Exercise/Aqua Aerobics

Advantages/Disadvantages

You don't have to know how to swim to get a vigorous workout in the water. You don't even have to get your head wet! As more people are discovering, exercising against water resistance in shallow water is a fine workout and great fun, especially with a group. Water exercise can be a social activity because you can carry on a conversation while working out. It is low impact, so joint problems are rare. The supportive effect of water buoyancy makes water exercise enjoyable and relaxing for individuals who have concerns about other forms of exercise. In chest-deep water, a person weighs only about 1/10th what he or she does on land. People who have arthritis or joint problems find that this buoyancy decreases stress to the joints, allowing a fuller range of motion than on land. It is easy to individualize intensity levels so that you get a good workout, whatever your level of fitness.

Water has at least 12 times the resistance of air and that number increases as movement speed increases. Thus, muscular conditioning improves and in a time efficient program as well. For example, biceps and triceps can be overloaded concentrically during the same exercise.

Hydrostatic (water) pressure pushes against the chest and body. This helps strengthen the breathing system and makes breathing on land easier. Hydrostatic pressure aids venous circulation and contributes to reduction in edema (swelling), which is especially helpful to expectant moms.

Water currents constantly challenge the trunk core muscles to maintain proper alignment when starting, stopping, and changing direction in the water. The abs have to work the entire time—a great plus.

Inclement weather is not a problem. Water exercise is cool, even on the hottest summer days, so heat stress is eliminated. It is also a comfortable indoor workout for rainy or cold winter days. If you are overweight and sensitive about exercising in public, the water covers you up so that you don't feel so self-conscious. Water exercise is also beneficial during pregnancy because of both decreased joint stress and decreased heat stress as compared to other forms of exercise.

The drawbacks are few. You need access to a pool at a time when you can have a lane separate from lap swimmers. It is probably best to first join a class to learn the exercises and activities. Then you can work out on your own.

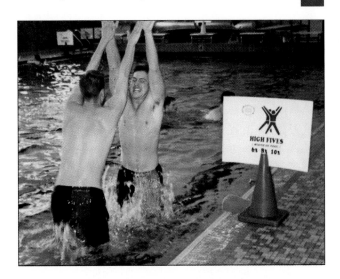

Nonswimming water workouts are one of the best forms of exercise because they build muscular strength and endurance as well as cardiorespiratory endurance.

What to Wear

A comfortable swimsuit is all that is required. Some people also like to wear pool shoes to protect their feet when doing water running and walking workouts.

Technique and Safety Tips

Workouts may have a muscle toning emphasis or an aerobic emphasis or combine the two. In constructing workouts, maintain muscle balance by exercising all major muscle groups. Particularly emphasize stretching tight muscle groups (i.e., lower back, hamstrings, calves) and toning weak areas (i.e., abdominals, upper body). To overload, keep in mind that, as in weight training, water adds resistance. The harder you push and pull, the more resistance you create and the more benefit you receive. In any activity, limit back hyperextension by keeping abdominals firm while exercises are being performed. In the water, as on land, workouts must maintain a training heart rate for 20 to 30 minutes to produce aerobic benefit. Training heart rates for swimmers appear to be about 10 percent lower than for land exercisers. This may also be true for other cardiorespiratory water exercise. To calculate an appropriate exercise intensity for water exercise, subtract 10 percent from your training pulse on land. Jogging in the water, aqua aerobics, and other vigorous activities can provide aerobic benefit if an adequate overload occurs. Several books that give examples of water exercises are available and are listed at the end of this chapter.

Whenever you exercise in the water, a few safety guidelines must be followed:

1. *Never work out in the water alone.* A lifeguard or workout partner, preferably one who can swim, should be present. Safety equipment, such as a life ring or reaching pole, should also be available.
2. *Shower before entering the pool.*
3. *Do not go into the deep water unless you can swim.*
4. *Don't mix water and electricity.* If you like to exercise to music, keep electrical equipment away from the water and make sure that all electric outlets have ground-fault circuit interrupters that shut off the electricity if it contacts water. Better yet, use battery-powered equipment.
5. *Do not enter the pool if you have an open sore, infection, or rash.*
6. *Do all exercises through a full range of motion with slow, controlled movements.* Swinging or flinging movements can injure joints.
7. *Maintain good body alignment in walking and jogging.* Keep abdominals tight and hips tucked under, and avoid excessive forward lean.

How to Begin and Progress

Water exercise workouts, like other aerobic programs, should incorporate a warm-up, conditioning period, and cool-down. The warm-up may be started on deck or in the water and may include a musculoskeletal (thermal) warm-up, stretching, and cardiorespiratory warm-up, transitioning smoothly into the conditioning bout. A thermal warm-up includes controlled movements using a gradually increasing range of motion and is designed to gradually increase muscle temperature. Prestretching exercises are designed to prepare muscles for activity and are generally held 5 to 10 seconds. A cardiorespiratory warm-up follows to transition the heart, lungs, and muscles gradually to an increased intensity level. Water exercise may involve many different activities—aerobic, muscle toning, and stretching. Recommendations on how to progress are given for the aerobic portion of the workout (i.e., water running) in terms of length of time at a training heart rate. Test your fitness using the 500-yard water run test described in Chapter 3. Then follow the appropriate Water Exercise Program. Stay on each level as long as necessary, don't skip levels. Go back a level if the next feels too strenuous. Progress slowly, listen to your body, and follow the FITT prescription factors. Monitor your THR or use the PRE.

Water Exercise Program

Fitness Category	Starting Level
Very low	1
Low	2
Average	3
Good	4
Excellent	5 or 6

Level	Vigorous	Easy	Sets	Total Time
1	1 min.	30 secs.	8–12	10–18 mins.
2	2 mins.	30 secs.	6–8	15–20 mins.
3	4 mins.	30 secs.	4–6	18–27 mins.
4	6 mins.	30 secs.	3–4	19–26 mins.
5	8–10 mins.	1 min.	3	26–32 mins.
6	continuous		1	30 min.

Follow the conditioning bout with a 5- to 10-minute cooldown combining a period of gradually decreasing intensity exercise with stretching for flexibility.

Variety

Exercise with friends or with music. After mastering the exercises with only water resistance, you may wish to add kickboards, pull buoys, or other water exercise equipment to increase resistance. Vary the exercises and activities so that you don't do the same workout 2 days in a row. For example, an aerobic workout may involve, on different days, running or walking widths, aqua aerobics, step aerobics, water games, deep water running, treading and kicking drills, or circuit training. There are so many different things to do in the water it is easy to add variety. Some examples of different types of workouts follow.

Muscular strength and endurance are built by performing repeats of exercises against resistance: side leg swings to tone inner thigh and outer hip, straight arm raises to tone deltoids, back leg swings to strengthen hamstrings and gluteus. A series of 8 to 12 exercises covering all major muscle groups can be performed 1 minute each and repeated two to three times for a thorough muscular workout.

Water walking involves walking in waist- to chest-deep water fast enough to produce a target heart rate. Good body alignment during walking and jogging is important. Walk tall with abdominals pulled in and buttocks tucked in to avoid leaning forward. It is also essential, for muscle balance, to vary the walking movements. Variations include walking forward, backward, or sideways and adding different arm variations such as forward pulls, breaststroke, or backstroke.

Shallow-water jogging is similar to water walking but is more intense, using a faster, bounding stride. A common error is running too much on the balls of the feet, which causes excessive calf tightness. Try to press your heel down to the pool bottom before pushing off on your toes.

Deep-water jogging is a nonimpact workout. Exercisers may wish to wear a flotation vest or belt and run, varying directions and arm movements. Deep water jogging without a flotation belt is strenuous.

Interval training alternates high- and low-intensity workout segments. This can allow even the most athletic exerciser to get a vigorous workout. For example, you might alternate four laps of shallow-water running with two laps of water walking.

Deep Water Running Guidelines. Deep water running can build muscle and cardiorespiratory endurance without risk of injury to knee and ankle joints. The only equipment needed is a flotation device, such as a belt or vest, to hold you in a comfortable position.

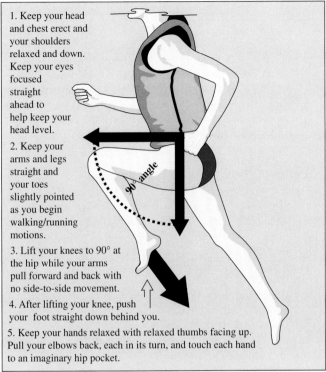

1. Keep your head and chest erect and your shoulders relaxed and down. Keep your eyes focused straight ahead to help keep your head level.

2. Keep your arms and legs straight and your toes slightly pointed as you begin walking/running motions.

3. Lift your knees to 90° at the hip while your arms pull forward and back with no side-to-side movement.

4. After lifting your knee, push your foot straight down behind you.

5. Keep your hands relaxed with relaxed thumbs facing up. Pull your elbows back, each in its turn, and touch each hand to an imaginary hip pocket.

90° angle

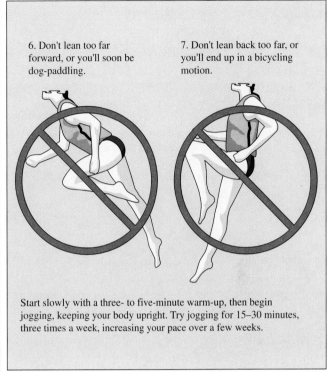

6. Don't lean too far forward, or you'll soon be dog-paddling.

7. Don't lean back too far, or you'll end up in a bicycling motion.

Start slowly with a three- to five-minute warm-up, then begin jogging, keeping your body upright. Try jogging for 15–30 minutes, three times a week, increasing your pace over a few weeks.

Water aerobics, like land aerobics, puts exercise to music. Workouts may be either choreographed or freestyle. Bench step workouts have also made the transition into the aquatic environment, with similar benefits as in land workouts.

Plyometrics are vigorous jumping and bounding exercises that increase muscle strength and power. They are also aerobic. Examples include high jumps in place, bounding across the pool, and a series of high two-foot hops. Because these are impact exercises, they can cause injury, are only for well-conditioned exercisers, and should be avoided if you have ankle, knee, or back problems. Water buoyancy lessens risk of injury, though.

In circuit training, a series of exercises are performed for a certain number of repetitions or a given amount of time (i.e., 1 minute each of side leg circles, jumping jacks, push-ups, forward kicks, etc.). Exercises may be written on numbered cards placed around the pool edge, and as each exercise is completed, participants move quickly to the next exercise station. Exercises may stress one fitness component or several. A set of 8 to 12 exercises can be repeated, or time at each station can be increased to produce overload.

Flexibility exercises are often used as a part of a water exercise program. A static stretch is held 20 to 30 seconds or more for each major muscle group to increase range of motion. Occasionally, it is fun to try a water game for variety. Examples include shallow-water polo, inner-tube water polo, water baseball, freeze tag, sharks and minnows, water basketball, or volleyball.

Common Discomforts

The most common discomforts water exercisers encounter are tight calves and blisters from running barefoot on the pool bottom. Blisters can be avoided by starting with only a few minutes of running in the pool and giving the feet time to toughen as you gradually progress in workouts. You could also wear pool shoes or clean sneakers during workouts. Calves tend to get tight because, due to buoyancy, most running and walking in the pool is done on the ball of the foot. Take care to stretch calves before and after the workout to maintain flexibility.

frequently asked questions

Q. Will carrying hand-weights, using walking poles, Powerbelts, and so on, while I fitness walk help to increase the intensity of my workouts? Will pumping my arms accomplish the same effect?

A. While the majority of healthy men and women can achieve a training heart rate by unaided walking, there are some people who may be too fit to achieve this threshold (i.e., young college students). Research shows that adding external weight to the body or involving the upper extremities during exercise can increase the intensity of walking.

For people who want to increase the overall intensity of their workout, or make walking more of a total body workout, there are a variety of reasonably priced adjuncts to consider, like weighted belts, gloves, vests, or walking poles. They are safe and effective and can increase CRE and weight control benefits of a regular walking program. See Table 4-2.

When using the walking equipment described in Table 4-3, be aware that 50 to 70 percent of the increase in oxygen consumption and caloric expenditure comes from swinging the arms to a greater degree. In one study for example, participants walked on a treadmill at 3.0 mph, VO_2 was 15.9 ml/kg/min. Walking at the same speed while swinging the arms to chin height required 17.8 ml/kg/min. The addition of 2-pound weights further increased the oxygen cost to 18.9 ml/kg/min. Thus 63 percent of the increase above normal walking was attributed to the exaggerated arm swim. Swinging the arms may serve as a good intermediate step for increasing walking intensity without being encumbered with extra equipment.

Q. I recently read that if I take 10,000 steps per day, I can achieve better fitness. Is this true?

A. Yes! Researchers estimate that it takes approximately 10,000 steps per day to reach the minimum public health guideline of accumulating 30 minutes of moderate activity most days of the week. (See Chapter 3.) Researchers stress "meets minimal health guidelines."

Participants in current research studies are using sophisticated pedometers worn on their waistbands to count the steps and miles they take per day. This includes routine activity in everyday activities plus any fitness walking they may do during the day. The goal of the research is to increase the activity levels of the American public by encouraging more people to move about at least 10,000 steps per day. Ten thousand steps is equivalent to about 5 miles. A mile can be anywhere from 1,800 to 2,200 steps depending on stride length and pace. Sedentary individuals typically walk only about 2,000 to 4,000 steps in a day, moderately active people take 5,000 to 7,000 steps per day, and active people take at least 10,000 steps per day. The 10,000 steps per day goal is applicable regardless of how much a person weighs or what his or her cardiorespiratory endurance fitness level is. A young fit person could accumulate steps through jogging or playing basketball, while an older person could meet the recommendation by walking. Thus, for improved health from moderate physical activity, Americans need to get up, get moving.

Pedometers are motivational, fitness experts contend. By keeping track of how many steps that have been taken, one can quickly check to see how many more steps must be taken to reach the goal of 10,000 steps that day. See the Internet Resources Section for information on pedometers.

Q. What is the Pilates Method of body conditioning?

A. The Pilates (pronounced puh-LAH-teez) Method was developed in the 1920s by physical trainer, Joseph H. Pilates. It is an exercise system that safely isolates and strengthens muscles without joint stress and without building bulk. It is a system of controlled exercises aimed at stretching and strengthening muscles of the back, buttocks, and abdomen for better improved posture, better balance, relief of aches/pains, increased flexibility. Pilates designed more than 500 specific exercises using five major pieces of unique apparatus. Instead of performing many repetitions of each exercise, more precise movements, requiring proper control and form are used. All Pilates movements must generate from the "powerhouse" or the "core" (the abdomen, lower back, and buttocks). Today's Pilates classes primarily use mat work, but classes featuring Pilates machines, which magnify resistance using springs and pulleys, are also available.

Conditioning sessions are done one-to-one with certified instructors or in closely supervised small groups. Instructors complete a rigorous certification program including extensive apprenticeship hours.

Mari Winsor's book, *The Pilates Powerhouse*, has brought the national spotlight to Pilates. It illustrates the exercises and concepts that make the workout an increasingly popular pursuit.

table 4-2   Pros and Cons of Walking Equipment

Walking Equipment	Pros	Cons
Weighted Vests	• Form fitting • Comfortable	• Minimal aerobic benefit • Expensive (compared to other equipment)
Ankle Weights	• Inexpensive • Good for leg rehab	• Minimal aerobic benefit • Potential for gait changes • Stresses knees
Wrist/Hand Weights	• Inexpensive • Easy to use • Moderate increase in intensity	• May elicit exaggerated blood pressure responses • No place to put the weight if you get tired
Walking Poles	• Excellent increases in intensity/caloric expenditure • Upper-body muscular endurance increases	• May elicit a pressor response due to gripping poles • Not adjustable, different height people need different poles • No place to put poles if you get tired
Powerbelts	• Excellent potential aerobic benefit • May increase muscular strength • Good for interval training • Resistance cords retract when not in use	• Higher levels may be too difficult to maintain • May elicit exaggerated blood pressure responses due to high degree of muscular effort

table 4-3   Heart Rate Increase, Oxygen Consumption, and Calorie Expenditures of Various Walking Equipment

Walking Equipment	Heart Rate Increases (bpm)	Oxygen Consumption (ml/kg/min)	Calorie Expenditures (% of increase)
Weighted Vests (5–10% of Body Wt)	3–7	1.3–2.5	3–10
Ankle Weights (1–3 lbs.)	4–6	1.5–3.0	5–10
Hand Weights/ Weighted Gloves (1–3 lbs.)	6–13	1.5–4.0	5–15
Walking Poles	10–15	4.5–5.5	20–25
Powerbelts			
Base unit	25–30	6.3–6.7	40–45
Powerpack 1	30–35	6.7–7.0	45–50
Powerpack 2	35–40	7.0–8.0	50–60
Powerpack 3	40–45	8.0–9.5	60–65

summary

The eight fitness activities in this fitness swimming chapter included: aerobic dance, bicycling, fitness walking, indoor exercise equipment, in-line skating, jogging, and water exercise/aqua aerobics. In each activity unit you found valuable information concerning taking part in the activity. Now you have the necessary tools to begin a program of aerobic activity—one you will enjoy and pursue for a lifetime. You will also have the satisfaction of knowing you are nurturing the most important habit you can adopt to safe-guard your health. The ball is in your court. Select an activity and go to it. We wish you well.

additional information resources

International Dance-Exercise Association (IDEA), 6190 Cornerstone Court East, Suite 204, San Diego, CA 92121–3773, (619) 535–8978 or (800) 999–IDEA.

National Dance-Exercise Instructor's Training Association (NDEITA), 1503 S. Washington Ave., Suite 208, Minneapolis, MN 55454, (800) 237–6242.

Dynamix Music Service, 733 W. 40th St., Suite 10, Baltimore, MD 21211, (800) 843–6499.

In-Lytes, 9400 Doral Ct., Louisville, KY 40220, (800) 243–7867 (call for a free catalogue) or (502) 495–0222.

Muscle Mixes, P.O. Box 533967, Orlando, FL 32853, (800) 52–MIXES or (407) 872–7576.

Power Productions, P.O. Box 550, Gaithersburg, MD 20884–0550, (301) 926–0707 or (800) 777–BEAT (call for a free catalogue).

The Workout Source, P.O. Box 55278, Sherman Oaks, CA 91413, (800) 552–4552.

Collage Video Specialists, 5390 Main St. N.E. Dept. 1, Minneapolis, MN 55421, (800) 433–6769.

Creative Instructors Aerobics Educational Videos, 2314 Naudain Street, Philadelphia, PA 19146, (215) 790–9767 or (800) 435–0055.

Billy Blanks Video Library 1–877–228–2326

Bicycle Federation of America, 1818 R. St. NW, Washington, D.C. 20009, (202) 332–6986. (Promotes bicycle transportation, recreation, and programs.)

The Bicycle Institute of America, 1506 21st St., NW, Washington, D.C. 20036, (800) 251–2453.

Bicycling Magazine, 33 E. Minor Street, Emmaus, PA 18049.

International Mountain Bicycling Association, P.O. Box 412043, Los Angeles, CA 90041, (818) 792–8830. (Promotes bicycle access to public lands and cyclist education.)

American Red Cross, National Headquarters, 431 18th St. N.W., Washington, D.C. 20006.

Aquatic Exercise Association (AEA), P.O. Box 1609, Nokomis, FL 34274, (813) 486–8600.

Aquatics International, 6151 Powers Ferry Road, Atlanta, GA 30339–2941.

Council for National Cooperation in Aquatics (CNCA), 901 W. New York Street, Indianapolis, IN 46223, (317) 638–4238.

International Swimming Hall of Fame, 1 Hall of Fame Drive, Ft. Lauderdale, FL 33316, (305) 462–6536.

United States Masters Swimming, 2 Peter Ave., Rutland, MA 01543, (508) 886–6631.

United States Swimming, 1750 E. Boulder St., Colorado Springs, CO 80909, (719) 578–4578.

United States Water Fitness Association (USWFA), John Spannuth, Executive Director, P.O. Box 3279, Boynton Beach, FL 33424.

YMCA of the USA, 101 N. Wacker Dr., 14th fl., Chicago, IL 60606, (312) 977–0031.

American Heart Association Walking Program, American Heart Association National Center, 7320 Greenville Ave., Dallas, TX 75231.

Heart and Sole Newsletter, National Organization of Mall Walkers, P.O. Box 191, Hermann, MO 65041.

North American Race-Walking Foundation (NARF), Box 50312, Pasadena, CA 91105–0312, (818) 577–2264.

Reebok Walking Program, Reebok International Ltd., 100 Technology Center Dr., P.O. Box 9116, Stoughton, MA 02072–9801.

The Rockport Walking Institute, P.O. Box 480, Marlboro, MA 01752.

Walkers Club of America, 445 E. 86th, New York, NY 10028.

The Walking Magazine, 11 Harcourt St., Boston, MA 02116, (617) 266–3322.

Aerobics Inc. (treadmills), (201) 256-9700.

Concept II (rowers), (800) 245–5676.

LifeFitness (Lifecycle stationary bikes, Lifestep climbers, Lifestride treadmills, Life rowers), (800) 877-3867 and (800) 735–3867.

NordicTrack (ski simulators, walkfit, treadmills), (800) 228–6635 and (800) 445–2360.

Precor (climbers, ski simulators, stationary bikes, treadmills), (800) 477–3267 and (800) 786–8404.

StairMaster, (800) 635-2936.

StarTrac (treadmills, climbers), (800) 228–6635.

Tectrix (climbers, stationary bikes), (800) 767–8082.

Tunturi (stationary bikes, climbers, ski simulators, treadmills, rowers), (800) 827–8717.

International In-line Skating Association (IISA)
Lake Calhoun Executive Center
3033 Excelsior Blvd, Suite 300
Minneapolis, MN 55416
1–800–FOR ITSA (367–4472)

In-line USA
419 Monterey Street
Morro Bay, CA 93442
1–800–685–6806

United States Amateur Confederation of Roller Skating
4730 South St.
P.O. Box 6579
Lincoln, NE 68506
(402)483–7551

In-line
2025 Pear St.
Boulder, Colorado 80302
(303)440–5111

Skate Great, Eden Prairie, MN.
Rollerblade, Inc. 1997
1-800-232-7665

American Running Association, 9310 Old Georgetown Road, Bethesda, MD 20814-1111, (301) 897–0197.

The Runner, Ziff-Davis Publishing Co., P.O. Box 2702, Boulder, CO 80321.

Runner's World Magazine, Box 366, Mountain View, CA 94042.

Silva Orienteering Services USA, P.O. Box 1604, Binghamton, NY 13902.

The Aquatic Exercise Association, Inc., P.O. Box 1609, Nokomis, FL 34274, (813) 486–8600.

IDEA Resource Library: Aqua Exercise, IDEA: The Association for Fitness Professionals, 6190 Cornerstone Court E., Suite 204, San Diego, CA 92121–3773.

U.S. Water Fitness Association, John Spannuth, Executive Director, P.O. Box 3219, Boynton Beach, FL 33424–3279.

AFA/Aquarobics, Inc., Box 5752, Greenville, SC 29606.

Aqua-Circuit, U.S. Games, Inc., P.O. Box 117028, Carrolton, TX 75011–7028, (800) 327–0484.

Dynamix Music Services, 711 W. 40th St., Suite 428, Baltimore, MD 21211, (800) 843–6499.

Fitness Wholesale, 895 Hampshire Rd., Stowe, OH 44224, (800) 537–5512.

Hydro-Tone Fitness Systems Inc., 16691 Gothard St., Suite M, Huntington Beach, CA 92647, (800) 622–TONE.

Resources for Walking Equipment: Wrist/hand/ankle Weights: any large department and sporting equipment stores

Weighted Vests: Smart Vest, Training Zone Concepts, Inc. Flint, MI 1-888-797-8378

Walking Poles: Exerstrider, Exerstrider Products, Inc. Madison, WI 1–800–554–0989

Powerbelts: Inergi Fitness, Norcross, GA 1–800–797–2358

Pedometers: Digi-Walker, www.digiwalker.com 1–888–748–5377

Accusplit Eagle 1–800–935–1996

Optimal Health Clicker 1–888–339–2067

 internet resources

American Council on Exercise

  http://www.acefitness.org

International Dance-Exercise Association (IDEA)

  http://www.ideasit.com

Billy Blanks Tae Bo

  http://www.Taebo.com

Bicycling links and resources

  http://www.cdc.gov/safeusa/bike/bike.htm

American Volkssport Association. Walking and hiking events sponsored by chapters throughout the United States.

  www.ava.org (800-830-9255)

Sierra Club. Hikes and walks sponsored by chapters in every state.

  http://www.sierraclub.org (415-977-5630)

Appalachian Mountain Club. Hikes and walks sponsored by chapters in the northeastern United States.

  http://www.outdoors.org (603-466-2721)

Walking Magazine

  http://www.walkingmag.com

Centers for Disease Control and Prevention

  http://www.cdc.gov/nccdphp/dnpa

Shape Up America

  http://www.shapeup.org

Analyze Your Physical Activity from Laurence Berkeley National Laboratory

  http://www.walkersurvey.org

Fitness equipment, treadmills, bikes, and more

  http://www.capecod.net/linray/cardio.html
  http://www.csafit.com/
  http://unigym.com/
  http://www.fitnessmart.com/Welcome2.html
  http://www.mgda.com/pb.html

http://www.hotnew.com/special.html
http://www.fitnesslink.com/program/home.htm
http://www.heartlinefitness.com/index.html
http://www.promaximamfg.com/index.htm
http://www.fitnesszone.com/
http://www.heathatoz.com
http://www.fitnesslink.com
http://www.razorskate.com
http://www.rollerblade.com
http://www.activeusa.com
http://www.getrolling.com
http://www.in-lineskating.about.com
http://www.skating.com
http://www.skatecity.com

Where to run/walk in different cities

  http://www.dada.it/rtp/links2.htm
  http://www.usaldr.org/ldrsites.htm

Aquatic Exercise Association Homepage

  http://youth.net/aea.html

Aquatic Exercise for people with multiple sclerosis

  http://www/orion.org/health/ms/aquatics.html

Aquatic Exercise Therapy

  http://www.agmc.org/lifeaq1.htm

Walking Magazine

  http://www.walkingmag.com

Centers for Disease Control and Prevention

  http://www.cdc.gov/nccdphp/dnpa

Shape Up America

  http://www.shapeup.org

Analyze Your Physical Activity from Laurence Berkeley National Laboratory

  http://www.walkersurvey.org

Exercise Across the U.S.A.

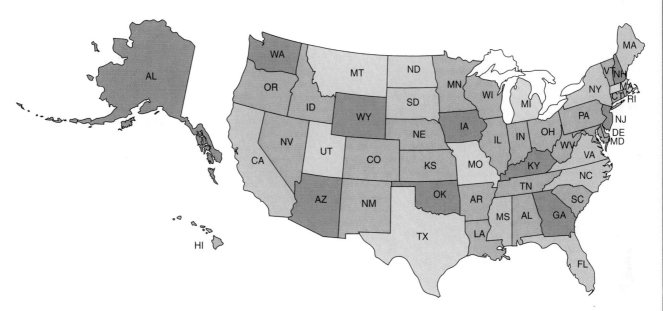

Exercise Across the U.S.A.

Directions:

1. Select a state to exercise across, or go for the coast-to-coast challenge and a grand total of 2,755 miles.

2. Record your exercise miles on the Exercise Across the U.S.A. log form.

3. If you wish, you may make the trip interesting by incorporating different activities to reach your total mileage goal. Many sports are easy to measure in miles, but if you prefer a different activity see the One Mile Equivalents chart, which is measured in minutes (estimated for a 143-pound person).

Exercise Across the U.S.A.
(Grand Total: 2,775 Miles)

Pick a State

Alabama 195 Miles	Hawaii 75 Miles	Massachusetts 25 Miles	New Mexico 340 Miles	South Dakota 379 Miles
Alaska 858 Miles	Idaho 302 Miles	Michigan 185 Miles	New York 285 Miles	Tennessee 439 Miles
Arizona 315 Miles	Illinois 212 Miles	Minnesota 273 Miles	North Carolina 396 Miles	Texas 661 Miles
Arkansas 227 Miles	Indiana 139 Miles	Mississippi 273 Miles	North Dakota 355 Miles	Utah 267 Miles
California 247 Miles	Iowa 310 Miles	Missouri 295 Miles	Ohio 225 Miles	Vermont 81 Miles
Colorado 371 Miles	Kansas 390 Miles	Montanta 546 Miles	Oklahoma 305 Miles	Virginia 340 Miles
Connecticut 80 Miles	Kentucky 351 Miles	Nebraska 400 Miles	Oregon 358 Miles	Washington 335 Miles
Delaware 36 Miles	Louisiana 177 Miles	Nevada 317 Miles	Pennsylvania 286 Miles	West Virginia 149 Miles
Florida 138 Miles	Maine 198 Miles	New Hampshire 76 Miles	Rhode Island 27 Miles	Wisconsin 254 Miles
Georgia 227 Miles	Maryland 215 Miles	New Jersey 72 Miles	South Carolina 207 Miles	Wyoming 348 Miles

One Mile Equivalents

Activity	Minutes	Activity	Minutes	Activity	Minutes
Aerobic dance	18	Gardening		Rowing	12
Basketball	13	Digging	15	Skiing	
Biking		Mowing	16	Cross country	13
Leisure	29	Raking	32	Downhill	16
Moderate	19	Golf (without cart)	21	Softball (fielder)	32
Racing	11	In-line skating	16	Stair climbing	9
Calisthenics		(use actual distance covered)		Swimming	12
(Sit-ups, push-ups, etc.)	25	Jumping rope	11	Tennis	16
Canoeing (leisure pace)	40	Karate	9	Weight training	15

Exercise Across the U.S.A. Log

State/distance _____   Activity(s) _____   Start date _____   End date _____

Month:		Month:		Month:		Month:		Month:		Month:	
1	17	1	17	1	17	1	17	1	17	1	17
2	18	2	18	2	18	2	18	2	18	2	18
3	19	3	19	3	19	3	19	3	19	3	19
4	20	4	20	4	20	4	20	4	20	4	20
5	21	5	21	5	21	5	21	5	21	5	21
6	22	6	22	6	22	6	22	6	22	6	22
7	23	7	23	7	23	7	23	7	23	7	23
8	24	8	24	8	24	8	24	8	24	8	24
9	25	9	25	9	25	9	25	9	25	9	25
10	26	10	26	10	26	10	26	10	26	10	26
11	27	11	27	11	27	11	27	11	27	11	27
12	28	12	28	12	28	12	28	12	28	12	28
13	29	13	29	13	29	13	29	13	29	13	29
14	30	14	30	14	30	14	30	14	30	14	30
15	31	15	31	15	31	15	31	15	31	15	31
16	Total	16	Total	16	Total	16	Total	16	Total	16	Total

Sample Training Schedule for Half-Marathon (Mini): 13.1 Miles

If you would like to train for a half-marathon (a distance of 13.1 miles) the following is a sample training program. The training schedule is approximately 18 weeks. Use the log sheet in Lab Activity 4–5 to record your workouts.

Monitor your daily resting heart rate upon waking. If it is 10 percent higher, reduce that day's workout and go easy. If pulse is 20 percent higher, cancel workouts until it is normal. You may have an overtraining condition or an illness coming.

Recommended Minimum Weekly Training Mileage

Week	Daily	Long Day	Weekly Total
1	2–3 miles × 2–3 days plus	3–6 miles	7–15 miles
2	2–3 miles × 2–3 days plus	3–6 miles	7–15 miles
3	2–3 miles × 2–3 days plus	4–7 miles	8–16 miles
4	2–3 miles × 2–3 days plus	4–7 miles	8–16 miles
5	2–3 miles × 2–3 days plus	5–8 miles	9–17 miles
6	3–4 miles × 2–3 days plus	6–9 miles	12–21 miles
7	3–4 miles × 2–3 days plus	5–8 miles	9–17 miles
8	3–5 miles × 2–3 days plus	6–9 miles	12–21 miles
9	3–5 miles × 2–3 days plus	8–11 miles	14–26 miles
10	3–6 miles × 2–3 days plus	7–10 miles	13–28 miles
11	3–6 miles × 2–3 days plus	9–12 miles	15–30 miles
12	4–6 miles × 2–3 days plus	7–10 miles	15–28 miles
13	4–6 miles × 2–3 days plus	10–13 miles	18–31 miles
14	4–6 miles × 2–3 days plus	8–11 miles	16–29 miles
15	4–6 miles × 2–3 days plus	11–14 miles	19–32 miles
16	4–6 miles × 2–3 days plus	8–11 miles	16–29 miles
17	3–4 miles × 2–3 days plus	4–7 miles	10–19 miles
18	2–3 miles × 2–3 days plus	13.1 miles	17–20 miles
19	Minimarathon	13.1 miles	

lab activity 4-3

Sample Training Schedule for Half-Marathon (Mini): 13.1 Miles

If you would like to train for a half-marathon (a distance of 13.1 miles) the following is a sample training program. The training schedule is approximately 11 weeks. Use the log sheet in Lab Activity 4–5 to record your workouts.

Monitor your daily resting heart rate upon waking. If it is 10 percent higher, reduce that day's workout and go easy. If pulse is 20 percent higher, cancel workouts until it is normal. You may have an overtraining condition or an illness coming.

Guidelines:

Monday	–	Easy Walk/Run (slower and a little shorter than usual)
Tuesday	–	OFF
Wednesday	–	Moderate Distance Walk/Run
Thursday	–	Moderate Distance Walk/Run
Friday	–	Moderate Distance Walk/Run
Saturday	–	Easy Walk/Run
Sunday	–	Long Walk/Run (Start out easy—time doesn't matter)

Week	Mon	Tue	Wed	Thur	Fri	Sat	Sun	Miles
1	3	0	4	3	4	4	5	22
2	3	0	4	3	4	3	5	22
3	3	0	4	0	4	4	5	19
4	3	0	4	4	4	3	6	24
5	3	0	4	4	4	3	6	24
6	3	0	4	0	4	3	6	20
7	3	0	4	4	4	3	7	25
8	3	0	4	5	4	3	7	26
9	3	0	5	0	5	3	9	25
10	3	0	6	0	5	3	8	25
11	3	0	5	0	0	0	Mini	(13.1)

lab activity @ chapter four

Nutrition Guidelines for Half-Marathon Training Program

Preevent

Three Days Prior to Event

- 60–70% of diet = carbohydrate (8–10 grams/kg - maximum)

Day of Event:

- Three hours prior: 200–350 grams of carbohydrate (May vary with individual—smaller person may require less)
- Thirty minutes prior: 50 grams of carbohydrate

Fluids:

- *Two hours prior:* 2–3 cups
  Fifteen minutes prior: 1–2 cups
- Preevent meal should be high in carbohydrate, moderate in protein, and low in fat/fiber, extra fluids
- Can use sports drink or complex carbohydrates
- Liquid meals appropriate alternative to conventional meal
- Don't try new foods—stay with familiar and well-tolerated foods

During Event

- Don't skip water stations
- Maintaining hydration key to enhancing performance
- Drink 1 cup of fluid every 15–20 minutes
- *Avoid:* caffeinated, alcoholic, and carbonated beverages
- A quick source of carbohydrate may be necessary if event lasts > 90 minutes (water bottle with sports drink, fig bars, sportsbar)

Postevent

- *Within thirty minutes of event:* 80–100 grams of carbohydrate
- *Every two hours (remainder of the day):* Consume a substantial amount of carbohydrate
- Continue to drink plenty of fluids until urine is pale
- Drink high carbohydrate beverages if not hungry
- Beer is *not* a good choice of carbohydrate immediately after the event—poor source of carbohydrate, has a dehydrating effect, and is a depressant

Conversion to Kilograms	
lb = pound	kg = kilogram
Weight in lbs ÷ 2.2 = kilograms	
Example:	
Male 160 lbs.	Female 120 lbs.
160÷2.2=73 kg	120÷2.2=55 kg

Carbohydrate Content of Some Foods			
	grams		grams
Medium Fresh Fruit =	15	6 oz. yogurt =	25
8 oz. milk =	12	(varies with brand)	
1/2 cup pasta =	15	1 slice bread =	15
1/2 cup rice =	15	depending on size bagle =	30–90
8 oz. sport drink =	20	2/3 cup dry cereal =	15
(varies with brand)			

Sample Training Schedule for a Marathon: 26.2 Miles

If you would like to train for a marathon (a distance of 26.2 miles) the following is a sample training program. The training schedule is approximately 27 weeks. Use the log sheet in Lab Activity 4-5 to record your workouts).

Monitor your daily resting heart rate upon waking. If it is 10 percent higher, reduce that day's workout and go easy. If pulse is 20 percent higher, cancel workouts until it is normal. You may have an overtraining condition or an illness coming.

Week	Mon	Tue	Wed	Thur	Fri	Sat	Sun	Miles
1	3	4	3	4	3	0	6	23
2	3	4	3	4	3	0	7	24
3	3	4	3	4	3	0	8	25
4	3	4	3	4	3	0	9	26
5	3	4	3	4	3	0	10	27
6	0	3	0	3 easy	3 easy	0	6 easy	15 (rest wk)
7	3	4	3	5	3	0	10	28
8	3	5	3	5	3	0	10	29
9	3	5	3	6	3	0	11	31
10	3	6	3	6	4	0	12	34
11	0	3 easy	3 easy	3 easy	3 easy	0	6 easy	18 (rest wk)
12	4	6	4	6	4	0	13	37
13	4	6	4	6	4	3	13	40
14	4	7	4	7	4	3	14	43
15	4	7	5	7	4	3	15	45
16	0	3 easy	3 easy	5 easy	3 easy	0	10 easy	24 (rest wk)
17	4	7	5	7	5	3	18	49
18	4	7	5	7	5	7	10	45
19	5	8	5	8	6	3	20	55
20	5	8	5	8	5	3	16	50
21	0	5 easy	3 easy	5 easy	3 easy	0	10 easy	26 (rest wk)
22	6	8	6	8	6	0	21	58
23	6	8	6	8	6	5	12	51
24	6	8	6	8	6	3	21	58
25	0	6 easy	3 easy	6 easy	3 easy	0	10 easy	28 (rest wk)
26	0	5 easy	4 easy	3 easy	0	2	26.2!!!	40+
27	0	0	walk 3	walk 3	3 easy	0	6 easy	12 rcvry wk

Source: Chuck Cornett (Road Runners Club of America) Orange Park, FL 32965, (904)264-7197

Name _____

Class/Activity Section _____

Date _____

lab activity
4–5

Log Sheet

(Make extra copies of this form as needed)

Week	Sun	Mon	Tues	Wed	Thurs	Fri	Sat	Total
1 Date: RHR: Distance/time: EHR: Location:								
2 Date: RHR: Distance/time: EHR: Location:								
3 Date: RHR: Distance/time: EHR: Location:								
4 Date: RHR: Distance/time: EHR: Location:								

Comments/Goals: _____

Log Sheet
(Make extra copies of this form as needed)

Name _____   RHR _____   THR _____

Week _____

Goals: _____
_____
_____

Date	RHR	Distance/time	HR (at end of workout)	Location	Comments
Sun					
Mon					
Tues					
Wed					
Thur					
Fri					
Sat					

Total _____

Name _____

Class/Activity Section _____

Date _____

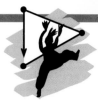

Using HealthQuest

Directions: **Insert HealthQuest 3.0 into your computer. Go to "Fitness."**
Read "Fitness introduction" then click on "Introduction" on left side of screen.
Click on "Topics." Click on "Key Articles."
Click on "Killer Workouts." Explore the four topics at this location and respond to the following questions.

1. *Aerobics and Step Aerobics.* What causes the "euphoric" high discussed at this site?

_____

_____

_____

_____

_____

_____

_____

_____

_____

2. *Krav Maga.* Discuss this exercise.

_____

_____

_____

_____

_____

_____

_____

_____

_____

3. *Kickboxing.* Click on "HealthGate: Kickboxing." In your opinion what were the three most important points of this article?

   a. _____

   _____

   _____

   _____

   b. _____

   _____

   _____

   _____

   c. _____

   _____

   _____

   _____

4. *Tae-Bo.* Click on "HealthGate: Tae Bo." List three benefits and three drawbacks of this activity.

   a. Benefits _____

   _____

   _____

   _____

   _____

   _____

   b. Drawbacks _____

   _____

   _____

   _____

   _____

   _____

Developing Flexibility and Muscular Fitness

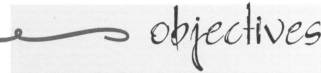 objectives

After reading this chapter, you will be able to:

1. Identify five benefits and five cautions for stretching.
2. Define two types of stretching.
3. Identify correct guidelines for flexibility development.
4. Identify five benefits and five cautions of resistance training.
5. Identify two differences between training programs for strength and programs for muscular endurance.
6. Describe three types of muscle contraction and give an example of each.
7. Define three principles of resistance training.
8. Identify correct safety guidelines for weight training.
9. Describe four out of five types of resistance training.
10. Define the chapter terms.

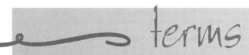 terms

- Agonist
- Antagonist
- Atrophy
- Concentric contraction
- Dynamic flexibility
- Eccentric contraction
- Fast-twitch muscle fiber
- Hypertrophy

- Isokinetic
- Isometric
- Isotonic
- Muscular power
- Progressive overload
- Proprioceptive neuromuscular facilitation (PNF)
- Repetition (rep)

- Repetition maximum (1 RM)
- Set
- Slow-twitch muscle fiber
- Static flexibility
- Stretch reflex
- Valsalva maneuver

At one time, physical fitness programs consisted almost entirely of strength and flexibility exercises. Then, in the 1970s, aerobic activities rose to prominence. As a result, strength and flexibility exercises were swept into the role of supplemental activities and added to the main workout only if time permitted. As people flocked to gyms for aerobics, they were exposed to weight training and began to value the benefits of muscular fitness. Today, as the emphasis on balanced fitness grows, muscular strength, muscular endurance, and flexibility assume new importance. They can enhance ability to perform daily tasks and athletic performance. Muscular fitness makes it easier to perform routine activities such as carrying groceries upstairs, lifting a child, or moving the couch. Flexibility enables us to reach, bend, twist, and perform movements without excessive tightness or stiffness. Enhanced muscular fitness allows us to perform vigorous activity with less risk of straining muscles or connective tissue, so it is important in the prevention and rehabilitation of injuries.

Flexibility

The ability to move your joints through their full range is an asset that can be maintained throughout life. As children, we are naturally flexible, but as we age, flexibility tends to decrease. Disuse, injury, excessive body fat, and muscle imbalances are common factors in this loss of range of motion. You can maintain youthful flexibility by incorporating stretching into your regular workouts.

The flexibility exercises in this section are grouped as follows: a basic fitness flexibility program with exercises for joggers, walkers, aerobic dancers, cyclists, swimmers, and water exercisers and examples of PNF partner-assisted stretches.

Benefits and Cautions

There are six main benefits to be gained from flexibility development:

- *It may decrease risk of injury.* When tight muscles restrict the natural range of motion of a joint, the slightest unusual twist can cause a strain or pull, such as a strained hamstring. Inflexibility also is a precipitating factor in overuse injuries such as tendinitis, because inelastic muscles transfer excessive stress to even less pliable connective tissue.
- *It counteracts age-related declines in flexibility.*
- *It decreases aches and pains.* Tight, inflexible muscles pull unevenly across joints, causing skeletal misalignment, poor posture, unnecessary fatigue, and

muscle and joint pain. Stretching can alleviate these problems.
- *It increases the ability to move freely and easily* and to perform activities such as bending down to tie your shoes, scratching your back, or turning to look back as you are driving.
- *It enhances athletic performance.* In racquetball, golf, tennis, volleyball, or swimming, greater range of motion and ability to apply force through that range of motion can give a winning edge.
- *It feels good.* Stretching reduces muscular tension, promoting relaxation.

If carelessly done, however, stretching can cause injury. You must be careful not to overstretch, particularly when muscles are cold and tight. Stretching is not a competitive activity, so don't try to imitate the most flexible person in your class. Injured areas should be stretched with great care and not into pain, which risks reinjury. If you feel pain during stretching, particularly joint pain, stop!

Types of Flexibility

There are two basic types of flexibility: static and dynamic. **Static flexibility** refers to the range of motion you can achieve through a slow, controlled stretch. **Dynamic flexibility** is the range of motion achieved by quickly moving a limb to its limits.

Static stretching techniques are those in which you slowly stretch a muscle to the point of tension and hold, such as in holding a sitting hamstring stretch. The stretching force is provided by gravity or the force of one limb pulling on another. When a muscle is stretched and held at a constant length, after a period of time there is a gradual loss of tension and muscle lengthening.

Dynamic stretching programs employ swinging or ballistic moves, such as a high forward kick. Ballistic exercises may be useful in preparation for athletic activities requiring such moves, but they do carry increased risk that a muscle or joint could be overstretched, resulting in muscle or tendon tears and joint injury. Also, ballistic exercises initiate the **stretch reflex,** a natural response that causes the stretched muscle to contract. This contraction is designed to protect the muscle from being overstretched, but it also limits flexibility gains. While both types of stretching can increase flexibility, static stretching is preferred in health-related fitness programs because it is highly effective and carries little risk of muscle or joint strain.

Principles of Flexibility Development

Both types of flexibility are specific to the joint; that is, flexibility in one leg does not guarantee identical flexibility in the other leg, and flexibility in the shoulders does not ensure flexibility in the lower back.

An individual's flexibility range for any particular joint is not only specific, but also partially genetically determined. You may have observed that some people seem to be naturally more flexible than others, even "double jointed" (they aren't really). Flexibility is determined by joint structure and elasticity of muscle and connective tissue. While you may not be able to change your genetics, you can improve your degree of flexibility within your genetically determined range of motion. People who have never been able to touch their toes may, for example, be able to get inches closer with practice but may never be able to wrap their palms around their feet without bending their knees.

Flexibility gains are proportional to the overload applied: to the frequency, intensity, and time (duration) of stretching.

- *Frequency:* Stretch at least 2 to 3 days a week and daily if possible. Greater flexibility is produced by more frequent stretching.
- *Intensity:* Low-intensity stretching is best. Progress at your speed. Stretching is not competitive. Flexibility changes from day to day, and some days you might not be able to stretch as far as you did the day before. Stretch slightly beyond the normal range of motion, to the point of tension, and hold. Do not force a stretch.
- *Time:* Many programs recommend a 10- to 30-second stretch, though holding up to 60 seconds in a cool-down stretch can increase flexibility retention.
- *Repetitions:* Three to four 10- to 30-second sustained stretches for each muscle group are recommended.

While less flexible individuals may envy those who can do splits with ease, keep in mind that, with flexibility, more is better only up to a point. There is concern (though no hard evidence) that excessive flexibility, unless accompanied by muscular strength, may increase joint laxity and susceptibility to injury. For this reason, it is wise to combine stretching with muscle strengthening for optimal fitness benefits.

Guidelines for Flexibility Development

Everyone can benefit from flexibility. To maximize results from the time invested, implement the following guidelines in your next stretching session:

- *Warm up before stretching.* An increase in muscle temperature produced by fast walking, slow jogging, jumping jacks, or other large muscle exercise will make stretching safer and more productive. You are sufficiently warmed up when you begin to sweat.
- *After warm-up, use stretching as preparation for activity.* While some feel that stretching during warm-up decreases risk of injury in the activity that follows, there is no evidence that this is true. Warm-up stretching is different from a planned program of stretching for general flexibility. Warm-up stretching can be limited to what is essential, avoiding overstretching. Stretch

muscle groups used in the activity, hold at the point of tension for 10 seconds, and do not push for flexibility increases. Any gains will be minimal due to the tightening effect of the workout that follows.

- *Stretch for flexibility during cool-down.* Muscles are warmest and most elastic at this point. Stretching is easier. More permanent changes in muscle lengthening occur with low-force, long-duration stretching if muscles are allowed to cool in a stretched position. Cooling muscles before releasing tension apparently causes muscle collagen (connective tissue), like stretched taffy, to stabilize toward its new stretched length.
- *Stop at the point of tension, not pain.* Stretching to the point of pain, or until muscles quiver, can risk overstretching injury.
- *Don't bounce.* A sustained stretch is more effective.
- *Incorporate 8 to 12 stretches into your program.* Flexibility is specific to a joint, so a well-planned program for general flexibility will contain one stretch for each major muscle group. Warm-up or cool-down stretching may contain fewer exercises because such stretching is activity specific and has different goals. Pay particular attention to body areas that are least flexible and stretch them more often.
- *Strive for muscle balance.* When stretching muscle on one side of a joint, stretch those on the other side as well; for example, if you stretch hamstrings, stretch quadriceps, too.

Flexibility Exercises for Basic Fitness

As part of a warm-up or cool-down, exercises A through F are important for runners, walkers, and aerobic dancers. Cyclists, swimmers, and water exercisers should add upper body stretches G through I. If time is limited, save stretching for the cool-down. For basic fitness flexibility, perform the full program of exercises in Figure 5-1. Hold each 10 to 30 seconds and repeat 3 to 4 times.

A. Hamstring stretch
    Keeping shoulders erect, press abdomen forward. Hold. Repeat with other leg.
B. Lower back/hip flexor stretch
    With hands behind thigh, press thigh toward chest. Keep extended leg straight. Repeat left.
C. Spinal twist (lower back and hip abductors)
    Sit with right leg extended, step left leg over right, and turn upper body toward left. Repeat on other side.
D. Quadriceps stretch
    With left hand, pull right heel toward buttocks. Keep shoulders up, abdominals tight, and hips tucked under to prevent back hyperextension. Omit if you have knee problems.

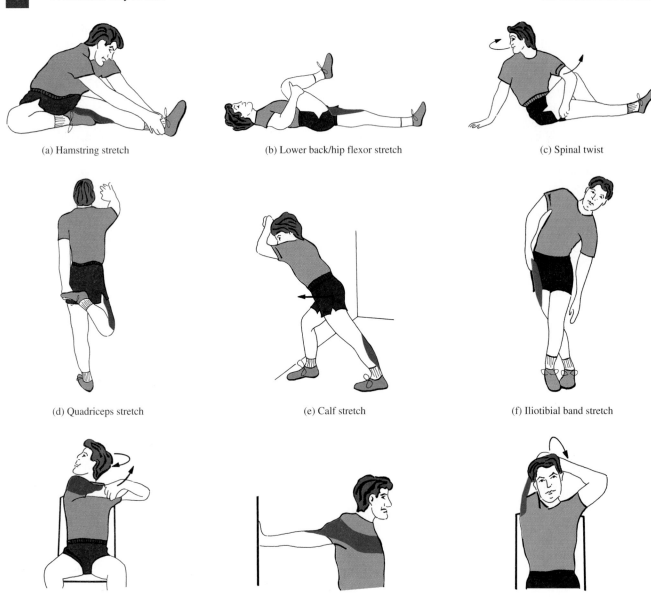

(a) Hamstring stretch   (b) Lower back/hip flexor stretch   (c) Spinal twist

(d) Quadriceps stretch   (e) Calf stretch   (f) Iliotibial band stretch

(g) Deltoid stretch   (h) Pectoral stretch   (i) Triceps stretch

figure 5-1   Flexibility exercises.

E. Calf stretch
Standing in forward lunge position, toes pointing forward, press heel toward floor. Repeat with other leg.

F. Iliotibial band stretch
Cross left foot over right, press hips to right. Repeat with other side.

G. Deltoid stretch
Cross right arm in front of body and pull it in toward midline with left hand.

H. Pectoral stretch
Place right hand on wall, elbow extended but not locked. Twist shoulders left. Repeat with left arm.

I. Triceps stretch
Pull left elbow behind head. Repeat right.

PNF Partner-Assisted Stretches

A type of static stretching called **proprioceptive neuromuscular facilitation (PNF),** a partner-assisted stretch often used by athletic trainers, is one of the most effective methods known for increasing flexibility. To perform a PNF stretch, you first perform a 10- to 30-second static stretch, then contract the muscle 6 seconds to produce fatigue, and then relax while a partner stretches your limb 10 to 30 seconds.

Be sensitive to your partner's needs and flexibility levels. Be sure to communicate when more/less resistance or pressure is needed throughout each exercise. Work with the same partner throughout the series. Switching partners can

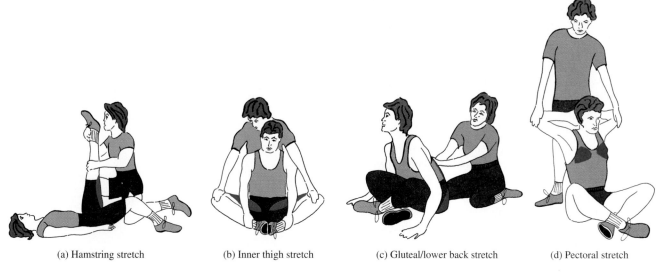

(a) Hamstring stretch   (b) Inner thigh stretch   (c) Gluteal/lower back stretch   (d) Pectoral stretch

figure 5-2   PNF partner-assisted stretches.

lead to injury because of unfamiliarity with the flexibility limits of the person being stretched. Some examples of PNF stretches are illustrated in Figure 5-2.

A. Hamstring stretch

Lie on your back and lift one leg into the air. Partner supports ankle and knee in a static stretch. Next, keeping knee extended but not locked, push against your partner as he or she resists. Stretch and then relax, as partner eases leg into a new stretch.

B. Inner thigh stretch

Sit with knees out and bottoms of feet together. Press down on knees in a static stretch. Next, partner kneels behind and resists on knees as you press them upward. Finally, relax as partner gently presses them toward the floor in a stretch.

C. Gluteal/lower back stretch

Sit cross-legged and stretch forward. Partner kneels behind you with hands on your upper back. Next, resist back against partner. Then, stretch forward as partner assists.

D. Pectoral stretch

Sit cross-legged with fingers interlaced behind your head and back supported by partner's thigh. Partner gently pulls your elbows back for 10 seconds and then resists as you attempt to pull them forward. Next, relax as partner gently stretches them back.

Muscular Fitness

Many people start muscular fitness programs to look better, feel better, shape and tone muscles, or increase lean muscle mass. At the same time, they increase muscular strength and endurance. In this section, we will examine benefits, muscle structure and function, general principles, safety, and specific exercise programs for muscular strength and endurance.

Resistance Training: Benefits and Cautions

An advantage of aerobic activities is their cardiorespiratory benefits. Resistance training can offer additional benefits, whether your goal is health-related fitness or improved athletic performance.

Weight Control. The more muscle a person has, the higher his or her metabolism and the more calories he or she burns, even at rest. This is one reason men can consume more calories without gaining weight than can women of equal size—the average male has roughly twice the muscle mass of the average female. Muscle is active, high-metabolic tissue, while fat is storage tissue. Resistance training increases muscle mass, so it makes weight control easier. While women do not appear to gain as much muscle as men do from weight training, when differences in body size are taken into account, gains are comparable. Over a 4- to 6-month period, a man may gain 4 to 6 pounds of muscle and a woman 2 to 3 pounds. Muscle is denser than fat and pound for pound takes up less space, so as muscle is gained, if fat is lost, the result is a loss of unwanted inches. While aerobic exercise and a nutritious low-fat diet are the quickest ways to reduce body fat, weight training does offer advantages in long-term weight control.

Weight Gain. For those who wish to gain weight, increasing lean muscle mass, not fat, is a desirable goal, and there is no better way than weight training. However, rate and quantity of muscle tissue gains vary from person to person because they are partially genetically determined. Those with a naturally tall, lean build tend to gain muscle slower than do those with a stockier build, and men gain faster than women. A weight-gain program is outlined in the weight-training section for those who wish to increase lean weight.

Appearance. Developing a lean, well-toned body is the main reason many people exercise. If you feel that you need to lose weight, but your body fat percentage is in the average range, reevaluate. Weight loss alone does not give a firm, well-toned appearance to flabby thighs or abdominals. Resistance training is the most effective way to shape and tone muscles, resulting in a trimmer appearance. Posture improves when agonist/antagonist muscles are in balance. Strengthening weak muscles and stretching tight, inflexible muscles helps develop good body alignment so that you move more fluidly and feel and look better.

Time Economy. Instead of doing 50 leg lifts without weights, you can cut your workout time by adding resistance. Lift a weight heavy enough to produce fatigue in 8 to 12 repetitions, and you will get more benefit in fewer lifts. For basic muscular fitness, a balanced resistance-training workout of 10 to 12 exercises takes approximately 30 minutes to complete. Despite what you may observe in the gym, more is not necessary. While body builders, competitive weightlifters, or other strength-event athletes will work out much more than this, keep in mind that they have different goals. Health-related fitness levels can be developed and maintained in much less training time than is needed for competition.

Energy. Performance and efficiency improve with resistance training—more work can be done with less effort as muscular strength and endurance increase.

Athletic Performance. Stronger muscles enable you to better control the forces of movement—self-generated and external, as well as your body position during activity. Improved muscular fitness contributes to skill-related components of balance, speed, power, coordination, and agility. All other things being equal, a strong person can run faster, jump higher, and throw a ball farther than can a weaker individual.

Injury Prevention. Aerobic exercises such as jogging and aerobic dance have the potential to cause injury through repetitive, forceful impact against unyielding surfaces. Strong, flexible muscles and connective tissue can better withstand the stress of many forceful landings during a workout. When ligaments, tendons, muscle, and bone are strengthened through muscular exercise, risk of injury is decreased. Many aerobic activities tend to develop strength in

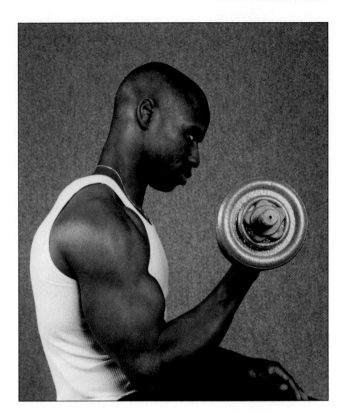

Resistance training is the most effective way to shape and tone muscles and is an important part of a balanced fitness program.

only a few groups of muscles, leaving others weak. For example, jogging strengthens quadriceps but leaves the hamstrings weak. Weak muscle groups are more susceptible to strains or pulls. A well-designed resistance-training program develops balanced, proportional strength in agonists (prime movers) and antagonists (opposing muscle groups). If injury does occur, it may be less severe and may heal more quickly if the muscle is well-conditioned. A carefully designed program can also rehabilitate injuries to regain normal (or better) strength levels. For more detailed information on injury prevention, see Chapter 9.

Bone Strength. Resistance exercises decrease the risk of osteoporosis. This is important not only for the elderly, but for young people as well. Osteoporosis may become a problem at age 50, but it starts much earlier—in the teens and twenties with poor exercise and eating habits that fail to build adequate bone density. The pull of muscles on bone in weight-bearing exercise stimulates development of increased bone density and preserves existing bone. Lifting heavy weights in a few repetitions may be more effective in increasing bone mass than is lifting a light weight many times.

Flexibility. Moving weights through a full range of motion, from full extension to full contraction, stretches and tones muscles. This is an important training technique to

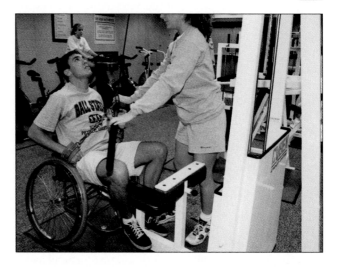

Resistance training benefits everyone. Greater muscular fitness improves performance of everyday activities and recreational and competitive sports.

master to maintain flexibility. Muscles become short and tight if exercises are performed repeatedly through only a partial range of motion.

Balance. Strong, fatigue-resistant muscles mean better balance during static and dynamic activities not only in athletics, but in functional activities for people of all ages. Studies have shown improvements in balance for elderly people participating in strength training. This may translate into decreased risk of falls and improved gait stability even for people in their 80s.

Cholesterol. Although little significant change in max VO_2 occurs in resistance training, studies have shown a significant reduction in total cholesterol and total cholesterol/HDL ratios after 3 to 4 months of weight training. The studies suggest that strength training may lower cardiovascular disease risk.

Psychological Benefits. While many people begin an exercise program to improve appearance, many other less visible but equally important effects may result. Benefits in the emotional dimension of wellness from regular exercise include feeling better, decreased stress, decreased depression, and enhanced self-esteem and self-confidence.

Social Benefits. In addition to offering physical and psychological benefits, lifting with a partner or friend offers social benefits. There are many more opportunities for conversation and interaction when you work out with someone than when you watch a movie.

Benefits at Any Age. Regardless of your age, you can benefit from resistance training. It is untrue that loss of strength is inevitable with age or that older people cannot gain strength. While the typical sedentary individual can lose up to 30 percent of his or her muscle mass between the ages of 20 and 70, this loss is more from atrophy due to disuse rather than to aging alone. Several studies including people in their 70s, 80s, and 90s participating in resistance training have shown that they increased muscle mass, more than doubled their strength, and improved their functional mobility and ability to perform daily living activities.

Disadvantages and Cautions. Although resistance training has many benefits, it does have disadvantages. Resistance training is not a complete exercise program because it does not develop cardiorespiratory endurance. As in any physical activity, injury is possible if you are careless or ignore safety procedures. You may have trouble accessing equipment. Also, you can expect some mild muscle soreness during the first week of your program.

Individuals with cardiovascular problems or high blood pressure should seek medical guidance due to the tendency of blood pressure to increase during strength training. Those who have hernias, arthritis, or lower back problems should also seek medical clearance. Individuals with these health concerns may benefit from resistance training but should be aware that they may need special exercise modifications.

Avoid use of hand and ankle weights during jogging, high-impact aerobic dance workouts, or other activities involving running and jumping. Ankle weights may distort proper form, increase stress to legs and feet, and increase risk of strains and sprains. While small increases in oxygen consumption and caloric expenditure do result from using light weights, the same effect can be produced with less risk by exercising longer or harder.

When used with controlled form and rhythm in a muscle toning or walking program, however, light weights are beneficial for increasing heart rate and muscular fitness in the upper body. All in all, resistance training offers few drawbacks and many major advantages for the time invested.

Muscle Function

Muscles are made of individual muscle fibers bound together and sheathed in connective tissue. They end in a tendon that connects the muscle to a bone. An example is the

Achilles tendon, which you can feel above your heel, connecting your calf to your foot. Muscle fibers can contract to shorten the muscle or relax and return to their resting length. They are also elastic. They can be stretched and will spring back to their resting length.

Muscle fibers are classified into different types based on their endurance, speed of contraction, and ability to exert force and increase in size. **Slow-twitch** (ST) **muscle fibers** have good endurance but low power. They are recruited mainly in endurance-type activities. **Fast-twitch** (FT) **muscle fibers** are able to contract quicker and stronger and increase in size better in response to training. Studies have shown that your ratio of FT to ST muscle fibers is genetically determined. Those born with more ST muscle fibers shine on long endurance-type activities. Those with more FT fibers find short-burst, anaerobic activities such as sprinting, jumping, and weight training easier. This may also partly explain why some people build muscle mass easier than others. While you cannot change a ST fiber into a FT fiber, FT fibers are preferentially recruited and developed by resistance training. Regardless of your genetic endowment, resistance training can improve and optimize your muscle performance. Keep in mind that muscle fiber type is only one of many factors that determine your ability to build muscular fitness.

Muscles cannot expand and push. Movement is produced as muscle contracts, shortens, and pulls on bones across a joint. As a muscle on one side of a bone contracts, muscles on the other side must relax to allow movement to occur. The contracting muscle that initiates movement is called the **agonist.** The opposing muscle is called the **antagonist.** In a biceps curl (Fig. 5-3), the agonist is the biceps, and the antagonist is the triceps. In a triceps extension, the roles reverse. What is the agonist in a hamstring curl? What is the antagonist?

Determinants of Muscular Fitness Gains

Gains in muscular fitness result from neurologic and muscular adaptations. Dramatic strength gains early in a program are often due to a "learning effect"—that is, you learn how to lift weights more efficiently. Your body represses its self-

protective reflexes and increases its ability to fully recruit muscle fibers when needed.

Your overall potential for development of muscular fitness is determined by many factors, including the types, number, and size of muscle fibers you possess and how well your muscular system can recruit them during muscular effort. The more muscle fibers you have, the larger they are, and the better your system is at activating them during muscular effort, the greater your strength. While the types and number of muscle fibers you possess is genetically determined, size and muscle fiber recruitment are a product of training.

Muscle Fiber Recruitment

When a muscle contracts, only the number of muscle fibers required for that momentary effort will shorten. Individual muscle fibers cannot contract partially. They either are working as hard as possible or not at all. This is called the *all-or-nothing principle*. For example, when a biceps curl calls for a 50 percent effort, all fibers in the muscle do not contract at 50 percent effort; rather, a portion of the muscle's fibers contract fully while the remainder rest. After these first muscle fibers contract, fatigue slightly decreases their ability to apply force. On each subsequent contraction, more fibers must be recruited to continue to lift the same weight. After several muscle contractions, enough fibers are fatigued that the muscle temporarily can no longer generate the same effort in what is called *temporary muscular failure*. Muscle fibers increase strength only if they are stimulated by intensity of effort. If your goal is to develop maximal muscular strength, try to recruit, or activate, as many muscle fibers as possible by working a muscle to a state of temporary muscular failure. If you are working for health-related fitness levels, a less intense effort is adequate.

Muscle Atrophy and Hypertrophy

Muscles adapt to the load placed upon them. When the load increases over time, muscular strength and endurance improve. When muscles are not used, they grow weaker, stiffen, and **atrophy** or shrink in size. A dramatic example of muscle atrophy occurs when a person has an injured limb in a cast for several weeks. When the cast is removed, the muscles of the affected limb are noticeably smaller. Increasing amounts of exercise over time are necessary to rebuild muscle strength, size, and flexibility.

When muscles are stimulated by an increased workload, they grow stronger and muscle fibers **hypertrophy** or increase in size. This increase occurs in both men and women and is proportional to muscle mass. The average man has about twice the muscle mass of the average woman, so hypertrophy in men is more pronounced.

Some women worry that they will develop big shoulders or massive, masculine musculature by weight training, and this myth is reinforced by televised images of women's

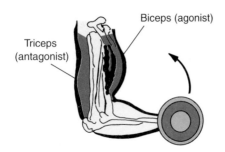

figure 5-3   Biceps curl demonstrating muscle function.

Biceps (agonist)

Triceps (antagonist)

bodybuilding competitions. Be assured that shoulder width, like hip width, is strongly influenced by genetics and that significant muscle gains require years of strenuous daily effort. They don't occur by accident, nor with a 30-minute muscle toning workout three times a week.

Types of Resistance Training Programs

Three basic types of muscle contraction are isometric, isotonic, and isokinetic. Different resistance programs have been developed for each type.

Isometric

Iso means "equal or constant" and *meter* refers to length. In **isometric** exercise, the muscle contracts but does not change length, and no movement occurs. If you pushed your palms together hard, your pectoral muscles would contract and try to shorten, but your arms would not move (Fig. 5-4). An advantage of isometric exercise is that it requires little or no equipment and can be done almost anywhere—for instance, while sitting at a desk. However, because resistance is applied at only one point in your range of motion, strength development is limited. Also, it is difficult to know how much force is being exerted, so strength gains are not as easy to observe as when equipment is being used. Four isometric exercises are illustrated in Figure 5-4. For additional exercises, consult the suggested readings at the end of this chapter. Caution: For these and other strength exercises, breathe throughout the exercise. Do not hold your breath during exertion, as this can produce a potentially harmful elevation in blood pressure.

Isometric Exercises

A. *Pectorals:* Press palms together at chest level for a count of five. Repeat five times.
B. *Upper back/triceps:* Clasp hands together at chest level. Pull outward for a count of five. Repeat 10 to 15 times.
C. *Inner thigh:* Sitting, place your knees outside the chair legs. Squeeze your thighs together for a count of five. Repeat 10 to 15 times.
D. *Outer hip:* Sitting, place your feet inside the chair legs. Press out for a count of five. Repeat 10 to 15 times.

Isotonic

Tonic refers to tone or tension, so in **isotonic** exercise as the muscle contracts, tension, or force, is controlled throughout the motion. Isotonic contractions may be either concentric or eccentric.

In a **concentric contraction,** a muscle shortens as it overcomes resistance. For example, a weight is lifted as the biceps contract during the lifting phase of a biceps curl. **Eccentric contraction** occurs when a muscle lengthens and contracts at the same time, gradually allowing a force to overcome muscular resistance; for example, the biceps contract eccentrically during the lowering phase of a biceps curl. Eccentric contraction is an important component of strength development because it makes up half of the muscular effort.

Advantages of isotonic exercise are that it strengthens through a full range of motion, the load is measurable, and a variety of isotonic programs are available. Calisthenics, free weights, or machines such as Universal or Nautilus use isotonic exercise.

Isokinetic

Kinetic means "motion," and in **isokinetic** exercise, speed of movement is controlled. If you apply great force or a light force, the resistance is adjusted to maintain a constant rate of contraction. The advantage of isokinetic work is that the load is controlled by the efforts of the user. The disadvantage is that it requires special machinery, such as Cybex or Orthotron, often used by athletic trainers for injury rehabilitation. You can get a sense of isokinetic movement by sweeping an arm through water. The harder you press, the more resistance you create.

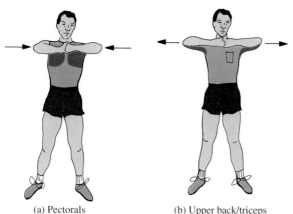
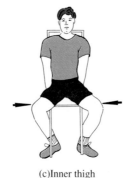
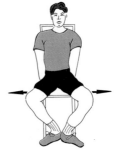

(a) Pectorals   (b) Upper back/triceps   (c)Inner thigh   (d) Outer hip

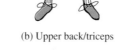

figure 5-4   Isometric exercises.

wellness flash

Muscular strength can be maintained with as little as one high-intensity resistance workout per week.

table 5-1   **Safety Guidelines for Resistance Training**

table 5-1 — Safety Guidelines for Resistance Training
1. Warm up before each workout and stretch afterward.
2. Use good technique—keep your abdominals tight, back straight, hips tucked under, knees relaxed.
3. Work each exercise through a full range of motion from full extension without lockout to full contraction.
4. Perform each exercise smoothly, with control. Do not swing the limbs or use momentum, Faster is not better.
5. Before you lift, inhale. Exhale on the exertion. Do not hold your breath.

Principles of Resistance Training

Principles of resistance training include progressive overload, specificity, and recovery.

Progressive Overload

Progressive overload is the most important principle of resistance training. To stimulate a muscle to increase strength or endurance, it must gradually be overloaded or forced to work at a higher than normal effort. Either the number of lifts performed or the amount of weight must gradually be increased. Increasing the number of repetitions increases muscular endurance. Increasing the weight lifted increases strength. General programs increase both until a desired maintenance goal is reached.

You must exercise two to three times per week to improve muscular fitness. To maintain strength, one intense workout is adequate.

Specificity

The speed of contraction, range of motion, amount and type of resistance, and number and type of exercise are a few of the variables that determine the results of strength training. If you desire a specific result, such as an increase in muscle mass, your program must be designed and executed to produce that result.

Recovery

Exercise stimulates the muscle to take in more protein and nutrients and undergo changes that increase its ability to forcefully contract. After a workout, you will be weaker, not stronger, due to fatigue. Improvement occurs during recovery, which gives the muscle fibers time to repair and grow. Strength workouts are best done with 2 to 3 days rest between sessions to allow recovery and improvement to occur.

Guidelines for Developing Muscular Fitness

In increasing muscular strength, endurance, or power, the key variables are resistance, repetitions, and speed. The purest example of strength is one maximal lift, and the closer a program comes to this, the greater the strength gains. However, risk of injury is high when working at or near maximal levels. Athletes working to develop strength often exercise at 80 to 95 percent or higher effort a few (three to six) times. Muscular endurance is enhanced by contracting repeatedly (i.e., one to two sets of 15 to 20 reps) with moderate (50 to 60 percent) effort.

There is some crossover effect between muscular strength and muscular endurance. Development of muscular strength also produces some increase in muscular endurance; for example, if you can lift a 100-pound weight five times, you can probably lift a 5-pound weight 20 times. However, muscular endurance does not enhance strength. If you can lift a 5-pound weight 20 times, you may not be able to lift a 100-pound weight even once. If you want to develop both muscular strength and endurance, a muscular strength program can pay double benefits.

Muscular power, a function of strength and speed, is the ability to apply force rapidly. Power is increased by performing a muscle contraction quickly as in plyometric exercises often used in athletics. While muscular power is not necessary for health-related physical fitness, it is an asset in many sports.

Optimal results can be obtained from any resistance-training program and risk of injury can be minimized if you follow the guidelines in Table 5-1.

Sequence

Ideally, work large muscle groups first, ending with small muscle groups. It is difficult to adequately exercise large muscle groups if you have already fatigued the smaller supporting muscles. The suggested order of exercises is hips/legs, torso, arms, abdominals (see the sample weight-training program).

Form

- Never sacrifice form for weight. After progressive overload, correct exercise form is the most important (and most neglected) factor in maximizing strength gains and minimizing risk of injury. Improvement is more rapid if correct technique, not only quantity of weight, is emphasized.

- Always work through a complete range of motion for flexibility and maximum strength gains. Move from full extension without lockout to full flexion.
- Keep your back straight and abdominals tight to protect your lower back.
- When doing standing exercises, keep your knees slightly bent and your hips tucked under to support your back.
- Avoid "cheating," a breakdown in exercise form that occurs when extra muscles are used to complete the exercise, decreasing the load to the prime mover. Cheating occurs when the load is too heavy or you are fatigued. Remember: Quality of work is more important than the amount of repetitions or weight lifted.

Rest Between Sets

A rest period between sets of an exercise should allow sufficient recovery so that good form can be maintained. This time will vary, depending on the intensity of lifting, with 1 to 2 minutes rest recommended between sets of a general program, and 2 to 4 minutes between sets of a strength program. To make efficient use of time, you may alternate exercises on different body parts—for example, legs, then arms—so that one muscle group is recovering while you are working another.

Muscle Balance

Muscles work in pairs, so it is important to strengthen muscles on both sides of a bone so that they pull evenly across joints and maintain body alignment. For example, if pectorals are stronger than upper back muscles, rounded shoulders result. When upper back muscles are strengthened, shoulders are naturally held erect. Tight lower back muscles opposed by weak, sagging abdominals pull the back into an exaggerated curve. This stresses lumbar vertebrae, increasing back fatigue and risk of lower back pain. Well-toned abdominals support the back, improve appearance, and prevent back problems. Resistance programs must be planned to develop proportional strength in the following muscle pairs: biceps/triceps, pectorals/trapezius-rhomboids, abdominals/lower back, hamstrings/quadriceps, gastrocnemius/anterior tibialis, and deltoids/latissimus dorsi (Figs. 5-5a and 5-5b).

Breathing

Exhale on the exertion; inhale on the release. Holding your breath while you strain against a closed epiglottis is called the **Valsalva maneuver.** This can elevate blood pressure dangerously and cause dizziness or fainting.

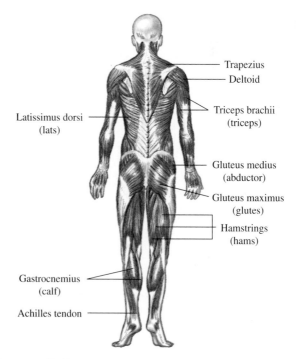

figure 5-5a   Major muscles of the body. Front.

Source: From John W. Hole, Jr., *Human Anatomy and Physiology*, 4th ed. Copyright;© 1987 Wm. C. Brown Publishers, Dubuque, Iowa. All Rights Reserved. Reprinted by permission.

figure 5-5b   Major muscles of the body. Back.

Source: From John W. Hole, Jr., *Human Anatomy and Physiology*, 4th ed. Copyright;© 1987 Wm. C. Brown Publishers, Dubuque, Iowa. All Rights Reserved. Reprinted by permission.

Speed of Movement

Exercising in a smooth, controlled manner maximizes strength gains and reduces injuries. Take 2 seconds to lift (concentric or shortening contraction) and 2 to 4 seconds to lower (eccentric or lengthening contraction). Control the movement; do not fling, swing, or kick. Jerky movements will cause excessive wear and tear on your joints. Also, when you use momentum to perform an exercise, you apply force and develop strength only through the first part of the movement. Lower a limb with the same control used to lift it. Do not drop weights with a crash. You are stronger lowering a weight than lifting it.

Resistance-Training Programs

There are many types of resistance-training programs. The type of program you select will depend on your goals and the type of equipment (if any) you plan to use. Regardless of the type of program you select, you can keep track of your progress with the Resistance-Training Log at the end of this chapter.

Weight Training

Weight training is a noncompetitive exercise program used to develop several health-related physical fitness components: muscular strength, muscular endurance, flexibility, and body composition. It differs significantly in its goals from the competitive sports of weight lifting and bodybuilding. Male, female, young, old, athlete, or fitness exerciser—all benefit from weight training. Beginners with low levels of muscular fitness benefit the most and will notice results more quickly than will experienced lifters. Weight training can build muscular fitness levels so that recreational, competitive, or daily activities are accomplished more easily, with less strain and fatigue.

Equipment

For beginners, it really doesn't matter what type of equipment is used. A beginner will improve on almost any type of program as long as an adequate overload is provided. Two major types of equipment used in weight training are free weights and machines. Both have advantages and disadvantages.

Free weights are far less expensive than machines, so you can have your own set at home. Free weights cost about $100 on sale, double that if you add a padded bench and rack. Machines can cost upward of $500 to $5,000. You have more variety of exercises on free weights than on machines because you have the freedom to lift in so many different positions. Lifting with proper technique is crucial. A wrong move can cause injury with any lifting but particularly with free weights. To lift free weights safely, you must have a skilled spotting partner who can handle the weight in case you start to lose control. For muscular fitness development,

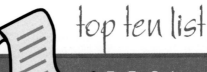

top ten list

Top Ten Resistance Training Mistakes to Avoid

Resistance training is a great way to shape and tone muscles. If done wrong, however, it can elevate blood pressure and cause back strain, sore knees, or ankle sprain. Also, training mistakes slow your progress. Here are the most common errors to avoid:

1. *Holding your breath during lifting.* This can cause a dangerous increase in blood pressure. Exhale on exertion, inhale on release.
2. *Lifting too heavy a weight.* If you can't lift it full range of motion with good form, lighten the load. Train, don't strain.
3. *Arching the back.* During the bench press or military press, this can strain back ligaments. Tighten abdominals and keep the back straight.
4. *Using momentum.* "Kicking" the weight up in the quadriceps extension or hamstring curl decreases the load through the full range of motion and slows progress. Bouncing or jerking a lift strains ligaments and indicates the weight is too heavy or you are getting too tired to lift smoothly.
5. *Doing reps too quickly.* Length of time a force is applied is a factor in muscle fitness. Lift for 2 to 4 counts, lower slowly, 2 to 4 counts for best results. Yes, it is harder than lifting fast. It takes fewer reps to get the same results as compared to lifting fast.
6. *Not using full range of motion.* Strength is built only in the range of motion used. If you stop before the "sticking point," you are building muscle imbalances.
7. *Not wiping off sweat.* Sweat makes your grip slippery.
8. *Going too deep in squats or leg press.* This strains knee ligaments. Don't go below 90 degrees.
9. *Letting ankles roll out when legs are loaded.* This can cause ankle sprain. Keep ankles straight in squats or toe presses.
10. *Working only "problem" areas.* Or, working the agonist, but not its opposing antagonist. In other words, working biceps but not triceps or abdominals but not the back. This causes muscle imbalances, increasing risk of injury.

free weights have an advantage over machines because they not only develop strength in the prime movers, but also develop balance and coordination by strengthening other muscles required to balance and control the weight.

Machines such as Nautilus and Universal are easy to use and safer than free weights because they guide your movements and control the weights. An advantage of Nautilus

table 5-2 — Safety Using Weights

1. Never attempt to lift more than you know you can handle. Work out—don't show off.
2. Always make sure that the weight pins, bars, or collars are secure.
3. Don't life weights alone. Always work with someone else.
4. Keep sweat wiped off your hands; it makes weights slippery.
5. When using free weights, work with a trained spotter.
6. Return all equipment to the proper place. Don't leave it lying around for someone to trip over.

equipment is that it prestretches the muscle and takes the joint through the full range of motion. Also, it provides variable resistance, adjusting the load for strength variations throughout a lift. Universal gives the exerciser more control over range of motion and allows people to work more closely together. Because of the cost of machines, it is best to start your machine-workout program at a health club or gym. Proper lifting technique is easier to learn on machines, and you won't need a spotting partner. Loads can be changed quickly, so the workout may take less time than with free weights. For safety, convenience, and time, machines have the edge. Whether you use free weights or machines, always follow the safety guidelines in Table 5-2 to minimize risk of injury.

Weight Room Etiquette

Be aware of and follow common weight room etiquette guidelines while working out:

- Wipe sweat off benches after use.
- Rerack weights when you are done.
- Don't lie around on the equipment chatting between sets if someone is waiting to use the machine. Let them work in between sets while you are resting.
- Don't drop or bang the weights together. This can damage the equipment and increases the noise level unnecessarily.

Program for General Conditioning

A conditioning program should develop balanced strength. Many muscle strains occur because of weakness in the pulled muscle or its opposing muscle. A general strength program prevents strength imbalances. If you exercised only problem areas, you would increase imbalances. Prime muscle movers, the muscle(s) mainly responsible for the joint movement, are listed and can be found in figures 5-5 a and b. The following exercises, listed in the order of large to small muscle groups, may be done on Universal (Fig. 5-6). Free weight exercises are also described and illustrated (Fig. 5-7). If you plan to use Nautilus equipment, your first workouts should include learning how to adjust and efficiently use the equipment.

Weight Training Exercises

A. Leg press

Prime movers: quadriceps, hamstrings, and gluteus maximus

On leg press, sit on seat, adjust position to last slot or to a 90-degree knee angle.

Place feet squarely on pedals, press out smoothly (do not lock knees), and return to starting position.

B. Leg extension

Prime movers: quadriceps

Sit on bench with both feet under the rollers. Toe in slightly. Do not lie back.

Extend your legs, hold 1 second, and return to starting position.

C. Hamstring curl

Prime movers: hamstrings and gluteus maximus

Lie face down on the bench, hook both heels under the rollers. Position knees at the pivot point where the rollers attach to the bench. Pull up to 90 degrees, hold for 1 second, and return to starting position.

D. Toe press

Prime mover: gastrocnemius

On leg press station, place feet squarely on pedals, press out to full leg extension without knee lockout. Press with toes from flat-footed position to foot extension and return.

E. Bench press

Prime movers: pectorals and triceps

Lie on bench, head next to the machine. The grips should be lined up approximately with the shoulders. Place your feet flat on the bench with knees bent and back flat. Press to extension and return.

F. Military press

Prime movers: deltoids and triceps

Sit on the stool or stand with abdominals tight, back flat, and knees slightly bent. With shoulders close to handles, extend upward with arms until they are straight but not locked and return.

G. Lat pull

Prime movers: latissimus dorsi

Grip bar directly above shoulders or at handles. Pull down until you are kneeling or sitting. From this position, pull down to chest or touch the back of shoulders and return.

H. Triceps press

Prime movers: triceps

Stand facing lat bar. With palms facing down, grasp the bar so that hands are shoulder-width apart. Keep elbows at waist. Press down to extension and return.

I. Biceps curl

Prime movers: biceps

Stand facing the weights, hold bar with both hands, palms up. Flex arms until the bar meets shoulders. Return to starting position. Keep back straight, abdominals firm.

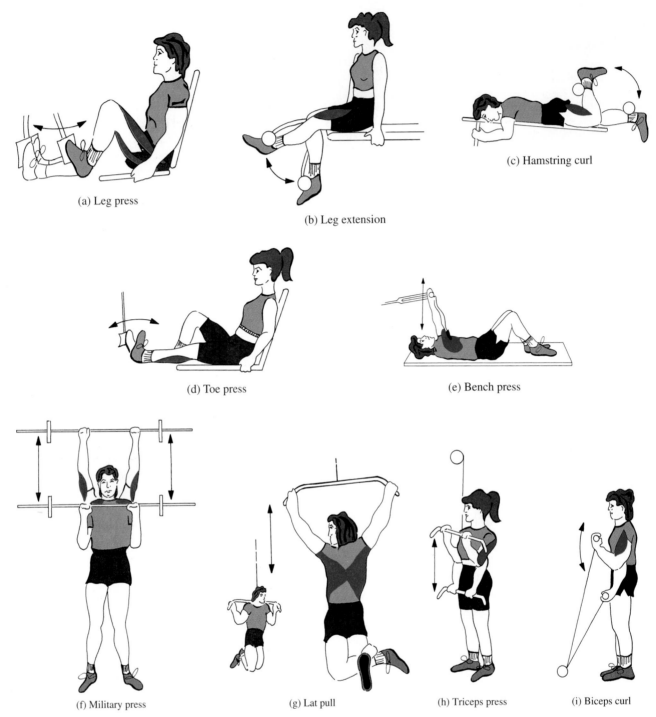

(a) Leg press

(b) Leg extension

(c) Hamstring curl

(d) Toe press

(e) Bench press

(f) Military press

(g) Lat pull

(h) Triceps press

(i) Biceps curl

figure 5-6   Weight training exercises.

Free Weight Exercises

These exercises (Fig. 5-7) may be done with a set of barbells or hand weights. Practice each move without weights before attempting weighted sets. Free weights provide additional challenge over machines because balance and coordination are developed in addition to strength. Strict attention to lifting form is critical because with free weights, a moment's carelessness can cause an injury. Always work with an experienced spotter in case you have difficulty. When possible, use power/squat racks with adjustable supports for added safety. To protect the back, you need to keep abdominals firm, back straight. Breathe continuously, do not hold your breath.

A. Squats

Prime movers: gluteus maximus, quadriceps, hamstrings
Start standing upright with the bar resting on your shoulders. Keep the head up, abdominals tight, back flat, feet a bit wider than your shoulders. With back straight, slowly lower hips until tops of thighs are parallel with the floor. Pause. Drive up with legs and hips to the starting position.

B. Lunge

Prime movers: gluteus maximus, quadriceps
Standing upright with the bar on the shoulders off the neck, abdominals tight, back flat, step forward (or backward) until the front thigh is parallel with the floor. The front knee should be over the ball of the foot. Keeping back straight, take a controlled step back to the starting position. Repeat with the opposite leg. This exercise requires considerable balance. You may wish to start first with dumbbells and progress slowly to use of a barbell.

C. Calf raise

Prime mover: gastrocnemius/soleus
Place bar on shoulders, position balls of feet on board and heels off board. Press up onto balls of feet, then lower with control. Knees straight tones gastrocnemius, knees bent tones soleus.

D. Bench press

Prime movers: pectorals and triceps
Lie with head and buttocks on bench, feet stabilized on ground. Grip about 4 inches wider than shoulders, palms under bar (pronated). Lower bar to chest. Focus eyes up to the sky, do not watch bar. Elbows should be directly under bar and forearms perpendicular to ground. Do not let bar slide to the neck. Press to extension, and return.

E. Supine flys

Prime movers: pectorals and biceps
Lie with head and buttocks on bench, feet stabilized on floor, and dumbbells close to chest. Move dumbbells directly overhead. Keeping elbows flexed, slowly lower dumbbells until chest is comfortably stretched. Keeping elbows out, wrists in, bring dumbbells back in an arc.

F. Military press

Prime movers: deltoids and triceps
Sit on bench or stand. With barbell on chest, press upward with arms until they are straight overhead but not locked, and return.

G. Bent over rowing

Prime movers: rhomboids, latissimus dorsi
Stabilize one knee and hand on a bench, opposite hand holds the weight and foot is flat on the floor. Pull elbow up and in toward the spine.

H. Triceps press

Prime movers: triceps
Standing with abdominals firm, feet apart for stability, grip the weight, palms up, and keeping elbows near the ears, slowly lower bar behind the head. Pause, then press until elbows are fully extended.

I. Biceps curl

Prime movers: biceps
Grasp bar, palms up, holding bar about thigh level. Bend elbows, moving bar in an arc toward shoulders. Pause, and slowly return to starting position.

J. Upright rowing

Prime movers: deltoid, biceps
With feet slightly wider than shoulder width, squat and grasp bar palms down, hands on top of bar. Stand using legs, not back, and let arms extend. Keeping bar close to chest, raise elbows toward ears, pulling bar high under chin. Slowly lower arms.

K. Shoulder shrugs

Prime movers: trapezius
Holding barbell or two dumbbells, raise shoulders toward ears, pause, lower shoulders.

How to Begin and Progress

A good general conditioning program would involve lifting one to two sets of 8 to 12 repetitions three times per week (for instance, M–W–F). A **repetition (rep)** is one lift; a **set** is two to a group of lifts.

The first week, a beginner should lift one set of 8 to 12 repetitions under the supervision of a trained professional. The first workouts should use light weights and concentrate on form, rhythm, and breathing. This will also minimize muscular soreness. The second week, an additional set can be added if desired, and the third week, a starting load can be established. Other weight training programs for goals of increasing muscular endurance, strength, or size are given in Table 5-3.

Establishing Your Workload

To establish your workload, for each exercise find the maximum amount of weight you can lift once with good form (one **repetition maximum** or **1 RM**). In a general

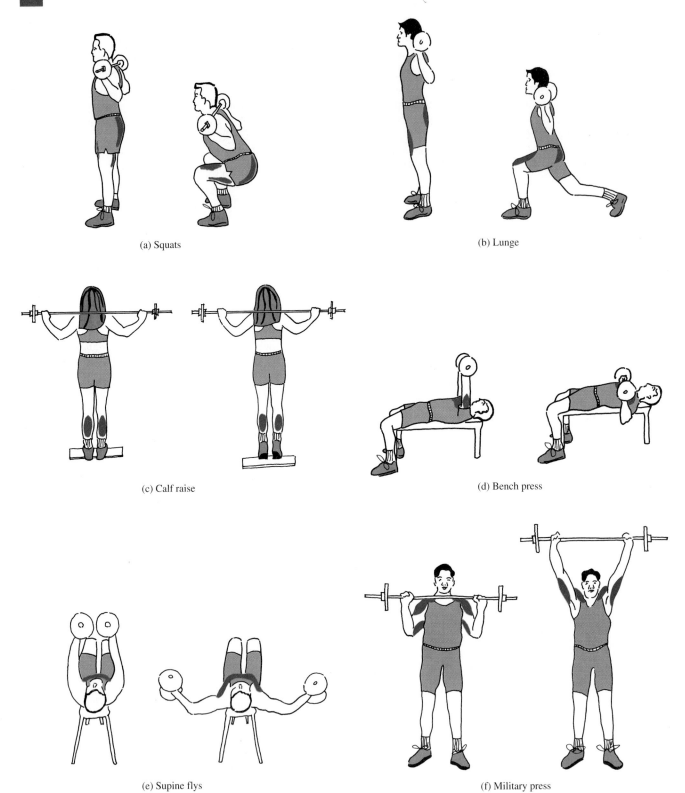

(a) Squats

(b) Lunge

(c) Calf raise

(d) Bench press

(e) Supine flys

(f) Military press

figure 5-7   Free weight exercises.

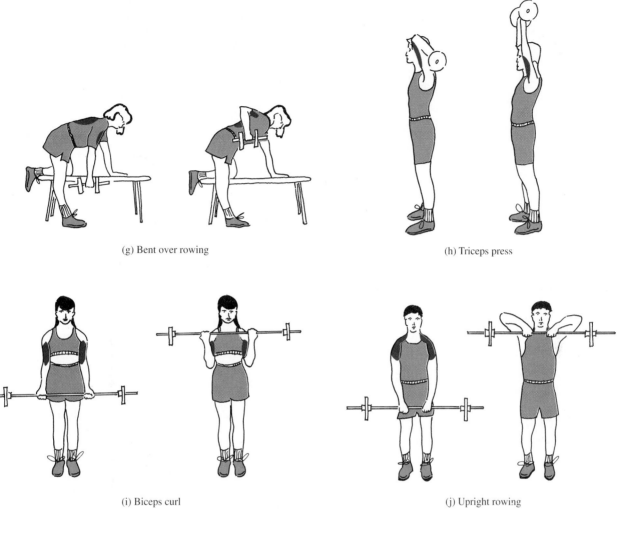

(g) Bent over rowing

(h) Triceps press

(i) Biceps curl

(j) Upright rowing

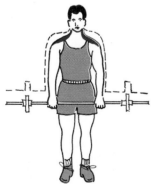

(k) Shoulder shrugs

figure 5-7   Free weight exercises. (*continued*)

table 5-3	Weight Training Goals and Programs			
	Muscular endurance	General conditioning	Muscle size (weight gain)	Muscular strength
Resistance (% of 1 RM)	50–60%	70–75%	70–80%	80–90%
Repetitions	15–20	8–12	5–10	4–6
Sets	1–2	1–2	3–5	1–3
Rest between sets (minutes)	1/2–1	1–2	1–3	2–4

conditioning program, seventy-five percent of that weight will be your workload. In the workout, lift to fatigue at each station. If you can do fewer than 6 reps, the weight is too heavy. If you can do 12 or more reps at that load, the weight is too light. Increase or decrease the load the next workout, if necessary. At the correct workload, the last 2 reps of each exercise should be difficult for you to do, and you should reach temporary muscular failure between 8 and 12 reps.

Increasing Your Workload

When you can do 12 reps, increase the amount of weight. If you can do at least 6 reps at the new weight, stay with that weight until you can do 12 reps. If, when you increase the weight you cannot do at least 6 reps, drop back to your old weight and increase the number of reps each time until you can do 15. You should then be able to increase the weight and do at least 6 reps. In general:

- Increase only one variable at a time (reps, sets, resistance).
- Increase reps or sets first, then resistance.
- When increasing resistance, decrease reps.
- To increase muscular endurance, increase the number of reps, sets, or decrease rest between sets.
- Increase the workload by no more than 5 to 10 percent each time.

Variety

You can incorporate variety into your workout by changing the workload, recovery period, number of sets, reps, rhythm, and number or order of lifts. Here are a few examples of different programs:

1. *General:* one to two sets of 8 to 12 reps at 70 to 75 percent 1 RM. Rest 1 to 2 minutes between sets.
2. *Strength:* one to three sets of 4 to 6 reps at 80 to 90 percent 1 RM. Rest 2 to 4 minutes between sets.
3. *Endurance:* one to two sets of 20 reps at 50 to 60 percent 1 RM. Rest 30 to 60 seconds between sets.
4. *Eccentric emphasis (negatives):* Lift for two counts, lower for eight. Some experts say that lowering the weight is more important to strength development

than lifting it. This does tend to promote more muscle soreness. Strength increases occur with eccentric lifting alone, and because you can lower more weight than you can lift, you may need to increase resistance.
5. *Supersets:* Work opposite muscle groups immediately (triceps/biceps, hams/quads).
6. *Continuous set:* Lift to muscular exhaustion at your regular weight, lower one plate and lift to exhaustion, and continue to lower weight as you fatigue. This is a type of muscular endurance program. It is supposed to increase muscular definition. It can be done with machines, but it is difficult with free weights.
7. *Pyramid:* Lift 6 reps at 70 percent 1 RM; 4 reps at 80 percent 1 RM; 2 reps at 90 percent 1 RM; 1 rep at 100 percent 1 RM. This program emphasizes strength.
8. *Split routine:* Work upper body one day and lower body the next day; or do pushers (i.e., quads, triceps) one day, pullers (i.e., hams, biceps) the next. You must work 6 days per week. This reduces total body fatigue but requires more time.
9. *Aerobic circuit:* A circuit is a group of exercises performed with little rest between each. Lighten weight to 40 to 60 percent of 1 RM. Lift quickly 30 seconds (20 lifts), recover for 30 seconds, while switching to the next station and setting the weight. Alternate a leg station with an arm station as you proceed through the circuit. As the goal is aerobic conditioning, you may also include a jump rope, bench step, jumping jacks, or jogging in place station. Begin with one set of 10 to 12 exercises and work up to three sets, maintaining a target pulse. This is designed to strengthen the heart as well as develop muscular endurance. Be careful to maintain good form—it is easy to get sloppy and hurt yourself in this workout because the lifting rhythm is so quick.
10. *Muscle size (weight gain) program:* A bulk-up of three to five sets of 5, gradually increasing to 10 reps at 70 to 80 percent effort should be performed for several months to increase lean weight.

Common Discomforts and Training Errors

After lifting for a few weeks, you may notice a buildup of callus on your palms. If it bothers you, lifting gloves will offer some protection. If you experience nausea or lightheadedness, stop and figure out the cause.

- Did you allow enough time since your last meal?
- Are you exhaling on the effort?
- Are you trying to progress too quickly?

If you experience pain, particularly joint pain, pay attention. It could be an early warning sign of injury. You may be lifting too heavy a weight or stressing your joints with poor form. Lifting too heavy a weight leads to poor form and increases risk of injury. Jerking, straining, holding your breath, using momentum, bouncing, and arching the back are problems that need to be corrected. Have a professional check your form periodically to make sure you are not falling into bad habits.

How to Shape and Tone Without Weights

There are many ways to develop muscular strength and endurance. While weight training is an excellent program, it is not always convenient. The programs described next can be done at home or while traveling. The abdominal, hip and thigh, or upper body programs require no special equipment. Partner exercises add a social dimension to a workout. Elastic resistance produces results without bulky equipment and is easy to take with you for exercise on a trip.

Abdominals, Hips, and Thighs

While weights add intensity to a workout, they are not always necessary when the goal is to shape and tone. Muscles develop firmness by working against a resistance, and that resistance can be your body weight. This program emphasizes muscular endurance rather than strength by increasing reps. Abdominals, in particular, benefit from a muscular endurance routine because their function is one of endurance—sustained contraction. If you would like a total body program, combine this with the upper body routine that follows.

These exercises (Fig. 5-8) will not burn calories like aerobic work will, so if you want to remove inches, diet and aerobic exercise are still important. Also, fat will not burn off only in the area exercised. While you can't spot reduce fat, say, in the thighs by doing leg lifts, you can spot tone flabby muscles. Be patient, and you may begin to see a difference in 8 to 12 weeks. You do not need to count repetitions. Select one exercise for each body area, and perform it for 1 minute. Start with one set and build up to two sets, 3 days a week. Variations are given to add variety to your program. If you wish to add intensity without purchasing weights, a sand-filled sock can be tied on as an ankle weight. You will want a mat or carpeted surface to work on.

Workout for Abdominals, Hips, and Thighs

A. Rectus abdominis
  1. Abdominal curl "crunch"
      Lie on back with knees bent, heels next to buttocks. Keep lower back on the ground, curl shoulders up 3 inches and return.
      Variations: Place one hand behind shoulders to support head, and reach other hand through knees. Do with feet raised or resting on a chair. Add resistance by moving hands from across chest to behind shoulders or by holding a 2-pound weight on each shoulder or behind neck. Do not pull or jerk on head.
  2. Reverse abdominal curls
      From the starting position in number 1, hold trunk steady and curl hips 1 to 2 inches off the ground; then lower slowly.
B. Oblique abdominal curl
      Start in the same position as for abdominal curls, but add a twist, first bringing right shoulder toward left knee and then left shoulder toward right knee.
      Variations: Cross right foot over left knee and twist right and then switch. Cross ankles, raise feet, and twist right and then left. Lay both knees to left, curl toward right hip, and then switch. To increase resistance, hold a 2-pound weight on each shoulder.
C. Outer hip (hip abductors)
  1. Lying side leg lift
      Lying on one side, head resting on arm and lower leg bent for balance, slowly raise and lower top leg.
      Variations: This can be done standing. Keep foot level and leg lifting directly to side, not toward front.
  2. Kneeling side leg lift
      Take a hands and knees position with one leg extended to side.
      Tighten abdominals, and round back to protect it. You may also support weight on one forearm if desired. Tense hip and raise and lower leg slowly no higher than 6 inches.
      Variations: Circle leg forward, then reverse.
D. Inner thigh (thigh adductors)
  1. Inner thigh lift
      Lying on left side, raise and lower left leg, keeping foot turned to side (not upward). Repeat right. To increase resistance, press gently on left calf with right foot as you raise and lower leg, or add an ankle weight.
  2. Plié
      Standing with feet 3 feet apart and knees bent, place hands lightly on inner thighs. Press thighs against hands, pulling in hard for a count of five. Repeat.

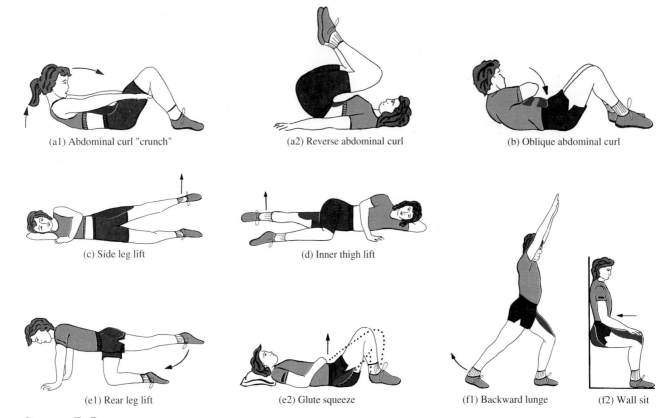

(a1) Abdominal curl "crunch"   (a2) Reverse abdominal curl   (b) Oblique abdominal curl

(c) Side leg lift   (d) Inner thigh lift

(e1) Rear leg lift   (e2) Glute squeeze   (f1) Backward lunge   (f2) Wall sit

figure 5-8   Abdominals, hips, and thighs.

E. Gluteus exercises
  1. Rear leg lift
     On hands and knees, hollow abdomen and round back to protect it. Extend right leg to the rear. Tense gluteus. Raise and lower leg slowly six to eight counts. Repeat left.
  2. Glute squeeze
     Lying on back with knees bent, squeeze gluteus hard, raising hips no more than 3 inches from floor. Do not arch back. Hold for a count of five, relax, repeat.
F. Quadriceps, hamstrings
  1. Backward lunge
     Keeping shoulders erect and weight centered over right foot, step back and touch lightly with left foot and then return to starting position. Repeat. Switch legs after 1 minute of reps.
  2. Wall sit
     Hold a sitting position with back against a wall for balance. Keep hips above knee level.

Upper Body

Upper body exercises can improve appearance by straightening rounded shoulders, firming upper arm muscles, and toning pectorals that underlie and support the breasts. You

do not need to count repetitions. Select one exercise for each body area and repeat for 1 minute. If you wish to increase resistance, bricks, books, or cans of food can serve as hand weights. Upper body exercises are illustrated in Figure 5-9.

Workout for Upper Body
  A. Push-ups (pectorals/triceps)
     These may be done standing, with hands against a wall and feet placed about 3 feet away from the wall (easiest), on the floor with knees bent (medium), or with weight supported on hands and feet (hardest). Keep abdominals firm and hips slightly flexed to support back. Lower to right angles of arms and then press back to arm extension.
     Variations: Keeping hands close emphasizes triceps. Keeping hands wide increases pectoral strengthening.
  B. Dips (pectorals/triceps)
     Dips are an alternative way to tone the same muscle groups as push-ups do. They may be done on a dip bar or using chairs. With weight evenly distributed between bars or two sturdy chairs, place a hand on each. Bend knees or extend legs so that

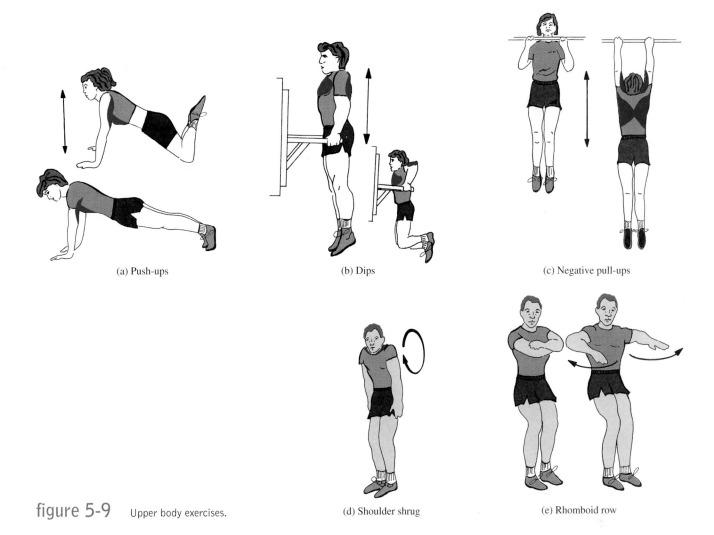

(a) Push-ups

(b) Dips

(c) Negative pull-ups

figure 5-9   Upper body exercises.

(d) Shoulder shrug

(e) Rhomboid row

weight is on arms, not feet. Bend arms to right angles and return to extension.

C. Negative pull-ups (latissimus dorsi/biceps)

Negative pull-ups offer the same benefits as full pull-ups for upper back and arms. Stand on a chair if necessary to grasp a pull-up bar with arms flexed. SLOWLY lower yourself to a count of five. As you gain strength over several weeks, try to start with a few full pull-ups and finish with negatives.

D. Shoulder shrugs (trapezius)

Shoulder shrugs can tighten upper back muscles to reduce rounded shoulders. Combine this with pectoral stretches for best results. Rotate shoulders in full circles—up-back-down—working to pull shoulder blades together.

Variations: Add resistance by holding a weight in each hand.

E. Rhomboid row (rhomboids)

Rhomboids are muscles that pull the shoulder blades back, down, and together. These also need to be strengthened to reduce rounded shoulders. With

arms slightly below shoulder level, elbows bent, pull elbows fully back, squeezing shoulder blades together, and hold for a count of five. Rest two counts. Repeat.

Elastic Resistance

Elastic resistance exercise was developed in the 1950s. It was originally used by .physical therapists who gave patients surgical rubber tubing to add resistance to rehabilitative exercise programs. Elastic bands and tubing are lightweight, portable, and readily available at fitness centers and medical supply companies. They are inexpensive but do not last forever and need to be replaced as they wear out. Safety tips are listed in the top ten list, "Tips for Elastic Resistance Exercise." They come in different strengths, based on thickness of the elastic. Thin bands are best for beginners and upper body work. Thicker bands are useful for lower body work. Two thin bands can be used in place of one thick band. The principles of form, rhythm, and breathing apply here as for any strength training program. Elastic resistance exercises are illustrated in Figure 5-10.

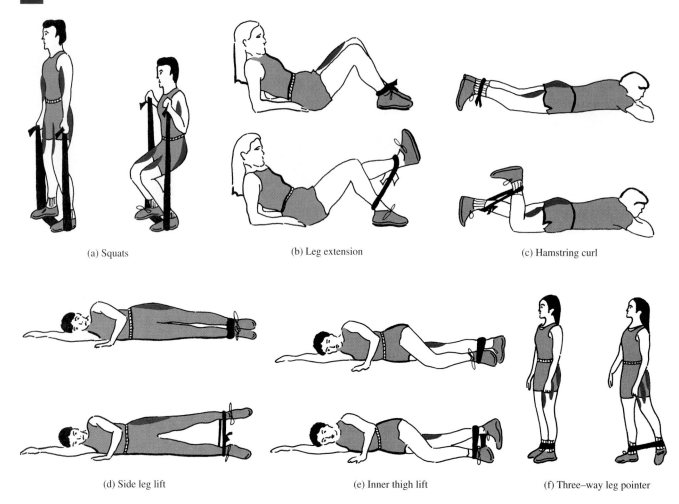

(a) Squats   (b) Leg extension   (c) Hamstring curl

(d) Side leg lift   (e) Inner thigh lift   (f) Three–way leg pointer

figure 5-10   Elastic resistance exercises.

Elastic Resistance Exercises

A. Squats (gluteus maximus, quadriceps, hamstrings, biceps)
   Step on the band with feet about shoulder width apart and hold ends of the band low enough to feel moderate tension. Slowly squat until hips are just above knees, bending elbows to maintain tension in the band. Return to standing.

B. Leg extension (quadriceps)
   Tie band around ankles. Lie back, knees bent and feet on floor. Keeping knees and thighs together, straighten knee, lifting the foot as high as possible. Release slowly and repeat. Change legs.

C. Hamstring curl (hamstrings, gluteus maximus)
   Place the band around ankles. Lie face down with arms under the chin or hands under hips. Bending knee, slowly lift one foot. Release slowly, maintaining some tension in the band. Repeat. Change legs.

D. Side leg lift (hip abductors)
   Place the band around both legs—around ankles is hardest, around knees easiest. Lying on right side, torso supported by arms, slightly bend lower leg for support. Keep hips facing forward, lift upper leg. Lower, keeping tension on the band, and repeat. Change sides.

E. Inner thigh lift (thigh adductors)
   Place band around left arch and right ankle. Lie on right side with trunk supported by arms. Lift bottom leg slowly, hold briefly, lower slowly, repeat. Switch sides.

F. Three-way leg pointer (gluteus maximus, gluteus medius, quadriceps).
   Place band around ankles. Place hand on wall for support. Keeping abdominals firm and back straight, pull foot back, return, side, return, forward, return. Repeat with other leg.

G. Toe press (gastrocnemius, soleus)
   Holding ends of band, place around ball of foot. With knee straight, slowly press through ball of foot from extension to flexion and back (gastrocnemius). To emphasize soleus, repeat with knee slightly bent.

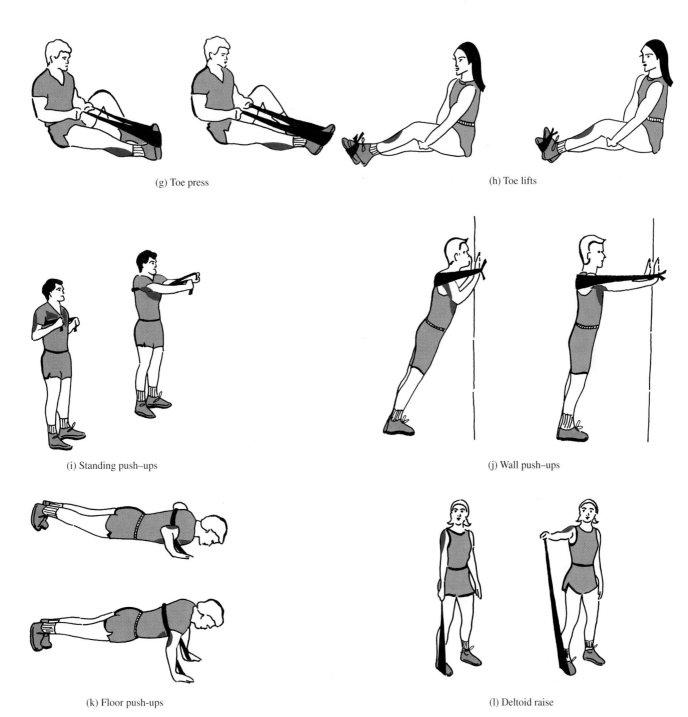

(g) Toe press

(h) Toe lifts

(i) Standing push–ups

(j) Wall push–ups

(k) Floor push-ups

(l) Deltoid raise

figure 5-10   Elastic resistance exercises. (*continued*)

H. Toe lifts (tibialis anterior)

   Tie band around arches. Place heels about 6 inches apart forward to back. Keeping one foot pointed, pull toes of the other foot back toward your face. Relax. Repeat on both feet.

I–K. Push-ups (pectorals and biceps)

   Three styles of push-ups are described here from easiest to most challenging. Use the style appropriate for your current strength level.

1. Standing push-ups: Wrap the band around your back and under your arms. Bend elbows and grasp ends of band. Extend arms forward, return slowly.

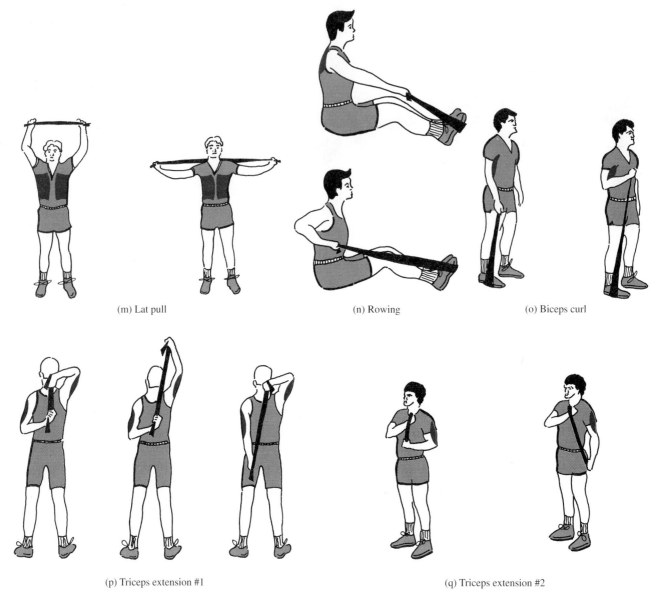

(m) Lat pull   (n) Rowing   (o) Biceps curl

(p) Triceps extension #1   (q) Triceps extension #2

figure 5-10   Elastic resistance exercises. (*continued*)

2. Wall push-ups: Tie ends of the band together, wrap around your shoulders and under palms, with hands about shoulder width apart. Place feet about 3 feet from the wall. Extend arms, return.
3. Floor push-ups: Trap ends of the band under hands. Keep abdominals tight and back straight to protect it as you bend and extend arms.

L. Deltoid raise (deltoid and triceps)
   Place one end of band under foot, hold the other end by your hip. Standing with good posture, lift arm to shoulder level, lower slowly.

M. Lat pull (latissimus dorsi)
   Hold band overhead, elbows extended but not locked. Pull arms apart to shoulder level. Be careful not to get hair caught in band.

N. Rowing (rhomboids)
   With band around arches, and knees extended, grasp band about mid-shin. Pull elbows back and try to bring shoulder blades together. Release slowly.

O. Biceps curl (biceps)
   Place one end of band under foot, grasp other end low, and keeping elbow at your side, curl right arm to shoulder. Slowly release.

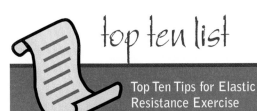

P. Triceps extension #1 (triceps)

   Standing with good posture, grasp both ends of band behind your back. Extend upper arm toward ceiling, pause, slowly release, pressing lower hand toward hip.

Q. Triceps extension #2 (triceps)

   Standing with good posture, grasp ends of band. Press lower hand toward hip, pause, slowly release. Do both arms.

Partner Resistance Exercises

Exercising with a partner can be both challenging and enjoyable. Partner communication and sensitivity to your levels of strength and fatigue are important. The partner must vary resistance for different muscle groups and increase resistance during the eccentric part of each contraction.

While many of these exercises can be done without equipment, to add variety, you may wish to try them using a towel to pull on (biceps curls) or a broomstick (overhead press). This is a balanced program of four lower-body and five upper-body exercises. Do not count reps. Perform each exercise for a minute and work up to two to three sets (Fig. 5-11).

Partner Resistance Exercises

A. Leg extension (quadriceps)

   Sit on a bench or chair. Move one leg from flexion to full extension and back as partner resists by pressing on front of lower leg.

B. Hamstring curl (hamstrings, gluteus)

   Lie face down while partner straddles your back and places a hand on each ankle. Bend knees and curl calves toward buttocks as your partner resists. Continue the resistance as you return to the starting position.

C. Inner/outer thigh press (thigh adductors and abductors)

   Sit, facing each other, legs forward, hands behind hips for balance. One partner places both feet inside the other's feet and presses outward as the other partner resists by pressing inward. Switch positions after six to eight reps.

D. Foot flexion (anterior tibialis)

   Sit with legs extended. Partner kneels and presses down on top of both feet as you flex them and then return to extension.

E. Overhead press (deltoids, triceps)

   Sit with hands at shoulder level, palms up. As partner resists, press up toward ceiling and then return to starting position.

F. Lat pull (latissimus dorsi)

   Sit and reach high overhead to grasp partner's hands. As partner resists, pull down to shoulder level and slowly return to starting position.

G. Elbow press forward (pectorals)

   Sit with elbows out and hands touching shoulders. As partner resists at the elbows, pull them in toward your midline and return to starting position.

H. Elbow press backward (rhomboids)

   Sit with elbows out or with arms crossed. Partner sits behind, pressing on your elbows as you press back, pulling shoulder blades together. As partner continues resistance, return to starting position.

I. Biceps curl (biceps)

   Stand, palms facing upward. Partner resists on your palms as you curl arm from extension to flexion and back. This may also be done holding a towel in one hand in front of body. Partner sits or kneels facing you, resisting on other end of towel as you curl your arm.

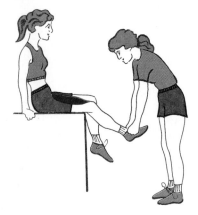

(a) Leg extension

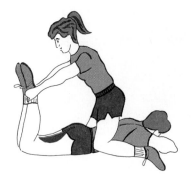

(b) Hamstring curl

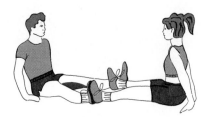

(c) Inner/outer thigh press

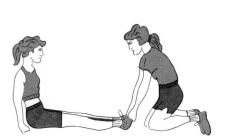

(d) Foot flexion

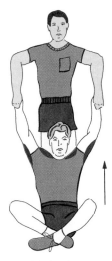

(e) Overhead press

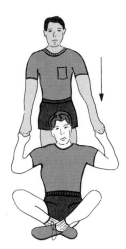

(f) Lat pull

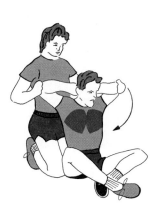

(g) Elbow press forward

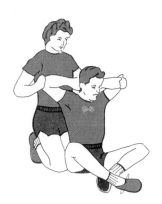

(h) Elbow press backward

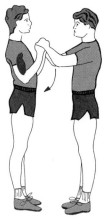

(i) Biceps curl

figure 5-11   Partner strength exercises.

frequently asked questions

Q. What are the advantages and disadvantages of stretching with a partner?

A. On the plus side, stretching with a partner adds a social element that makes it more fun. It's a good way to get to know your classmates if you stretch with different people. You can relax while your partner stretches you, so you may get a better stretch. On the minus side, you and your partner must communicate well to minimize risk of overstretching and it takes longer than stretching alone. A good compromise is to do a few partner stretches along with individual stretches.

Q. Which is better, free weights or machines?

A. It depends on your goals. A beginner will improve with overload from either system. Machines are safer and you don't need a spotter, but they are expensive to buy or you need access to a gym. With free weights, you need a spotter for safety, but they are inexpensive so you can have a set at home. Free weights allow a greater variety of exercises than machines and develop balance, timing, and muscular fitness, so many athletes prefer them. If you have access to both, start with machines, and as you gain strength, gradually work in a few free weight exercises to see which you like better.

Q. I just started a weight training program. How long until I see results?

A. Rate of improvement varies with individuals—some gain quickly, others more slowly. If you are lifting 2 to 3 days a week using a general program of 1 to 2 sets of 8 to 12 reps at 75 percent 1 rep max, you may begin increasing reps or load within 3 to 4 weeks. The most rapid gains are seen in the first 6 months, but people can continue to improve for

years. Other factors affecting rate of improvement include good nutrition, adequate recovery between workouts, and sufficient sleep.

Q. Should I take creatine to help build muscle mass? Is it safe?

A. Creatine supplements appear to enhance performance in repeated bursts of maximal activities like weight lifting. Research is ongoing to see if it really increases muscle mass or weight due to water retention. Potential adverse effects include muscle cramps, diarrhea and gastrointestinal pain, and dehydration and kidney dysfunction. Long-term effects on other sites including the brain, heart, liver, and reproductive organs are not known. Creatine is considered a dietary supplement and not a drug, so manufacturer's claims of performance and safety do not have to be substantiated by the U. S. Food and Drug Administration.

Q. I have been doing 100 abdominal crunches a day for 6 weeks and still my abdominals aren't flat. Why? They feel really strong and tight.

A. A layer of fat often overlays the abdominals, giving them a rounded appearance. Crunches will strengthen the abdominals, making them feel firm. If you are overweight, diet will help reduce the fat layer to get the results you seek. If you are normal weight, then check your posture— habitually standing with an overarched lower back will make the abdominals protrude even if they are firm.

Q. When I stop exercising, will my muscles turn into fat?

A. No. Muscle and fat (adipose tissue) are made up of different types of cells. Lack of exercise allows muscles to atrophy and turn flabby. Without exercise, a person burns fewer calories and may add pounds of fat. Muscle tissue can no more be turned into fat tissue than a cat can be turned into a dog!

summary

Muscular strength, muscular endurance, and flexibility exercises are a vital supplement to a regular program of aerobic exercise. They can enhance appearance by improving the shape, firmness, and tone of muscles. Enhanced posture, decreased risk of lower back pain, greater ease of movement, improved athletic performance, and more energy are benefits. While injury is possible in any exercise program if safety guidelines are ignored, sensible strengthening and stretching programs decrease risk of injury for those who participate in health-related fitness programs or athletics.

Sample Flexibility Program

Equipment needed:
None.

Purpose:
To experience a flexibility program.

Procedure:
Read the "Flexibility" section in Chapter 5, then complete these exercises.

Flexibility Exercises

Exercise	*Repetitions*
Hamstring stretch	_____
Lower back/hip flexor stretch	_____
Spinal twist	_____
Quadriceps stretch	_____
Calf stretch	_____
Iliotibial band stretch	_____
Deltoid stretch	_____
Pectoral stretch	_____
Triceps stretch	_____

Results:

1. What are three things you learned about flexibility training by doing this program?

2. What did you learn about your flexibility levels in different body areas?

3. What did you like/dislike about this type of program?

Resistance Training Log

Exercise	Seat/Pad	Date															
		Reps/Sets															
		Reps/Sets															
		Reps/Sets															
		Reps/Sets															
		Reps/Sets															
		Reps/Sets															
		Reps/Sets															
		Reps/Sets															
		Reps/Sets															
		Reps/Sets															
		Reps/Sets															
		Reps/Sets															
		Reps/Sets															
		Reps/Sets															
		Reps/Sets															
		Reps/Sets															
		Reps/Sets															

lab activity @ chapter five

Name _____

Class/Activity Section _____

Date _____

Weight Training Experience

Equipment needed:

Weight training machines or free weights.

Purpose:

To experience a weight-training program.

Procedure:

Read the "Weight Training" section then select one of the weight-training programs listed and perform the exercises using a weight that you can lift 8 to 12 repetitions for one to two sets. As this is an introductory session, use light weights and concentrate on correct form, rhythm, and breathing. If you want to perform and compare the two types of programs, rest 1 day between workouts for best results. If assigned by your instructor, track your weight-training program on the Resistance Training Log.

Weight-Training Exercises

(Choose one program)

Machines	Weight	Repetitions	Free Weight	Weight	Repetitions
Leg press	_____	_____	Squats	_____	_____
Leg extension	_____	_____	Lunge	_____	_____
Hamstring curl	_____	_____	Calf raise	_____	_____
Toe press	_____	_____	Bench press	_____	_____
Bench press	_____	_____	Supine flys	_____	_____
Military press	_____	_____	Military press	_____	_____
Lat pull	_____	_____	Bent over rowing	_____	_____
Triceps press	_____	_____	Triceps press	_____	_____
Biceps curl	_____	_____	Biceps curl	_____	_____

Results:

1. What are three things you learned about weight training by doing this program?

2. If you tried both types of weight training, how did they compare? Which did you prefer and why?

3. What did you learn about your strength levels in different muscle groups?

Elastic Band
Workout

Equipment needed:
Elastic bands.

Purpose:
To experience a strength-training workout with elastic bands.

Procedure:
Read the "Elastic Resistance" section in Chapter 5, then perform the exercises for 8 to 12 repetitions for one to two sets. As this is an introductory session, concentrate on correct form, rhythm, and breathing. See the handy pullout illustrating these exercises at the back of this text. If assigned by your instructor, track your program on the Resistance Training Log.

Elastic Band Exercises

Exercise	Repetitions
Squats	_____
Leg extension	_____
Hamstring curl	_____
Side leg lift	_____
Inner thigh lift	_____
Push-ups	_____
Deltoid raise	_____
Lat pull	_____
Rowing	_____
Biceps curl	_____
Triceps extension	_____

Results:

1. What are three things you learned about resistance training with elastic bands by doing this program?

2. What did you learn about your strength levels in different muscle groups?

lab activity
5–5

Exercises for Muscular Endurance, Shaping, and Toning

Equipment needed:

None.

Purpose:

To shape and tone muscles without weights.

Procedure:

Read "How to Shape and Tone without Weights", then perform the exercises for 15 to 20 repetitions for one to two sets. As this is an introductory session, concentrate on correct form, rhythm, and breathing. If assigned by your instructor, track your program on the Resistance Training Log.

Exercise	Repetitions
Abdominal curls	_____
Oblique abdominal curls	_____
Side leg lift	_____
Inner thigh lift	_____
Rear leg lift	_____
Backward lunge	_____
Wall sit	_____
Push-ups or dips	_____
Negative pull-ups	_____
Shoulder shrugs	_____
Rhomboid row	_____

lab activity @ chapter five.

Results:

1. What are three things you learned about strength training without weights by doing this program?

2. If you tried other programs, how did they compare? What did you prefer and why?

3. What did you learn about your strength levels in different muscle groups?

Partner Resistance Exercises

Equipment needed:

A partner, bench or chair, and towel to dry off sweat.

Purpose:

To experience a partner resistance-training program.

Procedure:

Read the section on "Partner Resistance Exercises" in Chapter 5, then complete these exercises.

Partner Resistance Exercises

Exercise	Repetitions
Leg extension	_____
Hamstring curl	_____
Inner thigh press	_____
Outer thigh press	_____
Foot flexion	_____
Overhead press	_____
Lat pull	_____
Elbow press forward	_____
Elbow press backward	_____
Biceps curl	_____

Results:

1. What are three things you learned about partner resistance exercises by doing this program?

2. What did you like/dislike about this type of resistance training?

lab activity
5–7

Changing Behavior Using the Transtheoretical Model

Using a highlighter, trace a path on the algorithm as you answer each question. Highlight your stage of change.

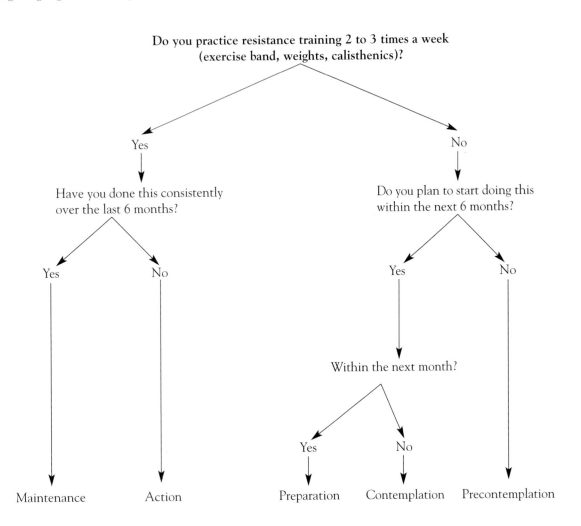

lab activity @ chapter five

Once you have identified which stage of change you are in, it is important to use the processes that will help you to progress to the next stage or remain in the maintenance stage.

In the box, write your stage of change from the previous page. List the processes that are most useful in that stage (see Fig. 2-2 in Chapter 2). Use *only* the processes that apply to your stage of behavior change. You may not need to use all six given. Under each process, give two specific behavior strategies (see Table 2-1 in Chapter 2) that could help you progress to the next stage—or maintain behavior, if you are in the maintenance stage.

The stage I am in is [   ].

Process 1.   _____

      Behavior strategy A.

      Behavior strategy B.

Process 2.   _____

      Behavior strategy A.

      Behavior strategy B.

Process 3.   _____

      Behavior strategy A.

      Behavior strategy B.

Process 4.   _____

      Behavior strategy A.

      Behavior strategy B.

Process 5.   _____

      Behavior strategy A.

      Behavior strategy B.

Process 6.   _____

      Behavior strategy A.

      Behavior strategy B.

Using HealthQuest

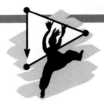

Measurement of Strength

In the HealthQuest Fitness module, click on Web Links, then click on Health and Human Performance Discipline Page. On the Discipline Page, click on Student Success Center, then click on "Assessment Activities". Scroll down Physical Activity Labs. The "Measurement of Strength Lab" includes tests of grip strength, back strength, bench press, and leg strength.

Evaluating Muscular Endurance Using Weights or Weight Machines

In the HealthQuest Fitness module, click on Web Links, then click on Health and Human Performance Discipline Page. On the Discipline Page, click on Student Success Center, then click on "Assessment Activities". Scroll down Physical Activity Labs. The lab "Evaluating Muscular Endurance Using Weights or Weight Machines" is an alternate way to evaluate muscular endurance and gives information on your muscular fitness using seven different lifts. Chapter 4 of this text also contains instructions and norms for evaluating muscular endurance using push-ups and abdominal curls.

Don't wait for your ship to come in. Row
out to meet it.
— H. Jackson Brown, Jr., ed. *Dad, a Father's Book of Wisdom*

Exploring Special Exercise Considerations

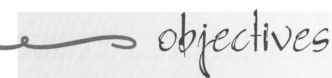

After reading this chapter, you will be able to:

1. Identify the physiological bases for differences in men's and women's exercise performance levels.
2. List the similarities in men's and women's responses to exercise.
3. Define *amenorrhea, oligomenorrhea, Kegel exercise,* and *stress incontinence.*
4. Identify correct recommendations for exercise during pregnancy.
5. Describe exercise addiction.
6. Describe how exercise impacts disease resistance.
7. Identify recommendations for safe exercise in hot and cold weather.
8. Identify the best replacement fluids to prevent dehydration during exercise in hot weather.
9. Identify the safe exercises from a list of safe and contraindicated exercises.
10. Identify the effects of a regular program of exercise on the aging process.

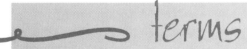

- Amenorrhea
- Contraindicated exercises
- Dysmenorrhea
- Endorphins
- Electrolytes
- Estrogen
- Exercise addiction
- Female athlete triad
- Hemoglobin
- Hyperthermia
- Hypothermia
- Kegel exercises
- Menarche
- Oligomenorrhea
- Stress incontinence

This chapter brings together several concerns related to exercise participation. Seven major areas are addressed: similarities and differences in men's and women's exercise performance, females and exercise, males and exercise, exercise addiction, environmental considerations, contraindicated exercises, and aging and physical activity.

Similarities and Differences in Men's and Women's Exercise Performance

While performance levels may differ, men and women respond to exercise in a similar manner. Although women have approximately 20 percent lower maximal oxygen uptake than men (due to smaller heart size), with exercise they show similar rates of improvement. Performance levels differ for several reasons. Due to hormonal changes during puberty, a woman adds fat because of estrogen, while a man's muscle mass doubles because of testosterone. In fact, women have half as much muscle tissue to move their weight and more inactive fat weight to carry. In addition, men's greater muscle mass gives them 30 percent to 40 percent greater strength. Women commonly have a smaller heart, a smaller thoracic cage, and lower blood volume than men, all of which may limit performance.

Women have fewer red blood cells than men and about 10 percent to 15 percent less **hemoglobin** (the oxygen-carrying component of red blood cells), so their blood has less oxygen-carrying capacity, which may limit endurance. Even though women are at a disadvantage in terms of physical performance, they benefit equally from aerobic exercise in terms of fitness improvement. Training effect benefits, such as loss of fat from deposit areas, increased bone density, and decreased exercise heart rates, are similar for men and women. When differences in body size are taken into account, fitness gains for men and women are *essentially* the same.

Some women fear that exercise will make them develop large or bulky muscles or a masculine appearance. This is not likely unless a woman is using anabolic steroids and spending many hours in extremely strenuous weight training. Potential for muscular development is genetically determined by levels of the sex hormone testosterone, and women have only one-tenth as much of this hormone as men. While women, like men, vary in their potential for muscular size development, what most women want from exercise is exactly what they will gain: decreased fat; increased lean body tissue; and firmer, toned muscles.

Females and Exercise

Once, the sight of a female training on the road or competing in a race was sufficiently unusual that people would stop and stare. As late as 1965, women were threatened with banishment from international competition if they ran races longer than 1.5 miles, and it was 1984 before the first women's Olympic marathon took place. As the interest in fitness as a lifestyle has grown, so has the number of women participants in aerobic activities and athletics. Now that large numbers of females have adopted a physically active lifestyle, research has provided us with new information concerning topics of special interest to women.

Menstruation

Is it safe to exercise during menstruation? Yes. Menstruation is only one small part of the ongoing female reproductive cycle. In the past, women sometimes used this as an excuse to avoid exercise, but now women are encouraged to lead a normal routine during all parts of the reproductive cycle. Menstrual cycle hormones affect heart rate; ventilation rate; basal body temperature; and blood hematocrit, the red cell portion of the total blood volume. How women experience menstruation varies greatly. Some feel no different than usual; some may experience abdominal and leg cramps, backache, or mood swings, particularly during the first two days of the menstrual flow.

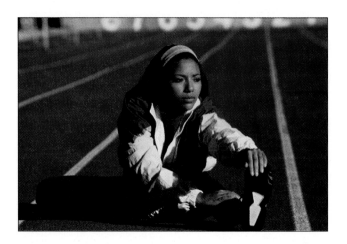

More women are discovering the joys of physical activity.

Dysmenorrhea, or painful menstruation, is probably neither caused nor cured by exercise. However, there is some evidence that enhanced fitness leads to a reduction in menstrual complaints, although this is still being researched. Some studies indicate that exercise decreases mood swings and relieves depression, anxiety, and irritability. Excess body water lost through perspiration can reduce weight gain due to water retention, relieving premenstrual bloating and edema. While there are no specific exercises that cure severe cramps, participation in a program of regular exercise has been shown to decrease the frequency of minor menstrual cramps. This is perhaps due to increased abdominal tone, increased circulation to the uterus, or increased levels of pain-relieving **endorphins.**

Menstruation should be treated as a normal physiological function, not an illness. As long as she is comfortable, a woman should continue her regular exercise program. For women who want to look and feel their best, exercise is beneficial at any time of the month.

Studies indicate that young girls who exercise vigorously may experience a delay in **menarche,** the start of their menstrual cycle, decreasing their risk of cancer later in life. While the average American girl experiences menarche between 11 and 12 years of age, those who train vigorously experience their first menstrual cycle at an average age of 15½, the same as the average age for menarche 100 years ago. This delay may be natural and even desirable, because it reduces the body's lifetime exposure to **estrogen,** a female sex hormone. The more menstrual cycles a woman has over her lifetime, the longer her exposure to estrogen and the greater her risk of cancer of the breast and reproductive organs. In addition, women who exercise tend to be leaner, thus producing less potent estrogen. In one study, women who had been athletic in high school and college as compared to sedentary women had half the incidence of breast and reproductive cancer in later life. In fact, a sedentary lifestyle is considered a primary risk factor for cancer.

Menstrual abnormalities, such as **oligomenorrhea** (infrequent or irregular menses) and **amenorrhea** (absent menses), occur in about 3 to 5 percent of the general population of women and in up to 10 to 25 percent of women athletes. In athletes, the prevalence appears high in sports that require greater intensity, frequency, and duration of training (e.g., distance running and swimming) or sports that emphasize low body weight or involve competition by weight class (e.g., dance, gymnastics, boxing, wrestling). Numerous factors, physiologic and psychologic, including change in diet or inadequate diet and physical and emotional stress, may affect menstruation abnormally (for example, stressors such as heavy athletic training and competition acting synergistically with other stressors in life). Weight loss and rate of weight loss (with extremely low body fat) have also been identified as probable causes of menstrual abnormalities. Some female athletes and other physically active women who are underweight and nonmenstruating are being diag-

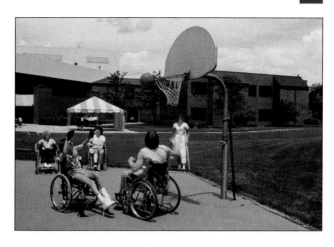

Everybody benefits from physical activity.

nosed as victims of the **female athlete triad.** This is a life-threatening syndrome marked by three disorders:

- disordered eating habits (inadequate food . . . energy intake insufficient to meet metabolic demands)
- amenorrhea
- osteoporosis

Societal pressure on females to have an unrealistically low body weight fuels this condition. Fitness professionals who work with physically active females should learn ways to prevent, recognize, treat, and reduce its risks.

Exercise-induced oligomenorrhea and amenorrhea are rare in women doing moderate amounts of exercise as part of a fitness program. They are more frequent among those whose menstrual cycles started late, past age 15, or who had a history of irregularity before starting exercise programs. Although no specific body fat percentage has been associated with the development of exercise-induced amenorrhea, the evidence suggests that decreased fat levels may lead to a decreased production of one form of estrogen. Thus, as fat percentages decrease, estrogen levels decline and the evidence of amenorrhea increases. Some scientists have suggested that the critical body fat level may be as low as 13 percent or that there may be no such critical level. If such a critical fat percentage does exist, it probably varies widely from individual to individual.

The focus of research is upon how all of the factors mentioned may affect the hypothalamus, thereby influencing the production of important regulatory hormones relative to menstruation and metabolism, including estrogen, epinephrine, and corticoids. Whatever the cause, exercise-induced amenorrhea is considered reversible. Normal menstrual cycles resume with as minor a change in lifestyle as a 10 percent decrease in exercise, improved nutrition, or a weight gain of 4 to 5 pounds. Also, exercise-induced amenorrhea does not seem to affect long-term fertility. While a woman with amenorrhea does not experience a regular menstrual cycle, it is still possible for her to ovulate and become

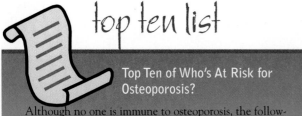

Top Ten of Who's At Risk for Osteoporosis?

Although no one is immune to osteoporosis, the following factors increase one's risk:

1. Female.
2. Postmenopausal.
3. Amenorrheic.
4. Small-boned.
5. Eating a diet low in calcium.
6. Drinking high quantities of alcohol and/or caffeinated beverages.
7. Eating a diet high in protein.
8. A sedentary lifestyle.
9. Smoking.
10. A family history of osteoporosis.
    Note: Some vegetarian diets also increase the risk.

pregnant. She should not rely on this for birth control and should continue her regular birth control method if pregnancy is not desired. Any active woman should be aware of her normal menstrual cycle and should discuss any irregularities with her physician to rule out such conditions as thyroid disorders, ovarian cysts, brain tumors, and pregnancy.

There is concern that low estrogen levels during amenorrhea accelerate bone mineral loss, increasing the risk of osteoporosis. Estrogen, exercise, and calcium must be present for a woman to build or maintain bone mass. An excess of one element will not make up for an absence of another. While people who exercise tend to have greater bone densities than do nonexercisers, loss of estrogen, regardless of age, may cause an irreversible loss of bone strength. A 20-year-old amenorrheic athlete can have the bone density of a 50-year-old. While bone density does increase with a resumption in normal estrogen levels, it does not appear to recover fully. If an amenorrheic athlete has a low estrogen level, lifestyle change and/or low-dose estrogen replacement therapy to prevent bone mineral loss should be discussed with a physician. In addition, a calcium intake of 1,500 mg/day (about 5 cups of milk) is recommended. See the top ten list for "Who's at Risk for Osteoporosis?"

Pregnancy

Is exercise advisable during pregnancy? How much? What are the benefits? Are there any limitations or cautions to keep in mind? Are some exercises better than others? Pregnancy is a natural and normal physiological function, not an illness. A pregnant woman is not fragile. She will be health-

ier and the pregnancy safer if she remains active. Any pregnant woman should obtain medical clearance from her physician before beginning or continuing an exercise program. General advice for a healthy woman having an uncomplicated pregnancy is to continue her regular exercise program, being careful not to get overtired. If she has not been exercising before pregnancy, this is not a time to begin a crash program. A 20- to 30-minute walk, 3 to 4 days per week, is a program a doctor might approve. Throughout pregnancy, to keep the effort aerobic, a woman should use the "talk test." She should be able to carry on a conversation while exercising without getting out of breath. In early pregnancy, if exercising seems to require more effort, decrease intensity and duration. Particular care should be taken to avoid overheating, which has been linked to increased risk of central nervous system abnormalities (such as spina bifida) in the baby. For this reason, steam rooms and saunas are contraindicated. Pregnant women also should be counseled not to undertake excessive physical activity in a hot climate to which they are not acclimated. A gradual weight gain, which is natural and desirable, is likely to increase stress to joints, ligaments, and muscles. Also, muscles and connective tissues become more lax as they gradually undergo hormonal changes. Increases in the pregnancy hormone relaxin help to facilitate the baby's birth but make the pregnant woman more susceptible to strains and sprains. Therefore, during late pregnancy and the early postdelivery period, vigorous increases in flexibility should not be pursued.

In the fifth to sixth months of pregnancy, due to increasing weight and joint flexibility, impact activities may become uncomfortable. At this time, many women switch to low- or no-impact exercises such as walking, swimming, or stationary cycling. While some women continue their normal exercise program to the day of delivery with no ill effects, don't feel guilty if you feel a need to cut back. Toward the end of pregnancy, if you fatigue easily and exercise seems to require more effort, it is natural to decrease the activity level. After the fourth month, it is not advised to do exercises that require lying on your back. This position can block the blood supply to the uterus (by compressing the aorta and/or the vena cava), re-

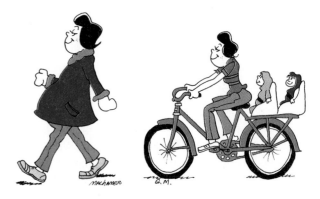

Exercise during and after pregnancy has many advantages.

table 6-1   ACOG Guidelines for Exercise During Pregnancy and Postpartum

1. Regular exercise (at least three times per week) is preferable to intermittent activity. Competitive activities should be discouraged.
2. Vigorous exercise should not be performed in hot, humid weather or when you have a fever.
3. Ballistic movements (jerky, bouncy motions) should be avoided. Exercise should be done on a wooden floor or a tightly carpeted surface to reduce shock and provide a sure footing.
4. Deep flexion or extension of joints should be avoided because of connective tissue laxity. Activities that require jumping, jarring motions, or rapid changes in direction should be avoided because of joint instability.
5. Vigorous exercise should be preceded by a 5-minute period of muscle warm-up. This can be accomplished by slow walking or stationary cycling with low resistance.
6. Vigorous exercise should be followed by a period of gradually declining activity that includes gentle stationary stretching. Because connective tissue laxity increases the risk of joint injury, stretches should not be taken to the point of maximum resistance.
7. Heart rate should be measured at times of peak activity. Target heart rates and limits established in consultation with a physician should not be exceeded.
8. Care should be taken to gradually rise from the floor to avoid a sudden drop in blood pressure. Some form of activity involving the legs should be continued for a brief period.
9. No exercise should be performed while lying on the back after the first trimester. This slows blood flow back to the heart and decreases its output. Also, avoid *motionless standing,* which may also decrease heart output.
10. Exercises that employ the Valsalva maneuver should be avoided.
11. Caloric intake should be adequate to meet not only the extra energy needs of pregnancy, but also of the exercise performed.
12. Maternal core temperature should not exceed 38°C (100.4°F).
13. Liquids should be taken liberally before and after exercise to prevent dehydration. If necessary, activity should be interrupted to replenish fluids.
14. Women who have led sedentary lifestyles should begin with physical activity of low intensity and advance activity levels gradually.
15. Activity should be stopped and the physician consulted if any unusual symptoms appear. (See Table 6-2.)

sulting in depression of the fetal heart rate. Throughout pregnancy, a woman needs to listen to her body and adjust exercise to maintain comfort. Specific pregnancy exercise guidelines from the American College of Obstetricians and Gynecologists are listed in Table 6-1. Also review Table 6-2.

There are many reasons exercise is important during pregnancy. The physiological changes of pregnancy place a great demand on the body. Labor and delivery are perhaps the most physically demanding events a woman will experience. Exercise can maintain optimal fitness, enabling a woman to control weight gain, improve muscle tone, improve posture, decrease backache, and decrease constipation. Exercise can also aid in increasing energy, increasing psychological well-being, managing stress, enhancing sleep at night, and regaining her prepregnancy figure.

While fitness is no guarantee of a quick labor or easy delivery, endurance and increased capacity to deal with the physical stress of childbirth are assets that come from fitness. A fit mother can enjoy a quicker recovery from childbirth and can regain her normal fitness and activity levels in less time than can the unfit.

Stress Incontinence

Stress incontinence, an involuntary leakage of urine when you laugh, cough, sneeze, or exercise, is a common problem, particularly in women over 30 who have given birth. During pregnancy and birth, these muscles become weakened and stretched. One solution is to wear a sanitary pad, but a better approach is to strengthen the perineal muscles that control this function. The pelvic floor is a hammocklike muscle

table 6-2   Reasons to Discontinue Exercise and Seek Medical Advice During Pregnancy

1. Any signs of bloody discharge from the vagina.
2. Any "gush" of fluid from the vagina.
3. Sudden swelling of the ankles, hands, or face.
4. Persistent, severe headaches and/or visual disturbance; unexplained spell of faintness or dizziness.
5. Swelling, pain, and redness in the calf of one leg (phlebitis).
6. Elevation of pulse rate or blood pressure that persists after exercise.
7. Excessive fatigue, palpitations, chest pain.
8. Persistant contractions (more than six to eight per hour) that may suggest onset of premature labor.
9. Unexplained abdominal pain.
10. Insufficient weight gain during the last two trimesters.

layer attached at the front and back of the pelvis. It supports the pelvic organs, including the bladder, uterus, and rectum. Kegel exercises, named after the Los Angeles physician who developed them, strengthen the pelvic floor muscles and may prevent or cure stress incontinence. As a side benefit, many women report increased pleasure during intercourse.

Kegel Exercise

Kegel exercises are done by contracting perineal muscles, which surround the bladder neck and vagina. To learn the exercise, when urinating stop and start the flow. Hold the contraction for 3 to 4 seconds during the stop phase. The muscle action you take to do this when urinating is the action you

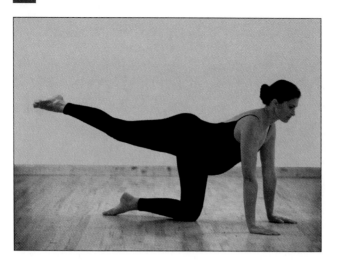

No exercise should be performed while lying on the back after the first trimester.

must take when doing Kegel exercises. You can do these exercises anytime—contract hard and then release. Do 10 in a row, and work up to five sets of 10 daily. These exercises should be done before, during, and after pregnancy.

Postpartum: Getting Back into Shape

Giving birth and coping with the demands of a new baby are both joyful and stressful for a new mother. The main problem in resuming exercise is not fatigue or shortness of breath, which might be expected, but finding someone to watch the baby while mother takes a well-deserved break. Postpartum recovery times vary greatly. If the delivery has been normal, walking is encouraged in the hospital the day after delivery. This can be continued when the woman returns home. Rest, good nutrition, and a progressive walking program will make recovery faster than will complete inactivity or resuming prepregnancy activity levels too soon. You should not rush into impact activities such as jogging or pursue flexibility increases until you have given loosened joints (due to the hormone relaxin) a chance to recover—6 to 16 weeks. Abdominal curls are important for toning overstretched abdominal muscles and preventing back problems. Also, do Kegel exercises to strengthen pelvic floor muscles.

A nursing mother needs to avoid fatigue and dehydration, which may reduce milk production. Drink eight or more glasses of fluid a day, and nap when the baby does to ensure adequate rest. Wear a good supportive bra, with pads to control leaks, and nurse before exercise for greater comfort. There is no conflict between nursing a baby and moderate exercise. Both help a mother regain her prepregnancy figure.

Breast Support

Does bouncing cause breasts to sag? Some believe that breast movement stretches the skin and ligaments that support the breasts. There is no evidence to support this claim; the main culprits are genetics and pregnancy. Still, a good bra makes exercise more comfortable by reducing breast movement during activity. The best designs flatten breasts to redistribute their mass across the chest wall. This results in less mass for gravity to affect. Racerback and crossback straps prevent slippage off the shoulder. Certain designs are more suited to small-breasted women, while others are more comfortable for large-breasted exercisers. A woman should try different styles to decide what is best for her. A good exercise bra should (1) limit breast movement; (2) have wide straps that do not slip off the shoulders; (3) have a wide band at the bottom to prevent the bra from riding up; (4) have no rough seams or uncovered fasteners to prevent chafing; and (5) be made of nonabrasive materials and be seamless, or at least have seams that do not cross the nipple area.

Males and Exercise

Participation in sports and physical activities no longer ends with graduation from high school or college. Large numbers of men are continuing or beginning lifetime exercise programs.

Exercise appears to lower the hormonal levels of males as it does of females. In one study, testosterone levels of men who ran 40 miles a week averaged 30 percent less than the levels of nonexercisers. The runners' levels were still in a normal range, and the effect was reversible. Sperm count and libido were not affected. While it may lower hormonal levels, overtraining is not associated with decreased fertility in male athletes unless accompanied by anorexic behavior and a high-stress lifestyle.

A more common male fertility problem results from constantly wearing tight undershorts. For the testicles to maintain normal sperm production, they must be a few degrees cooler than normal body temperature. Their position outside and slightly away from the body accomplishes this. When the testicles are overheated by consistently being held close to the body, sperm production temporarily decreases. A switch to boxer shorts solves the problem.

Male bicyclists have additional concerns. Males who ride for extended periods (i.e., 2 to 3 hours or more) have increased risk of reduced perineal (crouch) area circulation. It is caused by compression of the bike saddle. This can lead to pain; numbness; and, in severe cases, male impotence. Females are not exempt from this problem. Reduced perineal circulation in females may result in sexual and urinary tract dysfunction. Male bicyclists traveling over rough terrain may also experience pain and injury to the testicles. The following tips will help avoid these problems:

- Level the seat or point the nose downward to reduce pressure on the perineum.
- Lower the seat so the legs support more weight. (Knees should bend slightly at the bottom of the pedal stroke.)

- Avoid handlebar extensions because they place more body weight on the nose of the seat.
- Stand up and pedal every 10 minutes to encourage blood flow in the perineum.
- Rise out of the seat when going over bumps.
- Avoid crush injuries involving the top tube by riding a bike of proper size. The top tube of a mountain bike should be 3 to 4 inches below the crotch when standing over it; for road bikes, clearance should be 1 to 2 inches.
- Consider replacing a narrow racing-style saddle with a wider seat or a seat designed to reduce compression on the perineum. Special "male" seats are available.
- Switch to a recumbent bike.

Exercise Addiction

Exercising is unconditionally great for the body, the soul, and the mind, right? Almost but not quite. Even the most benign or beneficial elements can cause harm when taken to an extreme. Although exercise is highly recommended for health and vigor, it is not protected from this universal truth. When a commitment to exercise crosses the line to dependency and compulsion, it can create physical, social, and psychological havoc for those involved.

A "positive addiction" can be a healthy adaptation to the barriers to exercise in life because commitments to work, family, and other healthy pursuits must compete for time to work out. Sometimes the line between commitment and compulsion is crossed. There can be a negative side to exercise that gradually, insidiously takes over the positive. Other addictions such as compulsive gambling and compulsive shopping and substance abuse are discussed in Chapter 13.

Exercise addiction is not just another term for overtraining syndrome. Healthy athletes training for peak performance and competition can suffer overtraining symptoms, the short-term result of too little rest and recovery. **Exercise addiction,** on the other hand, is a chronic loss of perspective of the role of exercise in a full life. A healthy athlete and an exercise addict may share similar levels of training volume. The difference is in the attitude and the consequences. An addicted individual isn't able to see value in unrelated activities and pursues his activity even when it is against his best interest.

The exercise addict has lost balance allowing exercise to become overvalued compared to elements widely recognized as giving meaning to a full life (i.e., school, work, friends, family, community involvement). When emotional connections are passed up in favor of additional hours of training; when injury, illness, and fatigue don't

stop a workout; when all free time is consumed by training— *exercise addiction* is the diagnosis. Withdrawal symptoms like anxiety, irritability, and depression, which appear when circumstances prevent exercise, are the warning signs of addiction.

To the addict, there is no exception to the rule, "the more the better." Anything that interferes with the quest for more exercise is resented.

The paradox inherent in exercise addiction is the blurred boundary between what is healthy, admirable, and desirable, and behavior that is over the edge and dependent. The addict answers poor performance with more exercise and less rest. A healthy athlete looks at the big picture and adjusts training programs, allowing for rest and recovery among the training variables.

Remember that working out should always have an element of play. If exercising loses all aspects of fun, something has gone wrong. The most competitive athletes still love their sport. They love it because it gives pleasure and not because it has become a compulsive need. Take the self assessment in Table 6-3 to see if you are losing your perspective on exercise.

table 6-3 — Are You Addicted to Exercise?

Directions: Rate yourself as honestly as you can on the following checklist.

Yes	No	
___	___	1. I have missed important social obligations and family events in order to exercise.
___	___	2. I have given up other interests, including time with friends, to make more time to exercise.
___	___	3. Missing a workout makes me irritable and depressed.
___	___	4. I only feel content when I am exercising or within the hour after exercising.
___	___	5. I like exercise better than sex, good food, or a movie—there's almost nothing I'd rather do.
___	___	6. I work out even if I'm sick, injured, or exhausted. I'll feel better when I get moving.
___	___	7. In addition to my regular exercise schedule, I'll exercise more if I find extra time.
___	___	8. Family and friends have told me I'm too involved in exercise.
___	___	9. I have a history (or family history) of anxiety or depression.

Scoring: If you have checked "yes" on three or more of the statements, you may be losing your perspective on exercise.

Exercise and Disease Resistance

During exercise, 75 to 85 percent of the energy produced is released in the form of heat, producing an increase in body temperature. Much of this heat is dissipated at the skin, but body temperature still is elevated during exercise. This regular increase in body temperature, it is speculated, is inhospitable to some viruses and might decrease incidence of viral infections in exercisers. Moderate exercise also has been found to boost the immune system. However, overtraining leading to exhaustion might weaken the system and increase susceptibility to colds and minor infections. Studies on the relationship between the immune system and physical exercise have produced contradictory results. Nonexercisers who start a new program of intense exercise, exceeding their individual exercise limits or who exercise sporadically may experience weakened immunity for a brief period. Highly trained athletes may weaken their immune systems with acute, exhaustive exercise. Of course, psychological and emotional stress may play important roles here, too—whether it be the anxiety felt by the new, out-of-shape exerciser or by the athlete competing for a championship. Few people exercise so strenuously that they need to worry about any possible adverse effects on immunity. The problem for most Americans is too little exercise rather than too much. For anyone in doubt, a consistent and regular program of moderate exercise is a key component of overall health and well-being, including the immune system. However, the optimal level of exercise for each individual's immune system is unknown.

Should you exercise when you have a cold or feel ill? Many professionals recommend that you decrease the intensity and frequency of workouts or take some days off when you have a cold or feel one coming on. Illness affects lung and heart function as well as skeletal muscles. As a result, performance may be reduced. Some people find that exercising when they have a mild cold makes them feel better. Illnesses vary in severity and people react differently to them, so listen to your body. If you only have a minor head cold and otherwise feel fine, it is probably acceptable to work out. Avoid exercise to the point of exhaustion. Avoid exercise if you have the flu, have a fever, feel achy, feel extremely tired, are heavily congested, or have swollen glands. Exercise does not cure illness. The old adage that "you can sweat out a cold" with exercise is untrue. When you do recover from illness, do not start exercising at the same level as before. Give yourself a few days to build back to normal levels.

Environmental Considerations

Exercising in the Cold

Your friends think you're crazy, sharing a narrow roadway with cars that spray you with slush as you exercise on a chilly winter day. Walking, running, and cycling are more complicated in the winter. Still, there is something liberating about a good workout on an icy winter day. Cold weather workouts can be invigorating, comfortable, and safe if you follow these tips:

1. *Layer clothing:* Dress in several thin layers so you can remove or add a layer as needed. Wool and polypropylene clothing wick moisture away from the skin to keep you dry. The outer layer of clothing should be breathable and windproof.
2. *Avoid overheating:* Don't overdress or you'll overheat. You should feel a little cool until you warm up. Do

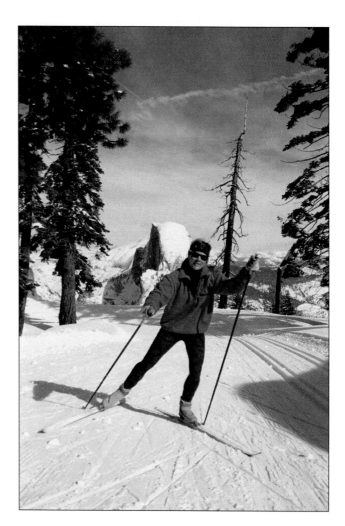

Cold weather workouts can be invigorating, comfortable, and safe.

Windchill Index

Wind speed in MPH	Actual Thermometer Reading (°F)											
	50	40	30	20	10	0	-10	-20	-30	-40	-50	-60
	Equivalent temperature											
Calm	50	40	30	20	10	0	-10	-20	-30	-40	-50	-60
5	48	37	27	16	6	-5	-15	-26	-36	-47	-57	-68
10	40	28	16	4	-9	-21	-33	-46	-58	-70	-83	-95
15	36	22	9	-5	-18	-36	-45	-58	-72	-85	-99	-112
20	32	18	4	-10	-25	-39	-53	-67	-82	-96	-110	-124
25	30	16	0	-15	-29	-44	-59	-74	-88	-104	-118	-133
30	28	13	-2	-18	-33	-48	-63	-79	-94	-109	-125	-140
35	27	11	-4	-20	-35	-49	-67	-82	-98	-113	-129	-145
40	26	10	-6	-21	-37	-53	-69	-85	-100	-116	-132	-148

(Wind speeds greater than 40 MPH have little additional effect)	Little danger (for properly clothed person)	Increasing danger	Great danger
			Danger from freezing of exposed flesh

figure 6-1   Windchill index.
Source: Ball State University Weather Station, Department of Geography.

> # wellness flash
> Up to 40 percent of body heat can be lost through the head.

take the windchill factor into account when preparing for your workout (Fig. 6-1).

3. *Avoid overexposure:* While frostbite is a possibility if you don't dress properly, there is no possibility that you will freeze your lungs or throat. If cold air bothers you, breathe through a bandanna. Frostbite can occur on outer body areas such as the fingers and toes when your skin temperature drops below 32°F. Frostbite can easily be avoided by covering exposed areas and by getting inside and warming up if any body parts feel numb or tingly. **Hypothermia** is a life-threatening condition in which body temperature drops to a dangerously low level. Medical attention should be sought immediately.

4. *Protect exposed parts:* Fingers and toes receive the smallest blood supply and experience winter's chill fastest. Mittens are more effective than gloves, which allow cold air to circulate around the fingers. On extremely cold days, it may be advisable to wear two pairs of socks or a thermal insole if the feet get too cold. Exposed ears or face can lead to windburn or chapping. To avoid discomfort, wear a hat and spread a thin layer of petroleum jelly on exposed skin areas.

5. *Work with the wind:* Plan out-and-back workouts, heading into the wind on the way out so you can return with the wind to your back. Not only will you appreciate the push when you're tired, but you'll be less likely to be chilled by your sweat during the return.

6. *Exercise with caution:* Winter weather changes the safety rules for outdoor exercise: Fewer daylight hours, icy roads, and snowy nights lower visibility for drivers. Exercise at midday as often as possible. Avoid high-volume traffic areas, wear bright clothing, and be prepared for potential hazards by remaining alert. Wear waffled or ridged shoe soles to provide extra traction on icy roads.

7. *Stay motivated:* Winter exercising demands greater personal motivation than exercising at any other time of the year. Winter holidays, less daylight, and poor weather can disrupt a routine. To maintain

enthusiasm, set realistic wintertime goals to work toward. Don't worry about your pace. Between the slick footing and the heavy clothing, it's prudent to run relaxed. Just go fast enough to stay warm.

8. *Be safe:* Tell someone your route and when you expect to be back. Better yet, go with a friend.

Don't hesitate to mix your usual exercise with other activities—cross-country skiing or sledding in snow country, aerobics, stair climbing, indoor cycling, or water exercise if you crave a break from the cold. Your heart will benefit as long as you stay in your training zone, and the cross-training will work new muscle groups.

Exercising in the Heat

Given a couple of weeks and plenty of water, the human body can adapt well to exercise in the heat. Hot-weather workouts make the body work harder than it does in cool weather. The heart must pump enough blood not only to fuel working muscles but also to carry heat to the skin to be dissipated, reducing work capacity. Drinking plenty of cold fluids is critical to maintain sweating, your body's air conditioning system. The body can acclimatize to heat but not to dehydration. Overexertion in hot weather, particularly when coupled with dehydration, can lead to heat cramps; heat exhaustion; heatstroke; or **hyperthermia,** a life-threatening condition in which the body's temperature rises to a dangerous level. Particularly susceptible are people who are over 40, are out of shape, are overweight, have heart disease, or have previously experienced heat injury. See Table 6-4 for symptoms and care of heat cramps, heat exhaustion, and heat stroke.

When performing endurance exercise, men and women have similar responses in adaptability to hot weather. Both genders are equally susceptible to heat stress, and both respond by acclimatization. Women seem to sweat less than men to maintain body temperature. This may indicate that women have a more efficient means of thermoregulation. However, with endurance training, women's level of sweating equals the level of sweating in men. To exercise safety when the weather is hot and humid, follow the Top Ten Guidelines for Hot Weather Exercise and postpone the workout when the Heat Safety Index is in the danger zone or above (Fig. 6–2).

Heavy Sweating During Exercise

One of the hazards of exercising in hot, humid weather is dehydration caused by excessive loss of body water in the form of sweat. Dehydration disturbs cellular fluid and electrolyte balance, thus interfering with muscular contraction. Water losses of as little as 2 to 3 percent of body weight have been shown to impair exercise performance, reduce the amount of time a person can exercise, reduce cardiac stroke volume (volume of blood pumped out with each heartbeat), and reduce cardiac output (the amount of blood pumped by the heart over time). Water loss can also interfere with the body's ability to regulate internal temperature, resulting in overheating, which can be deadly.

Sweat is primarily water, but a number of major **electrolytes** (essential minerals in the form of salts) and other nutrients may be found in varying amounts. Sodium, chloride, and potassium are the predominant electrolytes found in sweat. They help to maintain normal body fluid volume

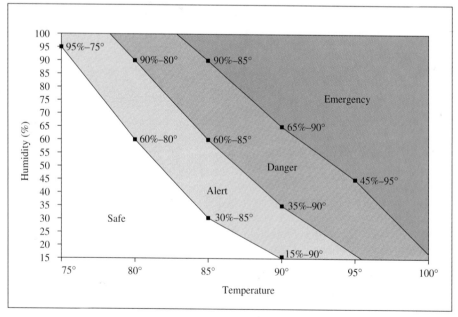

Heat Safety Index

figure 6-2   Heat safety index.
Source: Ball State University Weather Station, Department of Geography.

table 6-4   Heat Illnesses

Condition	Symptoms	Immediate Care
Heat cramps	Painful muscle spasms (calf is common) Sweaty skin Normal body temperature	Isolated cramps: Direct pressure to cramp and release, stretch muscle slowly and gently, gentle massage, ice
Heat exhaustion	Profuse sweating Cold, clammy skin Flu-like symptoms Dizziness Weak, rapid pulse Shallow breathing Headache Normal or slightly above normal temperature	Move individual out of sun to a well-ventilated area Place in shock position (feet elevated 12–18") Gentle massage of extremities Force fluids Reassure May apply wet towels Refer to physician or call EMS
Heat stroke (This is an extreme medical condition)	No perspiration Dry skin Very hot Temperature as high as 106°F Skin color bright red or flushed (African American—ashen) Rapid strong pulse Unresponsiveness (may be confused, stagger, or be agitated)	Transport to hospital quickly (call EMS) Remove as much clothing as possible without exposing the individual Cool quickly starting at the head and continue down the body (use any means possible—fan, hose down, pack in ice) Wrap in cold, wet sheets for transport Treat for shock (place in a semireclining position)

and are involved in nerve impulse transmission and muscle contraction (this includes the heart muscle).

Electrolyte Replacement

Is profuse sweating likely to create an electrolyte deficiency? No. This is not likely to occur, even during prolonged exercise, such as marathon running. This is not to say that electrolyte replacement is not important and that electrolyte deficiency is impossible. After prolonged exercise with heavy sweating, the body's stores of electrolytes are diminished and could eventually become deficient. However, with a normal diet, it is difficult to create an electrolyte deficiency.

Salt tablets are not recommended to replace lost sodium and chloride because these electrolytes are abundant in a normal diet. They may be prescribed for those who cannot replace them through normal dietary means. Keep in mind that diets high in sodium have been associated with high blood pressure. Citrus fruits, fruit juices, and bananas are foods recommended for electrolyte replacement.

Fluid Replacement: Water or Sports Drinks?

Rehydration (replacing body fluid volume) is critical to safe, effective exercise involving heavy sweating. For years, we were told that water is the best drink to replace fluids, because that is mainly what you lose when you sweat during a hard workout. But science is dynamic, and conventional wisdom sometimes becomes history in the light of new discoveries. New information, concerning exercise of *1 hour or more*, now gives the slight edge in fluid replacement to electrolyte-containing beverages such as the popular sports

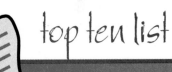

top ten list

Top Ten Guidelines for Hot Weather Exercise

1. Respect the heat. Hot, humid, sunny weather can be deadly.
2. Monitor weather conditions before exercising and adjust your workout accordingly. Postpone exercise when heat safety index is in the danger zone or above.
3. Drink plenty of fluids to avoid dehydration (see Fig. 6-3).
4. Weigh yourself before and after a workout. A sudden loss of weight may signal dehydration.
5. Wear loose-fitting clothing that allows air to circulate and expose as much skin to the air as possible to promote sweat evaporation.
6. Wear light colors because they reflect rather than absorb sunlight.
7. When acclimation to warmer weather in the spring, decrease exercise intensity and duration. Allow 2 weeks to acclimate to normal exercise levels.
8. Check with your doctor about the effects of any medications you take because some can reduce heat tolerance.
9. Do not wear vinyl or rubber sweat suits to lose body weight. They can lead to dehydration and death.
10. Stop exercising at the first sign of heat illness. See Table 6-4.

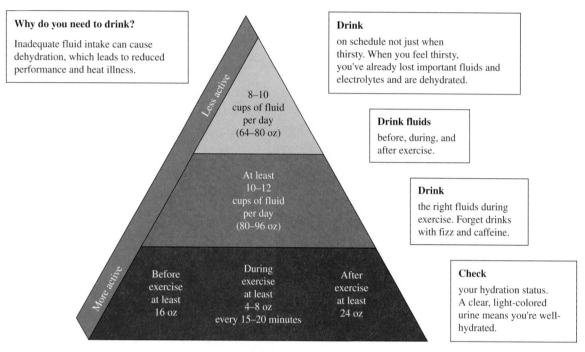

figure 6-3   Use the Fluid Pyramid as a guide to replenish body fluids lost during physical activity

wellness flash

If you lose as little as 1 percent of your body weight, you may be dehydrated and in serious need of fluids.

drinks. This is because fluids, containing electrolytes, are more readily retained in the body's tissues. Why? Because plain water tends to slightly increase urination so fewer fluids remain in the body's tissues. Also, when fluids taste good (as sports drinks do) they are more readily consumed. Thus the intake is increased. Due to these new findings, many commercial beverages have been produced to help in the process of rehydrating the body. These drinks are commonly known as carbohydrate-electrolyte replacement solutions (CES) or sports drinks. Other than water, the major ingredients in these solutions are carbohydrates in the form of glucose and/or sucrose and some of the major electrolytes. The glucose/sucrose content varies with the different brands, ranging from 1 percent to over 10 percent. Studies have shown that sports drinks containing carbohydrates boost endurance and energy as well as help to delay fatigue during exercise. Select

a sports drink carefully. Drinks with high carbohydrate concentrations are slow to empty from the stomach, interfering with rehydration, and can cause bloating and nausea. Avoid sports drinks containing carbohydrate concentrations higher than 8 percent (4 to 8 percent works best). Experiment during training to find out if you can handle one of these drinks. You should drink early and frequently during your workouts. Don't do anything new for competitive events. So if you are a competitive athlete or marathoner or if you are exercising for several hours at a time in hot humid weather, the fluid of choice for most effective rehydration or prevention of dehydration is a sports drink (not to exceed 8 percent carbohydrate concentration). Water is the next best fluid, followed by fruit juices diluted with 50 percent water. All three are preferable to caffeinated sodas. Caffeine acts as a diuretic, and the carbonation gives you a feeling of being fuller than you are. This information, which gives sports drinks a slight edge in terms of rehydration, does not mean that drinking water is not a good way to replace lost fluids. Water is still considered to be one of the most effective ways to rehydrate and works fine for the fitness exerciser and those exercising for less than 1 hour. Also, water is convenient and free.

Whatever you drink, drink it cold. Cold drinks are better than warm ones because they help cool down the core temperature of the body and empty from the stomach faster. Athletes/exercisers drink substantially more when fluids are cold. See the Fluid Pyramid in Figure 6-3 for fluid replacement guidelines.

Note: It is possible to drink too much and end up passed out because of hyponatremia, which can be life-threatening as it dilutes the electrolytes too much.

Contraindicated Exercises

A few stretching and toning exercises added to an aerobic program can promote balanced fitness by increasing flexibility in tight muscles and by strengthening weak ones. However, not all conditioning exercises commonly done in classes or seen on videotapes are good for everyone. These potentially harmful exercises are labeled *contraindicated exercises*.

By studying people with aches and injuries, fitness experts have learned that some common stretching and toning exercises should be avoided. Others should be modified for safety and effectiveness. Be aware of which commonly done high-risk movements you should avoid and which high-benefit, low-risk exercises to do instead. Here are some examples:

1. *Yoga plow:* Sometimes done as a back stretch, this exercise can injure discs, ligaments, and nerves in the neck and back. A better back stretch is a single- or double-knee tuck to the chest.

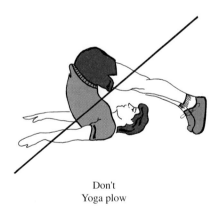

Don't
Yoga plow

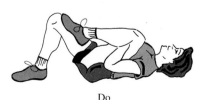

Do
Single-knee tuck to chest

2. *Knee tuck to chest:* Hyperflexing the knee by pulling it to the body with the arms or hands placed on top of the tibia places undue stress on the knee joint. The hand position should be changed to hug the thigh rather than the shin.

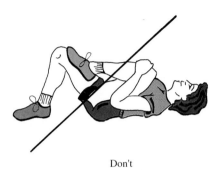

Don't

Single-knee tuck to chest

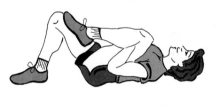

Do

Single-knee tuck to chest

3. *Head roll:* Hyperextension can injure discs in the neck. Safer neck stretches include half-head rolls to the front, turning the head side to side so that the chin touches the right and left shoulders, and touching an ear to each shoulder.

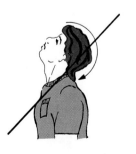

Don't

Head rolls

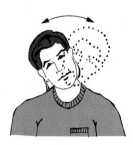

Do

Half-head rolls

4. *Hurdler stretch:* This stretch can cause groin pull, injure knee cartilage, and overstretch the medial collateral ligament—the one that helps stabilize the knee. It may also cause hip joint discomfort because the femur of the leg that is tucked behind is in a position of extreme rotation in the joint capsule. The alternate hurdler stretch safely stretches hamstrings.

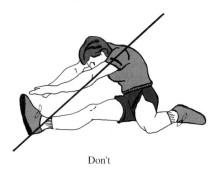

Don't

Hurdler stretch

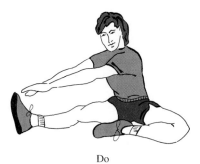

Do

Alternate hurdler stretch

5. *Full squat:* Excessive flexion or extension of the knee is dangerous. To strengthen the quadriceps, substitute half-knee bends for full squats, the duckwalk, deep lunges, and squat thrusts. Deep knee flexion exercises overstress knee ligaments and cartilage.

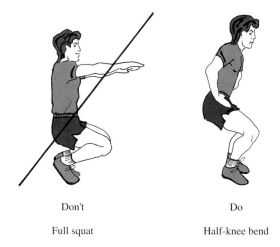

Don't   Do

Full squat   Half-knee bend

6. *Standing toe touch:* This exercise risks the straining of back ligaments. Limit forward flexion in a standing position. As your trunk dips below a 25 to 45 degree angle, the lower back muscles cease to work, and the posterior ligaments joining bone to bone must support the load.

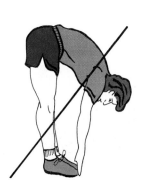

Don't

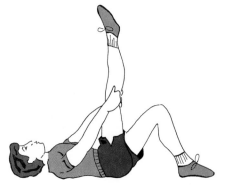

Do

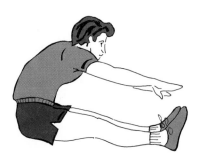

Do

7. *Leg stretches at a ballet bar (or other high object):* These may be potentially harmful. When the extended leg is raised 90 degrees or more and the trunk is bent over the leg, it may lead to sciatica problems, especially when the exerciser has limited flexibility. Substitute the back and hamstring stretches suggested in numbers 1, 4, and 6.

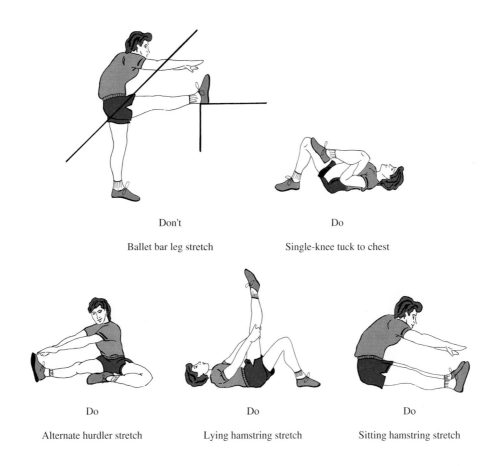

Don't

Ballet bar leg stretch

Do

Single-knee tuck to chest

Do

Alternate hurdler stretch

Do

Lying hamstring stretch

Do

Sitting hamstring stretch

8. *Leaning forward and twisting the trunk to the side:* These moves are particularly hazardous to the lower back, adding a shearing force to the stress on back ligaments. Avoid swinging hands and the trunk through the knees, windmill toe touches, waist circles, or elbow-knee lunges. There is no exercise you can do standing to tone your waist. The most effective exercise for reducing your waist is aerobic exercise and sensible nutrition. To tone oblique abdominals, the muscles that underlie the waist area, use twisting bent-knee abdominal curls. Lying on your back with heels close to your buttocks and crossing your arms across your chest (or with a hand touching each shoulder), curl the shoulders first toward the right knee and then toward the left knee.

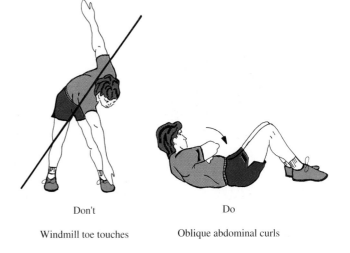

Don't

Windmill toe touches

Do

Oblique abdominal curls

9. *Double-leg lifts, straight-leg sit-ups, and low leg scissors:* These do little or nothing to tone the abdominals. They tighten hip flexors, which in most people are too tight already, causing lordosis (swayback). They may also cause lower back strain. The most effective exercise for toning abdominals

is bent-knee abdominal curls in which the lower back stays on the ground while the shoulders curl forward about 3 inches. To avoid jerking on the head or neck, cross your arms across your chest or behind your head with a hand touching each shoulder.

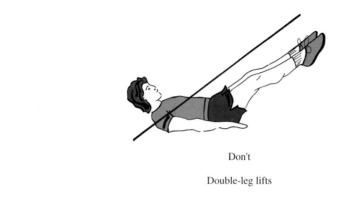

Don't

Double-leg lifts

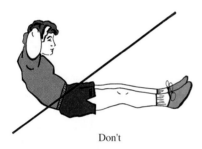

Don't

Straight-leg sit-ups

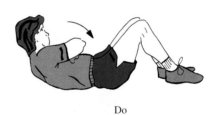

Do

Bent-knee abdominal curls

10. *The swan arch, prone double-leg raises, and yoga cobra:* These produce excessive back hyperextension and possible back strain. In a prone position, raise your right arm and the opposite leg a few inches off the ground and then switch; this will strengthen the back safely.

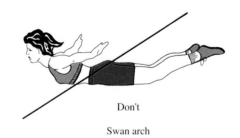

Don't

Swan arch

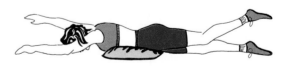

Do

Single arm/leg raises

11. *Donkey kicks or fire hydrants:* Done on hands and knees with the back hyperextended, these may strain the lower back. To protect the back, hold your abdominals tight, round your back, and raise your leg no higher than 6 to 12 inches.

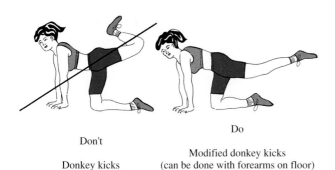

Don't

Donkey kicks

Do

Modified donkey kicks
(can be done with forearms on floor)

Your body is meant to move in many ways—to bend, twist, and stretch. Some people can do high-risk exercises for years with no ill effects. For others, after only a few repetitions, injury occurs. You may not know into which category you fit until it is too late. The problem is that some movements increase risks to muscles, joints, and connective tissue. While you may need to do deep squats if you are a competitive weightlifter or a yoga plow if you are in a yoga class, these moves don't offer any special benefit for the fitness exerciser. Low-benefit, high-risk exercises should be minimized in programs designed to emphasize personal fitness. Follow these general rules when exercising:

1. Do not hyperflex the knee.
2. Do not hyperextend the knee, neck, or lower back.
3. Do not apply a twisting or lateral force to the knee.
4. Avoid holding your breath during exercise.
5. Avoid stretching long/weak muscles (i.e., abdominals) and avoid shortening already short/strong muscles (i.e., hip flexors). See common muscle imbalances in Chapter 9 Table 9-2.
   a. Most people should avoid aggravating common postural faults: forward head, dorsal kyphosis (rounded upper back), medial rotations of the thigh, and pronation of the foot.
   b. Most people need to stretch the chest muscles, hip flexors, calves, hamstrings, lower back, and medial thigh rotators.
6. Avoid stretching any joint to the point of pain.
7. Be especially careful when using passive stretches with another person (unless the person is a physical therapist).
8. Avoid movements that place acute compressional forces on spinal discs, such as extending and rotating the spine simultaneously (i.e., trunk and neck circling and double-leg lifts).
9. Avoid movements that cause joint impingements or cartilage damage, such as arm circles in the palm-down position.
10. If the nature of your sport regularly requires the violation of good mechanics (baseball catcher assuming a deep squat position or gymnast performing double-leg lifts), make certain that the muscles are as strong as possible to endure the stress.

Aging and Physical Activity

Is your body older than you are? Scientist and well-known physical educator T. K. Cureton estimated that middle age begins for the average person at age 26, because at that age he or she has the physical capacity our ancestors did when they were 40. When we retire, we are expected to slow down and take it easy. This often produces disastrous results as atrophy and disuse take their toll. Disorders such as cardiovascular disease, hypertension, and Type 2 diabetes don't have to be the natural consequences of aging. We now feel that they are more related to physical inactivity. The body adapts to whatever load is placed on it, and the ability to do work is reduced if the load lessens. However, attitudes are changing. Older adults, encouraged by their doctors and by research

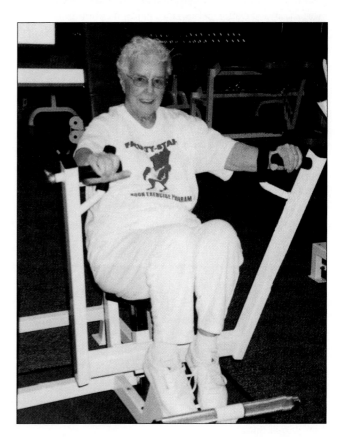

You don't stop playing because you grow old. You grow old because you stop playing.

revealing the benefits of exercise, are biking, swimming, jogging, lifting weights, and walking in ever-increasing numbers. We know that older adults (even up to age 100) are remarkably responsive to exercise, reaping health benefits. As the health-conscious baby-boom generation matures, they are likely to redefine the concept of aging.

Aging and Performance

Some say, "Growing old isn't so bad, if you consider the alternative." James Dean's "Live fast, die young, and leave a good-looking corpse" does have its proponents, but they are quickly weeded out of the genetic pool. I think a lot more of us would choose to die young, as late as possible. At birth, we each have a 70-plus-year warranty, but the maintenance is up to us. Just like any machine, the human body grows less efficient as it ages. The decline in aerobic fitness among the sedentary is about 1 percent for every year after 25. Decreases in strength, flexibility, and endurance and increased body fat proportion with age are often accepted as a natural part of the aging process. These changes may be common, but they are not inevitable. The most significant factor contributing to declines in physiological capacity at any age is *lack of regular exercise*. The "use it or lose it" rule applies. Unused muscles atrophy, lose elasticity, and grow weak. Ligaments and tendons shorten and tighten, decreasing range of motion and causing aches and pains as they pull across joints. As muscle tissue atrophies, basal metabolism drops, resulting in an increase in body fat even when a person is not eating enough to maintain adequate nutritional levels.

Other adverse changes that occur with aging can also be favorably affected by exercise. For example, exercise can enhance insulin sensitivity, reduce blood pressure, and improve psychological well-being.

To develop optimal bone strength and mass and to ward off osteoporosis, women need adequate amounts of calcium in the diet, estrogen in the bloodstream, and weight-bearing exercise in their lifestyle. Exercise acts synergistically with estrogen to develop bone strength. Inactivity accelerates bone mineral loss and increases risk of osteo-

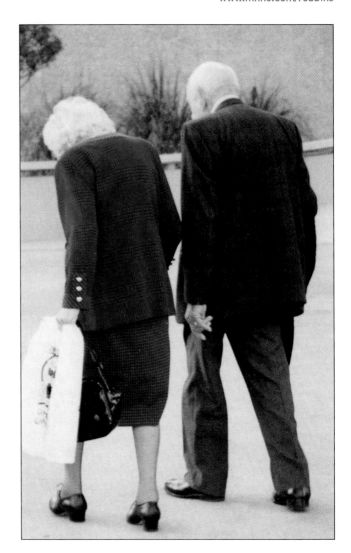

Postmenopausal women can increase their bone density 2 to 8 percent a year by regularly doing weight-bearing and resistance exercise.

porosis. Bone mass begins to decline gradually after the age of 30. The decline is hastened by menopause. While exercise alone cannot prevent osteoporosis, it may help premenopausal women build their bone densities so they enter menopause ahead of the game. Weight-bearing exercise, such as running and walking, builds bone mass before this age and slows its decline afterward. Ideally, women should exercise early in life to build bone and later in life to keep it strong. Exercise has been shown to increase mineral content of vertebral and arm bone. Weight-bearing and other resistance exercise that stresses the bone help to increase bone content. It is better increased by a combination of aerobic and weight-training exercises than it is by weight training alone. Once osteoporosis has developed, women should still be encouraged to exercise, except while a fracture is healing. Men also are affected by osteoporosis, but at later ages than women. Studies show that men and women 60 and older who train with weights, exercise bands, and resistance ma-

wellness flash

Research on centurians revealed findings in opposition to all previous thoughts on aging. Rather than "the older you get the sicker you get," a new conclusion was determined. It is, "The older you get the healthier you've been." The study found that attaining old age is not a process of declining health, but of avoiding disease. Centurians are far more likely to have a near lifetime of excellent health followed by a quick decline before death.

chines several times a week can quickly double their total body strength. See the exercise band photo. This helps fight osteoporosis by keeping skeletons sturdy. Also, such strength gains have major implications for maintaining independence in later years. Muscle weakness can advance to the stage where an elderly individual cannot do common activities of daily living. Household tasks such as getting out of a chair, sweeping the floor, or taking out the trash may become impossible. Reduced functional ability may then increase the chance of nursing home placement. Life-long exercise may also help protect the elderly against falls and the devastating effects of hip fractures. It's never too late to start exercising. Starting late in life is far preferable to not starting at all.

While aging is unavoidable, declines in functional capacity with age are not inevitable. How you age is largely up to you. Cardiologist George Sheehan has said that growing older isn't so bad; it is inactive people who give aging a bad name. Biological aging can be significantly slowed by regular exercise. As much as 50 percent of the functional decline seen in aging is related to disuse and can be prevented with regular aerobic exercise. Older adults who engage in an aerobic exercise program can slow this decline and may even have the same aerobic capacity as that of a sedentary person 25 or more years younger.

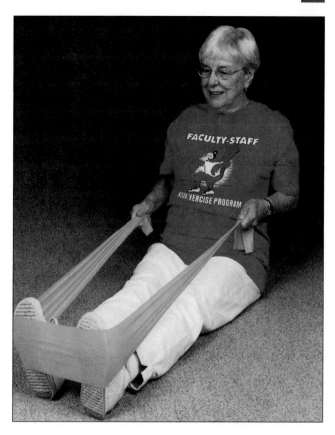

Use the exercise band routine found at the back of this book. Proper strength training offers numerous benefits to people of all ages and fitness levels.

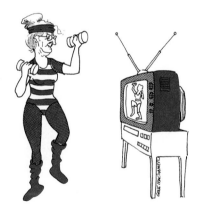

Exercise slows the aging process

As one physician observed, "So many things we think are linked to aging . . . actually have to do with lifestyle. Exercise produces a 40-year age offset. A fit person of 70 is the equal of an unfit person of 30 in regard to bones, muscles, heart, brain, sex, and everything else. I see an immense energy in old people who continue [exercise]." Exercise intensity appears to be the key to greatest benefit. A group of master athletes (ages 40 to 75) studied over an 18-year period showed no significant decline in aerobic capacity if they maintained training intensity. *For most elderly fitness exercisers, however, an exercise intensity of 50 to 70 percent maximal heart rate reserve is considered adequate.*

The effect of true nonpreventable aging involves a gradual loss of the speed and vigor with which we do activi-

ties, but it should not prevent us from doing them. As one older runner observed, "I can do everything I used to. It just takes longer to do it and longer to recover."

Exercise is adult play. At what point was our childhood eagerness to get out and romp replaced by hours of sitting in front of the TV watching others play? Whether aging is an extension of a full and active life or a gradual wasting away is determined by how you choose to live your life.

Does Exercise Increase Life Span?

While the length of your life may have a strong genetic component, study after study has shown that exercise helps lower the risk of major chronic diseases and premature death. Research conducted at the Cooper Institute for Aerobics Research in Dallas found that exercise of *moderate* intensity improved the overall *quality* of life (e.g., enhanced the ability to perform daily tasks, helped with weight control, enhanced psychological well-being) and perhaps increased the *quantity* of life by postponing a heart attack or stroke. A second study, part of the famous ongoing research of male Harvard alumni, reported that exercise of moderate intensity improved the quality of life but that it took

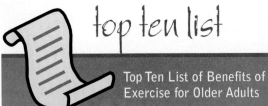

Top Ten List of Benefits of Exercise for Older Adults

1. Helps maintain the ability to live independently and reduces the risk of falling and fracturing bones.
2. Increases energy and helps the individual perform daily routines with greater ease.
3. Helps control joint swelling and pain associated with arthritis.
4. Helps maintain healthy bones, muscles, and joints.
5. Enhances cardiorespiratory function and improves peripheral circulation, and decreases the risk of arteriosclerosis and other circulatory problems.
6. Reduces constipation.
7. Reduces symptoms of anxiety and depression and fosters improvements in mood and feelings of well-being.
8. Helps people with chronic, disabling conditions improve their stamina and muscle strength.
9. Reduces the risk of dying from coronary heart disease and of developing high blood pressure, colon cancer, and diabetes.
10. Improves a person's posture, decreases backache, enhances appearance, and helps control weight.

exercise at a *vigorous* intensity level to add years to one's life. The Harvard men who had expended at least 1,500 calories a week in vigorous physical activity had a 25 percent lower death rate than did sedentary men. Vigorous activity was defined as fast walking; jogging; playing singles tennis; swimming; and performing heavy, sustained household chores. Studies such as these illustrate that any exercise has health benefits, but more exercise, enough to give your heart and lungs a real workout, is better. While a healthful lifestyle is no guarantee to a longer life, it does stack the odds in your favor.

Are you ever "too old" to begin exercise? No! While the overall impact you can make on the quality of your life is greater if you start exercising young and continue throughout life, there is no age at which the benefits of exercise stop. The older you are, the more you need exercise. Instead of searching for the "fountain of youth," Ponce de Leon would have been better off to dock his ship and remain on land—to start a walking program. The "Top Ten List of Benefits of Exercise for Older Adults" identifies the benefits of exercise for older adults.

 ## frequently asked questions

Q. *Can I work out when I have a cold or upper respiratory infection?*

A. It depends. Studies suggest that *moderate* exercise training (at 70 percent HRR) during an upper respiratory infection (URI) does not appear to extend the length or increase the severity of the illness. However, exercising during a URI should be considered carefully. Use the following guidelines to decide if it is OK for you to exercise during a cold or URI.

• If you are not experiencing extreme tiredness, malaise, fever, or swollen lymph glands, you may safely exercise at a lower intensity level than that of your regular workouts.

• Also, perform a "neck check." Assess cold symptoms and classify them as either above or below the neck. If symptoms are "above the neck" (i.e., runny nose, sneezing, or scratchy throat), you may exercise at a lower intensity. Exercise is not advised when you have "below the neck" symptoms (i.e., fever, aching muscles, productive cough, vomiting, or diarrhea).

• If you begin feeling better during the workout, increase intensity of the workout accordingly.

Q. I have asthma. Can/Should I exercise?

A. Yes. Years ago, everyone thought strenuous physical activity was dangerous if you had asthma, but now we know better. Exercise is not only safe if done properly, it's an integral part of treatment. Regular workouts will make you stronger and more energetic and reduce your risk of heart disease, diabetes, and other health problems. What's more, your asthma is likely to improve. Studies have shown that physically fit people have fewer attacks, need less medication, and lose less time from work or school. Follow these recommendations:

• Exercise regularly. Acute attacks are more likely if you exercise only occasionally.

• Carry medication during workouts and avoid exercising alone.

• Warm-up and cool-down slowly to reduce the risk of acute attacks.

• When starting an exercise program, choose self-paced endurance activities, especially those involving interval training (short bouts of exercise followed by a rest period).

frequently asked questions (continued)

Increase intensity of cardiorespiratory endurance exercise gradually.

- Cold, dry air can trigger or worsen an attack. Drink water before, during, and after a workout to moisten your airways. In cold weather, cover your mouth with a mask or scarf to warm and humidify the air you breathe. Swimming in a heated pool is an excellent activity choice for people with asthma.
- Avoid outdoor activities during pollen season or when the air is polluted. Avoid exercise in dry or dusty indoor environments.

Q. Is exercise beneficial or harmful for people with arthritis?

A. Beneficial. It is better to be active. For years, arthritis sufferers shunned physical activity, thinking it was bad for them. Today, experts believe the opposite. While rest is important, inactivity only leads to weaker muscles, stiffer joints, less energy, and weight gain—all of which can worsen the symptoms of arthritis. Many experts recommend aerobics, range-of-motion and flexibility exercises, and strength training. To keep exercising with arthritis follow these tips:

- Maintain a healthy weight. This will lessen impact on the joints.
- Wear good exercise shoes, and replace them often.
- Consider orthotics, which will help correct the body's biomechanical imbalances.
- If pain is experienced for more than 1 hour postexercise, cut back on exercise.
- Discouraging as it may sound, consider reducing mileage or exercising on alternate days, substituting low-impact workouts such as swimming, biking, or walking.

summary

Exercise is meant to be enjoyed throughout life. Regardless of gender or age, the body improves with use and degenerates with disuse. People don't wear out; they rust out. For greatest benefit from an exercise program, it is helpful to be aware of special concerns, such as how to safely exercise in hot and cold weather and how to avoid high-risk exercises. You have learned in this chapter that women respond to exercise the way men do but perhaps a little slower and to a lesser extent. This means training principles are approximately the same, regardless of gender. You have also learned that sports drinks are slightly more strongly recommended than is water for rehydrating the body after prolonged exercise and profuse sweating. Sports drinks contain electrolytes, which enhance fluid retention, contain carbohydrates, delay the onset of fatigue, and boost energy, and they taste good, which increases the likelihood that we will drink more when working out. Water is also a fine rehydrater, especially for the fitness exerciser. As you adjust to a physically active lifestyle, you will find that the benefits far outweigh the effort involved. Exercise will become a habit, and you will begin to look forward to your workout as an important part of your day.

Let the words of Don Ardell inspire you to maximize your potential . . . to be the best you can be! "Excellence ain't easy. If it were, everyone would be doing it and it would be ordinary. Know that, in lots of ways, the deck is stacked against anyone who wants to excel. Do it anyway."

internet resources

American Alliance for Health, Physical Education, Recreation, and Dance
http://www.aahperd.org/

American College of Sports Medicine
http://www.al.com/sportsmed/index.htm

Shape Up America
http://www.shapeup.org

Fitness World
http://www.fitnessworld.com

National Association of Governor's Council on Physical Fitness and Sports
http://www.fitnesslink.com/Govcouncil

Fitness Link
http://www.fitnesslink.com

Cooper Institute for Aerobics Research
http://www.cooperinst.org

Access America for Seniors
http://www.seniors.gov

Exploring Special Exercise Considerations Challenge

1. Your sister's gynecologist just told her she is pregnant. Knowing you are taking a college fitness/wellness course, she asks you for advice concerning the fitness walking program she began 2 months ago to help her get back into shape and lose a few pounds. Give her three or four tips.

2. At dinner, two of your friends were debating whether to use a popular sports drink to replace the sweat they expected to lose in the July 4th 12-mile run, which they estimated would take *more* than 1 hour to complete. The July 4th festivities are tomorrow with the race beginning at noon in Old Town and ending at the top of Heartbreak Hill. What advice would you give them?

3. Your grandparents (age 65) were advised by their neighbor to stop that "foolish" exercising, to slow down, and to start acting their age. They ask you your opinion of this advice. What can you tell them about the benefits of staying physically active?

4. In Speech 101, your topic for the final exam speech is "The Difference Between Men's and Women's Exercise Performance Levels. Are They More Alike Than Different?" List three similarities and differences you want to highlight in your speech.

5. Your friend signed up for a fitness class, and, while he was demonstrating one of the workouts, you noticed he was doing standing toe-touches with his legs crossed and double leg lifts. Explain to your friend why those two exercises are contraindicated (not advisable) and give him safe alternatives for them.

6. Take the "Are You Addicted to Exercise?" self-assessment in the chapter. How many "yes" statements did you check? _____ Discuss your assessment score.

7. Have a friend you think may becoming addicted to exercise take the "Are You Addicted to Exercise?" self-assessment in the chapter. How can you help a friend who may becoming addicted to exercise?

Changing Behavior Using the Transtheoretical Model

Using a highlighter, trace a path on the algorithm as you answer each question. Highlight your stage of change. Continue the activity on the back of this sheet.

Do you drink at least 8 eight-ounce glasses of water every day?

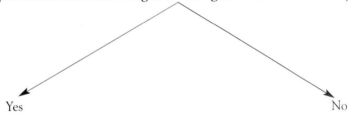

Yes   No

Have you done this consistently over the last 6 months?   Do you plan to adopt this practice within the next 6 months?

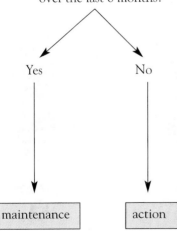 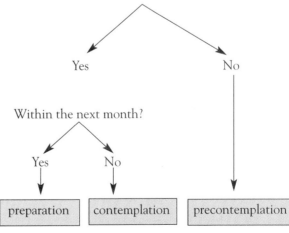

Yes   No   Yes   No

Within the next month?

Yes   No

| maintenance | action | | preparation | contemplation | precontemplation |

Once you've identified which stage of change you are in, use the processes that are most useful in progressing to the next stage—or remaining in maintenance.

In the box, write your stage of change. Then, list the processes that are most useful in that stage (see Fig. 2-2 in Chapter 2). Use only the number of processes that apply to your stage of behavior change. You may not need to use all six. Under each of the processes that you use, give two specific behavior strategies (see Table 2-1 in Chapter 2) that could help your progress to the next stage—or maintain, if you're in the maintenance stage.

The stage I am in = [   ] .

Process 1.   _____

        Behavior strategy - a.

        Behavior strategy - b.

Process 2.   _____

        Behavior strategy - a.

        Behavior strategy - b.

Process 3.   _____

        Behavior strategy - a.

        Behavior strategy - b.

Process 4.   _____

        Behavior strategy - a.

        Behavior strategy - b.

Process 5.   _____

        Behavior strategy - a.

        Behavior strategy - b.

Process 6.   _____

        Behavior strategy - a.

        Behavior strategy - b.

Maximizing Your Heart Health

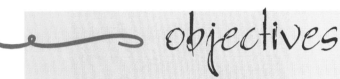

After reading this chapter, you will be able to:

1. Identify the five primary heart disease risk factors.
2. Identify the seven secondary heart disease risk factors.
3. Identify the controllable and uncontrollable risk factors for coronary heart disease (CHD).
4. Define *arteriosclerosis, atherosclerosis, angina pectoris, myocardial infarction,* and *stroke*.
5. Identify the symptoms of a heart attack and stroke.
6. Identify the role of cholesterol and saturated fats in the development of atherosclerosis.
7. Explain the roles of HDL and LDL in heart health.
8. Explain why smoking cigarettes increases heart disease risk.
9. Identify normal blood pressure range and the blood pressure reading that indicates hypertension.
10. Identify the cholesterol reading that indicates high blood cholesterol.
11. Recognize the personality traits of Type A behavior that increase heart disease risk.
12. Recognize five of eight heart disease risk factors that are positively affected by exercise and identify the two trends that will affect cardiovascular disease in the future.

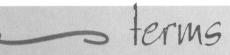

- Angina pectoris
- Arteriosclerosis
- Atherosclerosis
- Cardiovascular disease
- Cholesterol
- Collateral circulation
- Diabetes mellitus
- High-density lipoprotein (HDL)

- Homocysteine
- Hot reactors
- Hypercholesterolemia
- Hypertension
- LDL cholesterol receptors
- Low-density lipoprotein (LDL)
- Myocardial infarction
- Plaque
- Primary risk factors

- Risk factors
- Secondary hypertension
- Secondary risk factors
- Stroke
- Systolic pressure
- Triglycerides
- Type A, B, and C emotional behavior

The number one killer in America is not cancer, accidents, or AIDS. It is heart disease (Fig. 7-1). Make no mistake, cancer and other diseases are real threats, but cardiovascular diseases kill almost twice as many victims as all other leading causes of death. The tragedy is compounded because cardiovascular diseases are often inaccurately perceived as diseases of the elderly. On the contrary, based on data from the Framingham Heart Study (Chapter 1); approximately 45 percent of heart attack victims are under the age of 65, and 5 percent are under the age of 40. Adolescents, those aged 12 to 17, are not exempt from the grim heart disease picture either. Now it is revealed that most teenagers (63 percent) already have two or more risk factors for heart disease. The American Heart Association revealed that one in six teenagers and one in three people in their 20s showed evidence of atherosclerosis. This information was obtained from autopsies of young accident victims. This is alarming information and confirms that the disease process starts early in life. These diseases demand attention because they are killing too many Americans in the prime of their lives. Don't become complacent! The way you are living your life now determines your future heart health. Many coronary heart disease deaths are preventable. You can reduce your chances of developing coronary heart disease by assessing your current level of risk and by learning ways to reduce those identified risk factors. We realize that education and behavior change are the keys.

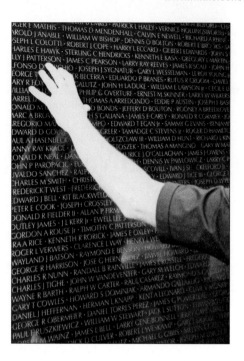

More Americans die each year from heart disease than would have been killed in 10 Vietnam wars.

Read the "Top Ten Ways to Protect Your Heart." This chapter will provide you with valuable information about each of the items and guide you toward maximizing your heart health.

Impact of Cardiovascular Disease

Cardiovascular disease (CVD) accounts for nearly 41 percent of deaths in the United States according to the American Heart Association (AHA) statistics. In other words, 1 out of 2.4 Americans who die each year does so from CVD. How do the death rates from cancer, accidents, and AIDS compare to that from CVD? See Figure 7-1. **Cardiovascular disease** (from *cardio* meaning "heart" and *vascular* meaning "blood vessels") is a condition in which either blood flow through the heart and body is impeded or the electrical impulse of the heart muscle is interrupted. Common forms of CVD include heart attack, stroke, high blood pressure, angina pectoris, irregular heartbeat, congestive heart failure, rheumatic heart disease, and congenital heart disease. More than one in five Americans suffers from these related disorders. See Figure 7-2 to see the toll taken by these various forms of CVD. Studies show that lower educational levels are directly associated with increased incidence of death from heart disease. Look at Figures 7-3, 7-4, 7-5, 7-6 and 7-7. What is the leading cause of death for each group?

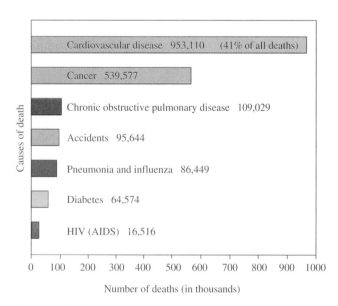

figure 7-1   Leading causes of death for men and women in the United States, (1997 estimates). There is no question about it, heart disease continues to be a serious health threat.

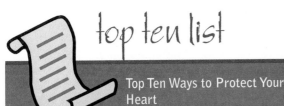

Top Ten Ways to Protect Your Heart

1. Exercise regularly. Aim for 30 minutes 5 days per week. Performing aerobic exercise regularly helps protect coronary arteries by reducing heart rate, blood pressure, cholesterol level, and body fat.
2. Maintain blood pressure level within normal limits.
3. Maintain blood cholesterol levels within acceptable limits.
4. Don't smoke.
5. Keep your weight within reasonable limits. Weighing too much (especially if you carry the extra pounds in your waistline) raises the risk of heart attack.
6. Keep blood sugar (glucose) level close to normal.
7. Don't let your triglyceride level exceed 200 mg/dl (or 100 mg/dl if you have other coronary risk factors).
8. Control stress and hostility. Learn and practice stress management strategies and how to diffuse anger/hostile behaviors.
9. Know the early warning symptoms of angina pectoris and the symptoms of a heart attack and stroke.
10. Be aware of your genes. If several close blood relatives have had a heart attack before age 60, your risk rises substantially. Accordingly, the need to control the primary risk factors for coronary heart disease is heightened.

Note: In addition to the "Top Ten Ways to Protect Your Heart", eat healthy. This will provide added protection against coronary heart disease. Recommendations include: reduce homocysteine levels by eating five servings of fruits and vegetables and six servings of grains per day. Also, consuming foods high in antioxidants (vitamin C, E, and beta carotene) helps prevent heart attacks by preventing LDL oxidation (which increases clotting and plaque rupture).

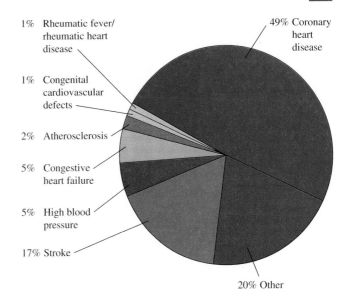

figure 7-2 Percentage breakdown of deaths from cardiovascular diseases.
United States: 1997
Source: CDC/NCHS and the American Heart Association.

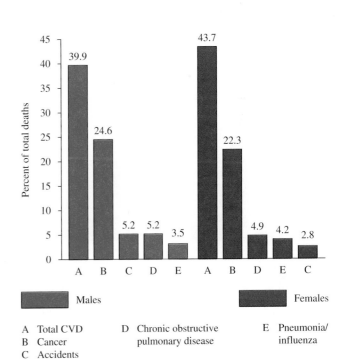

figure 7-3 Leading causes of death for white males and females.
United States: 1997
Source: CDC/NCHS and the American Heart Association

Heart attack, the most prevalent form of CVD, is still the single largest killer of American men and women (about one of every five deaths). The cost of CVD in 2000 was estimated by the AHA at $326.6 billion. This figure includes the costs of physician and nursing services, hospital and nursing home services, medications, and lost productivity resulting from disability. While costs for treatment of CVD are spiraling upward, the death rate for these diseases appears to be declining. Advances in medical treatment and education and healthy lifestyle changes can be credited for the declining death rate. However, don't become too complacent about these facts. We still have a long way to go. Cardiovascular

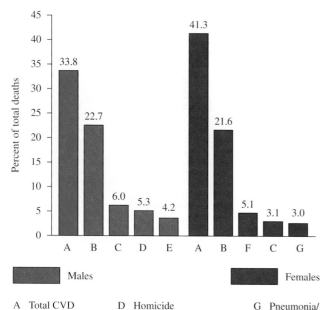

A Total CVD
B Cancer
C Accidents
D Homicide
E HIV (AIDS)
F Diabetes mellitus
G Pneumonia/
   influenza

figure 7-4   Leading causes of death for African American males and females.
United States: 1997
Source: CDC/NCHS and the American Heart Association.

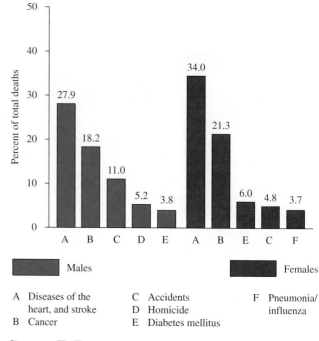

A Diseases of the
   heart, and stroke
B Cancer
C Accidents
D Homicide
E Diabetes mellitus
F Pneumonia/
   influenza

figure 7-5   Leading causes of death for Hispanic males and females.
United States: 1997
Source: CDC/NCHS and the American Heart Association.

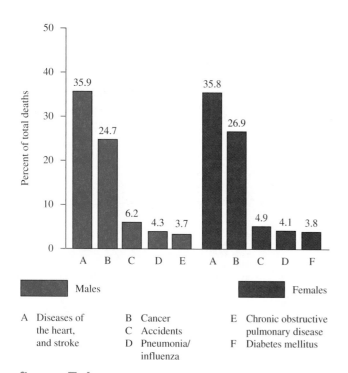

A Diseases of
   the heart,
   and stroke
B Cancer
C Accidents
D Pneumonia/
   influenza
E Chronic obstructive
   pulmonary disease
F Diabetes mellitus

figure 7-6   Leading causes of death for Asian/Pacific Islander* males and females. Unites States: 1997
*Note: This is a heterogeneous category that includes both high-risk (South Asian) and low-risk (Japanese) people. More specific data are not available.
Source: CDC/NCHS and the American Heart Association.

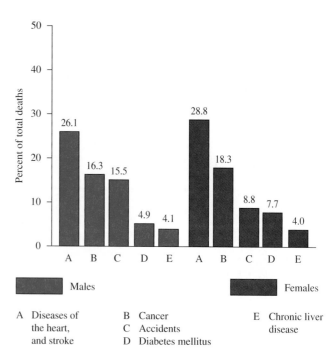

A Diseases of
   the heart,
   and stroke
B Cancer
C Accidents
D Diabetes mellitus
E Chronic liver
   disease

figure 7-7   Leading causes of death for American Indian/Alaska native males and females.
United States: 1997
Source: CDC/NCHS and the American Heart Association.

disease is the *number one* health concern in the United States. It is a killer; someone still dies every 33 seconds, more than 2,600 Americans die each day of CVD.

Coronary Heart Disease (CHD)

The heart is a muscle that works all the time. It never stops beating. Each day, the average heart beats 100,000 times and pumps about 2,000 gallons of blood. Besides providing oxygen and other nutrients to all tissues of the body, the heart must supply itself with oxygen. It has a separate circulatory system, which nourishes only the heart muscle. This system has two coronary arteries, each about the size of a pencil, that subdivide and encircle the entire heart muscle (Fig. 7-8). What is commonly known as "hardening of the arteries" is **arteriosclerosis,** a general term for the thickening and hardening of arteries. Some hardening of arteries normally occurs as we age. Coronary heart disease is most commonly the result of atherosclerosis. **Atherosclerosis** (*athero* from the Greek work for "paste" and *sclerosis* for "hardness") is a type of arteriosclerosis. It is a progressive condition in which deposits of cholesterol and other lipids, along with cellular waste products, accumulate on the inner walls of coronary arteries. This buildup is called **plaque.** As the condition progresses, the inner walls of blood vessels become more and more inelastic and clogged and may become hardened and

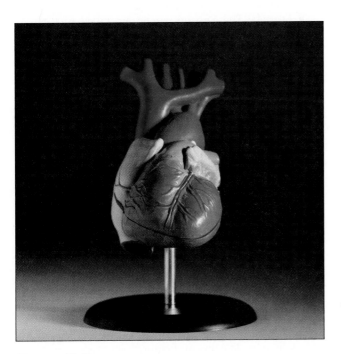

figure 7-8   If your heart beats 72 times per minutes, by the time you turn 65, your heart will have beat about 2.5 billion times.

blocked. Sometimes, a blood clot forms on the plaque buildup and blocks the entire artery. A heart attack or stroke may result.

There are a variety of causes of atherosclerosis, many of which are related to unhealthy lifestyle choices. One theory attributes atherosclerosis to minor injuries of the inner wall of coronary arteries, which create a roughened region where debris and materials in the blood can attach. Thus begins the atherosclerotic buildup. What injures the lining of our coronary arteries? High blood cholesterol levels, excessive dietary cholesterol and saturated fat, high blood pressure, your reaction to perceived emotional stress, and nicotine are often responsible. All are influenced by lifestyle. Besides causing damage to the smooth lining of our blood vessels, lifestyle factors also contribute to excess plaque in the bloodstream. Atherosclerosis does not suddenly develop at age 65. It is a long, progressive process beginning in childhood.

Angina Pectoris

Atherosclerosis may lead to **angina pectoris,** or chest pain. This pain occurs when a coronary artery becomes partially blocked, causing an oxygen debt in the heart muscle. Often, angina pectoris is brought on by sudden exertion or vigorous exercise when the blood flow to the heart is insufficient to meet its oxygen demands. The American Heart Association estimates that over 6 million people suffer from angina pectoris with 350,000 new cases occurring each year.

Myocardial Infarction

Myocardial infarction, or heart attack, results when one or more of the coronary arteries is partially blocked by atherosclerotic deposits called plaque. When one of the deposits suddenly breaks open, a blood clot (thrombus) forms and chokes off the supply of blood to the heart muscle.

The portion of heart muscle beyond the blockage is deprived of oxygen, resulting in injury or death of that portion of the heart muscle. If a damaged area is large enough or in a vital area of the heart, the individual will die. However, many people do survive a heart attack and are capable of living productive lives (Table 7-1).

table 7-1 — Warning Signs of a Heart Attack

"Classic" or more common signs:

- Uncomfortable pressure, fullness, squeezing, or pain in the center of the chest lasting more than a few minutes or that goes away and comes back.
- Pain spreading to shoulder, neck, jaw, arms, or back.

Less common signs:

- Atypical chest pain, stomach or abdominal pain.
- Nausea or dizziness.
- Shortness of breath and difficulty breathing.
- Unexplained anxiety, weakness, or fatigue.
- Palpitations, cold sweat, or paleness.

Not all of these signs occur in every heart attack. If some of these symptoms do occur, don't wait. Get help immediately!

Source: American Heart Association. 1997 *Heart and Stroke Facts Statistical Update.*

A number of studies have shown that, in some damaged hearts, new blood vessels develop to nourish the area that is being starved of oxygen and other nutrients. This is called **collateral circulation.** Everyone has collateral blood vessels, which are microscopic and closed under normal conditions. However, in some people with coronary heart disease, these seem to enlarge and form a detour around the blockage to provide alternate routes for the blood. Exercise appears to be one practical way to increase myocardial oxygen demand, which in turn may stimulate the development of collateral vessels. In some cases, coronary angiography (X ray) has revealed increased collateralization after exercise training.

Stroke (Brain Attack)

A **stroke** occurs when blood flow to the brain is interrupted either by a blockage (ischemic stroke) or by a burst blood vessel (cerebral hemorrhage). The brain needs a continuous supply of oxygen-rich blood to function. When a blood clot interrupts the flow of oxygen, the brain does not receive the nourishment it needs, and brain cells die. Stroke, primarily caused by atherosclerosis, is the *third* leading killer of Americans (behind heart attack and cancer). On the average, someone suffers a stroke in the United States every 53 seconds or every 3.4 minutes, someone dies of one. See Table 7-2 for the warning signs of stroke. It is the chief cause of serious disability and a major contributor to later-life dementia. A stroke can result in paralysis of one side of the body, loss of ability to speak or to understand the speech of others, loss of memory, and behavioral change. Because brain cells can't heal, modification of risk factors is important in the prevention of this disease that affects 600,000 Americans every year, killing about 160,000. It is not solely a disease of the elderly;

table 7-2 — Most Common Warning Signs of Stroke

- Sudden numbness or weakness of face, arm, or leg, especially on one side of the body.
- Sudden confusion, trouble speaking or understanding.
- Sudden trouble seeing in one or both eyes.
- Sudden trouble walking, dizziness, loss of balance or coordination.
- Sudden severe headaches with no known cause.

more than 28 percent of stroke victims are under age 65. Your risk of stroke increases with these factors:

- *Hypertension:* If you have high blood pressure, you are two to four times more likely to have a stroke than is someone with normal blood pressure. It is the most important risk factor for stroke.
- *Heart disease:* Sometimes, blood clots forming in the heart can move up to the brain and block blood flow.
- *Gender:* About 19 percent more men than women have strokes.
- *Diabetes:* Those with diabetes have almost double the risk of stroke.
- *Age:* The incidence more than doubles in each decade after age 55.
- *Race:* African Americans have nearly twice as many fatal strokes as whites and more than twice as many as other minorities. Hypertension and sickle-cell anemia are the suspected causes.
- *Lifestyle:* These factors can be controlled: high-fat, high-cholesterol diet; alcohol or cocaine abuse; smoking; and sedentary lifestyle.

Risk Factors

Risk factors are the conditions, situations, and behaviors that increase the likelihood that an undesirable outcome (injury, illness, or death) will occur. The risk is established by multiple scientific studies. A risk factor does not cause the undesirable outcome 100 percent of the time, but of those people who engage in the behavior (or experience the condition), a certain number of them will experience the undesired outcome. The stronger the risk factor's link with a negative outcome, the more likely it is that an individual will experience the undesired result.

The riskiness of various behaviors is determined in part through epidemiological research, which involves studying large populations to investigate the causes and control of diseases. The famous Framingham Study is an example of this type of research. Research studies on animals and humans, in which conditions are carefully set up to test hypotheses, are often needed to confirm relationships among behaviors, conditions, illness, and death. Over time, clearer and clearer pictures emerge about the degree of danger or risk in a particular situation until health experts can say, "If you do this, chances are good that this will occur."

Coronary heart disease (CHD) researchers have identified several risk factors that may lead to the development of atherosclerosis. The more risk factors you possess, the greater your chances are of developing coronary heart disease. While no one can accurately predict whether you will have a heart attack, you can estimate your odds by evaluating your risk factors. Take the *Are You At Risk?* test in Lab Activity 7-1 to determine your risk and how to reduce it.

Primary risk factors are linked directly to the development of CHD; they increase the possibility of having a heart attack. *All primary risk factors are controllable.*

Controllable Factors

1. Inactivity
2. High blood pressure
3. High blood lipid level
4. Cigarette smoking
5. Obesity

The **secondary risk factors** for heart disease contribute to the development of coronary heart disease but not as directly as the primary risk factors.

Controllable Factors	Uncontrollable Factors
1. Stress	3. Age
2. Emotional behavior	4. Gender
	5. Race
	6. Positive family history
	7. Diabetes mellitus

Notice that some of these secondary risk factors are *controllable*. The choices you make or the way you live have a profound impact in reducing these risk factors. If you possess several uncontrollable risk factors, it is imperative that you adopt a healthy lifestyle as soon as possible.

Primary Risk Factors

1. Inactivity

Countless studies have linked inactivity to coronary heart disease. A surgeon general's report confirmed that physical inactivity is a major health problem in the United States. The report warns couch potatoes, "Beware, sitting around is hazardous to your health." Additionally, the Centers for Disease Control and Prevention (CDC) in Atlanta has named physical inactivity as our nation's most common cardiac threat. Why? Because only 15 percent of Americans engage

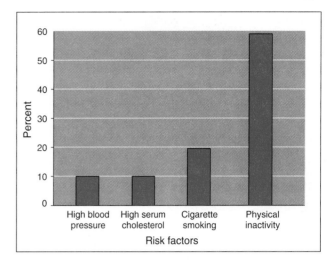

figure 7-9 Estimated percentage of U.S. population having selected risk factors for coronary heart disease. More Americans are at risk for heart disease because of physical inactivity than because of any other manageable risk factor.

in physical activity at intensity levels recommended for fitness and health benefits. This leaves close to 85 percent of our population either entirely sedentary or not active enough to reap health benefits. Consequently, it is not surprising to learn that approximately 250,000 deaths (12 percent of deaths) every year in the United States can be attributed to lack of exercise. Many experts believe today's best buy in the prevention of heart disease is *exercise* (Fig. 7-9).

In yet another ongoing inquiry into the relationship between physical activity and mortality, the Harvard Alumni Study continues to produce results that have led its director Dr. Ralph S. Paffenbarger to conclude that "There's no doubt whatever that insufficient activity will shorten your life." Even exercise of moderate intensity (brisk walking or gardening) is beneficial in improving health and well-being. It is vigorous exercise (using the FITT prescription), however, that produces the greatest health benefits and is linked to increased longevity.

The American lifestyle is sedentary. We no longer have to hunt and grow our food, build our homes, or walk to school and work. Our ancestors did not have to build physical activity into their daily lives; it was a part of their lifestyle. Modern conveniences and technology have eliminated physical activity from our lives. The culprits are the automobile, television (with remote control), elevators, escalators, riding lawn mowers, portable telephones, as well as computers and computer games. You can probably add more to this list.

Vigorous physical exercise is essential to a healthy cardiovascular system. Equally important, however, is overall lifestyle and how long you have been exercising. News from the U.S. surgeon general's report provides strong support for physical activity in the prevention of heart disease,

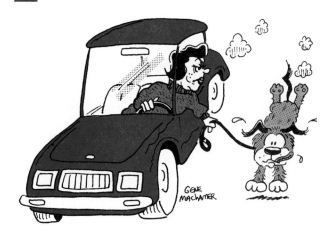

Americans are ingenious at avoiding activity. Dr. Steven Blair compares the dangers of sedentary living to smoking one pack of cigarettes a day. "Improving low fitness seems to be as important as stopping smoking in terms of reducing the risk of dying," he said.

high blood pressure, high cholesterol, diabetes, obesity, and cancer. The report recommends 30 minutes of moderate-intensity physical activity on most days of the week. This would include dancing, playing volleyball and basketball, gardening, and brisk walking. The old saying, "Use it or lose it!" is true. You don't have to run marathons to be physically active. Small increases in daily activity can significantly burn up excess calories, make the heart muscle a stronger and more efficient pump, lower blood pressure, alleviate stress, increase HDL levels, and build self-confidence.

The American Heart Association reports that regular vigorous exercise protects against coronary heart disease and even improves the survival rate after a heart attack. That is life insurance that money cannot buy. The most important thing you can do to improve your health and well-being is to *exercise*.

Health benefits appear to be proportional to the amount of activity, rather than to intensity of the exercise. If health maintenance is the goal, the surgeon general suggests a minimum of 150 calories expended per day in physical activity (about 30 minutes a day).

To increase longevity, Ralph Paffenbarger suggests expending between 300 and 500 calories a day (about 3,500 calories per week). This he calls the Longevity Zone and it represents roughly an hour of exercise per day.

Ride your bike, walk to school, play tennis instead of watching others doing these activities. Park at the back of the parking lot instead of right next to the building. There are many ways to add activity to your daily life. Remember, it doesn't have to be exhausting!

2. High Blood Pressure (Hypertension)

Blood pressure is the force exerted by the heart while pumping blood through the body. It is also the pressure of blood against the arterial walls.

There are two blood pressure levels, recorded as two separate numbers in fraction form (for example, 120/80). When the heart contracts and pumps blood into the arteries, the pressure increases. This is the **systolic,** or pumping, **pressure,** recorded as the upper number. The **diastolic,** or resting, **pressure** is the force of the blood against the arteries when the heart relaxes between beats. It is recorded as the lower number. Both the systolic and diastolic numbers are important. High levels of either or of both mean greater risk for heart attack and stroke. Average blood pressure is 120/80, and the acceptable range is 90/60 up to 139/89. High blood pressure, **hypertension,** is acknowledged as blood pressure equal to or greater than 140/90. Doctors once called this level of blood pressure *borderline* or *mild* hypertension. This language is falsely reassuring—mild weather is pleasant, but mild hypertension is not. The new term *Stage 1 hypertension* describes it better. Even *high normal* calls for lifestyle changes and monitoring. Look at the four stages of hypertension listed in Table 7-3.

High blood pressure causes the heart to overwork. Over a period of time, the overworked heart weakens, enlarges, and has a difficult time keeping up with the demands of the body. High blood pressure also causes blood vessels to become inelastic, severely reducing the amount of blood flow to the body's vital organs. Decreased levels of oxygen and other nutrients can produce heart, brain, and kidney damage. Remember, high blood pressure also leads to heart attacks and strokes.

One in four American adults has high blood pressure, and in 90 percent of the cases there is no known cause. However, factors that can increase your chances of developing high blood pressure are heredity, cigarette smoking, male

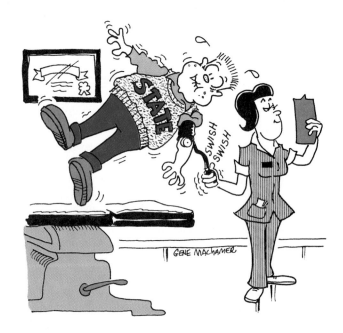

Have your blood pressure checked regularly.

table 7-3   Blood Pressure Stages

Category	Systolic/Diastolic	Recommendation
Normal	less than 130/85	Recheck in 2 years.
High normal	130–139/85–89	Recheck in 1 year; begin lifestyle modifications.
Hypertension		
Stage 1	140–159/90–99	Confirm in 2 months; begin lifestyle modifications.
Stage 2	160–179/100–109	Medical evaluation; begin treatment within 1 month
Stage 3	180–209/110–119	Medical evaluation; begin treatment within 1 week.
Stage 4	210/120 and over	Immediate medical evaluation and treatment.

gender, age, African American, obesity, sensitivity to sodium, heavy alcohol consumption, use of oral contraceptives, and a sedentary lifestyle. In a small number of cases, hypertension is caused by a specific condition, such as kidney disease, a tumor of the adrenal gland, or a defect of the aorta. This is called **secondary hypertension.** The cause of secondary hypertension can be identified and treated successfully.

How do you know if your blood pressure is too high? The only way of knowing is to have it checked. You cannot feel high blood pressure—and usually there are no symptoms until complications develop. You can be hypertensive for years and be unaware of the damage occurring; of those with high blood pressure, over 32 percent do not know they have it. Even warning signs associated with advanced hypertension may go unnoticed but may include headaches, sweating, rapid pulse, shortness of breath, dizziness, and visual disturbances. It is imperative that you know your blood pressure, because high blood pressure, while it cannot be cured, can be controlled or prevented by specific lifestyle changes: See the "Top Ten Nondrug Approaches for Preventing or Managing Hypertension."

3. High Blood Lipid Profile (Cholesterol and Triglycerides)

Research has firmly linked high levels of cholesterol and other blood fats to the development of arterial plaque, a major cause of atherosclerosis and coronary heart disease. **Cholesterol** is not a true fat but a waxy substance found in the bloodstream. Because it is soluble in fats rather than in water it is classified as a lipid, as fats are. About 80 percent of total body cholesterol is manufactured in the liver, while 20 percent comes from dietary sources—mainly from foods of animal origin.

Cholesterol is not all bad. It is needed by the body for cell structure and for the manufacture of hormones and in the digestive process. The problem with cholesterol is that your body makes most of what it needs, and the normal American diet adds much more. Most people consume 400 to 500 milligrams of dietary cholesterol per day. As a result, one-half of all adult Americans have cholesterol levels high enough to require treatment. Health experts recommend

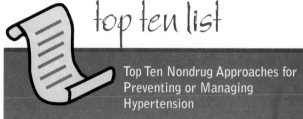

top ten list

Top Ten Nondrug Approaches for Preventing or Managing Hypertension

1. *Maintain a healthy weight.* Losing even 5 or 10 pounds, if you are overweight, can reduce blood pressure.
2. *Exercise regularly.* Exercise helps you lose weight and keep it off.
3. *Do not smoke.* Smoking does not cause hypertension but does promote heart disease. A hypertensive who smokes is at serious risk.
4. *Keep your sodium intake low (below 2,400 milligrams daily).* Many people are salt-sensitive, meaning that salt (sodium chloride) elevates their blood pressure.
5. *Avoid alcohol or if you drink alcohol, do so in moderation.* Drink no more than one drink daily if you are a woman or two if you are a man.
6. *Eat a well-balanced diet rich in fruits, grains, and vegetables.* This will help you cut back on the consumption of fats and high calorie foods and lose some excess weight. Reduce caffeine intake.
7. *Increase your calcium intake.* Calcium has been linked to reduction in blood pressure. A daily consumption of 800–1,500 milligrams is recommended. (One glass of milk has approximately 300 mg.)
8. *Increase your intake of potassium.* Studies have documented a blood pressure lowering effect of increased potassium intake in people with mild hypertension. Do not exceed 6,000 mg. Per day. (Bananas are high in potassium.)
9. *Increase fiber intake.* Plant fiber has been observed to lower blood pressure in hypertensive individuals by an average of four to eight points.
10. *Practice a stress management technique such as meditation,* or one of those discussed in Chapter 8. Harvard Medical School studies have confirmed the value of stress management in the reduction of high blood pressure.

that we keep dietary cholesterol consumption to less than 300 milligrams per day (less than 200 if you have high blood cholesterol). **Hypercholesterolemia** is the term for high cholesterol levels in the blood.

Ninety-five percent of the fats in the body are in the form of triglycerides, a true fat stored in the fat cells and found in the blood. Both high cholesterol and triglycerides increase the risk of developing atherosclerosis.

When evaluating your blood lipid profile for risk of heart disease, there are two factors to consider: (1) the total amount of cholesterol/triglycerides found in the blood and (2) the way cholesterol/triglycerides are transported in the bloodstream.

Total Amount of Lipids. Knowing your total cholesterol level provides you with a *rough* estimate of your heart disease risk. Blood cholesterol is measured by analyzing a small blood sample in a laboratory. Total cholesterol level includes the amount of cholesterol carried by high-density lipoprotein, low-density lipoprotein, and very low-density lipoprotein. The National Heart, Lung, and Blood Institute relates blood cholesterol level to heart disease risk as illustrated in Table 7-4. A reading above 200 milligrams per deciliter of blood (mg/dl) indicates increased risk of developing heart disease.

Transportation of Lipids. Like oil and water, cholesterol and blood do not mix. Cholesterol must attach to a protein molecule to be carried through the bloodstream. This combination is called a *lipoprotein*. A lipoprotein analysis gives a more accurate picture of your heart disease risk than does total cholesterol alone. A lipoprotein analysis breaks down the total cholesterol into its components, or lipoproteins, of which there are two main types—one that protects and one that damages coronary arteries:

1. **Low-density lipoprotein (LDL).** LDLs are considered "bad" because they carry a large amount of cholesterol. The lower density of the lipoprotein allows it to easily attach to the inner wall of the blood vessel, thus accelerating the atherosclerotic process. A *high* LDL cholesterol level increases your risk for heart disease (Table 7-4). It is recommended that LDL levels should be kept below 130 mg/dl. See

Figure 7-10. Cigarette smoking, emotional stressors, and diets high in saturated fat have been shown to increase the LDL level. Very low-density lipoproteins (VLDL) are even more dangerous.

2. **High-density lipoprotein (HDL).** HDL is considered to be a "good" form of cholesterol because of the dense structure of the lipoprotein. It is thought that HDL acts as a garbage collector in clearing away plaque and other debris as it flows through the bloodstream to the liver to be excreted from the body. The higher your HDL cholesterol level, the better and the more protection from heart disease it provides. See Table 7-4. HDL levels above 35 mg/dl are recommended. See Figure 7-11. How can you increase your level of HDL?
   - Exercise regularly
   - Don't smoke
   - Reduce weight and/or maintain a normal weight
   - High-fiber and low-fat diets may also increase the HDL cholesterol level
   - Use monounsaturated fats (i.e., olive oil, canola oil, sunflower oil) as primary fat, while keeping total fat intake low.

Alcohol consumption has received attention as a protective factor against heart attack because it is thought to raise HDL cholesterol in the blood and it might help prevent clotting that leads to plaque buildup inside arteries. "*Moderate*" consumption of alcohol (one drink for women per day

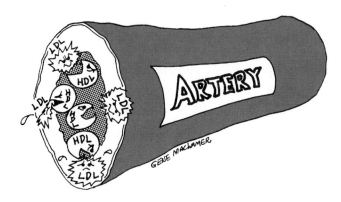

HDL cholesterol clearing away plaque in arteries.

table 7-4	Cholesterol		
Risk	Total Cholesterol (mg/dl)	LDL (mg/dl)	HDL (mg/dl)
Desirable	<200	<130	>60
Borderline High	200–239	130–159	NA
High	≥240	≥160	<35

Source: National Heart, Lung, and Blood Institute U.S. Department of Health and Human Services. Note: The levels apply to anyone 20 years of age or older.

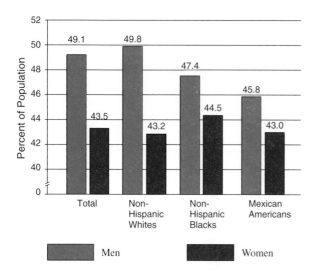

figure 7-10   Estimated age–adjusted (2000 standard) prevalence of Americans age 20 and older with LDL cholesterol of 130 mg/dl or higher by race and sex.
United States: 1988–91
Source: NHANES III (1988–91), CDC/NCHS and American Heart Association.

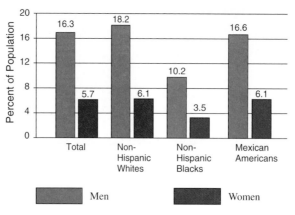

figure 7-11   Estimated age–adjusted (2000 standard) prevalence of Americans age 20 and older with HDL cholesterol of 35 mg/dl or lower by race and sex.
United States: 1988–91
Source: NHANES III (1988–91), CDC/NCHS.

or two drinks for men per day) is the amount associated with a reduction in the rate of heart attacks. The following amounts are examples of one drink:

- 1½ oz. of bourbon, scotch, vodka, gin
- 4 oz. wine
- 12 oz. beer

Consuming more than two drinks a day is known to damage the heart. A protective effect of alcohol consumption has not been proven, but many adverse effects are well documented. Besides causing automobile accidents and social disruption, excess intake of alcohol can raise blood pressure and triglyceride levels and cause diseases of the liver, pancreas, and nervous system. Even though alcohol consumption above moderate levels adversely affects blood pressure and triglycerides and can damage the heart, alcohol is still *not* considered a primary or secondary heart disease risk factor. To put the benefit of moderate drinking in proper perspective, the reduction in heart disease risk is comparable to what you might achieve by exercising regularly or by cutting blood cholesterol levels through a low-fat diet.

Scientists believe that the ratio of total cholesterol to HDL cholesterol is a better indicator of risk for cardiovascular disease than the total value alone. To determine your ratio, take a laboratory blood test that will reveal your total cholesterol and HDL cholesterol levels. Next, divide the total cholesterol level by the HDL cholesterol level to find the ratio. For example, if the total cholesterol were measured to be 160 and the HDL cholesterol 40, your ratio would be four (160 ÷ 40 = 4). This would place you at lower than average risk, as you can see in Table 7-5. A 4.5 or lower ratio (total

cholesterol/HDL cholesterol) is excellent for men, and 4.0 or lower is best for women.

Average HDL levels in adult Americans are about 45 to 65 mg/dl, with women averaging higher than men. The female sex hormone, estrogen, tends to raise HDL levels, which may explain why premenopausal women are usually protected from heart disease. Studies suggest that HDL levels above 70 may protect against heart disease, while those below 35 signal coronary risk. In summary, if you have a cholesterol reading of 200, with HDL at 80 and LDL at 120, you are considered at low risk for heart disease. On the other hand, even if you have a total cholesterol level well under 200, if your HDL level is under 35, you would still be considered at increased risk of developing CHD.

There is genetic variability in how efficiently (or inefficiently) a person metabolizes dietary saturated fat and cholesterol. Some people can eat almost anything and their blood cholesterol levels remain stable. Others find that even a small amount of dietary fat makes their blood cholesterol levels increase. Most of us are somewhere in between on this spectrum.

Drs. Michael Brown and Joseph Goldstein won the Nobel Prize in Medicine in 1985 for their discovery of **LDL cholesterol receptors.** Located primarily in liver cells, these receptors bind and remove cholesterol from the blood. The more cholesterol receptors you have, the more efficiently you can remove cholesterol from the blood. The number of cholesterol receptors is, in part, genetically determined. Lifestyle factors also influence the number. A diet high in saturated fat and cholesterol produces what Brown and Goldstein termed "double trouble." It not only saturates the receptors, it also decreases their number—a bad combination. Only about 5 percent of the population has genetically high cholesterol levels that remain elevated regardless of lifestyle.

table 7-5 — Ratio of Total Cholesterol and HDL Cholesterol to Risk of CHD

Risk of Heart Disease	Ratio of TC/HDL-C Men	Ratio of TC/HDL-C Women
Very low	under 3.43	under 3.27
Low	4.97	4.44
Moderate	9.55	7.05
High	more than 23.39	more than 11.04

Source: The Wellness Encyclopedia, University of California, Berkeley.

Triglycerides are manufactured in the body to store excess fats. They are also known as *free fatty acids*, and in combination with cholesterol, they accelerate the formation of plaque. Triglycerides are carried in the bloodstream by very low density lipoprotein (VLDL). These fatty acids are found in poultry skin, lunch meats, and shellfish. However, they are mainly manufactured in the liver from alcohol, starches, and refined sugars (honey included). Alcohol, starches, and sugars are not fat, but the body can convert them into fats and them dump those fats into the blood stream. Ways to lower triglycerides include:

- Decrease alcohol and sugar consumption.
- Reduce weight, if overweight.
- Reduce consumption of animal fats in the diet (poultry skin, lunch meats, shellfish).
- Get regular aerobic exercise.
- If necessary, take prescribed medications.

As a general rule, you should keep your triglyceride level below 200 mg/dl of blood. However, some reports indicate trigyceride levels over 100 should be cause for concern. See Table 7-6.

You should know your cholesterol level and have it checked annually, especially if you have a positive family history of heart disease. The best way to do this is to have a 12-hour fasting blood test that is analyzed by a reputable laboratory. The over-the-counter tests that don't require fasting are not as reliable. The National Heart Savers Association states that only 8 percent of Americans know their cholesterol level and more than 50 percent have a level that is too high. Since cholesterol levels are greatly influenced by diet and lifestyle, follow these guidelines to reduce high levels:

- A diet rich in cholesterol—or worse, one rich in saturated fat (saturated fat is highest in vegetable oils such as tropical and palm, and in meat and high fat dairy products) and trans fatty acids (hydrogenated oils in many crackers, cookies, cakes, pies, pastries)—can increase your blood cholesterol level. Keep total fat less than 30 percent of total calories per day and dietary cholesterol below 300 mg per day. This small

table 7-6 — Triglycerides

Normal	Less than 200 mg/dl
Borderline High	200–400 mg/dl
High	400–1,000 mg/dl
Very high	above 1,000 mg/dl

modification in dietary fat can reduce cholesterol levels by 10 percent to 15 percent. (See Chapter 10 for other dietary strategies that affect heart health.)
- Reduce body weight if overweight. Weight reduction alone can lower cholesterol and triglyceride levels.
- Lowering your stress level also helps offset high cholesterol. See Chapter 8.
- Increase daily aerobic exercise. Try to walk more, use escalators and cars less, be a participant rather than a spectator.
- Reduce alcohol, sugar, and caffeine consumption.
- Increase consumption of fiber-rich foods, such as: oatmeal, dried beans and peas, whole grain breads and cereals, raw fruits and vegetables.
- Take your medication, if prescribed.

4. Cigarette Smoking

Cigarette smoking is a primary risk factor. Nicotine increases heartrate and blood pressure and constricts blood vessels. Carbon monoxide also creates cardiovascular stress by impairing the transport of oxygen in the blood. About one in five deaths from CVD is attributable to smoking. Tobacco useage begins early. Of adults who smoke, 80 percent started before they turned 18. See Figure 7-12. Every cigarette package is required by law to carry a consumer warning. One such warning is "Cigarette Smoking Can Kill You."

Even Ann Landers, the nationally syndicated columnist, gives warning: "Beware, cigarettes are killers that travel in packs." In 1998, four million humans (one every 7 seconds) died because of tobacco. Numerous studies have proven that cigarette smoking causes oral cancer, lung can-

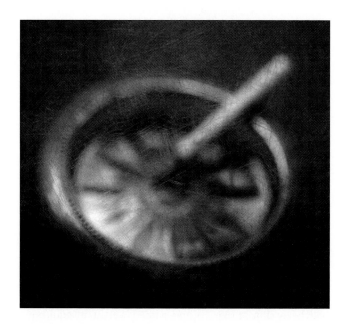

Every cigarette a person smokes reduces his or her life by 11 minutes. Each carton of cigarettes thus represents a day and a half of lost life. Every year of smoking a pack a day shortens life by almost 2 months. Smoking in the teenage years causes permanent genetic changes in the lungs and forever increases the risk of lung cancer even if the smoker quits.

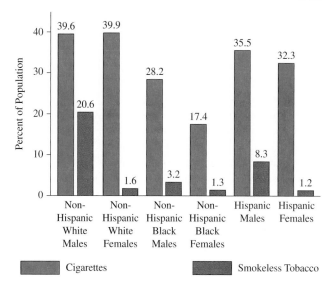

figure 7-12   Percentage of high school students smoking cigarettes or using smokeless tobacco within the last 30 days by race and sex. United States: 1997

Source: Morbidity and Mortality Weekly Report, Vol. 47, No. SS-3, Aug. 14, 1998 (Youth Risk Behavior Survey, 1997).

2000 Heart and Stroke Statistical Update, American Heart Association

cer, and emphysema, and in women it is linked to cervical cancer, early menopause, and damage to the fetus during pregnancy. It also leads to the development of wrinkles in men and women. The number of Americans killed each year from smoking is greater than the number killed during World War II and the Vietnam War combined. No level of smoking is safe!

The American Heart Association reports that smokers have more than twice the risk of heart attack of nonsmokers. Even limited smoking (four to five cigarettes per day) increases CHD risk. Also, smoking increases the risk of developing peripheral vascular disease (narrowing blood vessels in the arms and legs), which may lead to the development of gangrene and eventually amputation.

Passive smoke, synonymous with secondhand smoke, is the cigarette smoke inhaled by nonsmokers from environmental air. Research has shown there are plenty of reasons to worry about secondhand smoke:

1. Nonsmokers may be *more* susceptible to heart and vascular damage from secondhand smoke than smokers are, even though they absorb much smaller doses of the smoke's toxins. That is because smokers develop compensatory responses to some of the adverse cardiovascular effects of cigarette smoke—but nonsmokers do not get the "benefit" of these adaptive responses.
2. Repeated exposure to secondhand smoke causes permanent damage to the heart and arteries.
3. The cardiovascular system is extremely sensitive to the chemicals in secondhand smoke (i.e., carbon monoxide, nicotine, and hydrocarbons).
4. Carbon monoxide, a substance in secondhand smoke (and in inhaled cigarette smoke), damages the smooth inner lining of blood vessel walls. This accelerates the atherosclerotic buildup. Carbon monoxide, higher in the blood of smokers but also found in nonsmokers, decreases the amount of oxygen carried in the blood. It also reduces the heart's ability to use the oxygen it does receive.
5. Even low levels of secondhand smoke increase the stickiness of blood platelets in nonsmokers, making it more likely that a clot will form in the narrowed arteries, which can ultimately lead to a heart attack.
6. Cigarette smoking (as well as secondhand smoke) *decreases* the HDL levels in the bloodstream (the "good" type of cholesterol). Both cause heart rate and blood pressure to rise.
7. Secondhand smoke (and smoking) worsens the damage done by free radicals (i.e., destructive oxygen compounds) to heart muscle cells.
8. When a heart attack occurs, prior exposure to secondhand smoke worsens the damage and makes the outcome more serious.
9. Nonsmokers who live with smokers or work where environmental smoke is present have between 58 percent and 91 percent higher risk of dying from heart disease than do other nonsmokers.

10. Heavy smoking in the same workplace or study area gives the nonsmoker the equivalent of mainstream smoking two to three cigarettes a day.

11. Secondhand smoke is a human carcinogen, killing about 3,000 nonsmokers a year through lung cancer. Smoking is everyone's business!

12. The population burden associated with passive smoking and heart disease is estimated to be 60,000 deaths annually in the United States. The simplest and most cost-effective control measure to reduce cost is to *mandate* smoke-free workplaces, schools, and public places.

While studies show that smoking has declined by more than 42 percent since 1965, this downward trend appears to be leveling off, and smoking may be on the upswing again, especially among college students. Smoking promotes heart disease. A nonsmoker should not begin to smoke. Smokers should stop *now*. Ninety percent of smokers who quit do so on their own!

5. Obesity

Obesity has escalated to epidemic proportions in the United States and is continuing to increase at an alarming rate. See Figures 7-13 and 7-14. Obesity is uncomfortable; increases the burden on the vital organs, especially the heart, and is directly linked to coronary heart disease.

It is especially risky to have excess body fat in the waist and abdominal area. The distance around the waist and body mass index (BMI) are recommended ways to estimate one's body fat. A high-risk waistline is 35 inches or more for women, 40 inches or more for men. See Chapters 3 and 11 for instructions on how to measure BMI. Skinfold calipers

(discussed in Chapter 3) more accurately measure percent of body fat. The CDC considers anyone above 30 pounds over target weight to be obese.

Over one-half of the U.S. population is obese or overweight. Childhood obesity rates have doubled since the late 70s with 25 percent of 12 to 19 year olds (one in four teens)—significantly overweight. Hypertension is nearly six times higher in overweight people aged 20 to 44, and high cholesterol levels are twice as frequent in the obese. Ninety percent of people with Type 2 diabetes are overweight. Obesity, considered a chronic disease, causes more than 300,000 premature, preventable deaths per year.

In addition, obesity puts women in particular at increased risk of heart disease. A study conducted by the Harvard Medical School of 115,000 women ages 30 to 55 found that of all the women in the 8-year study who developed heart disease, 40 percent had no other risk factors except being 20 percent or more over their ideal weight. Women who had been slim at age 18 and gained weight in adulthood seemed to be at increased risk. The first step in medical treatment for these conditions is usually weight reduction. Obesity is controllable and can be reversed. You can eliminate the obesity risk factor by maintaining reasonable weight (see Chapter 11). Even modest weight reduction (5 to 10 percent of body weight) can help reduce your risk of CVD and stroke.

Physical inactivity is a major factor in the development of obesity in men, women, and children. Watching too much television is one of the main culprits. The number of television hours watched per person in this country averages about four per day. Americans should limit TV viewing to about 1 hour a day to prevent physical and mental inactivity. Of course, consuming more calories than are used in daily activity also contributes to obesity.

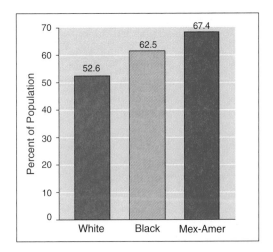

figure 7-13   Prevalence of overweight.

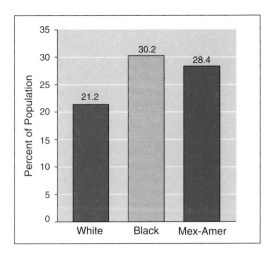

figure 7-14   Prevalence of obesity.

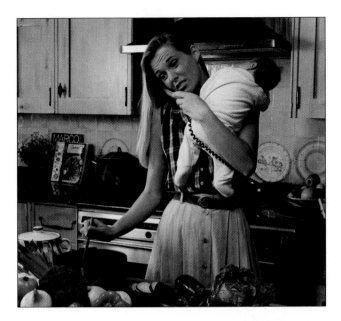

Performing several tasks at the same time is an excellent example of how hectic life in the twenty-first century has become.

Secondary Risk Factors

These are factors associated with increased risk of heart disease, though not as directly as the primary risk factors.

1. Stress

Stress is unavoidable. It includes happy, wonderful, and positive events as well as sad, destructive, and negative ones. For example, the death of a family member and the birth of a child, while perceived differently, are stressors that produce the same physiological response in the body. Job stress may be particularly unhealthy. High blood pressure is three times more common among people who have jobs with high demands but little control (assembly line worker, waitress). Stress has been found to cause a rise in heart rate, blood pressure, and blood cholesterol, and it can lead to excessive smoking or eating—all linked to coronary heart disease. The type of stress is not that important. Indianapolis 500 race car drivers have higher cholesterol levels after they race than before. Tax accountants have increased cholesterol around April 15. Students have higher cholesterol levels during exams. Stress causes chemical wear and tear on the body by releasing stress hormones into the bloodstream (adrenaline). Large amounts of stress hormones are found in the bloodstreams of people who react to stressful situations with hostile and angry behavior. However, low levels of stress hormones are found in the bloodstreams of people who react normally to stressful events. How you react to stress seems to be the critical factor. You should recognize

stress in your life (the positive and the negative) and learn to handle the stressful situations in a healthful manner. Coping with stress successfully is vital in today's hectic, in-the-fast-lane lifestyle. Exercise, relaxation techniques, and behavioral modification have been found to be excellent methods for reducing stress. We need to change the way we look at stressful situations. Problems are to be solved, not worried about. Read more about ways to reduce stress in Chapter 8.

2. Emotional Behavior

Several studies have linked emotional behavior to increased risk of heart disease. There are basically three **emotional behavior** patterns—**Type A, B, and C.** The Type A individual exhibits aggressiveness, competitiveness, and impatience and is easily annoyed. Type As demonstrate a high degree of time urgency—a tendency to do two or three things at the same time. These behaviors may lead to angry, cynical, and hostile behavior. The Type B individual is more relaxed, noncompetitive, patient, and slow to anger. A third emotional behavior pattern, Type C, has been identified recently. Type Cs are actually classified as Type As but they learn to cope with emotional stress by using the five Cs: control, commitment, challenge, choices in lifestyle, and connectedness. Such people welcome change, considering it a challenge. They are committed to goals, gaining confidence as a result (see Chapter 8). Type Cs are called *"hardy" stress resisters*.

Early studies identified Type A people as the ones at greater risk of having heart attacks. However, more recent research indicates it is only when the Type A exhibits the behaviors of *hostility* and *anger* that a serious risk is apparent. These behaviors arouse the fight-or-flight response, significantly elevate blood pressure, overstimulate the production of stress hormones, and have been documented to increase coronary artery atherosclerosis. The other Type A behaviors do not seem to be as significant but may be factors in overall poor health and may eventually lead to hostile, angry reactions to stress. Type Bs with these negative behaviors will also suffer adverse health consequences. Twenty percent of apparently healthy people suffer extreme surges in blood pressure when confronted with the challenges of everyday life. They are called **hot reactors** because their systolic blood pressure can rise from 120 to a deadly 300 when stressed. They often go untreated until felled by a stress-induced heart attack or stroke. Hot reactors can be found in all emotional behavior types.

We are not born with hot reacting, angry, and hostile behaviors. These behaviors are learned and, for the sake of our health, we can unlearn them. Learning to modify Type A personality behaviors, especially hostility, anger, and hot reacting, is not difficult, and doing so may add years to your life. How does a "hostile heart" become less angry and cynical—and become a "trusting heart"?

Carry a notebook and record every time you feel angry and/or hostile. Once you have done this for a while, you will start to recognize the situations that provoke these reactions and be able to head off the troublesome behavior. Other suggestions follow:

1. *Stop angry, cynical thoughts.* Every time you have a cynical thought, think to yourself, "STOP!" This is called *thought stopping* and is an effective behavior modification technique when practiced regularly.
2. *Practice laughing at yourself.* Once you realize how silly your anger is in many situations, laughing at yourself will quickly replace fuming.
3. *Be empathetic.* Put yourself in the other person's shoes. Often the other individual is a victim of circumstances, too.
4. *Reason and understand your anger.* There will be times when anyone would be angry in that same situation, but you must say, "I have this trait, and it is bad for my health." Decide if the situation warrants your attention and if you have an effective response. If not, take a "time out" from the situation.
5. *Learn to relax.* Practice the excellent "stress busters" in Chapter 8.
6. *Practice patience and trust.* Instead of getting irritated while standing in a line, concentrate on a relaxing word (such as "quiet") until your anger subsides. Trust that others are not out to cheat you.
7. *Become a good listener.* Pay attention to what others are saying and do not interrupt. This may help you understand the situation better *before* you jump to an angry response.
8. *Live as if you have a serious disease.* You will soon see that the little problems that once riled you up aren't really so important.
9. *Learn to forgive.* Compassion is the strongest medicine for anger. Blame leads to anger; forgiveness heals.

3. Age

Being older has some advantages (wisdom and experience), but protection from CHD is not one of them. As you age, your risk for developing heart disease increases. This does not mean that coronary heart disease is *only* a disease of the old. You don't just suddenly drop dead one day at age 45 from a "heart attack." At any age and certainly at age 18, you have atherosclerotic plaque in your arteries. It accumulates over time, and by the time you've gained "age," you've also increased the private stash of cholesterol in your arteries. There is little that can be done to stop the calendar. Adopting a healthy lifestyle early in life may add years to your life and life to your years.

4. Male Gender

Males have a higher risk of coronary heart disease and stroke throughout their lives than do females. Even after menopause,

when women's death rate from heart disease increases, it is less than men's. The increased male risk is not clearly understood. Some credit the increased risk to the male sex hormone testosterone, which triggers production of low-density lipoproteins, thereby clogging blood vessels. Others say a male's lifestyle may be the culprit. We do know that a female's hormonal makeup is protective until menopause. Female hormones signal the liver to produce more "good" cholesterol (HDL) and make blood vessels more elastic than male's blood vessels, especially during childbearing years.

It is imperative that males modify other risk factors to protect their cardiovascular systems. (i.e., increase physical activity, maintain a healthy weight, don't smoke, keep blood pressure and cholesterol levels at recommended levels, manager stress, and modify emotional behaviors).

5. Race

According to the American Heart Association, African Americans have the greatest risk of all races for heart attack and stroke. It is estimated that due to high blood pressure African Americans have more than 60 percent greater chance of death and disability from strokes than do whites (Fig. 7-15). One explanation for this higher incidence is that many African Americans share a mutation in a gene that helps control blood pressure. A hereditary intolerance to sodium may also account for the danger. African Americans and Mexican Americans risk of diabetes and obesity is twice that of any other ethnic groups in the United States. Social and economic stresses may also contribute to increased cardiovascular disease risk. It is paramount that early heart health intervention and education programs be supported for African-American populations. Also, being aware of these risks, African Americans should adopt a healthy lifestyle early. See the Diversity Issues Box for additional population information.

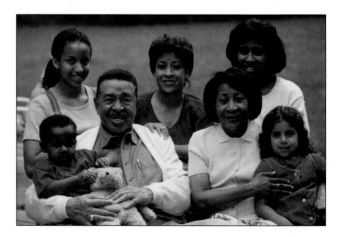

African Americans have increased risk for heart attack, stroke, and diabetes.

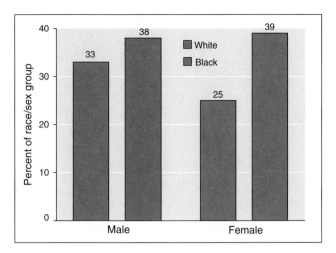

figure 7-15 Estimated percentage of population with hypertension by race and sex in U.S. adults. Hypertensives are defined as persons with a systolic level ≥140 and/or a diastolic level ≥90 or who reported using antihypertensive medication.

Heart disease and stroke risks are high among Mexican Americans, American Indians, and native Hawaiians, also. Again, this increased risk is due to higher rates of obesity and diabetes.

6. Positive Family History

A family history of heart disease in brothers, sisters, parents, or grandparents increases your risk of developing coronary artery disease. Tendencies toward high blood pressure, stroke, peripheral blood vessel disease, rheumatic fever, high blood lipid levels, obesity, and early heart attack appear to be somewhat hereditary. This is why your physician is so interested in your family history. A family's lifestyle also may contribute to heart disease and stroke. For example, family members may be overweight, smoke, eat large amounts of cholesterol and saturated fat, or be physically inactive. You should find out as much as possible about your family's medical history. You can be alerted early to a possible risk and take preventive measures.

7. Diabetes Mellitus

What do blindness, gangrene, kidney failure, heart attack, and stroke have in common? They can all result from diabetes, which eventually strikes one in three people in the United States.

Diabetes mellitus (which includes both Types 1 and 2) is a condition characterized by the body's inability to produce enough of the hormone insulin or to use it properly. The body's ability to process sugars (glucose) is slowly destroyed and sugar-laden blood soon begins to damage the circulatory system. In the normal digestive process, sugars, starches, and other foods are changed to a form of sugar called *glucose*. The bloodstream carries glucose to the body

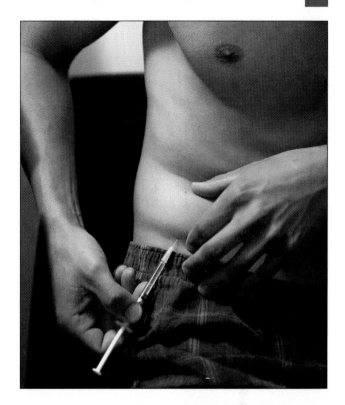

Diabetes increased at an alarming rate in the United States in the past decade—rising 70 percent among people in their 30s. Health experts are blaming the wired-up, couch potato culture of the 1990s.

cells. There, with the help of insulin, a hormone produced in the pancreas, it is converted to quick energy for immediate use or stored for future needs. In diabetes, this normal process is interrupted. Glucose accumulates in the blood until some of the surplus is eliminated by the kidneys, passing it off in the urine. Too much sugar in the urine and in the blood are classic signs of diabetes.

Diabetes is found in two forms. In insulin-dependent diabetes (IDDM), also known as Type 1 or juvenile onset, the pancreas makes little or no insulin. The diabetic must receive insulin injections every day to stay alive and must carefully watch his or her diet and exercise regularly. (See Fig. 7-16.) It occurs most often in children or young adults. Symptoms develop rapidly, usually within a period of months or even weeks.

More common (85 to 90 percent of diabetics) is non insulin-dependent diabetes (NIDDM), also known as Type 2 or adult onset, in which the pancreas makes insulin but either the amount is insufficiently released or the body cannot properly use what is available. This type of diabetes can often be controlled without insulin injections through other medications, diet, and weight management. This form of the disease usually occurs in people over 40 years old and is associated with aging and obesity. New data however shows a dramatic rise of Type 2 in children and young adults making

diversity issues

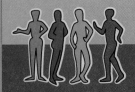

Who Smokes?

	Men	Women
All	27.1%	22.2%
White	27.3%	23.9%
African American	32.3%	22.3%
Hispanic	25.4%	13.9%
Asian/Pacific Islander	20%	11.7%
American Indian/ Alaska Native	41%	29.8%

Studies show that smoking prevalence is several times higher among those with less than 12 years of education than it is among those with more than 16 years of education.

Who Has High Blood Pressure (HBP)?

- Men have a greater risk of HBP than do women until age 55. Beyond age 55, the percentage of women is higher.
- African Americans, Puerto Ricans, and Cuban and Mexican Americans are more likely to suffer from HBP than are whites.
- Compared to whites, African Americans develop high blood pressure at an earlier age, and it is more severe at any decade of life.
- Death rates for HBP in 1997 were 14% for white males and 12.8% for white females; 50.0% for African American males and 40.6% for African American females.
- 36.7% of African American males and 36.6% of African American females have HBP.
- 25.2% of white males and 20.5% of white females have HBP.
- 22.8% of Cuban American males and 15.5% of Cuban American females have HBP.
- 24.0% of Mexican American males and 22.4% of Mexican American females have HBP.
- 15.6% of Puerto Rican males and 11.5% of Puerto Rican females have HBP.
- 9.7% of Asian American and Pacific Islander men and 8.4% of Asian American/Pacific Island women have HBP.
- HBP is 2 to 3 times more common in women taking oral contraceptives, especially in obese and older women, than in women not taking them.

Who Is Physically Inactive?

- People with lower incomes and less than a 12th-grade education are more likely to be sedentary.
- Regular exercise is more prevalent among men (44%) than women (38%).
- African American women, the less educated, overweight persons, and the elderly are the most inactive groups.
- In general, whites are more likely to exercise or play sports regularly than are African American or Hispanics.
- Non-Hispanics are more likely to exercise or play sports regularly (41%) than are Hispanics (35%).

Who is Overweight (BMI of 25.0% or higher = Overweight; 30.0% or higher = Obese)

- For whites, 61.5% of men and 46.8% of women are overweight; 20.8% of men and 23.2% of women are obese.
- For African Americans, 58.4% of men and 68.3% of women are overweight; 21.3% of men and 38.2% of women are obese.
- For Mexican Americans, 69.3% of both men and women are overweight; 24.8% of men and 36.1% of women are obese.
- For Cuban Americans, 57.5% of men and 52.0% of women are overweight, 12.8% of men and 17.8% of women are obese.
- For Puerto Ricans, 60.5% of men and 58.5% of women are overweight; 12.2% of men and 24.6% of women are obese.
- For Asian/Pacific Islanders, 10.8% of men and 10.1% of women are overweight.

Source: American Heart Association, *1997 Heart and Stroke Facts Statistical Update* (National Center, 7272 Greenville Ave., Dallas, TX 75231–4596).

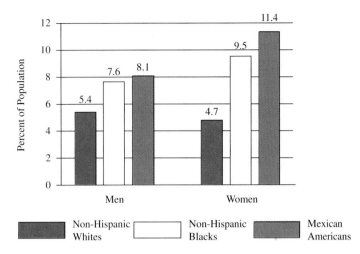

figure 7-16 Age-adjusted (2000 standard) estimated prevalence of physician-diagnosed diabetes in Americans age 20 and older by sex and race.
United States: 1988–94

Source: Prevalence of Diabetes, Impaired Fasting Glucose, and Impaired Glucose Tolerance in U.S. Adults, The Third National Health and Nutrition Examination Survey, 1988–1994, *Diabetes Care,* Vol. 21, No. 4, April 1998.

the term "adult-onset diabetes" obsolete. Because the onset of Type 2 is gradual, the disease may go undetected for years. Diabetes seriously increases the risk of developing cardiovascular disease. More than 80 percent of people with diabetes die of some form of heart or blood vessel disease. Part of the reason is that diabetes affects cholesterol and triglyceride levels by producing a different kind of LDL that is even worse for the arteries than is ordinary LDL. This accelerates atherosclerosis. Even so, Type 2 diabetes can be delayed or averted by weight management and physical activity. One condition shared almost universally by Type 2 diabetics is obesity. Not all obese people become diabetic, but 90 percent of people with Type 2 diabetes are overweight or obese. The risk of diabetes is two times greater in people who are mildly overweight (20 percent above ideal weight), five times greater in the moderately overweight (20 percent to 30 percent above ideal weight) and *ten* times greater in the obese (30 percent above ideal weight).

The surge in youth obesity in this country has paralleled a rise in childhood Type 2 diabetes. At one time Type 2 diabetes was almost unheard of in children. They almost always had Type 1. A new advisory from The American Academy of Pediatrics and the American Diabetes Association calls for diabetes testing of overweight children with any two other risk factors starting at age 10 or at puberty, if it comes earlier.

Many people know their blood pressure and their cholesterol levels, but few know their glucose level, a simple sugar found in the blood. A substantially elevated glucose level is the chief diagnostic sign of diabetes. Unfortunately, far too few people are properly tested. As a result, researchers say that nearly half of the estimated 16 million people who have diabetes don't know it.

But detecting even a minimally elevated glucose level has become important, too, according to the new guidelines issued by the American Diabetes Association (ADA). That's because this signals a metabolic disorder called *insulin resistance,* which affects up to 30 percent of adults. Insulin resistance greatly increases the risk of developing diabetes and almost surely raises the risk of hypertension, coronary heart disease, stroke, and possibly cancer.

There is another reason why public health experts are urging wider glucose testing. It is the only way to catch diabetes early. The disease usually causes no symptoms for a decade or more, even though it is silently festering this entire time. That's 10 to 12 years that diabetes quietly eats away at your vision, injures your kidneys and nerves, and sets the stage for heart disease. This is damage that's preventable if only people learned sooner that they have Type 2 diabetes.

According to the ADA's new guidelines, all people age 45 and older should have their fasting blood-glucose level tested at least every three years. Several groups of people are at greater risk and should be checking for diabetes at least once a year. Get tested, starting at age 35, if you:

wellness flash

Diabetes causes about 86,000 amputations nationwide each year. The ailment can deaden nerves in the arms and legs, allowing sores, and infections to develop into gangrene.

- Are overweight, especially with extra belly fat.
- Have a brother, sister, or parent with diabetes.
- Are not White (i.e., African American, Hispanic, and Native American).
- Had a baby weighing more than 9 pounds or had gestational diabetes (diabetes during pregnancy).
- Have an HDL cholesterol of 35 or less or a triglyceride level of 250 or more.
- Have hypertension or take antihypertension drugs.
- Had a minimally elevated glucose level on a previous test.

Two readings of *126 mg/dl or more* on a fasting blood-glucose test, taken on different days, means you have diabetes. Less-elevated reading, from *110–125*, indicate impaired fasting glucose, which means you are insulin resistant and face a sharply increased risk of diabetes. Regardless of your glucose level, you are probably resistant if you have low HDL, high triglycerides, high blood pressure, or excessive abdominal fat.

Certain lifestyle changes such as:

- Regular moderate exercise
- Losing weight
- Stopping smoking
- Eating a high-fiber diet
- Eating a diet low in sugar and other sweets

can improve insulin resistance; they may also help improve the associated HDL, triglyceride, and blood pressure prob-

wellness flash

Every 90 seconds someone is diagnosed with diabetes. The disease kills 180,000 Americans each year.

lems. Those steps can also help people who have Type 2 diabetes (and sometimes even Type 1) control their glucose level.

Symptoms of both types can include

- hazy vision
- excessive thirst
- frequent urination
- frequent hunger
- a weight loss or weight gain
- dry skin
- a tired washed-out feeling
- slow healing wounds
- itching, tingling, or numbness in the extremities
- frequent vaginal or skin infections
- combinations of these symptoms.

Unless detected and controlled, diabetes can ultimately lead to stroke, heart disease, kidney failure, blindness, amputation of limbs from gangrene, and death. See Table 7-7. According to the American Diabetes Association, the disease

table 7-7   Complications of Diabetes

Over time, untreated or poorly controlled diabetes can cause debilitating, even life-threatening complications.

		What Happens	Complications
	Eyes	The small blood vessels of the retina become damaged.	Decreased vision and ultimately blindness. Diabetes is the leading cause of blindness in people 20 to 74.
	Blood vessels	Plaque builds up and blocks arteries in major organs, such as the heart and brain. The walls of blood vessels are damaged so that they cannot transfer oxygen normally.	Poor circulation causes wounds to heal poorly and can lead to heart disease, stroke, gangrene of the feet and hands, and infections. Diabetics suffer 2 to 4 times the usual rate of CVD.
	Kidneys	Blood vessels thicken; protein leaks into urine; blood isn't filtered normally.	Poor kidney function; kidney failure. Nearly one-half of new cases of end-stage kidney disease stem from diabetes.
	Genitals	Poor circulation in blood vessels in genitals can lead to impotence.	Eighty percent of diabetic men suffer from impotence.
	Nerves	Nerves are damaged because glucose isn't metabolized normally and blood supply is inadequate.	Leg weakness; reduced sensation, tingling, and pain in the hands and feet; chronic damage to nerves. Nerve damage and poor blood vessel circulation may lead to leg amputations.

is a leading cause of death in this country and diabetics are 2 to 4 time as prone to heart attack and stroke as are nondiabetics. Assess your risk of developing diabetes by completing "Are You at Risk for Diabetes?" Lab Activity 7-4.

Treatment for Blocked Coronary Arteries

As you have discovered, most of the risk factors linked to coronary heart disease can be controlled. The way you live, the choices you make, can have a profound impact on the health of your cardiorespiratory system. When coronary arteries do become blocked, usually the first treatments prescribed are diet modification (low fat) and exercise therapy. These are two major areas of one's life that, if maximized, can have positive results. When these methods are unsuccessful, the following procedures may be required.

Drug Therapy

This involves drug treatment affecting the supply of oxygen to the heart muscle or the heart's demand for oxygen. Some drugs (coronary vasodilators) cause the blood vessels to relax, enlarging the opening inside them. Blood flow then improves and more oxygen reaches the heart. Nitroglycerine is the most commonly used drug in this category. Another category of drugs slows down the heart rate or reduces blood pressure, thus decreasing the heart's need for oxygen, reducing its workload.

Angioplasty (or Balloon Angioplasty)

The American Heart Association describes this treatment as a nonsurgical procedure that improves the blood supply to the heart by dilating a narrowed coronary artery. The blocked part of the coronary artery must be identified before this technique is performed. During this process (cardiac catheterization), a doctor guides a thin plastic tube (catheter) through an artery from the arm or leg into the coronary arteries. A liquid dye, visible in X rays, is injected into the catheter and X-ray movies are taken as the dye flows through the arteries. Doctors can identify obstructions in the arteries by tracing the flow of the dye. Once obstructions are identified, another catheter having a balloon tip is inserted inside the first; the balloon tip is inflated at the obstruction site. This compresses the plaque and enlarges the opening of the blood vessel. The balloon is deflated and both catheters are removed. The process injures the vessel wall, causing the area to grow new cells. Some people grow too many cells, reclogging the artery. About 25 percent of the people who have this technique have renarrowed arteries within 6 months. The introduction of stents (cylinders that prop the arteries open) has substantially reduced the

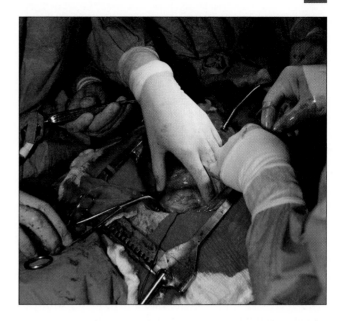

The cost of cardiovascular diseases and stroke was an estimated $326.6 billion. This figure includes health care expenditures and lost productivity for the year 2000. Each year these costs increase.

risk of arteries closing again. However, the reclosure risk is still 10 to 20 percent within the first year.

Coronary Bypass Surgery

This is a surgical technique in which doctors take a blood vessel from another part of the body (usually the leg) and use it to detour around a blockage in the coronary artery. Blood flow to the heart is restored.

New Techniques

What follows are new techniques under research and showing great promise:

1. *Enzyme therapy:* In this nonsurgical process, enzymes are injected into the blockage, dissolving it.
2. *Laser beam treatment:* This is used to break up the plaque, after which the particles of debris are vaporized.
3. *Vaccination:* Because a virus has been identified in the blocked arteries of heart patients during autopsy, a vaccine might be given early in life (like the polio vaccine) to treat some forms of coronary artery disease.
4. *Insertion of a cancer gene:* A gene that slows cancer growth may also help prevent heart patients' arteries from reclogging after angioplasty. The retenoblastoma gene is inserted into an ordinary cold virus, it is genetically modified so it cannot spread, and then angioplasty is performed with the virus-coated balloon. The gene does its work until the virus dies; both then become inactive. Reclogging has been reduced in early trials.

The Future . . . Focus on Lifestyle

The cost of treating cardiovascular diseases in this country is staggering. Many scientists believe we will be more successful if we focus on prevention rather than rely on expensive, high-tech treatments. "An ounce of prevention is worth a pound of cure" will, in all likelihood, be the slogan of the twenty-first century. Heart disease prevention in our future will focus primarily on lifestyle changes and approaches that involve "mind and body" concepts. Many scientists are already substantiating these trends in their research and medical practices.

One example is Dr. Dean Ornish, cardiologist, clinical professor of medicine at the University of California at San Francisco, and pioneer in the treatment of coronary heart disease. He found that after treating his patients with the current, recommended medical procedures—medication, angioplasty (balloon technique), and coronary bypass surgery, all expensive and dangerous—most did not stay well. Despite the procedures, some died and many returned for further treatment. He began to question the wisdom of such dramatic medical care for coronary heart disease. He found it interesting that lifestyle factors could trigger all mechanisms known to cause CHD. The lifestyle choices we make each day, such as about what we eat, how we respond to stress, how much we exercise, and whether we use tobacco, have a profound impact on our heart's health. With this concept in mind, he developed a plan that focused on lifestyle. His new program, "Reversing Heart Disease," is having significant success in reducing atherosclerosis without medication or surgical procedures. The program involves the following lifestyle changes:

1. A special diet is recommended. The Reversal Diet is 10 percent fat, 70 to 75 percent carbohydrate, 15 to 20 percent protein, and 5 milligrams of cholesterol per day. In comparison, the typical American diet is 40 to 45 percent fat, 25 to 35 percent carbohydrate, 25 percent protein, and 400 to 500 milligrams of cholesterol per day. The Reversal Diet allows, but does not encourage, moderate alcohol consumption (less than 2 oz. per day). It excludes caffeine, allows moderate use of salt and sugar, and is not restricted in calories.
2. Smoking is prohibited.
3. Thirty minutes a day or one hour every other day of moderate exercise is prescribed.
4. Stress management methods are prescribed every day. These include yoga stretches, progressive relaxation, abdominal breathing, meditation, and imagery.
5. Psychological support should be enhanced. This involves increased time spent talking about feelings with friends and family and participating in spiritual and religious activities.

Mind and Body Connection

The traditional risk factors explain only a portion of the known causes of heart disease. Why do some people develop heart disease and others do not? Clearly, all the risk factors are important, but could there be something more? Are there common psychological—and perhaps even spiritual—factors that lead to or prevent coronary heart disease? Is there an unconscious connection between mind, body, and spirit that would explain the unknown causes of heart disease?

Scientists are beginning to examine these questions: Is laughter good for you? Can prayer bring down blood pressure? Does a bad marriage or divorce suppress your immune system? Does listening to others lower blood pressure? Is a cynic more likely to have heart trouble? To each of these questions there is a scientist able to answer "YES!" and provide data to back it up. There is a whole field of mind/body research tapping into the interaction between our immune systems and our bodies, mind, moods, and spirit. Just as we learned the importance of exercise and nutrition to our health, we are discovering ways to go deeper into inner wellness. Ponder these studies that support the mind/body concept:

- Norman Cousins, author, philosopher, and former professor at the Department of Psychiatry and Biobehavioral Sciences at UCLA Medical School, (now deceased) found that laughter heals because it replaces fear and stress with serenity and homeostasis. He taught others to never underestimate the capacity of the human mind and body to regenerate, even when the prospects seemed most dismal. His research confirmed that positive emotions boost health.
- Larry Scherwitz, professor of psychology at the University of California, found that people who overuse the self-centered pronouns "I," "me," or "mine" are twice as likely to have heart attacks. These people are hostile, have a low level of trust in others, and put their self-centered interests and pleasures ahead of others.
- Redford Williams of Duke University found that cynics, being full of contempt for other people, and angry hostile people have more than their share of heart trouble.
- Many scientists have developed psychological tests to measure levels of anger that bring on heart attacks. Studies linking social support (i.e., loving family, happy marriage, one or two close friends, support groups) to vitality, longevity, lowered blood pressure, and healthier immune systems confirm that emotions may regulate health. These head and heart factors are powerful medicine.
- Dean Ornish, M.D., is convinced that one cause of blocked coronary arteries stems from three kinds of loneliness (or isolation): (1) we feel isolated from

ourselves, (2) we lack "connectedness" and intimate relationships with others, (3) we have a cosmic loneliness of the spirit (or higher part of ourselves). He feels that isolation leads to chronic stress and to illnesses such as heart disease, and that real intimacy and feelings of connectedness with others can be healing. He argues that the ability to be intimate with ourselves, with others, and with a higher spirit—within ourselves—is the key to emotional health and essential to the health of our hearts as well.

- Mind/body connection authority, Jon Kabat-Zinn, author of *Full Catastrophe Living*, advocates meditation as a technique to bridge the gap between the mind and the heart to improve health, ease pain, and reduce stress.

- Another authority on the mind/body connection, Bill Moyers, author of *Healing and the Mind*, explored the latest research in the field of medicine known as psychoneuroimmunology. He found evidence supporting the ways in which thoughts, feelings, and emotions influence our health. Moyers documents the importance of mind/body interactions in the prevention and the treatment of illness.

 ## frequently asked questions

Q. Is it really OK to eat eggs two or three times a week even though I'm on medication to keep my cholesterol down?

A. Yes, it is. Research shows that two or three eggs weekly are not apt to raise blood cholesterol. The real villain is saturated animal fat, found in whole milk, fatty meat, cheese, and butter. A Harvard study of 120,000 men and women found that a daily egg did not boost the risk of heart disease or stroke. Eggs are rich in choline, needed for proper brain functioning, and the antioxidant lutein, believed to help protect eyes from macular degeneration.

Q. What is homocysteine, and how is it related to CHD?

A. **Homocysteine** is an amino acid in the blood and a natural by-product of protein metabolism. The consumption of protein from meat or vegetable sources (such as soy) starts a series of biochemical reactions that ultimately leads to the production of homocysteine. Studies have shown that too much homocysteine in the blood is related to a higher risk of CHD, stroke, and peripheral vascular disease. Additionally, evidence suggests that homocysteine may have an effect on atherosclerosis by damaging the inner lining of arteries and promoting blood clots. A high homocysteine level is considered to be the "new" risk factor for CHD and to be in the same league as cholesterol.

Homocysteine levels in the blood are strongly influenced by diet, as well as genetic factors. The dietary components with the greatest positive effects are folic acid and vitamins B6 and B12. Folic acid and the B vitamins help break down homocysteine and thereby lower concentrations in the blood. Also, studies reveal that low blood levels of folic acid are linked with higher risk of fatal CHD and stroke.

Along with diets high in protein and low in B vitamins, heavy smoking has been linked to high homocysteine levels. Heavy smokers, have up to 50 percent higher homocysteine levels than nonsmokers. Homocysteine levels above 15.8 micromoles/liter have a threefold greater risk of heart attack than those with lower levels.

Although evidence for the benefit of lowering homocysteine levels is lacking, people with high risk should be strongly advised to be sure to get enough folic acid and vitamins B6 and B12 in their diet. Foods high in these nutrients include green leafy vegetables, fruits, and grain and cereal products fortified with folic acid.

It has been suggested that laboratory testing for homocysteine levels can improve the assessment of CHD risk. It may be particularly useful in people with a personal or family history of CVD, but in whom the well-established risk factors (inactivity, smoking, high blood pressure, high blood pressure, obesity) do not exist.

Q. Why does exercise prevent heart disease?

A. Here's at least part of the answer. In addition to lowering blood pressure, cholesterol, and body fat, certain components in the blood stream called cytokines act either to promote atherosclerosis (atherogenic) or prevent it (atheroprotective). Research published in the *Journal of the American Medical Association* studied the effect of long-term exercise on those blood factors. The participants worked out for an average of 2 1/2 hours per week for 6 months. After the exercise program, production of the atherogenic blood factors fell by 58.3 percent and the level of atheroprotective factors rose by 35 percent. In any individual, the amount of change was proportional to the level of activity. In other words, those participants who exercised more, enjoyed more of the beneficial effects in their blood levels. Those who exercised less had a smaller response. It appears that with every extra minute you exercise, your body is producing more protection and less destruction of your arteries. Although there is likely an upper limit (or point of diminishing returns), this study gives you one more reason to exercise.

frequently asked questions

Q. Don't more women die from breast cancer than heart disease?

A. No. Across nearly all racial and ethnic groups, heart disease is the number 1 killer of women just as it is the number 1 killer of men.

Q. I know my HDL and LDL. Why don't they add up to my total cholesterol?

A. Certain blood fats known as triglycerides also figure into the equation:

Total cholesterol = HDL + LDL + (triglycerides ÷ 5)

LDL is not measured directly, but derived as follows:

LDL = total cholesterol − HDL − (triglycerides ÷ 5)

Q. How often should I have my blood cholesterol measured?

A. Adults should be screened at *least* once every 5 years, but more frequently if the total cholesterol is elevated, if HDL is low, and/or they have other cardiac risk factors.

Q. How many people in the United States adhere to a lifestyle that reduces their risk of coronary heart disease?

A. It is somewhat difficult to pinpoint the exact number but findings from the Nurse's Health Study (involving more than 80,000 women) may give us some insight. The study revealed that women in this low risk category make up only

3 percent of the population . . . a pitifully low number. The study confirmed that the risk of heart disease can almost be eliminated if we follow a few rules. The heart-healthy lifestyle defined in this study involves:

- Engaging in moderate-to-vigorous physical activity for at least half an hour per day.
- Not smoking.
- Eating healthy and consuming a diet:
  - low in saturated fat (found in animal products) and trans fat (found in cookies, crackers, pies, cakes, donuts, candy, margarine)
  - high in fiber
  - high in folate (found in green leafy vegetables, orange juice, fortified cereals, legumes, and whole grains)
  - high in omega-3 fatty acids (found in fish)
  - low in glycemic foods (found in sweets, etc., which raise glucose levels)
  - averaging at least half a drink of an alcoholic beverage a day
- Avoid being overweight (a body mass index of 25 or under).

summary

Heart disease is the number 1 killer in the United States. Extensive studies have identified twelve factors that increase the risk of developing coronary heart disease. These factors lead to the development of atherosclerosis. The most significant factors are inactivity, high blood pressure, high blood lipid profile, cigarette smoking, and obesity. These five are labeled *primary* and can be controlled. There are seven additional contributing factors labeled *secondary*. The first two of these are controllable. They are stress and emotional behavior (especially negative emotional behaviors, such as hostility and anger). The other five secondary risk factors, which cannot be controlled, are age, male gender, race, positive family history, and diabetes. The more risk factors you have and the longer they are present, the greater the chance you have of developing heart disease. By age 20, you already have fatty deposits present in your coronary arteries. If your risk of CHD is low, keep up the good

work by maintaining a healthy lifestyle. However, if your coronary risk is high, now is the time to act. You can't do anything about heredity, sex (gender), or age. However, you can choose to act on those risk factors under your control.

If the coronary arteries become blocked due to advanced atherosclerosis, there are several treatments available. These include exercise and diet modification, drug therapy, angioplasty, and coronary bypass surgery. The cost of treating CVD continues to spiral upward every year. To counter this trend, many scientists are convinced that preventing CVD through lifestyle change is the key to maximizing heart health.

Adopting a healthy lifestyle early in life can add years to your life and life to your years. In addition, great discoveries await us as the field of mind and body research gains wider acceptance in the quest for increased well-being.

additional information resources

American Diabetes Association, Inc.
Two Park Avenue
New York, NY 10016
(212) 683–7444

American Heart Association
7272 Greenville Avenue
Dallas, TX 75231–4596
(800) AHA-USA1

www.americanheart.org

National Diabetes Information
Clearinghouse
Box NDIC
Bethesda, MD 20205
(301) 496–7433

National Heart, Lung, and Blood
Institute Information Center
4733 Bethesda Avenue, Suite 530
Bethesda, MD 20814–4820
(301) 251–1212

http://www.nhlbi.nih.gov

National Stroke Association
1565 Clarkson Street
Denver, CO 80218
(303) 839–1992

The Juvenile Diabetes Foundation International
23 East 26th Street
New York, NY 10010
(212) 889–7575

 # internet resources

http://www.ama-assn.org
American Medical Association—Access to full-text articles from medical journals

http://www.healthfinder.gov
Healthfinder, U.S. Government

http://www.medscape.com
Medscape—A commercial collection of full-text journal articles

http://healthlink.stanford.edu/with health news
AFAA/Your Body

http://www.afaa.com/your_body/yourbody.html
American Heart Association

http://www.americanheart.org
American Lung Association

http://www.lungusa.org/asthma
Cardiology Compass

http://www.cardiologycompass.com
Centers for Disease Control and Prevention

http://www.cdc.gov.cdc.html
Cooper Institute for Aerobics Research

http://www.cooperinst.org
Dietary Approaches to Stop Hypertension (DASH)

http://dash.bwh.harvard.edu
Franklin Institute Science Museum/The Heart: An On-line
Exploration

http://www.fi.edu/biosci/heart.html
Healthy People 2010

http://www.odphp.osophs.dhhs.gov/pubs/hp2010/
HeartInfo—Heart Information Network

http://www.heartinfo.org
Medline (This vast, government-operated database of medical journal abstracts is open to anyone)

http://www.nlm.nih.gov/databases/medline.html
National Institute for Health

http://www.nih.gov
National Stroke Association

http://www.stroke.org
New England Journal of Medicine

http://www.nejm.org
St. John's Cardiovascular Research Center

http://www.heartct.humc.edu
Shape Up America

http://www.shapeup.org

http://www.health.gov/healthypeople
Healthy People 2020

Are You at Risk?

Your chances for developing heart disease depend on a variety of habits and risk factors. Smoking, physical activity, stress management, blood pressure, and cholesterol are important prognosticators for heart disease. Read the question, and circle the most appropriate response as it relates to your lifestyle. Finally, add the points associated with your response to obtain your total score and your risk of developing heart disease.

1. Do you smoke cigarettes?	Yes	12
	No	0
2. Do you use other tobacco products (pipe, cigars, chewing, snuff)?	Yes	3
	No	0
3. Do you usually exercise vigorously at least three times per week for 20 to 30 minutes?	Yes	0
	No	10
4. How would you describe your lifestyle?	Sedentary (inactive)	6
	Somewhat active	2
	Very active	0
5. What is your blood pressure?	High 140/90 +	9
	Normal or low	0
	Don't know	2
6. What is your total cholesterol?	High 240 mg/dl+	9
	Normal	0
	Don't know	2
7. Has anyone in your family ever been told they had any form of heart disease (parents or siblings #55 years)?	Yes	5
	No	0
8. Have you ever had any of the following?		
a. Pain or discomfort in chest and surrounding areas?	Yes	2
	No	0
b. Unaccustomed shortness of breath with mild exertion?	Yes	2
	No	0
9. What is your gender?	Female	0
	Male	4
10. Have you ever been told you have diabetes?	Yes	4
	No	0

11. Have you suffered a personal loss or misfortune in the past year that had a serious impact on your life? (i.e., job loss, disability, separation/divorce, jail term, or the death of someone close to you)	No Yes, 1 serious loss or misfortune Yes, 2 or more	0 1 2
12. Do you feel you handle everyday stress well?	Yes No	0 2
13. Would you describe yourself as a Type A person (i.e., aggressive, competitive, time-conscious)?	Yes No	4 2
14. If you are male, what is your age? If you are female, what is your age?	Under 40 40+ Under 50 50+	1 3 0 3
15. What is your race?	White African American Hispanic Other	0 3 1 1
16. How would you describe your weight?	Normal/below Normal to +30 lbs. +30 lbs. or more	0 1 2
17. Do you consume meat, eggs, cheese, butter, whole milk, and fried foods?	0 to 5 times/week to 10 times/week daily 2 to 3 servings/day over 3 servings/day	0 2 3 6
	Your Total Score	_____

Scoring

Scores of 0 to 16

Your risk is **low** for developing heart disease at this time. Evaluate your risk every year since risk factors such as blood pressure, cholesterol levels, and age change from year to year. If you have any uncontrollable risk factors, you would be wise to modify other risk factors to protect your cardiorespiratory system.

Scores of 17 to 29

Your risk is **average** or moderate. Your score indicates there is room for improvement on some risk factors. If you have any uncontrollable risk factors, it is imperative that you modify other risk factors to protect your cardiorespiratory system.

Scores of 30+

You have a **high** risk of developing heart disease. You should take action **immediately** to modify all controllable risk factors.

Evaluation of Are You at Risk?

After completing the *Are You at Risk?* assessment, answer the following questions:

1. List the factors you identified that contribute to your risk of coronary heart disease.

2. List at least five personal lifestyle changes you can make to lower your risk for heart disease. Be specific; don't say, "Eat better," for example.

3. Take the *Are You At Risk?* assessment for a parent or friend. What is his or her score? What advice would you give to help to lower his or her score?

4. List **your** personal controllable risk factors. How can you make changes in each one to become more heart healthy?

5. List **your** personal *uncontrollable* risk factors.

6. Some physicians are refusing to treat people when they discover that they smoke or don't exercise or have diets high in fat. Discuss how you feel about this decision.

lab activity
7-3

How to Mend a Broken Heart

Read the opening scenario concerning Rob on page 2 in your text. You were the physician on call when he was brought in. Complete a medical history on this patient and answer his wife's questions.

1. List Rob's four primary risk factors for heart disease given in the scenario.

2. List Rob's two secondary risk factors for heart disease.

3. What three or four lifestyle changes will you tell Rob to make to reduce his heart disease risk?

Rob's wife has read the chart. She is distraught and has several questions for you. Please respond.

4. "Doctor, I really don't understand some of the words used on the chart. What is angina? Myocardial infarction? What is atherosclerosis, and will it ever go away?"

lab activity @ chapter seven

5. "I saw that his cholesterol was 280, his HDL level was 28, and his LDL level was 174. His cholesterol and HDL ratio was 10, and his triglycerides were 325. What do each of these mean? What is normal or desirable for each?"

   a.

   b.

   c.

   d.

   e.

6. "Rob doesn't want to quit smoking—he's smoked for 20 years. Why is smoking bad for his heart?"

7. "A nurse said Rob needs a special exercise program to aid in recovery. Won't exercise strain his heart? What good will it do?" (Give three benefits.)

8. "Rob enjoys having an occasional beer. Will he have to give this up?"

Are You at Risk for Diabetes?

Directions: Answer the questions in Part I to evaluate your risk for developing diabetes. Complete Part II to learn more about diabetes and the connection it has to heart disease.

Part I

Yes	No	
_____	_____	1. I am overweight (Body-mass index greater than 27. To calculate your BMI, multiply your weight in pounds by 705; divide the result by your height in inches, then divide that result by your height in inches again.) What is your BMI? _____.
_____	_____	2. I get little or no exercise.
_____	_____	3. I have a parent with diabetes.
_____	_____	4. I am African American, Hispanic American, or Native American.
_____	_____	5. I am over 40 years of age (counts as one "yes" answer; if over 65 years of age, counts as two "yes" answers.
_____	_____	6. I am a women who had diabetes during pregnancy or delivered a baby weighing more than 9 pounds.
_____	_____	7. I have a brother, sister, or parent with diabetes.
_____	_____	8. I have high blood pressure and/or high cholesterol.
_____	_____	9. I had a minimally elevated glucose level on a previous test (110–125 mg/dl)

Scoring: Each "yes" answer you have increases your risk of developing diabetes.

Part II

1. How many "yes" answers did you have? _____

2. Discuss your potential risk for developing diabetes. _____

_____

_____

_____

lab activity @ chapter seven

3. List the warning symptoms of Type 1 and Type 2 diabetes. _____

_____

_____

_____

_____

4. Discuss the difference between Type 1 and Type 2 diabetes. _____

_____

_____

_____

_____

5. What can you do to prevent or reduce your risk of developing diabetes? _____

_____

_____

_____

_____

6. Why is diabetes such a serious disease? _____

_____

_____

7. Why does diabetes increase the risk for heart disease? _____

_____

_____

_____

_____

8. What segments of the U.S. population are at increased risk of diabetes?_____

_____

_____

_____

_____

9. How does diabetes affect the eyes, blood vessels, kidneys, genitals, and nerves?_____

_____

_____

_____

_____

_____

lab activity 7-5

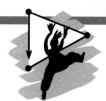

Using HealthQuest

Directions: Insert CD. When the table of contents screen appears, click on "Cardiovascular Health." Click on "Wellness Activities," then "Heart Attack Risk:"

I. Read "Introduction."

   1. What is the number one killer in America? _____

   2. Why is heart disease a national concern? _____

II. Assess yourself. Answer the questions on the self-assessment.

  A. "Risk Assessment":

     1. What was your risk on the "Risk Assessment" section? _____

     2. What was your total number of points? _____

     3. Discuss your findings. _____

     4. What were your weaknesses? _____

  B. "Knowledge Inventory":

     1. What was your "Knowledge Inventory" ranking? _____

     2. What was your score in this section? _____ Discuss the findings. _____

     3. What were your weaknesses?

  C. Additional Feedback:

     1. Do you agree that high blood pressure, smoking, and high blood cholesterol are the three most important risk factors for heart disease? _____ Why or why not? _____

     2. Discuss how physical inactivity influences an individual's risk for heart disease. _____

     3. List three lifestyle behaviors that you could change or implement that would reduce your heart disease risk.

     _____

     _____

lab activity @ chapter seven

> **Happiness is an inside job.**
> —H. Jackson Brown, Jr., ed. *Dad, a Father's Book of Wisdom*

Coping with Stress

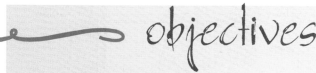 *objectives*

After reading this chapter, you will be able to:

1. Define the terms *stress, stressor,* and *stress response.*
2. Explain the three stages of the stress response.
3. Define and give examples of eustress, distress, and optimal stress.
4. Explain how perception and control are involved in stress.
5. On the Life Event Stress test, measure the amount of life changes you have encountered this year and be able to predict your susceptibility to a stress-related illness.
6. Explain the difference between daily hassles and daily uplifts and how each affects overall health.
7. Describe six harmful effects of too much stress.
8. Contrast Type A, Type B, and Type C personality.
9. Describe a hot reactor's behavior and the health consequences of this behavior.
10. List five Type A behavior modification techniques.
11. List five strategies for managing stress.
12. Define and list three benefits of the relaxation response.

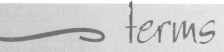 *terms*

- Autogenic training and imagery
- Biofeedback training
- Catecholamines
- Daily hassles
- Daily uplifts
- Distress
- Eustress
- Fight-or-flight response (Alarm Reaction Stage)
- General Adaptation Syndrome (GAS)

- Hatha Yoga
- Hot reactors
- Meditation
- Mindfulness meditation
- Optimal stress
- Progressive relaxation
- Psychoneuroimmunology
- Psychosomatic disease
- Reframing
- Relaxation response
- Stage of exhaustion

- Stage of resistance
- Stress
- Stressors
- Stress Response
- Transcendental meditation (TM)
- Type A personality
- Type B personality
- Type C personality

Lisa was the oldest child of three and the first in her family to go to college. Living on campus was wonderful—it meant new friends, open visitation in the residence hall, and no curfew hours. But, by the end of the school year, her life had changed for the worse.

Her G.P.A. was barely above a "C" average, which was far below her high school performance. There never seemed to be enough hours in the day to keep up with all the reading. Also, she felt exhausted most of the time and had trouble waking up for early classes. It was no wonder: The "action" never settled down on her hall before 12:30 or 1:00 A.M. The parties on the weekends were awesome. There were so many she couldn't decide which one to go to so she went to them all. She would stay out partying until 6 A.M., grab a bite, and then sleep all day. With all the partying, fast food, and beer, her waistline also began to slip, 15 pounds worth! Then, just before final exams, her parents announced that they were getting a divorce. Had her college expenses created a financial burden on the family budget and contributed to the divorce? She felt guilty and partially responsible for her parent's problems. Now she would have to move back home and work full-time at the local discount store to help pay for college. Would it be possible to finish the nursing degree by taking night classes? Antonio, her boyfriend was pressuring her to drop out of school so they could get married. He complained that she devoted too much time to school work and not enough to him. Her mother would now have to go back to work and would expect her to help take care of her younger brothers and assist with the household chores. Feeling fatigued and stressed out, she wondered, with work and family obligations, when would she study? Would she have any time for herself? Was she the only one in college with such problems? How complicated her life had become.

This scene just described is not that uncommon on the typical college campus. The many challenges faced by college students can be stressful and can cause feelings of anxiety. Stiff competition for grades, career choices, selection of classes, test anxiety, sense of loss of family and home, balancing work and school, peer pressure, inadequate sleep, poor nutritional habits, low physical fitness levels, and increased social involvements contribute to high levels of stress. Clearly, college is a stressful environment, one that makes demands on you physically, socially, intellectually, and emotionally. It's no wonder that you sometimes feel anxious, irritable, and stressed out. Contrary to what many college students believe, stress does not "evaporate" after

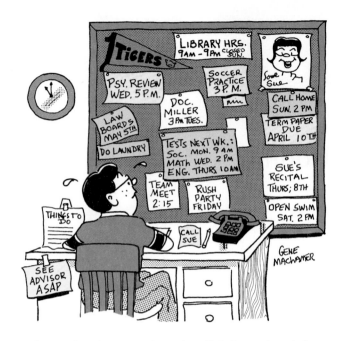

College students have many demands on their time and must plan wisely.

graduation. The pace of life seems to be accelerating. Federal Express overnight service is no longer quick enough—the letter needs to be faxed immediately. Receiving one telephone call at a time is not enough; now, with call waiting, two or more can be received at once. Even the traditional places of refuge in the twenty-first century—the car and the home—are transformed into offices away from offices, with fax machines and computers in the home and cell phones, fax machines, and the Internet in the car. With cellular telephones and laptop computers, work stress never ends. We often do not have time to recover from one stressful situation before we face another one.

No one is exempt from stress. This is good because a certain amount is beneficial for an optimal level of health and achievement, and it helps us cope with emergency situations. Figure 8-1 illustrates how the "right" amount of stress improves health and performance, but how our health and well-being can be adversely affected by excessive stress. Too much stress ultimately exhausts the body's ability to adapt; vital organs wear out, and various illnesses may appear. This is especially true when stress is perceived to be negative or harmful. Stress is a normal part of life, so why do so few people understand it or how to manage it? Improvement in the quality of life is dependent on *balancing* the demands made upon you and developing effective ways to *manage* stress.

What Is Stress?

Dr. Hans Selye, one of the foremost authorities on stress, defined **stress** as the "nonspecific response of the human organism to any demand made upon it." It is the response of the body to any type of change and to any new, threatening, or exciting situation. *Nonspecific* means that the body reacts the same regardless of the cause. **Stressors,** factors causing stress, can be pleasant or unpleasant, either real or imagined, and can be of different types. All cause the body to adapt. For example, *physical* stressors include illness, accidents, injury, heat, cold, and noise. *Psychological* or *emotional* stressors involve parenting, deadlines, poverty, final exams, work overloads (school or job), rejection, depression, holidays, divorce, and marriage.

Dr. Selye described the ways in which we react to stress as either *eustress* (good) or *distress* (bad). In both cases, the physiological response is the same. In the case of **eustress,** which refers to happy, pleasant events (holidays, getting married, etc.), health and performance improve even as stress increases. On the other hand, **distress** refers to unpleasant or harmful stress (flunking an exam, breakup of a relationship, etc.) under which health and performance begin to decline. **Optimal stress** is a point at which eustress and distress are intense enough to motivate and physically prepare us to perform optimally yet not intense enough to cause the body to overreact or to sustain harmful effects. Figure 8-1 illustrates this concept. Optimal stress gives the athlete the competitive edge and the public speaker the enthusiasm to project with charisma. Overstress results in poor performance and produces overreaction, poor concentration, test anxiety, and health problems. When experiencing positive stress, individuals feel in control. Negative stress causes out-of-control feelings.

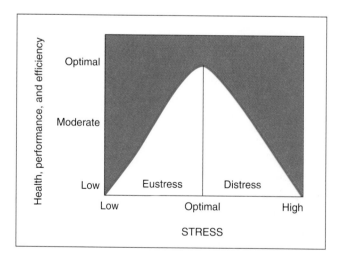

figure 8-1   Optimal stress and the relationship to health and performance. Everyone has a point at which the "right" amount of stress improves performance, health, and efficiency.

Regardless of the cause, the adaptation (reaction) to stress is both psychological and physiological and leads to what Dr. Selye called the **General Adaptation Syndrome (GAS).** Today, the GAS is called the **Stress Response.**

The Stress Response—a Three-Stage Process

Hans Selye summarized the Stress Response in a three-stage process:

1. **Fight-or-flight response (Alarm Reaction Stage):** The body prepares to cope with a stressor. The response is a warning signal that a stressor is present. Physiological and psychological responses appear. This is a primitive survival mechanism that today is rarely needed. See Figure 8-2.
2. **Stage of resistance:** The body actively resists and attempts to cope with the stressor. In this stage, the stress response is channeled into the specific organ system most capable of suppressing it. It is this adaptation process that contributes to stress-related illness. The specific organ system becomes aroused and, if prolonged, it may fatigue and begin to malfunction. Headache, forgetfulness, colon spasms (constipation or diarrhea), asthma, anxiety attacks, and high blood pressure are examples of prolonged arousal.
3. **Stage of exhaustion:** Adaptation energy is exhausted and signs of fight-or-flight reappear. During the exhaustion phase, the organ system involved in the repeated stress response breaks down. Disease or malfunction of the organ system or even death may occur. For example, high blood pressure (caused by excessive stress) promotes kidney and heart damage, which can kill the individual if allowed to continue.

Fight-or-Flight (Alarm Reaction)

The body responds to stress, whether emotional or physical (real or perceived), by activating a series of mechanisms collectively known as the fight-or-flight response. This response, a part of our physiological makeup since the beginning of time, prepares us to either fight or to flee to safety by pumping powerful stress hormones and steroids into the bloodstream (Fig. 8-2). The fight-or-flight response has many benefits. Early humans, faced with daily life-and-death situations, relied heavily on this response for survival. The caveman or -woman could escape the jaws of a hungry lion (stressor) by swiftly running (the fight-or-flight response in action). These mechanisms work best where the danger is clear, well-defined, and short-term (acute not chronic).

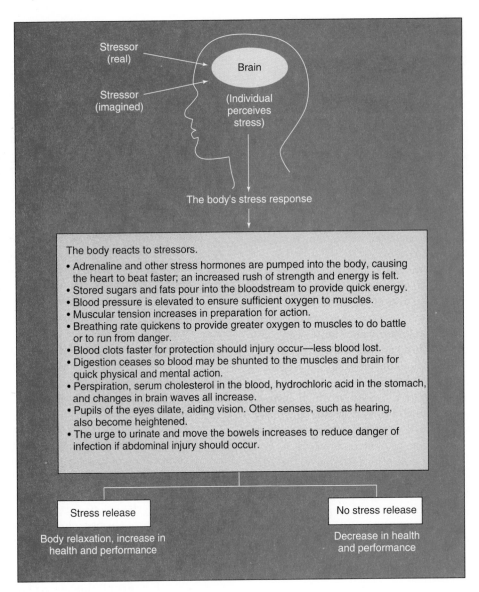

figure 8-2   Physical reactions to stressors.

Many examples of the fight-or-flight response can be found even in today's world. Imagine this scenario: You are crossing the street on your way home when suddenly you see a car fast approaching you. Instinctively, your muscles tense, and you jump back on the curb with such force that you fall back into a newspaper stand and cut your head, which quickly stops bleeding. The fight-or-flight response saved your life (the quick backward jump and the cut that stops bleeding). Other examples of the response, normally described as "superhuman" acts, are in reality the fight-or-flight response in action. Perhaps you can add others to this list:

- A person lifts an automobile off an injured individual at an accident scene.
- A paraplegic rescues a woman drowning in an apartment complex swimming pool.

- After having both arms ripped off by a farm machine, a young farmer manages to telephone for help by dialing 911 with a pencil clenched in his teeth.
- A mother knocks down a locked bedroom door to rescue her children from a burning house.
- A student outruns a mugger on a dark corner of campus.

These are only a few examples that have required action to prevent or minimize physical harm. A few minutes after the frightening event (acute stressor), the individuals return to their normal physiological state. Other stressors, the kind you encounter every day, such as noise, arguments, keys locked inside the car, missed deadlines, traffic tickets, or any new situation that causes us to adapt, have the same potential for eliciting the fight-or-flight response. Ironically, the

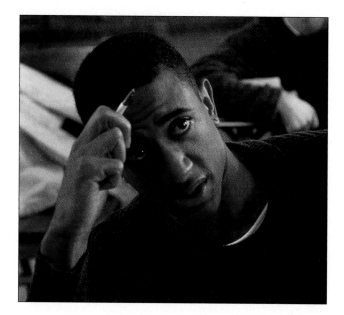

Chronic arousal of the fight-or-flight response causes chemical wear and tear on the body.

strains and hassles of life in a civilized world have transformed this life-saving mechanism into a potentially life-threatening one.

Physical and emotional stress (too much to do, breakup of a relationship, public speaking, etc.) may be either acute or chronic. We are designed to cope with acute stress much better than with chronic stress. Unfortunately, physical and emotional stress in modern times tends to be chronic rather than acute. The pace of life accelerates every year. Constant hurrying, common to today's lifestyle, is associated with the chronic arousal of the fight-or-flight response. We often do not have time to recover from one stressful situation before we face another one.

Innate physiological stress responses (Fig. 8-2) have evolved over the centuries to help us survive danger and prepare us for swift action whether or not it is needed. However, the buildup of unused stress products produces excessive wear and tear on the body and may even increase the rate of aging. When stressors inappropriately provoke the fight-or-flight reaction many times a day, the body repeatedly responds as if experiencing real emergencies. The fight-or-flight response is often appropriate and should not be thought of as always harmful. It is a necessary part of our physiological makeup, a useful reaction to many situations in our current world. However, we need to learn how to avoid triggering the stress response except in real emergencies.

Stage of Resistance

The longer our bodies stay in a chronic "on guard" resistance stage, the more likely we are to experience ill effects. Today, we don't have much opportunity to physically play out the fight-or-flight response in acute stress situations because today's stress is mostly chronic. Though we chronically evoke the fight-or-flight response, modern society does not accept the fight naturally associated with it. For example, you do not run away from or hit your boss when he or she reprimands you. Our innate reactions have not changed, but society has. The response is turned on, but we do not use it appropriately. As a result, the body remains in the resistance stage for longer periods. Our sedentary lifestyles decrease the outlets for fight-or-flight hormones that are pumped into the body. The length of time that a stressor is with you is an important factor. Stress becomes harmful when it is prolonged and perceived as negative to the recipient.

Learning stress management skills is important in coping with the stresses of life. People who have learned these skills may still overreact to a stressor but will relax more quickly to their resting physiological state than will people who have not learned these skills.

Stage of Exhaustion

The exhaustion stage of the stress response can ultimately result in death if not countered. Thankfully, it is not often reached. If our bodies are successful in resisting stress, exhaustion does not follow. We usually adapt to the stress and make whatever adjustments are necessary to cope, whether the stress is physical or psychological. Learn and practice regularly one or more of the stress management skills described in this chapter to reduce the unhealthy stress in your life.

Perception and Control

Individuals may respond differently to the same stressor. Whether a particular stressor causes a negative reaction depends on whether the person perceives that stressor as being negative. This concept was confirmed by the research of Dr. Richard Lazarus who asserted that we are, after all, thinking, cognitive creatures. We are able to assess the positive and negative consequences of any situation or threat. One person may *perceive* a stressor as threatening, and as a result, experience a full-blown fight-or-flight response. Another may encounter the same event and not perceive it as a threat. We are different, and each of us perceives stressors in a different light. How do you perceive snakes, announcement of an exam, competition, being cut off in traffic, being called in to see the boss, a doctor's appointment, being called on to contribute to class discussion, a professor requesting to speak with you after class? These situations do not bother some individuals but are agonizing to others.

In reality, most people's problems have to do with *faulty perception*—that is, unnecessarily seeing a situation as hopeless, harmful, or negative. Fortunately, we each have the power to develop cognitive skills to cope with faulty

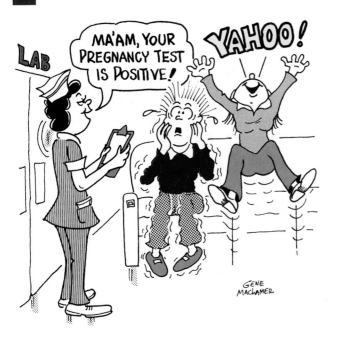

We perceive stressors differently.

perception. As Duke Ellington put it, "A problem is a chance to do your best." Before gearing up to fret, fight, or flee, ask yourself, "Does a threat really exist? Is the issue important to me? Can I make a difference?" If the answer to any of these questions is "no," do not waste your energy. It is not worth it. Some situations are truly threatening and deserve high energy stress responses. When the threat you perceive in a situation is real, go ahead and gear up. You can then benefit from the energy generated by your natural stress response by applying it to the situation at hand.

Control is another important factor in the total stress picture. You are in much greater control over your stress than you realized. Managing stress means empowering yourself to take control rather than relinquishing the control to events, to other people, to your environment, or to the calendar. People who handle stress best tend to control their lives and look for active solutions to the problems and circumstances of their lives. You are responsible for allowing stressful situations to raise your blood pressure and heart rate. We can all recall events that made us angry one time but did not even faze us the next. Why is this? It is because we *allowed* ourselves to become upset. Perhaps the situation was complicated by nasty weather, lack of sleep, or a buildup of particular events. The bottom line is this particular time we *allowed* the event to provoke an angry response. This does not need to be the case. You cannot control what other people say or do, but you can change how you react to what others say or do. Whether to allow stressful events to provoke physiological reactions, such as increased muscle tension and nervous stomach, is your decision. By taking charge, you can decide whether to be an overstressed, nervous wreck or a calm, collected person.

Other ways to gain control over your life include:

- Make healthy lifestyle decisions—getting proper amounts of exercise and adequate sleep. Not smoking, eating nutritionally, and not overindulging on alcohol allow you to exert control.
- Learn and implement time management skills. Getting organized helps spread stress out instead of having it pile up. See Strategy 3b in this chapter.
- Learn when to say "no." Only you know when to take on added duties and assignments and when your "plate is full" and must say "No sorry, not at this time. I have too many irons in the fire." This puts you in charge of your precious time.
- Regularly practice relaxation techniques and employ often the other stress-coping strategies found later in this chapter. Commit to restoring a sense of control, and reduce symptoms of stress in your life.

Remember, only you can decide if you want to manage your stress. It is your responsibility to exert control of your life. The key to surviving and even thriving on stress is self-control. Take charge of you—for you.

Harmful Effects of Stress

Stressors (i.e., all events, emotions, or situations, good or bad) cause you to react and force you to adapt. We are constantly adapting to new things, things we like and things we don't like. This adaptation to the stresses of life isn't harmful unless you are overloaded with too much in a short time—too many life change events and hassles, especially the ones perceived as undesirable or uncontrollable. In today's society, stress has increased dramatically. In essence, your fight-or-flight responses stay aroused 24 hours a day, 7 days a week. Having more stress than one can cope with can lead to a psychosomatic disease.

A **psychosomatic disease** (*psych* refers to the mind, *somatic* refers to the body) is a physical ailment that is mentally induced. The mind and the body are an interrelated whole—what affects one ultimately affects the other. **Psychoneuroimmunology** is a specialized branch of medicine that studies the mind/body connection. Examples of psychosomatic conditions are hypertension, stroke, cardiovascular disease, ulcers, life-threatening gastrointestinal problems, migraine headaches, tension headaches, cancer, allergies, asthma, hay fever, rheumatoid arthritis, and backache. These "stress" diseases, as they are frequently called, are not "all in the mind" as some people believe. They are real and can be diagnosed.

One of the stress diseases best studied is cardiovascular disease. Chronic stress contributes to hypertension and increases harmful blood clotting causing heart attack or stroke. Stress has been associated with increased risk of abdominal obesity and insulin resistance (a precursor for diabetes), risk factors for cardiovascular disease. Stress hormones damage the arterial lining and make unhealthy arteries more prone to spasms, which occlude blood flow. Stress may lead to unhealthy changes in sleep, eating, and exercise habits, and increased use of harmful substances such as caffeine, alcohol, tobacco, and other drugs—all of which may contribute to cardiovascular disease. Stress may interact with personality variables such as hostility, feelings of isolation, low self-esteem, and emotions such as anger and depression to increase artery disease.

While most digestive problems are not caused by stress, it exacerbates these disorders. Examples are gum disease, ulcers, nervous stomach and nausea, irritable bowel syndrome, chronic constipation, chronic diarrhea, and inflammatory bowel.

Chronic stress causes the musculoskeletal system to brace for fight-or-flight. This can create painful muscular tension or worsen existing muscular problems. Areas most vulnerable to such problems include muscles of the jaw, head, neck, shoulders, and back.

Prolonged stress decreases the strength of the immune system and lowers the body's resistance to disease. It can also contribute to autoimmune disorders such as rheumatoid arthritis, multiple sclerosis, and lupus. The stressful consequences of living in modern society—constant job insecurity, inability to make deadlines because of family and school obligations, running a single-parent family, living in poverty—take their toll and can lead to some devastating mind/body diseases.

Too much stress contributes to a number of psychological disorders including depression, anxiety, phobias, and addictions. Behavior manifestations of excess stress include disordered eating, excessive drinking, irritability, insomnia, and nervous habits such as nail biting.

Stress is responsible for two-thirds of doctor's visits and plays a role in another major killer—cancer. How is stress related to cancer? In addition to depressing the immune system, according to some studies, stress increases the incidence of smoking, alcohol consumption, and promiscuous sexual behavior, all associated with increased risk for developing certain kinds of cancer.

Managing stress in our lives means adapting and changing as circumstances demand and learning to *listen*. Listen to our bodies, our feelings, and our relationships and be *aware* of the common signs of stress. See Table 8-1. You are not alone if you need to begin practicing the healthy self-care strategies found later in this chapter. Sure, a few weeks in a crisis mode won't kill us but if you are experiencing five or more of the symptoms of stress (or feel particularly "stressed out") you may be headed toward developing a serious psychosomatic disease.

Measuring Your Stress

In 1967, two psychiatrists at the University of Washington School of Medicine, Thomas H. Holmes, M.D., and Richard H. Rahe, M.D., observed that certain life events coincided with illness. According to the doctors, change, whether for "good" or "bad," causes stress, leaving humans more susceptible to disease. Even simple changes, such as in eating habits, job routine, and housekeeping duties, can increase one's susceptibility to stress-related diseases. After studying medical histories and personal biographies of patients, the doctors found a curious link between life-changing events and illnesses such as heart disease, ulcers, and psychiatric problems (depression, anxiety, etc.); they developed a list of life changes that range from minor to severe and assigned points to each one based on the amount of stress evoked. The list includes both the positive, such as a vacation trip or marriage, and the negative, such as trouble at work or most stressful—the death of a child or spouse. The original test was revised recently to keep pace with the new millennium. Take a few moments to complete the *Life Event Stress Test*, identifying those events that have occurred in your life during the past year. See Table 8-2. The total score on this self-test offers some insight into one's risk for illness as a result of recent life events. Stressful change in itself won't necessarily harm you, that depends, at least in part, on how well you handle stress. Lab Activity 8-1 is an excellent evaluation of your score on this self-test.

The test can be an effective tool when used to anticipate major life events so that you can *control* the stress they produce. No one would suggest we get rid of holidays, vacations, weddings, and family reunions. But we should take all life changes, including these positive ones, into account when planning our lives. Scheduling predictable life events such as marriage or recreation provides you with some control over them and is helpful in reducing stress. Realizing there are certain life events you cannot control is equally important in stress reduction. Remember, change is inevitable; that's what living is about. But keep in mind that you can plan ahead for change and regulate the timing of many events (stressors) to prevent them from draining much of your adaptation energy. Spread change over time. When you feel in control, you perceive stressful situations as much less stressful; thus, there is less chance of provoking a stress-related illness. Change in life situations alone may not be enough to cause illness. When these changes are perceived as distressing and result in chronic and prolonged emotional and physiological wear and tear, your risk of illness increases. Some people are more vulnerable to certain types of stress than others. If you would like to find out what type of stress you are most susceptible to and how well you cope with stress take the *Measuring Your Stress and Coping Skills* test in the Lab Activities section (8-5). This test also measures coping skills for dealing with stress.

Establishing coping strategies such as the ones discussed later in this chapter is a positive way to block the development of a stress illness. Well-timed social support is probably the best coping mechanism we have. When you are experiencing many life changes but have family and friends with whom you can discuss your problems, you probably will avoid a stress illness. Another individual experiencing fewer life changes but with less support may become ill.

table 8-1   Common Signs of Stress

Check the signs of stress that you have experienced lately. Stress affects many dimensions of your life.

Physical

_____ Headaches	_____ Allergy flare-up, rashes, hives
_____ Asthma attack	_____ Muscle twitches or eye twitches
_____ Constipation and/or diarrhea	_____ Heart pounding, racing, or beating erratically
_____ Abdominal pains	_____ Restlessness
_____ Acne flare-up	_____ Fatigue
_____ Excessive dryness of hair or skin	_____ Tension
_____ Frequent colds, flu, low-grade infections/herpes flare-ups	_____ Overeating/overdrinking
_____ Chest pain	_____ Sleep disorders (sleeping too much, sleeping too little)
_____ Digestive upsets	_____ Trembling hands
_____ Neck, back, or shoulder pain	_____ Weight change
_____ Excess perspiration	_____ Teeth grinding, foot tapping

Emotional/Social/Behavioral

_____ Feeling depressed, the "blues"	_____ Mood swings
_____ Feeling nervous, anxious, fearful	_____ Isolation
_____ Feeling burned out	_____ Crying spells
_____ Feeling that life is out of control	_____ Resentment
_____ Feeling that you are being rushed	_____ Little joy
_____ Questioning your personal worth	_____ Loneliness
_____ Feeling sensitive to criticism	_____ Lashing out
_____ Often feeling suspicious	_____ Irritability
_____ Nagging	_____ Clamming up
_____ Accident prone	_____ Trouble getting along with others
	_____ Loss of sex drive

Mental

_____ Disorganization (losing things, making dumb mistakes)	_____ Negative attitude
_____ Daydreaming about escaping	_____ Confusion
_____ Difficulty making small decisions	_____ Lethargy
_____ Focus on unimportant details while not completing more important jobs	_____ Whirling mind
_____ Restlessness, poor concentration	_____ No new ideas
_____ Worrying	_____ Boredom
_____ Forgetfulness	_____ Spacing out
	_____ Dull senses
	_____ Negative self-talk

Spiritual

_____ Emptiness	_____ Intolerance
_____ Loss of meaning	_____ Looking for magic solution
_____ Doubt	_____ Loss of direction
_____ Unforgiving	_____ Cynicism
_____ Martyrdom	_____ Apathy
_____ Lack of intimacy	_____ Needing to "prove" self
_____ Fewer contacts with friends	

table 8-2   Life Event Stress Test

Directions: To get a feel for the possible health impact of the recent changes in your life, think back over the past year and circle the "stress points" listed for each of the events that you experienced during that time. Then total your points. Your score is termed your life change units (LCU). This is a measure of the amount of significant changes in your life to which you have had to adjust. In other words, your LCU is a measure of the stressors you have encountered this past year.

Life Change Event

Health

An injury or illness which:		due to marriage	41
kept you in bed a week or more, or sent you to the hospital	74	for other reasons	45
was less serious than above	44	Change in arguments with spouse	50
Major dental work	26	In-law problems	38
Major change in eating habits	27	Change in the marital status of your parents:	
Major change in sleeping habits	26	divorce	59
Major change in your usual type and/or amount		remarriage	50
of recreation	28	Separation from spouse:	
Work		due to work	53
Change to a new type of work	51	due to marital problems	76
Change in your work hours or conditions	35	Divorce	96
Change in your responsibilities at work:		Birth of grandchild	43
more responsibilities	29	Death of spouse	119
fewer responsibilities	21	Death of other family member:	
promotion	31	child	123
demotion	42	brother or sister	102
transfer	32	parent	100
Troubles at work:		**Personal and social**	
with your boss	29	Change in personal habits	26
with coworkers	35	Beginning or ending school or college	38
with persons under your supervision	35	Change of school or college	35
other work troubles	28	Change in political beliefs	24
Major business adjustment	60	Change in religious beliefs	29
Retirement	52	Change in social activities	27
Loss of Job:		Vacation	24
laid off from work	68	New, close, personal relationship	37
fired from work	79	Engagement to marry	45
Correspondence course to help you in your work	18	Girlfriend or boyfriend problems	39
Home and family		Sexual difficulties	44
Major change in living conditions	42	"Falling out" of a close personal relationship	47
Change in residence:		An accident	48
move within the same town or city	25	Minor violation of the law	20
move to a different town, city, or state	47	Being held in jail	75
Change in family get-togethers	25	Death of a close friend	70
Major change in health or behavior of family member	55	Major decision regarding your immediate future	51
Marriage	50	Major personal achievement	36
Pregnancy	67	**Financial**	
Miscarriage or abortion	65	Major change in finances:	
Gain of a new family member:		increased income	38
birth of a child	66	decreased income	60
adoption of a child	65	investment and/or credit difficulties	56
a relative moving in with you	59	Loss or damage of personal property	43
Spouse beginning or ending work	46	Moderate purchase	20
Child leaving home:		Major purchase	37
to attend college	41	Foreclosure on a mortgage or loan	58
		Total Score _____	

Scoring:

Score	Rating	Implication for Illness
≤ 249	Low Stress	37% chance of getting a stress-related illness in the next year or two. Consider yourself fortunate.
250–500	Moderate Stress	51% chance of getting a stress-related illness in the next year.
≥501	High Stress	80% change of getting a stress-related illness in the next year.

Source: Miller and Rahe, "Life Changes Scaling for the 1990s." *Journal of Psychosomatic Research*, Vol. 43, 1997. With permission from Richard Rahe, M.D. and Elsevier Science.

Daily Hassles and Uplifts

Studies by Richard Lazarus and colleagues suggest that it is not only the major "life events" that have a negative impact on health, but other factors called *daily hassles*, and these may be even more harmful. **Daily hassles** are the events or interactions in your daily life that you find bothersome, annoying, or negative in some way. These irritating demands include common problems such as losing things, time demands/deadlines, exams (i.e., preparing for, taking), relationship problems, traffic jams, arguments, and family concerns. Lazarus and colleagues found that the greatest toll from stress may not come from a divorce, loss of a job, or other traumatic changes, but from an accumulation of the minor, frequent annoyances we experience daily. Having too many things to do, roommate problems, not enough sleep, parking problems on campus, and money difficulties were the most frequently reported hassles of students at Ball State University. Examine the "Top Ten Hassles of College Students" to see how the hassles in your life compare.

Everyday hassles can be the "straw that broke the camel's back" when they are added to your life at a time when it is already overloaded with stressful events. The average person is as likely to be "nibbled to death" by everyday hassles as to be overwhelmed by tragedies. The way you handle daily hassles to a large degree depends on your score on the Life Event Stress Test. When scores are high (i.e., you are overstressed), you are more likely to react to daily hassles with less tolerance and a shorter fuse. For example, after Akiko's mother died of cancer, she had to leave college in her first year and enroll at the local community college in her hometown because she was needed at home to care for her younger brothers. On top of this, she lost her billfold (with driver's license and credit cards) on the first day of classes at the new school. The hassles of too many things to do, losing the billfold, caring for the home and her brothers, and keeping up at school were overwhelming. Frustration boiled over into stress and anger and she soon became ill. As with any stressor, the way you perceive it is critical. What constitutes a hassle or an uplift varies greatly from person to person. Concern about weight may not be a hassle to you but may be a real problem to another for whom physical appearance is a top priority.

The counterpart to daily hassles are **daily uplifts.** These are positive events that make us feel good. Fridays, payday, going shopping, and having a date were the uplifts most often listed by students at Ball State. Research has shown that these little daily uplifts can reverse the negative effects of daily hassles. An appropriate balance between hassles and uplifts may be the important ingredient in your overall health and well-being. These daily uplifts may protect you from stress-related illnesses.

List the events in your everyday life that you find bothersome. How many of them can you eliminate? How

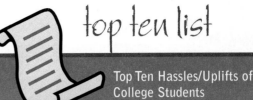

top ten list

Top Ten Hassles/Uplifts of College Students

Hassles
1. Misplacing or losing things
2. Troubling thoughts about your future
3. Not getting enough sleep
4. Money problems (overspending/bills)
5. Social obligations
6. Concerns about weight and physical appearance
7. Too many things to do (registration of classes, exams, getting low grades, extracurricular groups, everyday chores)
8. Concerns about meeting high standards (not living up to expectations, getting low grades)
9. Being lonely (relationship issues)
10. Child care problems

Uplifts
1. Being visited, phoned, or sent a letter
2. Visiting, phoning, or writing someone
3. Having fun (socializing, partying, being with friends)
4. Completing a task
5. Recreation (sports, games, etc.)
6. Hugging and/or kissing (relating well with spouse or lover)
7. Getting enough sleep
8. Being complimented
9. Having someone to listen to you
10. Eating out

many will you have to deal with in some manner? List the daily uplifts you find enjoyable. Can you find ways to add to this list? How does your list compare to the "Top Ten Uplifts" list?

Type A Behavior and Stress

We all know people who have the "hurry-up-itis" syndrome. They always are rushed, never have enough time, usually need more than 8 hours a day to complete a day's work, could not survive without their cell phone or laptop computer, and appear to be doing four or five things at one time. The woman who impatiently pushes ahead of you in line at the grocery, the young man who honks the horn of his automobile indicating for you to hurry up, or the friend who constantly looks at his or her watch all exhibit Type A behavior.

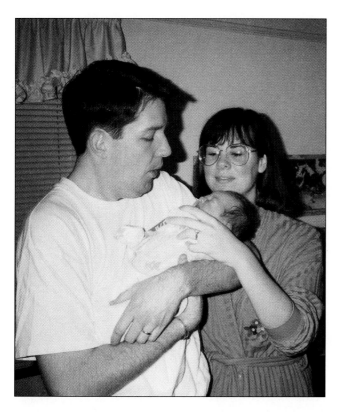

Everyday hassles (such as not getting enough sleep) won't end with college.

The **Type A personality** is described as competitive, ambitious, driven, impatient, workaholic, and *always* rushed. Type As put big demands on themselves to accomplish more in less time. They have little time for or interest in hobbies or leisure pursuits and have few intimate friends. The key problem with Type A behavior is stress. Type As put themselves under constant pressure and their bodies react by producing extra amounts of stress hormones.

The **Type B personality** is the opposite—relaxed, casual, unaggressive, and patient. Most Type Bs build time in the day for absorbing activities such as exercise, hobbies, and friendship. They speak more softly, are less obsessed with success, and tend to deal more effectively with stressful situations.

Type A behavior was identified and named in the late 1950s by two cardiologists, Drs. Meyer Friedman and Ray Rosenman. Their research led many to believe that the individual who exhibits Type A behavior is prone to developing coronary heart disease, with increased risk of suffering a heart attack. However, research suggests that it may be the personality behaviors of hostility, cynicism, and anger that are the major culprits that increase the risk of heart disease. People exhibiting hostility, cynicism, and anger in response to stress produce greater amounts of hormones that damage the cardiorespiratory system. These traits are also related to atherosclerosis and higher diastolic blood pressure. The problem is that the components of Type A behavior can be harmful because they often lead to the development of hos-

tile, angry behavior. This is especially true in the case of chronic hurrying, a hallmark characteristic of Type A behavior. Chronic hurrying, synonymous with Type A behavior and life in the twenty-first century is especially stressful when we want to hurry but are stuck in situations where all we can do is wait, such as heavy traffic and long lines. The frustration boils over into stress and *anger*. Type Bs exhibiting angry, cynical, and hostile behaviors suffer the same negative effects as Type As.

Do you become enraged when a car in front of you cuts you off? Do you find it intolerable to wait in lines? Do you lash out with gestures, raised voice, and increased heart rate when someone does something that seems incompetent, messy, selfish, or inconsiderate to you? These are examples of angry, hostile behavior. While the debate connecting Type A and illness continues, the evidence is stacking up in favor of a positive connection—even without the hostility, cynicism, and anger. This means that just being a Type A person may have some health risks attached.

The Hot Reactor

Another example of how the combination of angry behavior and stress can be lethal has been discovered by Robert S. Eliot. He has found that 20 percent of apparently healthy individuals are prime candidates for stress-related heart attacks or strokes because of the extreme reactions they demonstrate in response to daily stress. He labeled these people **hot reactors** because, when stressed, they produce astronomical amounts of powerful adrenalinelike chemicals called **catecholamines** that damage the cardiovascular system and disrupt the electrical rhythm of the heart. Abnormally high blood pressure and dangerous heart muscle lesions are the results of the massive doses of these stress hormones being released into the bloodstream. (Systolic readings can raise from 120 to a deadly 300.) Additionally, anger can trigger an acute myocardial infarction (heart attack) when atherosclerotic plaque ruptures and the resulting clot blocks an artery. So, venting anger by "blowing off steam," losing your cool, and lashing out can be dangerous to your health. Many people ask, "Isn't it better to express anger—to let it out rather than bottle it up inside?" Now you know, the answer is NO! It is healthier to diffuse these harmful feelings by using the techniques described in Chapter 7 on page 246.

Hot reactors are guilty of faulty perception. They perceive nearly every stressor as a life-and-death issue and constantly perceive a loss of control in their daily lives. Daily challenges at work or school (deadlines, friendly competition, dealing with the kids, disagreement with a neighbor) trigger an overblown fight-or-flight reaction. The fight-or-flight reaction is a human response meant to be used only in real life-or-death situations. Squandering doses of these powerful hormones on mundane situations (i.e., missing a green light, standing in a checkout line, and running out of

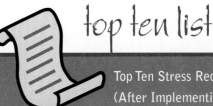

top ten list

Top Ten Stress Reduction Tips
(After Implementing the Five Stress Management Strategies Outlined in this Chapter)

1. Remind yourself you are not the general manager of the universe. Someone else has that job and he doesn't need any help.
2. Live within your budget, and don't use credit cards for ordinary purchases.
3. Simplify and unclutter your life. Start with cleaning out your wallet or purse, then a desk drawer, then a closet.
4. Allow extra time to do things and get places.
5. Listen to relaxing tapes while driving, working, or thinking.
6. Do something for the kid in you everyday. Set aside time to play and laugh.
7. Worry constructively and only about things you can control. Don't sweat the small stuff. It's all small stuff.
8. Weed out trivia. Write down important things, forget unimportant details. Don't overburden your memory.
9. Live in the present. Clear your mind of unpleasant experiences and emotions. Let it go!
10. Every night, think of one thing for which you are grateful.

SLOW DOWN!

dental floss) is a characteristic of a hot reactor. Hot reactors may be either hard-driving Type As or more placid Type Bs.

Constant stress causes many people to bristle with aggressiveness, hostility, cynicism, and anger. Our increasingly complex world fosters the development of the Type A personality. We reward the student who excels in the classroom, the winning athlete, the "superwoman" (with career and family), the youngest-ever CEO, the secretary who never takes a break, the executives who talk business over lunch, and the college student who works, carries a full load of classes, is an A student, and volunteers at church. Our society provides a rich environment for Type A personality development. Recognize your behavior pattern. Are you a Type A person or a Type B? Are you hostile and angry or a hot reactor?

Life-threatening overreaction to stress is neither innate nor inevitable. People are not born with this trait. They learn it, and they can unlearn it. Reframing is an excellent way to calm hot, angry reactions to stress. Read more about reframing later in this chapter. Take a few minutes now to read the "Top Ten Stress Reduction Tips." You can take charge and be in control of your life. Ask yourself, "Is this situation worth dying for?" Stop sweating the small stuff and, remember, it is all small stuff! Assess your reaction to stress by taking the behavior quiz in Table 8-3.

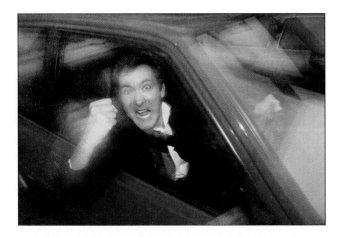

Releasing anger—lashing out—can be deadly.

Type A Behavior Modification

Okay, so you are a Type A. What can you do about it? We know that many Type A behaviors are learned and that the most severe Type As can learn to modify their behavior and successfully control hot, angry, and hostile reactions to stress in a more healthful way. Try these behavior modification suggestions:

1. Every day find time to be alone. It recharges your batteries. Everyone can spare 15 minutes or so a day to calm down and reflect on happy memories.
2. Practice relaxation techniques daily, especially meditation.
3. Develop a sense of humor about life. *He or she who laughs lasts.*
4. Laugh more.

table 8-3   Quiz to Identify Your Type A, Angry/Hostile, Hot Reactor Behavior

Answer **yes** or **no** to the following statements:

Part I: Are You a Type A?

Yes No

1. I hate to wait for anyone or anything.
2. I often interrupt others when they are speaking.
3. I am usually rushed. There's never enough time in the day.
4. I feel guilty when I have nothing to do or when I play.
5. I get impatient when others perform tasks that I can do faster.
6. I eat faster than most of my friends.
7. I feel stretched to my limits at the end of the day.
8. I think about other things during conversations.

Scoring:

Part I: Statements in this section demonstrate Type A behavior. If you said "yes" to *three* or more of these statements, you probably fall into the Type A category.

Part II: Are You Too Angry?

Yes No

1. I am quick tempered.
2. When driving, I get irritated at drivers who cut me off or drive too slowly. I frequently blow my horn, tailgate, and try to pass them.
3. I have been so mad that I have thrown things or slammed a door.
4. I remember irritating incidents and get mad again.
5. I fly off the handle.
6. I react with gestures, raised voice, and increased heart rate when someone does something incompetent, messy, inconsiderate, or unfair or after an irritating encounter.
7. I get angry when I am slowed down by other's mistakes.
8. I think cashiers will shortchange me if they can.
9. I feel my anger is justified. I feel an urge to punish people—plot to get back at them.
10. I frequently feel irritated when I stand in line or drive in heavy traffic.
11. I like to have the last word in an argument.
12. In a checkout express line, if the person in front of me has more items than the limit, I get frustrated.
13. I feel annoyed when I am not given recognition for doing good work.
14. When I am angry, I keep things inside, pout, and sulk.
15. When I get angry, I say nasty things.

Scoring:

Part II: Statements in this section demonstrate angry/hostile/cynical/hot reactor behavior. Even one "yes" response to any of these statements is too many and may be raising your risk of heart disease. Have a friend or loved one who knows you also check the statements for you. Was there a change in any of the answers to the statements?

5. Spend more time with friends and make these friendships more intimate.
6. Anticipate stresses and regulate their number and timing when possible.
7. Maintain a flexible schedule. Don't schedule appointments and activities unnecessarily.
8. Learn to say no and to protect your precious time.
9. Delegate more.
10. Listen to others without interrupting.
11. Avoid irritating, competitive people.
12. Allow extra time to do things and to get places.
13. Carry a paperback with you to read while waiting in lines or for appointments.
14. Develop a caring attitude (most people are doing the best they can).
15. Learn to savor food instead of grabbing fast food and eating "on the run."
16. Purposely choose the longest line in which to do your business (at the bank, at the checkout in the grocery store, in a fast-food restaurant, or in a discount department store).
17. Discontinue polyphasic behavior (doing two or more things at once).
18. Practice smiling for a whole day.
19. Build a time each day for exercise or another absorbing activity.
20. Read a good book.
21. Spend an entire afternoon in a museum or art gallery.

The Stress-Resistant Hardy Person

Have you ever imagined what George Washington or any of our other founding fathers would think about our modern, high-tech, fast-paced world? They might be surprised by computers, fax machines, television with global news, heart transplants, over-crowded calendars, never-ending deadlines, and chronic shortages of time. Certainly, they would agree that we have just cause to feel overwhelmed by our daily schedules and would be glad not to be participating in the twenty-first century with us. Yet we all know some people who, in spite of it all, seem relatively insulated from the potential negative effects of their hectic pace. Their lives are as full as ours, but they seem to carry on, taking "everything in stride"—often with a sense of enjoyment and fun. Who are these effective copers? Are they born this way or are they bred—learning strategies for coping with stress that protect them from being overwhelmed and feeling stressed-out?

Two psychologists, Dr. R. Flannery of Harvard University Medical School and Dr. S. Kobasa, independently researching these questions discovered that, even when highly stressed, many individuals manage lower incidence of physical illness, lower amounts of anxiety and depression, and increased longevity. These stress-resistant individuals were labeled "hardy." They have strong immune systems and are optimists. The same study found that people lacking "hardiness" were more prone to illness in the face of stress. They are pessimists with weak immune systems. A hardy soul is a Type A who has been relabeled a **Type C personality** because of the five unique personality traits he or she possesses for adapting to life stress. We call the Type C traits *The Five Cs:*

- *Control:* Control is the opposite of helplessness. The hardy person has a sense of internal control (influence) over life events and their outcomes. They take daily hassles in stride. They think ahead, plan, and make lists of what needs to be done. They seek active solutions to problems. Do you feel "in control" of your life? If not, what plan can you implement that will help you gain more control?
- *Commitment:* Commitment is the opposite of alienation and is typified by meaningful involvement in life (i.e., with one's family, job, and community.) The hardy person has a sense of purpose in life and sets short- and long-term goals. Rearing one's children, having friends, participating in community projects, having religious values, reaching career goals, and working to complete your degree are examples of personal commitments that help us unstress. List one or two goals to which you have made a commitment.
- *Challenge:* The hardy person perceives life change as a potential opportunity and a challenge rather than a threat. They continue to learn from positive and

negative experiences. Hardy people are highly confident in their ability to do their work. They accept setbacks as a part of life and as an opportunity for growth. They are positive thinkers and view bad situations as temporary and changeable.
- *Choices in lifestyle:* Hardy individuals make lifestyle choices that enhance health and reduce stress. They reduce use of caffeine, nicotine, alcohol, and sugar and incorporate aerobic exercise and relaxation activities into their lives. How much caffeine do you consume every day? Do you practice any of the relaxation techniques found in this chapter? Sydney J. Harris said it best: "The time to relax is when you don't have time for it."
- *Connectedness:* Hardy people develop a social network that includes helping and being helped by others. They have developed a sense of "connectedness" to others. They are actively involved with others. Studies show that social interaction is important. It may lower pulse rate and blood pressure, enhance the immune system, and boost the production of endorphins. When you're in a caring relationship with another person, these health benefits accrue. Do you have one or more close friends to whom you feel "connected" (i.e., sharing troubles, ambitions, and desires) or whom you can count on for emotional support?

Research on the hardy, stress-resistant Type C personality has made it clear that the five interrelated traits of control, commitment, challenge, lifestyle choices (personal health practices), and connectedness (social support) are important factors that buffer us from the ravages of our modern lifestyles and help us to adapt and even flourish in the face of them. How many of these hardiness traits do you possess? The Lab Activity 8–3 *Becoming Stress Resistant and Hardy* will help you strengthen these traits in your life. Can you think of two ways you can apply the knowledge of these five traits to your life, bolstering your "hardiness" rating?

Building Skills for Stress Management

Relaxation training is being recommended, in combination with medication, nutrition, and exercise, not only to reduce stress but to treat chronic pain and illness, such as heart disease, high blood pressure, diabetes, infertility, and cancer. Relaxation is also being used in easing depression, painful AIDS symptoms, headaches, and back pain. The concept of relaxation as "good medicine," once dismissed by scientists, is accepted now, thanks to the work of several pioneers in the mind/body field.

As you have learned, when an individual is stressed, the body responds with an outpouring of hormones to prepare him or her to either fight or to take flight (the stress response). Performance and work decline when you feel stressed out. When relaxed and feeling in control, the mind and body function efficiently and effectively. Dr. Herbert Benson of the Harvard Medical School and founder of the Mind/Body Medical Institute at New England Deaconnes Hospital in Boston, discovered that, with effort and training in the use of meditation, we can learn to quiet down and summon at will the healing changes in body chemistry called the **relaxation response.** Benson found that the relaxation response was the body's built-in defense mechanism against the harmful effects of the inappropriate elicitation of the fight-or-flight response caused by everyday living.

The innate physiological changes produced by the relaxation response, which we can elicit to counteract stress, include the following:

- Decreased oxygen consumption and metabolic rate, lessening strain on the body's energy resources
- Increased intensity and frequency of alpha brain waves associated with deep relaxation
- Reduced blood lactates (substances in the blood associated with anxiety)
- Decreased anxiety, fears, and phobias and increased positive mental health (i.e., less anxiety and greater feeling of control)
- Significant decreases in blood pressure in hypertensive individuals (which remained lowered throughout the day)
- Reduced heart rate and slower respiration
- Decreased muscle tension
- Increased blood flow to arms and legs
- Improved quality of sleep

Dr. Redford Williams, director of the Behavioral Medical Research Center at Duke University, found that angry, hostile people suffered more heart disease than calm ones. Dr. Williams, like Benson, believes relaxation and other stress-management techniques are critical ways to reduce negative emotions.

Dr. Jon Kabat-Zinn, another stress pioneer, is known for using stress-reduction programs, especially mind/body interactions and mindfulness meditation, to help patients suffering from chronic pain and stress-related disorders at the University of Massachusetts Medical Center. While traditional meditation involves training the mind on a single point of focus, such as a word or phrase, mindfulness meditation (i.e., nonmantra meditation) involves nonjudgemental awareness of whatever a person happens to be experiencing at the time—and learning to experience it calmly, whether it is pleasant or unpleasant. Kabat-Zinn describes *mindfulness* as waking up and living in harmony with oneself and the world. He encourages his patients to cultivate some appreciation for the fullness of each moment they are alive.

He asserts that it is important to be "in touch" with each moment so that we may live our lives with greater satisfaction, harmony, and wisdom. What he's talking about is conscious attention to behavior. Mindfulness meditation is not an attempt to escape from problems or difficulties. On the contrary, it is a willingness to go nose-to-nose with pain, confusion, and loss. For example, people using mindfulness meditation to cope with chronic pain would not try to distract themselves from the pain but would experience the pain without fear or anxiety (emotions that make the pain more intense). Like Benson, Kabat-Zinn has found that meditation is a way of slowing down enough so that we can get in touch with who we are, a true mind/body approach to managing the stresses in our lives.

You can't change the complexities of life, but you can develop strategies that enable you to cope more effectively. You can learn to relax, to quiet down the mind and body (so you can get "in touch" or "connected to" your inner thoughts, feelings, goals, and values), and successfully manage the stress in your life. Review behavior change in Chapter 2 and Table 8-4 to assess your current stage of behavior change relative to stress management.

Practice the relaxation techniques in this chapter to find the ones that you feel most comfortable using and that work best for you. For best results, set aside some time every day for relaxation. By following the five stress management strategies in this chapter, you will be well on your way to becoming a stress hardy person. Enjoy!

table 8-4   **Tips for Behavior Change— Managing Stress**

Stages of Change: In What Stage Are You?

1. Precontemplation: "Stress is no problem for me"
2. Contemplation: "I wish I could get control of my stress level"
3. Preparation: "I am going to start working on managing my stress"
4. Action: "I am actively taking steps to control my stress"
5. Maintenance: "I have been able to control my stress level for this entire year"

Process of Change:

After identifying your current stage, try using some of the following selected processes and behavior strategies that are appropriate for your particular stage—facilitate your transition into the next stage.

- Consciousness raising: assess your level of stress (Life Event Stress Test)
- Social liberation: identify stress management self-help groups/workshops on campus
- Emotional arousal: read about long-term ill effects of stress on the body
- Self-liberation: keep a diary of daily stressors, reactions, and coping skills used
- Countering: do deep breathing exercises when feeling stressed
- Helping relationships: use stress management support group in your residence hall

Strategy #1 Exercise

Get physical. Regular exercise is an excellent method for reducing stress, mental and physical tension, anxiety, and aggressive feelings. Exercise allows us to play out the instinctive fight-or-flight response, to use the muscles that are tensed for action, and to reduce the adrenaline being pumped into the bloodstream. A number of studies suggest that exercise reduces the intensity of the stress response, shortens the time it takes to recover from stress, and helps ward off illness in people experiencing stress. While stress increases blood pressure and platelet stickiness (the factor that increases clotting), exercise reduces these. Regular exercise also helps reduce abdominal obesity, improves insulin sensitivity, and slows the progression of artery disease.

Exercise is a natural way to relax and renew energy. When hassles and problems begin to pile up in the office or at school, change into your workout clothes and take a vigorous run, a swim, or a brisk walk. The effect is amazing. Headaches, tension, anxiety, aggressiveness, and irritability are diminished. Because research supports the value of exercise in reducing stress, many physicians recommend exercise to their patients instead of medications such as tranquilizers. Vigorous exercise increases the release of endorphins, brain chemicals that may alleviate harmful effects of stressors by producing a more relaxed state. Besides better stress management, other psychological benefits of exercise, documented by research, are increased self-esteem, increased alertness, and decreased depression and anxiety. Although aerobic vigorous exercise is best, even a relaxing walk can do wonders to relieve tension. Play tennis or racquetball, golf, dance, bowl, swim, rake leaves, garden, bike, or do whatever. Enjoy physical activity. It is the healthiest thing you can do for yourself, and it's inexpensive.

Strategy #2 Relaxation Techniques

2.a Meditation

Meditation is a mental exercise that affects body processes, producing physical benefits. The purpose of meditation is to gain control over your attention—to internally quiet down, allowing *you* to choose what to focus upon and to block out distracting thoughts.

Meditation originated in the Eastern cultures of India and Tibet and was exported to the Western world by the Maharishi Mahesh Yogi. The Maharishi popularized the **transcendental meditation (TM)** method. In recent years, TM, as well as other forms of meditation, have been subjected to a battery of scientific studies. Especially revealing and conclusive were the findings conducted at the Harvard School

wellness flash

Research has shown that the practice of meditation reduces atherosclerosis already established in coronary arteries.

of Medicine by Dr. Herbert Benson and at the School of Medicine, University of California, San Francisco, by Dr. Dean Ornish. They found that meditation was a simple yet powerful, easy-to-learn, nonchemical stress reducer that produced the relaxation response. They call meditation the "universal stress antidote" and assert that it is compatible with modern medicine. Other experts agree that meditation is now mainstream. They feel that the proficient meditator develops a sense of wholeness and is able to face stress, pain, and illness with equanimity and triumph over his or her problems. Meditation is merely a discipline for training the mind to focus, for developing greater calm, relief, and understanding. This, in turn, leads to a greater sense of control and happiness.

To bring the relaxation response benefits into your everyday life, learn to meditate. Meditation, recognized as one of the most powerful antidotes for stress, should be practiced for 10 to 20 minutes, twice a day. Soon you will be enjoying the relaxing periods of stillness and quietness of the mind that meditation produces. (Use Lab Activity 8-2 for additional practice.) Meditation involves the following four essential elements:

1. *A quiet, comfortable environment.* A place where you will not be disturbed is essential. However, once you become experienced, you will be able to meditate almost anywhere.
2. *A comfortable position.* A position that will allow you to remain in the same position for approximately 20 minutes is necessary to avoid any undue muscular tension. Lying down or sitting in an overstuffed chair may cause you to break your focus and fall asleep.
3. *Focusing your attention on something repetitive or unchanging such as a mantra, a mental device, or the breath.* For starters, you can keep it simple by focusing on your breathing, feeling it as it moves in and out. Use your breath as an anchor to bring you back when your attention is disrupted. A mantra is a silently repeated word, phrase, sound or thought such as *one, love, peace* or *omh.* The mantra should be easy to pronounce and short enough to repeat silently as you exhale. A mental device is an unchanging object such as an object in the room where you meditate. Gaze at the object fixedly. Select any one of the three methods to help you maintain your focus, to shut out outside stimuli, and

to keep you calm. The method may vary but the relaxation benefits do not.

4. *A calm, relaxed attitude.* Relax. Try not to try. Let it happen. The harder you try, the more tense you get. Disregard outside noise and thoughts. When distracting thoughts and noise intrude—it is normal that they will occasionally—calmly return focus to the slow, steady repetition of the mantra or the mental device.

2.b Autogenic Training and Imagery

Autogenic means "self-generating" or "self-induced." The **autogenic training and imagery** technique uses mental concentration exercises to bring about sensations of warmth and heaviness in the limbs and torso and then uses relaxing images to expand the relaxed state. Both meditation and autogenic training lead to the relaxation response. Many who find meditation too easy and boring enjoy autogenic training because of the switches of focus from one part of the body to another and the use of imagery. Autogenic training has been successful in the treatment of chronic and lower back pain. Otherwise, the physiological and psychological benefits are similar to meditation.

Autogenic training should be done with eyes closed while you are either lying down or in a seated position. Whatever position you choose, be sure that you are relaxed and comfortable. Eliminate muscle tension in any part of the body by changing position slightly. Practice 10 to 30 minutes, one or two times a day, to become skillful at this technique.

The six steps to autogenic training follow:

1. Concentrate on heaviness of arms and legs, beginning with dominant side.
2. Concentrate on warmth of arms and legs, beginning with dominant side.
3. Concentrate on warmth and heaviness of heart and chest.
4. Concentrate on breathing rhythm.
5. Concentrate on warmth of abdominal area.
6. Concentrate on coolness of forehead.

After the six stages of autogenic training have been mastered, transfer body relaxation to mind relaxation by using images of relaxing scenes, such as the following:

- Sinking into a mattress
- A sack of sugar melting away in the rain
- Floating out to sea
- A feather floating in the sky
- A soaring bird
- Clouds drifting by
- Ocean surf splashing on the sand
- A warm, relaxing fire burning in the fireplace
- A sailboat drifting on a calm lake

Use images you find relaxing. They may be different than those of your friends.

2.c Jacobson's Progressive Relaxation

Edmund Jacobson, a physician, designed for his tense patients a series of exercises called **progressive relaxation** that emphasize the relaxation of voluntary skeletal muscles—that is, the muscles over which you have control. He taught his patients to contract a muscle group and then relax it, progressing from one muscle group to another until the entire body was relaxed. The idea was to learn to recognize tenseness and be able to consciously relax whenever it was needed. This method of relaxation, named after its developer, does not produce the relaxation response. However, if practiced regularly, it is beneficial in helping people relax. It has been used in the treatment of insomnia and psychological conditions such as poor self-concept, depression, and anxiety.

There are many routines of contract-relax exercises for progressive relaxation. Try the progressive relaxation routine in this chapter (Table 8-5) that begins at the head and ends at the feet or develop your own routine. With practice, you will be able to eliminate the contraction phase and focus on relaxation.

table 8-5 **Progressive Relaxation Routine**

1. Lie on your back on the floor in a quiet place with the lights dimmed. Remove shoes. Let feet relax and rotate outward. Arms should be beside body, palms turned upward.
2. Proceed slowly over the body, tensing a muscle group and then relaxing it. Stop if cramping or pain develops.
3. Face: Squint eyes, wrinkle nose, make a face, and then relax. Open mouth wide, stick out tongue. Close mouth and clench teeth. Now relax.
4. Neck: Nod head downward to touch chin to chest. Relax.
5. Head: Try to touch right ear to right shoulder and left ear to left shoulder. Relax and center head over torso.
6. Shoulders: Shrug shoulders up toward ears; pull shoulders down from ears; press hard against floor. One at a time. Relax.
7. Hands and arms: Squeeze fingers together, making a fist. Relax. Raise right arm, bending at elbow, and "make a muscle" with biceps. Relax. Repeat with left arm. Relax. With arms on floor, stiffen both arms, making a fist. Relax.
8. Back: Try to squeeze shoulder blades together. Relax. Press lower back area into floor. Relax.
9. Abdomen: Suck in abdominal muscles. Relax.
10. Buttocks: Contract buttock muscles. Relax.
11. Thighs: Contract thigh muscles, one at a time and then both at the same time. Relax.
12. Calves: Flex toes back toward head and then extend or point toes away from head, using right leg and then left leg. Relax.
13. Toes: Curl toes under, first right foot and then left foot. Relax.
14. Be aware of relaxed state of body.

2.d Abdominal Breathing

Most of us breathe in short shallow breaths, expanding only the chest, especially when we're under stress. This is called *thoracic breathing* and is not the proper way to breathe. It does not allow the lungs to fill and empty completely, and it can increase muscle tension.

During stressful situations, it is even more important to breathe from the abdomen. This method allows more oxygen to enter the body and relaxes the muscles. You can practice the steps described in this chapter at almost any time or in any place, even on the telephone, in class, or at a meeting. Practice at least once a day so that it becomes natural when you use it in stressful or fatiguing situations. This procedure has produced excellent results for many (Table 8-6).

table 8-6	Abdominal Breathing

1. Inhale and exhale fully through mouth.
2. Inhale slowly and push out your abdomen (stomach) as though it was a balloon inflating. Move your chest as little as possible.
3. Exhale *slowly* and allow stomach to flatten.
4. Repeat the pattern. On each "in" breath, let belly inflate, and on each "out" breath, let it flatten.
5. Each "out" breath is an opportunity to rid body of tension.

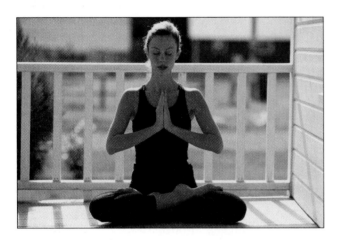

Yoga is a relaxing form of exercise.

2.e Hatha Yoga

The most familiar form of yoga is **Hatha yoga,** or physical yoga. It is a discipline that involves the use of various exercises or postures (called *asanas*) in combination with proper breathing rhythm to remove tension and inflexibility in the body. It also improves muscular strength, muscular endurance, and body alignment. Hatha yoga should not be associated with religious or spiritual groups. The physiological and psychological benefits of Hatha yoga have been thoroughly researched, confirming it to be an excellent form of exercise and an aid to improving the health and well-being of those who practice it.

2.f Massage

When you are bombarded with too much stress, the muscles in the neck, shoulders, and back can become tight and stiff to the point of pain. Without relaxation, these muscles can become chronically tight and can cause much distress. One of the most enjoyable ways to relieve this condition is to have a massage.

There are two popular forms of massage:

1. *Swedish massage*, the most familiar form, involves kneading and rubbing the muscles to increase relaxation and circulation.
2. *Shiatsu*, originating in Japan and China, is a technique that is a form of acupressure. Pressure is applied with the thumbs or fingers along acupuncture meridians. The idea is to restore balance so that the "chi" energy (an energy believed to be linked to the life force) flows freely and in a balanced manner.

Massage given by a spouse or friend can be just as pleasant. You can even massage yourself when tight neck and shoulder muscles are tense. Put on your favorite music and enjoy.

2.g Biofeedback Training

Biofeedback training is a technique in which machines measure certain physiological processes of the body. The machines then convert this information to an understandable

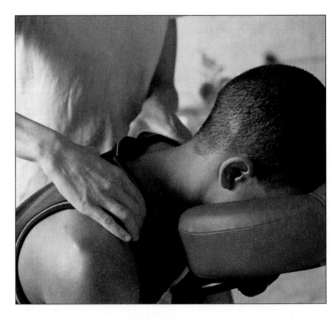

Massage is one of the most enjoyable stress relievers.

form and feed it back to the individual. This process allows a person access to biological information not usually available to one's consciousness. Proponents of biofeedback believe that by mentally recognizing involuntary biological responses such as heart rates, you can control them. With feedback training, stressors are not removed, but the response to them is controlled. Control of physiological arousal is an important step in stress management. A major drawback of biofeedback is the cost and availability of the machines and the lack of trained professionals to operate them.

Strategy #3 Lifestyle Change

3.a The Impact of Diet

Proper diet is an important part of your stress-management program and an area in which you can definitely exert *control*. A nutritious diet will help you look and feel good, plus it will strengthen your immune system. Many feel that poor diet can increase your susceptibility to stress by causing fatigue and irritability. This is especially true for individuals who are eating too many meals away from home, missing meals, or eating on the run. Unfortunately, there are no miracle foods to boost energy and reduce stress. The best advice for surviving the stress of modern life is to eat three nutritious meals a day and follow these guidelines to help keep you from feeling irritable and uptight:

1. Reduce (below 250 milligrams per day) or eliminate the caffeine in your diet. Caffeine is a stimulant and magnifies the effects of stress (see *caffeine* in Chapter 13). Also, avoid or minimize the use of stimulating drugs (i.e., diet pills and oral decongestants) that may cause added agitation.
2. Limit foods containing sugar, especially if you have been skipping meals. It robs the body of B-complex vitamins and may induce anxiety and failure to cope with stressful situations.
3. Limit your intake of sodium because excessive fluid buildup leads to discomfort and increased stress. Too much sodium (salt) can also increase blood pressure due to the fluid buildup.
4. Limit alcoholic beverage consumption. Alcohol makes people feel relaxed and less stressed while drinking it, but it leaves them feeling more tired the next day.

3.b Time Management

Insufficient time appears to be the plague of the twenty-first century. College students frequently complain about the lack of this precious commodity. How well you manage your time plays a large role in how much pressure you feel. You should manage your time as if your life depended on it, because it does. The goal of time management should not be the elimination of leisure time (relaxation, etc.); rather, it should be the elimination of life's real time wasters. Use *Time Management*, Lab Activity 8-6, to practice this important stress-management lifestyle strategy. Also, review the Top Ten Tips on How to Reduce College Stress by Improving Studying and Test-Taking Skills. Time management experts suggest these time-saving tips:

1. Analyze how you spend time and then evaluate that use of time. Keep a diary. You may find you are wasting too much time.
2. Learn to set short- and long-range goals. Write them down. This helps you plan for today and for the future.
3. Learn how to set priorities. Not everything you do is number one on your list of importance. With goals in mind, you will know how to prioritize your activities. Items on the "Do" list must get done; items on the "Maybe" list are those you would like to take care of today, if possible; and those on the "If Possible" list are those you would like to do if the activities of the first and second lists are completed.
4. Use a planner calendar to schedule your priorities into your day, week, and year. This will help you organize and simplify your life by keeping track of important dates, appointments, and meetings. A planner calendar is productive. By systematically planning your day, you can more clearly see what needs to be done. Minor tasks need no longer overshadow major ones. A few minutes of planning can control hours of chaos. A planned day allows you to schedule stress-reducing breaks and rest periods and to have time for family, friends, personal development, and hobbies. Gaining control over your life reduces stress.
5. Take 5 to 10 minutes at the end of the day to evaluate how well you managed your time. How many of your goals did you check off today? Good time managers use this technique daily to assess time wasted, reprioritize goals (even dumping some), and maintain progress for achieving their short- and long-range goals.
6. Adopt the following time-saving strategies:
   - Learn how to stop being inefficient. This is an art that anyone can learn. Go through mail one time only. Start a task with the intention of completing it now. Don't look it over and put it aside for later. You have wasted time looking it over the first time.
   - Know your limits. Don't allow too many demands to be made "on your time." You can say, "No!" Learn to delegate certain activities to others when possible.
   - Practice quick relaxation tricks frequently throughout the day. Get up and go for a drink of water. Give yourself a massage to the neck, shoulders, and forehead. This energizes you to complete tasks more efficiently.

3.c Alcohol, Drugs, and Cigarettes

Alcohol is a powerful depressant drug that temporarily masks but doesn't solve your problems. It can increase stress by creating new problems—hangovers, arrests, traffic violations, fights, and accidents. Taking illegal drugs can only increase your stress. Why risk ruining your physical and mental health and the stress of being arrested? Do not smoke cigarettes or use other tobacco products (snuff, chewing tobacco). Nicotine is a stimulant that increases stress.

3.d Get Plenty of Restful Sleep

Take care of yourself. Most people need 7 to 9 hours of restful sleep each night. Getting enough sleep can make you more alert, less irritable, and better able to cope with stressful situations. Cumulative sleep loss has debilitating and even fatal effects. Poor judgment and other declines in cognitive performance lead to increased risk of accident and injury when sleep is short-changed. Quality of life decreases dramatically if fatigue dominates the day. When short on sleep people tend to overeat and underexercise. Good sleep is as important as regular exercise and good nutrition to help cope with life's stresses and to keep the body functioning in top form physically, mentally, and spiritually. You know if you are getting enough sleep if you wake up in the morning before the alarm goes off, feel re-

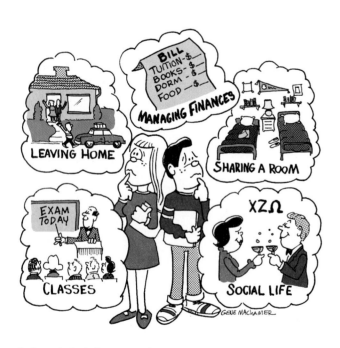

College students face many stresses.

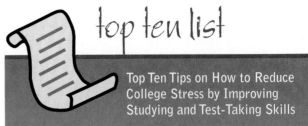

freshed and rested, and are alert throughout the day. Review the guidelines in Table 8-7 if you have concerns about the quality of your sleep.

3.e Develop Satisfying Relationships

Having close friends with whom to share the joys and sorrows of living is a huge asset in protecting your health.

table 8-7	Improve Your Quality of Sleep

To improve your quality of sleep implement the following helpful guidelines:
- Stick to a regular schedule for sleeping, waking, and eating.
- Avoid frequent daytime naps—they may disrupt sleep at night.
- Develop a soothing bedtime routine.
- Create a dark, quiet, and comfortable place to sleep.
- Get adequate exposure to bright light each day. Get outside as much as possible, especially at midday during short winter days.
- Exercise regularly—but not within a few hours of bedtime. Don't overtrain, though, this has the opposite effect on sleep.
- Check your medications. Many contain ingredients that can cause insomnia (i.e., pain relievers, decongestants, asthma/cold/antihistamine medications, exercise and diet aids)
- Acknowledge the sources of stress in your life and devise a plan to eliminate the ones you can.
- Practice relaxation techniques.
- Modify your lifestyle. Reduce or eliminate caffeine, tobacco, and alcohol, especially before bedtime. While alcohol may help people fall to sleep, it usually produces a light restless sleep, often causing the individual to awaken suddenly during the night, unable to sleep again.

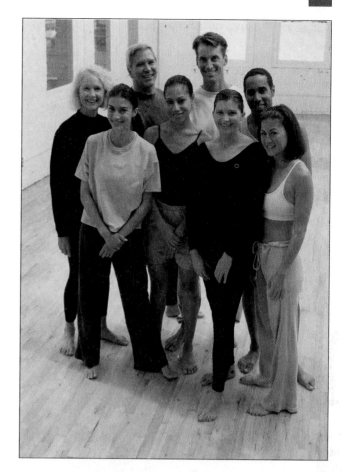

Social support enhances the immune system.

Unhappiness, depression, and feelings of isolation can be caused by lack of close emotional bonds with friends, a spouse, or family members. Intimate relationships and social support can become a powerful life-support system when internal resources have fallen short. Social support can directly provide reinforcement for healthy behaviors and indirectly buffer disappointments that would otherwise lead to excessive stress. Friends are not just nice, they are a necessity. You have to be *a friend to have a friend.* Make the effort. It's good health and happiness insurance.

3.f Learn When to Seek the Help and Support of Others

There will be stressful situations you will not be able to deal with alone. Don't be embarrassed to seek professional help. Developing a variety of support groups such as family, friends, coaches, counselors, or physicians can be helpful. Talking to someone gives a different perspective on worries and concerns.

3.g Balance Work and Play

Plan for regular recreation (or a time for yourself) and make that time inviolate. It is your special time. Let nothing else interfere. This can include learning to do nothing (loafing) at times and feeling okay about it.

Strategy #4 Reframing

Reframing means consciously reinterpreting a situation in a more positive light. It is a way of looking at life in a positive manner. This makes you better able to deal with problems when they come. Is the glass half empty or half full? Viewing yourself as a sick person because you have asthma is different, for example, than perceiving yourself as a healthy person who also happens to have asthma. In the case of the driver who cuts you off in traffic, you might tell yourself, "Maybe she had some emergency." This is an excellent way to diffuse anger and negativism. See if you can learn to "reframe" life's stumbling blocks into challenges. Look at the bright side of each situation. Learn to be an optimist. Good things happen to people who expect them. Remember, you are in control of you. Positive emotions and laughter play an important role in keeping well and fit. Optimists have higher hardiness scores (and stronger immune systems), whereas pessimists are more likely to resort to anger and hostility. Laughter and its subtle companion, humor, can provide psychological relief from tension, anxiety, anger, hostility, and emotional pain. Laughing is like "internal jogging"—it causes endorphins (pain-relieving chemicals) to be released in the brain. Laughter is a natural tranquilizer with no negative side effects. Scientific evidence is beginning to support the biblical axiom that "a merry heart doeth good like a medicine."

Strategy #5 Create a Memory Bank

Happiness comes from noticing and enjoying the little things in life. Take five minutes of your day, every day, to savor the special experiences of your life. Store these in your memory bank. When you look back over your day (and your life), what special memories do you fondly recall: Roasting marshmallows over a campfire, watching the sunset, smelling a rose, the glow after a satisfying workout, birds singing early in the morning, a beautiful morning sunrise, newborn animals, a hug that said "I care"? What can you do today to increase your store of pleasant memories?

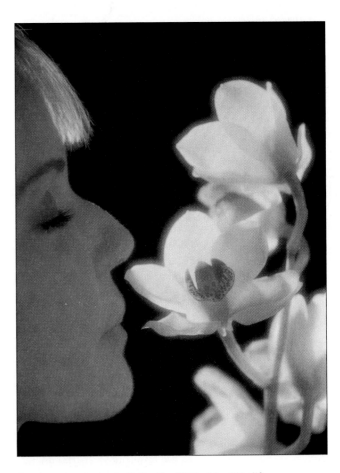

Reframing: Is the glass half empty or half full?

Create a memory bank. Notice the "little things" in life.

frequently asked questions

Q. Can spirituality uplift your health?

A. Modern medicine, with its high-tech wizardry, can do wonders for the body but little for the soul. And, until recently, medical research avoided spirituality.

In the past decade, a growing number of researchers have put spirituality and religion under the microscope. The research so far suggests that having a spiritual dimension in your life may help you get healthy when you are sick and stay healthy when you are well.

Studies have linked religion and spirituality with a reduced risk of disease, faster recovery from surgery, and a lower overall death rate. There are several plausible explanations for a faith-health link: religion and spirituality may encourage healthy habits and help reduce stress, perhaps by promoting social support; an optimistic outlook; and deep relaxation during prayer, meditation, or other relaxation technique.

Q. I sleep five to six hours a night and don't feel tired during the day. Am I getting enough sleep?

A. Probably not. Roughly 5 percent of people claim that's all the sleep they need to function well during the day. But getting so little slumber may harm your health even if it doesn't impair your performance. Without enough sleep:

- your ability to learn; your problem-solving, speaking, and writing skills; your reaction time; and your stamina can decline.
- you are more likely to become tense and moody and to have trouble getting along with others.
- the body's immune system may weaken. People who report daytime sleepiness have worse overall health and higher mortality rates than well-rested people.
- the risk of developing insulin resistance increases. This may predispose people to diabetes, high blood pressure, coronary heart disease, stroke, and possibly cancer.
- weight gain and reductions in muscle mass may occur due to inhibited nocturnal surges of growth hormone.

Q. What is Tai Chi? Is it a beneficial form of exercise?

A. Tai Chi is an ancient Chinese exercise form that combines relaxed, slow movement with a calm, alert mental state. The practitioner keeps his or her body relaxed and upright, focusing throughout the exercise sequence on natural diaphragmatic breathing. The Chinese have long touted Tai Chi's medical benefits, practicing it for health, vitality, relaxation, and self-defense. Medical research has begun to confirm that Tai Chi practice has a positive effect on health by:

- reducing diastolic and systolic blood pressure.
- improving strength and balance.
- improving emotional health (i.e., reduced tension, depression, anger, improved general mood).
- possibly positively impacting on the immune system.

Q. The nation seems to be in the midst of an anger epidemic. Why is this?

A. Bad tempers are everywhere. The media reports incidents of road rage, airplane rage, cell phone rage, grocery store rage,

parking lot rage, and youth sports activities rage. Leading social scientists confirm that the nation is in the middle of an unsettling and deadly anger trend. This all-too-frequent display of rage is described as a fuming, unrelenting sense of anger, hostility, and alienation that simmers for months, even years, without relief. Eventually, all it takes is a triggering incident, usually minor, for the hostile person to go ballistic. Why?

- Stress is a hallmark of the anger epidemic, and the major contributing factors are lack of time and intrusive technology. Cell phones, pagers, and so on allow us to be interrupted anywhere, at any time. This constant accessibility and compulsive use of technology fragments what little time we have, adding to our sense of urgency and overload.
- Multitasking. People feel the need to constantly do several things at the same time (i.e., drive and talk on the phone).
- High expectations and entitlement. Pressure to achieve more and live the "good life." People feel they are entitled to fulfillment, at any cost because of materialism and consumerism.
- Lack of manners. Rude and selfish behavior has increased and so has anger at the bad behavior of others.
- Lack of connection. Families are not doing things together the way they use to. Social support also has diminished.
- Media. Television programs (talk shows such as *The Jerry Springer Show*; crime shows such as *NYPD Blue* and *The Practice*; even shows such as *Dateline* and *20/20*) continually show examples of rage outbursts, almost convincing the viewing public that it's okay or at least normal.
- We feel it's normal. We are exposed to more violence, which makes it mainstream.

Q. What is reflexology and how does it help manage stress?

A. Reflexology is an ancient healing art that has been practiced by the Indian, Chinese, and Egyptian cultures for thousands of years. Patients and practitioners of reflexology believe that massaging or applying pressure to certain points on the body, especially the hands, feet, and ears, can alter the function of an organ or an entire body system. By identifying "meridians" similar to those used in accupressure, reflexologists believe they can alter energy pathways to specific structures, which in turn reduces stress and cures illness. This possibility makes reflexology an attractive approach to medical care that does not involve surgery or drug therapy.

Reflexology is promoted as a comprehensive therapy that can tone and relax the body, reduce stress, and maintain or restore function in every organ system. Reflexology can be administered without special equipment and in any setting by a variety of practitioners, including doctors of chiropractic and naturopathic medicine and trained reflexologists.

summary

Stress is unavoidable. Optimal levels of stress improve health and performance, but excess levels, especially when chronic and perceived as negative, can be hazardous to your health. Major life events—death of a spouse, marriage, and divorce, for example—are significant stressors. Other more frequent stressors are daily hassles (i.e., missed sleep, rush-hour traffic, losing things). We learn to cope with major life events and daily hassles in a variety of ways. Some are healthy; some are not. Healthy stress-management strategies include exercise, relaxation techniques, lifestyle changes, reframing, and creating a memory bank. Hassles can be countered with the giving and receiving of daily uplifts (i.e., compliments, hugs, and getting enough sleep).

Three stress-coping behavior types—Types A, B, and C—have been identified. Type As are described as rushed, competitive, and impatient. These behaviors often lead to angry, hostile, and cynical reactions when the individual is stressed, which are, in turn, the lethal risk factors for coronary heart disease. Type Bs are more relaxed than Type As but if they demonstrate anger and hostility, they also will develop negative health consequences. Hot reactors perceive every stressor as a life-or-death situation and may be either Type A or Type B. Type Cs are often referred to as "hardy." Type Cs possess The Five Cs: They accept challenges, feel they are in control of their lives, have a strong commitment or purpose in life, make healthy lifestyle choices, and have a strong sense of connectedness to others.

Your wellness is dependent on how well you balance the stress in your life, how well you can modify your angry and hostile behavior, and how successfully you take charge of your life. As one wise person said, "If you can't fight and you can't flee, flow."

additional information resources

Benson, Herbert, M.D. *Timeless Healing: The Power of Biology of Belief*. New York: Simon and Schuster, Inc., 1996.

Birkel, Dee Ann. *Hatha Yoga: Developing the Body, Mind and Inner Self*. Dubuque, Iowa: Eddie Bowers Publishing, Inc., 1999.

Chopra, Deepak, M.D. *Ageless Body, Timeless Mind*. New York: Harmony Books, 1993.

internet resources

American Psychological Association
http://www.apa.org

Association for Applied Psychology and Biofeedback
http://www.aapb.org

Center for Anxiety and Stress Treatment
http://www.stressrelease.com

Duquesne University Stress links
http://the-duke.duq-duke.duq.edu/special/stress.htm

The Humor Potential
http://www.stressed.com

The Humor Project
http://www.humorproject.com

National Institute of Mental Health
http://www.nimh.nih.gov

Psych Central: Dr. John Grohol's Mental Health Page
http://www.grohol.com

Stress Free NET
http://www.stressfree.com

Stress Less
http://www.stressless.com

Yang Style Tai Chi
http://www.chebucto.ns.ca/Philosophy/Taichi

Evaluation of the Life Event Stress Test

After completing the *Life Event Stress Test* (Table 8–2, p. 275) in this chapter, answer the following questions:

1. What was your score? _____

2. What was your rating? _____

3. Discuss the results of this test in terms of its implication for you having a stress illness this year. List at least four or five factors that influence this implication.

4. Describe one of the relaxation techniques (Strategy #2) you would enjoy practicing on a regular basis. Why did you select this one?

5. List and discuss *three* stress management strategies you could incorporate into your current lifestyle. How will you do so? Be specific.

lab activity
8–2

How to Meditate and Experience the Relaxation Response

Meditation is recognized as a valuable antidote for stress. This powerful mind/body approach is a natural, nonchemical, inexpensive method to help you calm down and gain greater control over your life. Meditation relieves stress by lowering the level of powerful stress hormones that inhibit immune function and interfere with our natural healing processes. Meditation increases body-mind relaxation by calming feelings of panic, fear, and pain. Learning to meditate is a do-it-yourself, self-help project. You do not need a guru, special lessons, an expensive club membership, or an expert to help you learn how to meditate. You can't simply wish to be a more relaxed person; meditation is a skill that takes commitment and practice. For meditation to be helpful, plan now to incorporate meditation into your daily schedule so that you, too, may profit from its numerous benefits.

Read the following helpful meditation guidelines before you begin:

1. The best times to meditate are before breakfast and before dinner. Do not meditate directly after a meal. After eating, the blood is diverted toward the stomach area, aiding the digestive process. This diversion inhibits complete relaxation.

2. Find a quiet room and sit in a comfortable chair. A straight-back chair is best because you do not want to be so comfortable that you fall asleep. Rest your arms on the arms of the chair or in your lap.

3. Wear nonrestrictive clothing while meditating or loosen the clothes you are wearing.

4. Relax all your muscles as best you can, without forcing it. Focus on your breathing.

5. The goal is to meditate for 20 minutes but don't worry about meditating for a full 20 minutes at first. As you become more comfortable with the process, you will be able to progress up to 20 minutes or more, twice a day.

6. Do not smoke cigarettes or drink coffee, tea, or colas before meditating. These substances are stimulants and will not promote relaxation.

7. It would be helpful to disconnect the telephone. Also, *do not* set the alarm clock for 20 minutes.

8. Relax and enjoy this time. Your problems will be there when you're finished. However, they will seem less distressing to you after meditation if you commit yourself to the time necessary to do it.

9. Don't come out of the meditative state too abruptly.

10. Practice regularly. It takes practice to learn to sit still, meditate, relax, and calm the mind. Be patient. You won't discover the benefits unless you practice every day.

lab activity @ chapter eight

The four guidelines involved in learning how to meditate are as follows:

1. *Find a quiet environment.* Find a quiet room and sit in a comfortable chair. A straight-back chair is best because you don't want to be so comfortable that you fall asleep.

2. *Choose a comfortable position.* It is best to close your eyes (unless you are using a mental device). There should be no tension in your forehead or eyes. Breathe easily and naturally through your nose. Rest your arms on the arms of the chair or in your lap.

3. *Focus your attention on something repetitive or unchanging such as a single word, phrase, sound, thought, or prayer (called mantras).* A fixed gazing at an unchanging object or image may also be used. For starters though, you can keep it simple by focusing on just your breathing, feeling it as it moves in and out. Use the breath as an anchor to bring you back when your attention is disrupted. As you gain experience you may wish to select and use a mantra that you can focus on silently. The mantra should be easy to pronounce and short enough to repeat silently as you exhale. Focusing your attention on your breath, on a mantra, or on an unchanging object merely helps to block out distracting thoughts and sounds that will interfere with the meditative process. Relax all your muscles as best you can, without forcing it. Focus on your breathing. Now silently repeat the mantra very, very slowly, without a break on every exhale. Many meditators like to use as a mantra a word, such as *one, love, calm,* or *peace,* as they slowly exhale. Use whatever feels comfortable to you.

4. *Maintain a calm, relaxed attitude.* Do not force yourself to relax or watch yourself relax; the rhythm of the mantra (or the fixed gazing) will be interrupted and so will your relaxation period. It is normal for distracting thoughts to occur; do not worry about them—let them pass on when this happens. Return your focus to the repetition of the mantra, the mental device, or the breathing rhythm.

Continue to meditate for approximately 20 minutes. It is recommended that you meditate twice a day for 20 minutes each time.

When you stop meditating, give your body time to adjust. Keep your eyes closed for 1 minute and let regular thoughts return. Next, open your eyes and focus on the objects in the room. Take several deep breaths. Stretch while seated. When you feel ready, stand and stretch.

Meditation Log Sheet

Practice meditating for 1 week. Use the following log to record the time of day, the location, the length of time, and comments about the meditative session. Make copies of this log form as needed.

Week:

Sunday	Time of Day	Location	Length of Meditation	Comments
Monday				
Tuesday				
Wednesday				
Thursday				
Friday				
Saturday				

lab activity 8–3

Becoming Stress Resistant and Hardy

List two ways your "hardiness" can be strengthened in each of the following categories:

1. *Control:* Do you feel you are in control of your life? List at least two ways you gain more control. (Example: Plot out the courses you need to complete your degree, semester by semester.)

2. *Commitment (task involvement):* How can you build commitment in your life (i.e., family, friends, studies, work, community)? List at least two ways to improve commitment. (Example: I will complete my nursing degree by 20__.)

lab activity @ chapter eight

3. *Challenge:* Do you see change and/or setbacks as challenges instead of stumbling blocks? Give at least two examples that have occurred recently or list two strategies you can use in the future. (Example: So I didn't do well on this anatomy pop quiz. . . . Now I know that I need to study daily for this course.)

4. *Choices in lifestyle:* How healthy is your current lifestyle? List at least two improvements you can make in your lifestyle. (Example: I will get at least 8 hours of sleep every night for 2 weeks.)

5. *Connectedness:* Do you have anyone you can count on for emotional support? Do you feel *connected* with at least one other person or group? Do you have close friends and family? List at least two ways to improve connectedness. (Example: Twice a week I will either telephone or write a note to a friend to keep in touch with friends I rarely get to see.)

lab activity
8-4

Relaxation

There are many ways to relax—meditation, progressive relaxation, autogenic training, and imagery. Hatha yoga, massage, abdominal breathing, and flotation tanks are excellent tension relievers. You cannot simply wish to become a more relaxed person. Becoming relaxed is a *skill* that takes *commitment* and *practice*! Make the commitment now!

Choose any relaxation technique in Strategy #2 in Chapter 8 and practice it for 20 minutes every day for 1 week. Then respond to the following questions. Before you begin, rate your current ability to relax. How good are you at relaxing? Mark the line where you would rate your current skill:

Very Poor	Poor	Average	Good	Excellent

1. How often do you practice relaxation now? Circle one: . . . never . . . once in a while . . . every day. Explain: (i.e., why don't you practice relaxation, what method do you use, how often do you practice?)

2. Do you believe you could benefit by improving your ability to relax? Explain your response.

3. Which relaxation technique did you choose to practice? Why did you select this technique? Describe your experience with this technique (i.e., how you felt before and after).

4. Did this technique help you feel relaxed? Why or why not?

5. Is this a skill you feel you can use to manage the stress in your daily life? Explain.

6. Would you like to try any of the other techniques? If so, which and why?

7. Do you think relaxation is important in the management of your stress? Why or why not?

8. Take the Life Event Stress Test (Table 8-2). What was your score? _____ What was your implication for illness?

9. What role does diet play in the total stress picture of your life? List *three* ways you can improve the diet-stress connection in your everyday life.

10. List the top *three* daily hassles and top *three* daily uplifts in your life.

Measuring Your
Stress and Coping Skills

This is a four-part test. The first three parts are designed to give you an indication of how vulnerable you might be to certain types of stress and to make you aware of how they might affect you. The last part of the test will provide you with information on how to cope with stressful situations. (Source: Daniel Girdano/George S. Everly, *Controlling Stress and Tension: A Holistic Approach,* © 1979, pp. 62, 67, 108–109. Adapted by permission of Prentice Hall, Englewood Cliffs, New Jersey.)

Part I

Choose the most appropriate answer for each of the 10 questions.

	a. Almost always true	b. Usually true	c. Usually false	d. Almost always false
1. When I can't do something "my way," I simply adjust and do it the easiest way.	___	___	___	___
2. I get upset when someone in front of me drives slowly.	___	___	___	___
3. It bothers me when my plans are dependent upon others.	___	___	___	___
4. Whenever possible, I tend to avoid large crowds.	___	___	___	___
5. I am uncomfortable when I have to stand in long lines.	___	___	___	___
6. Arguments upset me.	___	___	___	___
7. When my plans don't flow smoothly, I become anxious.	___	___	___	___
8. I require a lot of space in which to live and work.	___	___	___	___
9. When I am busy at some task, I hate to be disturbed.	___	___	___	___
10. I believe that it is worth waiting for all good things.	___	___	___	___
Total score				___

Scoring
For 1 and 10, a = 1, b = 2, c = 3, d = 4; for 2 through 9, a = 4, b = 3, c = 2, d = 2. This test measures your vulnerability to stress from being frustrated or inhibited. Scores in excess of 25 seem to suggest some vulnerability to this source of stress.

Part II

Check or mark the letter of the response
that best answers the following 10 questions.
How often do you . . .

	a. Almost always	b. Very often	c. Seldom	d. Never
1. find yourself with insufficient time to complete your work?	___	___	___	___
2. find yourself becoming confused and unable to think clearly because too many things are happening at once?	___	___	___	___
3. wish you had help to get everything done?	___	___	___	___
4. feel your boss/professor expects too much from you?	___	___	___	___
5. feel your family and friends expect too much from you?	___	___	___	___
6. find your work infringing on your leisure hours?	___	___	___	___
7. find yourself doing extra work to set an example to those around you?	___	___	___	___
8. find yourself doing extra work to impress your superiors?	___	___	___	___
9. have to skip a meal so that you can get work completed?	___	___	___	___
10. feel that you have too much responsibility?	___	___	___	___
			Total score	___

Scoring

a = 4, b = 3, c = 2, d = 1. This test measures your vulnerability to overload; that is, to having too much to do. Scores in excess of 25 seem to indicate vulnerability to this source of stress.

Part III

Answer each question as it is generally true for you.

	a. Almost always true	b. Usually true	c. Usually false	d. Almost always false
1. I hate to wait in lines.	___	___	___	___
2. I often find myself racing against the clock to save time.	___	___	___	___
3. I become upset if I think something is taking too long.	___	___	___	___
4. When under pressure I tend to lose my temper.	___	___	___	___
5. My friends tell me that I tend to get irritated easily.	___	___	___	___
6. I seldom like to do anything unless I can make it competitive.	___	___	___	___
7. When something must be done, I'm the first to begin even though the details may still need to be worked out.	___	___	___	___
8. When I make a mistake it is usually because I've rushed into something without giving it enough thought and planning.	___	___	___	___
9. Whenever possible, I try to do two things at once, such as eating while working or planning while driving or bathing.	___	___	___	___
10. When I go on a vacation, I usually take along some work to do just in case I get a chance.	___	___	___	___
			Total score	___

Scoring

a = 4, b = 3, c = 2, d = 1. This test measures the presence of compulsive, time-urgent, and excessively aggressive behavioral traits. Scores in excess of 25 suggest the presence of one or more of these traits.

Part IV

This scale was created largely on the basis of results compiled by clinicians and researchers who sought to identify how individuals effectively cope with stress. This scale is an educational tool, not a clinical instrument. Its purpose, therefore, is to inform you of ways in which you can effectively and healthfully cope with the stress in your life. At the same time, through a point system, it will give you some indication of the relative desirability of the coping strategies you are currently using. Simply follow the instructions given for each of the 14 items listed. Total your points when you have completed all of the items.

1. Give yourself 10 points if you feel that you have a supportive family. _____

2. Give yourself 10 points if you actively pursue a hobby. _____

3. Give yourself 10 points if you belong to some social or activity group (other than your family) that meets at least once a month. _____

4. Give yourself 15 points if you are within 5 pounds of your ideal body weight, considering your height and bone structure. _____

5. Give yourself 15 points if you practice some form of deep relaxation at least three times a week. Deep relaxation exercises include meditation, imagery, and yoga. _____

6. Give yourself 5 points for each time you exercise 30 minutes or longer during one average week. _____

7. Give yourself 5 points for each nutritionally balanced and wholesome meal you consume during one average day. _____

8. Give yourself 5 points if you do something just for yourself that you really enjoy during an average week. _____

9. Give yourself 10 points if you have some place in your home that you can go in order to relax and/or be alone. _____

10. Give yourself 10 points if you practice time management techniques in your daily life. _____

11. Subtract 10 points for each pack of cigarettes you smoke during one average day. _____

12. Subtract 5 points for each evening during an average week that you take any form of medication or chemical (including alcohol) to help you sleep. _____

13. Subtract 10 points for each day during an average week that you consume any form of medication or chemical substance (including alcohol) to reduce your anxiety or to calm you down. _____

14. Subtract 5 points for each evening during an average week that you bring work home—work that was meant to be done at your place of employment. _____

Total score _____

Scoring
Now calculate your total score. A perfect score would be 115 points or more. If you scored in the 50 to 60 range, you probably have an adequate collection of coping strategies for most common sources of stress. You should keep in mind, however, that the higher your score, the greater your ability to cope with stress in an effective and healthful manner.

Time Management

I. Lifetime and Yearly Goals

Read the time management strategies in Chapter 8 (Strategy 3.b). Complete sections A and B before proceeding to parts II and III.

A. *Setting lifetime goals.* List three to five goals you wish to accomplish in your lifetime. Next, prioritize them by numbering them from 1 to 5:

-
-
-
-
-

B. *Setting yearly goals.* List three to five goals you wish to accomplish this year. Next, prioritize them by numbering them from 1 to 5:

-
-
-
-
-

Keep Part I to review at a later date.

II. Daily Time Study Log

Analyze how you spend your time by keeping a daily log for 1 week. Record at half-hour intervals the activities you do. At the end of each day, use a highlighter to identify the times of the day you feel were wasted. Then plan for tomorrow about how to correct the wasted time and how to be more productive. Make copies of this form as needed.

7:00 A.M.	7:00 P.M.
7:30 A.M.	7:30 P.M.
8:00 A.M.	8:00 P.M.
8:30 A.M.	8:30 P.M.
9:00 A.M.	9:00 P.M.
9:30 A.M.	9:30 P.M.
10:00 A.M.	10:00 P.M.
10:30 A.M.	10:30 P.M.
11:00 A.M.	11:00 P.M.
11:30 A.M.	11:30 P.M.
Noon	Midnight
12:30 P.M.	12:30 A.M.
1:00 P.M.	1:00 A.M.
1:30 P.M.	1:30 A.M.
2:00 P.M.	2:00 A.M.
2:30 P.M.	2:30 A.M.
3:00 P.M.	3:00 A.M.
3:30 P.M.	3:30 A.M.
4:00 P.M.	4:00 A.M.
4:30 P.M.	4:30 A.M.
5:00 P.M.	5:00 A.M.
5:30 P.M.	5:30 A.M.
6:00 P.M.	6:00 A.M.
6:30 P.M.	6:30 A.M.

III. Weekly Goals

A. *Set goals:* Think through the entire week and list the specific goals you wish to accomplish (or tasks you wish to complete) this week. Schedule into the week your appointments, obligations, and other responsibilities. Be sure to leave time for work projects, schoolwork, exercise, time with family and friends, and play/recreation/time for you (i.e., watching TV, socializing).

-

-

-

-

-

B. *Prioritize:* To beat the negative effects of stress, you have to learn to prioritize. Not everything on your list can be number one. Prioritize the week's tasks now by numbering them from 1 to 5.

C. *Complete a weekly evaluation:* After completing the *Daily Time Study Log* in Part II, evaluate how successfully you managed your time this week. Explain in a few sentences how you did. What goals/tasks did not get completed? Should these be eliminated or reestablished on next week's list? Explain.

IV. Daily Planning

The goal of time management is not to eliminate leisure time (time for self, family, friends, etc.); it is to eliminate life's real time wasters and redundancies.

A. *Analyze your time and set goals.* After completing a week of the *Daily Time Study Log* in Part II (analyzing how you spend your time) and establishing *Weekly Goals* in Part III, you are ready to begin daily planning. Look over the goals and tasks you have prioritized for the week. Include any of these you want to check off today. Write the goals/tasks that must get done today on the must do list (no more than five items on this list). This way you are more likely to get all the things done, and you will feel a greater sense of accomplishment and control. The ones you would like to take care of today put on the *maybe* list; and those you would like to complete if all items are completed on the first and second lists put on the *if possible* list. Be sure to schedule into the day appointments, meetings, study time, exercise, recreation (and/or time to do nothing), and errands. Make extra copies of this form as needed.

B. *Prioritize and schedule priorities into your day.*

Must do:

-
-
-
-
-

Maybe:

-
-
-
-
-

If possible:

-
-
-
-
-

C. *Evaluation.* A good time manager takes 5 to 10 minutes each day to evaluate how he or she did.
   1. How did you do today? Explain in a few sentences.

   2. Did you check off everything on the *must do* list? List what did not get checked off. Will it be added to tomorrow's list?

   3. How did you do on the *maybe* and *if possible* lists?

   4. How many hours today did you feel were unproductive or wasted? Why? Explain in a few sentences.

   5. Were you able to say "no" or to "delegate" any chores that would have made too great a demand on your time? Describe.

lab activity
8-7

Using HealthQuest

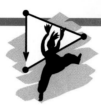

Directions: Insert HealthQuest CD. Click on "Stress Management and Mental Health" on the Table of Contents. Read "Introduction". Go to "Tutorial".

A. Click on "Audio Tapes and Videos".

  1. Try "Deep Breathing". Do you feel this method of relaxation can improve your ability to relax?

  _____Explain your response. _____

  2. Try "Progressive Relaxation." Do you feel this method of relaxation can improve your ability to relax?

  _____Explain your response. _____

B. Now click on "Stress Challenge".
  1. Complete the "Build your Day's Schedule".

  2. Select a lunch partner.

  3. Click on "Alarm Clock" and begin the day. Go through the day selecting each "What will you do?" And then pick your first reaction to each stressor. Continue until you reach the end of the day.

  4. Go to "Feedback Screen".

    4.1 How many positive coping skills did you exhibit? _____

    4.2 How many negative coping skills did you exhibit? _____

    4.3 What was your average stress level? _____

  5. Go to "Feedback" and discuss the feedback information.

  6. Click on "What do you think?" Respond to the following: _____

    6.1 How did the way you respond compare to your normal response to stress? _____

    _____

    6.2 What does your stress score indicate to you? _____

    _____

    6.3 How do you feel about this information? _____

    _____

    6.4 How could you improve your reaction to stressful situations? _____

    _____

Changing Behavior
Using the Transtheoretical Model

Using a highlighter, trace a path on the algorithm as you answer each question. Highlight your stage of change. Continue the activity on the back of this sheet.

Do you consistently practice relaxation techniques (meditation, progressive relaxation, yoga, etc.)?

Yes   No

Have you done this consistently over the last 6 months?

Do you plan to start doing this within the next 6 months?

Yes   No   Yes   No

Within the next month?

Yes   No

| maintenance | action | preparation | contemplation | precontemplation |

lab activity © chapter eight

Once you've identified which stage of change you are in, it is important to use the processes that are most useful in progressing to the next stage-or remaining in maintenance.

In the box, write your stage of change. Then, list the processes that are most useful in that stage (see Fig. 2-2 in Chapter 2). Use only the number of processes that apply to your stage of behavior change. You may not need to use all six. Under each process that you use, give two specific behavior strategies (see Table 2-1 in Chapter 2) that could help you progress to the next stage-or maintain, if you're in the maintenance stage.

The stage I am in = [   ] .

Process 1.   _____

    Behavior strategy -a.

    Behavior strategy -b.

Process 2.   _____

    Behavior strategy -a.

    Behavior strategy -b.

Process 3.   _____

    Behavior strategy -a.

    Behavior strategy -b.

Process 4.   _____

    Behavior strategy -a.

    Behavior strategy -b.

Process 5.   _____

    Behavior strategy -a.

    Behavior strategy -b.

Process 6.   _____

    Behavior strategy -a.

    Behavior strategy -b.

An ounce of prevention is worth a ton of cure.
—Anonymous

Preventing Common Injuries and Caring for the Lower Back

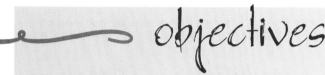

After reading this chapter, you will be able to:

1. Identify four main reasons injuries occur.
2. Give three tips for avoiding an overuse injury.
3. Explain how muscle weakness and inflexibility contribute to injuries.
4. Identify four common muscle imbalances.
5. List and explain the general recommended treatment for common injuries (P.R.I.C.E.).
6. Describe the basic causes and treatment of ankle sprain, blisters, bursitis, chafing heel spur syndrome, iliotibial band syndrome, muscle cramp, muscle soreness, muscle strain, patellofemoral syndrome, plantar fasciitis, shin splints, side stitch, stress fracture and tendinitis.
7. Identify the four symptoms of injury that indicate the need for medical attention.
8. Explain two vital components of rehabilitation needed to resume activity safely without injury.
9. Identify the two most important keys to preventing lower back pain.
10. List and describe six of the eight exercises recommended to reduce the risk of lower back pain.

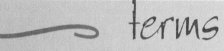

- Blisters
- Bursitis
- Cramp
- Heel spur
- Iliotibial band syndrome
- Intervertebral disc
- Ischemia
- Ligament
- Orthotics
- Overpronation
- Overuse
- Patellofemoral syndrome
- Plantar fasciitis
- P.R.I.C.E.
- Pronation
- Shin splint
- Side stitch
- Sprain
- Strain
- Stress fracture
- Supination
- Tendinitis
- Tendons

ou walk into your first jogging class, eager to improve your fitness. You have not exercised regularly and you hope this class will help you get into shape. Your instructor begins with a warm-up and an easy jog around campus. After your run, you feel great and invigorated. The next morning, you wake up and your whole body aches. You don't remember having been run over by a truck. "What should I do now? Withdraw from class? Stay in bed? Buy stock in Ben-Gay? When will I be able to move again?"

Participation in fitness activities offers many benefits. These benefits far exceed the risk of injury. When you exercise, you intentionally use certain muscles to increase their strength and endurance. As your body adapts to these efforts, you may experience minor aches and soreness. Physical activity also carries some risk of overuse or injury. Fortunately, many of these discomforts are minor, and you will be able to continue or quickly resume your workouts. Everybody is built differently and varies in physical potential, so "listen to your body" to safely improve your personal fitness level—and avoid the pain of injury. This chapter discusses how to prevent injuries, how to recognize their signs and symptoms, and what treatments are recommended. It also examines how to maintain a healthy back, because chronic back pain is a common problem. Finally, factors that affect the musculature of the spine and how to avoid lower back injury are covered.

Injury Prevention

Prevention is the key to reducing the frequency of injuries. Ninety percent of injuries include slow wear and tear, strains, sprains, and inflammations. Understanding the causes of injuries allows you to stop minor problems before they turn you into the "walking wounded." Prevention is far more conducive to wellness than any patch and repair job. There are four main reasons injuries occur:

1. *Overuse:* doing too much too soon or too often, causing a breakdown at the weakest point—ankle, Achilles tendon, shin, knee, or back.
2. *Footwear:* wearing improper or worn-out shoes.
3. *Weakness and inflexibility:* muscles so weak or tight that the slightest unusual twist strains them.
4. *Mechanical problems:* the result of biomechanical/anatomical problems (the way the foot hits the ground, body build, etc.) or using poor form while exercising.

An individually adjusted workload, well-made and well-kept shoes, supplemental toning and stretching exer-

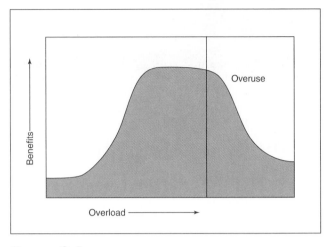

figure 9-1   Overload and overuse. Overload is good to a point; overuse can cause injury.

cises, and mechanical improvements will prevent the majority of injuries.

Overuse

To improve or maintain fitness, you must over-load, or push, beyond normal demands. Overload following the F.T.I. formula in Chapter 3 is necessary and good to a point, but you must be able to recover between workouts. The goal is to exercise so that you improve but not so much that you cause **overuse,** excessive overload leading to injury or illness (Fig. 9-1). Overuse problems commonly occur at the beginning of a new exercise program and account for the majority of injuries. It is estimated that between 25 and 50 percent of athletes visiting sports medicine clinics have sustained overuse injuries. The first 2 months of a new program are the most critical. The body and muscles must be given time to gradually adapt to the new demands.

Set realistic goals early in a fitness program. Your instructor will help you determine an appropriate entry-level conditioning program and progression. Gradually increase your exercise intensity and duration to attain your personal goals. For example, if you have never participated in aerobics, your first goal may be to perform 10 minutes of continuous aerobic exercise, although other members of the class may work out 25 or 30 minutes. Try not to compete or compare yourself with your friends who may be able to exercise for a longer duration or at higher intensity. You will be able to catch up in time, but if you attempt to keep up with them before your body is ready, you risk an overuse problem.

A good rule of thumb to follow when building your program is to increase the duration of the workout no more than 10 percent weekly. A beginner should not jump from a 20-minute workout up to 40 minutes. Also, do not increase both intensity and duration during the same week. This principle holds true in aerobics, lap swimming, water exercise, bi-

| table 9-1 | Symptoms of Overtraining, Overuse, and Chronic Fatigue |

Signs in your Training

- Persistent soreness and stiffness in joints, tendons, or muscles
- Labored breathing during a workout of normal intensity
- Performance decline, or cutting sessions short
- Recovery takes longer
- Persistent lethargy, fatigue, and unusual disinterest in exercise

Signs in your life

- Increased tension, anger, irritability
- No interest in activities you usually do
- Poor concentration (general clumsiness, tripping, poor auto driving)
- Not sleeping well

Signs in your health

- Increased infections and colds
- Increases of six to eight beats per minute in morning resting pulse
- Swelling or aching lymph glands in neck, underarm, or groin area
- Skin eruptions in nonadolescents
- Constipation or diarrhea
- Loss of appetite
- Chronic thirst
- Cuts and scars take a long time to heal
- Inexplicable weight changes, either up or down
- Anemia or amenorrhea (in women)

cycling, fitness walking, and jogging. Studies show an increasing injury rate with increasing weekly jogging distance beyond 20 miles per week. Many fitness buffs and athletes have a feeling of invulnerability. They think their bodies can adapt to increased exercise workloads without any problem. Realize that more is not always better. By allowing your body to gradually adjust to new exercise demands, you will greatly reduce the risk of suffering an overuse injury. See Table 9-1 for symptoms of overtraining, overuse and chronic fatigue.

Consider alternating an impact activity with a low impact or nonimpact activity. This alternation allows the muscles a period of rest and recovery and switches the demands to a new muscle group. It is repetitive stress on the body that causes problems. Some people enjoy alternating activities because it adds variety and develops total body fitness better than any single activity. It also allows specific muscles and joints a chance to rest and recover. For example, water exercise or bicycling is a good supplement to an impact exercise such as jogging.

It is crucial that you listen to your body during and after exercise. After a great workout, if you feel a little soreness, it should gradually decrease over the next hour. However, if you develop excessive soreness or pain, cut back in your next workout, try a different activity, or take a day off.

The importance of rest is often overlooked. When you are fatigued you are most susceptible to injury.

If you are getting the right amount of exercise, you should look good, feel good, and be alert and productive. Too much exercise, like too little, can be unhealthy. After a workout, you should get enough rest to be fully recovered by the next workout. Rest is probably the most neglected aspect of fitness. Fitness does not occur during exercise alone, but from the proper combination of training and recovery. Exercise provides the overload that stimulates that improvement. During the rest period between workouts, the body makes adaptations to the demands made upon it. When the recovery is adequate, you will begin the next workout feeling strong and energetic. If you feel tired and washed out, rest will do you more good than exercise. Pay attention to your water intake. Dehydration can be a major contributor to fatigue. Drink 8 to 10 glasses of water daily—and more if you exercise in a hot climate. Also keep in mind that exercise isn't the only source of overstress. Other aspects of daily life such as poor nutrition; emotional tension; job, social, or family problems; and lack of sleep can contribute to chronic fatigue.

There is a difference between the pain of injury and the pain of hard effort. The concepts of "no pain, no gain" and "going for the burn" are useful in athletics, but inappropriate for fitness exercisers whose goal is health, not athletic performance. Pain is the body's natural way of informing you that something is wrong. Pain may be localized or generalized. However, pain is a subjective response, and each individual will tolerate it differently. Do not try to exercise through pain or injury. Previous injury is a strong risk factor for future injuries. Allow time for healing and correct mechanical problems before resuming activity.

Footwear

While many injuries are due to overuse, it is only part of the problem. Wearing improper or worn-out shoes places added stress on your hips, knees, ankles, and feet—the sites of up

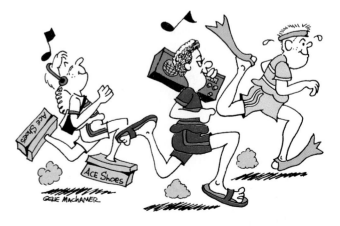

Improper footwear increases risk of injury.

to 90 percent of sports injuries. The feet are the most abused and neglected part of the body. Good footwear is the best investment you can make in an exercise program. Each time your foot hits the ground when jogging, the force of impact is three to five times your body weight. Your feet, ankles, shins, knees, hips, and lower back must absorb a tremendous amount of stress. If the stress is too great, breakdown occurs at the weakest link in the chain. A well-fitted pair of shoes is the first line of defense against impact injuries.

Shoes should provide good shock absorption, support, and stability yet maintain a reasonable degree of flexibility. Your foot will naturally roll inward from outer heel contact to big toe pushoff when you jog; therefore, the heel counter (the rigid plastic insert in the shoe's heel) must be firm to prevent excessive heel movement. The bottom of the shoe must have good traction to prevent slipping. Shoes are manufactured to be used for a certain number of miles, and they can lose their cushioning ability even if the uppers still look good. Each step compresses the sole, causing it to flatten and gradually lose shock absorbability. Exercise shoes typically lose about one-third of their ability to absorb shock after 400 to 500 miles of use. The upper part of the shoe stretches and weakens, decreasing lateral support. This happens so gradually you may not notice it until you try on a new pair of shoes. With less cushioning and support, there is a greater chance of injury. If you wear the shoes 5 to 10 hours a week during exercise (walking, jogging, aerobics, etc.), you should probably replace them every 6 months to retain adequate cushioning. Runners would be well-advised to keep a log of their mileage as a reminder of when to buy new shoes.

Weakness and Inflexibility

Sit down with your feet extended in front. Slowly reach toward your toes. Can you touch them without bending your knees? Many exercisers who neglect flexibility exercises cannot pass this test for minimal flexibility. Their legs are too tight, and this increases susceptibility to muscle and tendon injuries. Aerobic activities are great for the cardiorespiratory system, but they alone do not develop balanced fitness. They tend to shorten and tighten muscles used repetitively, leaving opposing, relatively unused muscles weak. This can lead to muscle imbalance. If some muscles are too tight, joint movement is restricted. Table 9-2 lists some common muscle imbalances. The solution to this problem is to stretch the tight muscles and strengthen the weak ones. Flexibility is one of the most important factors in injury prevention.

Incorporate a basic stretching routine into each workout, preferably during the cool-down. (See Chapter 5 for recommended strength and flexibility exercises.) Stretch gently, placing only slight tension on the muscles. Hard stretching or bouncy movements may activate the stretch reflex. This causes the muscle to involuntarily contract and shorten—exactly the opposite of what you're trying to do—

table 9-2   Common Muscle Imbalances

The rule of thumb in avoiding injuries is to *stretch* the muscles that are tight and *strengthen* the opposing muscles that are weak.

Tight	Weak
gastrocnemius (calf)	tibialis anterior (shin)
quadriceps (front of thigh)	hamstrings (back of thigh)
erector spinae (lower back)	abdominals (stomach)
pectorals (chest)	rhomboids (upper back)

to protect itself from injury. Concentrate on event-specific exercises. For example, if you are a swimmer, you will want to spend additional time stretching the shoulders and arms. If jogging or aerobics is your activity, concentrate on stretching the hamstrings, quadriceps, lower back, and calf. Abdominal curls are an important supplement to any fitness workout. Strong abdominals and a flexible lower back are critical in preventing lower-back problems.

Mechanics

Structural weaknesses, mainly affecting the legs, knees, ankles, and feet, are often revealed when a beginner starts a new exercise program or when overuse occurs. Biomechanical difficulties often arise in the feet. The foot is a marvelous structure of 26 bones, with almost double that number of ligaments and muscles. It strikes the ground about 80 to 90 times a minute during exercise. When a weak foot pounds the ground several thousand times a day, the potential for injury is great. Slight **pronation** of your foot is natural—that is, your foot will roll inward slightly after the outer edge of the heel strikes the ground. All bodies are not created equal, so different foot types, gait styles, and body mechanics vary in susceptibility to injury. For example, knock knees or flat feet may cause **overpronation**—too much inward roll when the foot should be pushing off (Fig. 9-2). This twists foot, shin, and knee and can cause tendinitis, plantar fasciitis, or knee strain. Observing the wear pattern on your shoes can help you select a shoe designed for your specific mechanics. Set your shoes on a flat surface. If they tilt inward and if there is excessive shoe wear on the inside of the forefoot, your feet may overpronate. If, on the other hand, the outside of the shoe is overstretched and tilts outward, and there is excessive wear on the outside of the shoe, your feet may supinate too much. **Supination** is insufficient inward roll of the foot upon contact. People with high arches and tight Achilles tendons tend to supinate. When the foot hits the ground, it does not roll inward enough to absorb the shock of impact, increasing the risk of shin splints, stress fractures, iliotibial band syndrome, tendinitis,

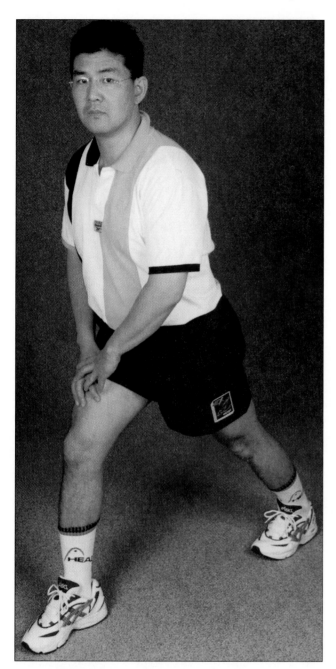

Good calf flexibility reduces risk of Achilles tendinitis, plantar fasciitis, and shin splints.

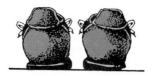 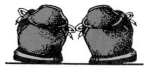

Supination   Overpronation

figure 9-2   Supination and overpronation.

trained to help you select a proper shoe. If discomfort persists, you may want to consult a physician or podiatrist who will check your foot mechanics. He or she may prescribe **orthotics,** shoe inserts molded to your foot, to correct abnormalities. These allow the foot to operate mechanically efficiently. They are highly effective for alleviating excessive foot pronation/supination.

Regardless of your body type, pay attention to form when participating in any aerobic activity. Participants in aerobic dance, water exercise, bicycling, and step aerobics and even those using stair climbing and cross country skiing machines need to understand the proper mechanics of each activity. In this way, many injuries and discomforts can be avoided. You will find technique and safety tips for a variety of aerobic activities in Chapter 4. You may also want to refer to the "Contraindicated Exercises" listed in Chapter 6.

The body is a marvelous mechanism. Considering its complexity, it is a wonder it doesn't break down more often. Exercise is vital to maintain wellness. Illness and injury are less common in those who maintain peak performance through regular exercise than it is in those who exercise sporadically. Even when injuries do occur, few are debilitating. Many simply cause some inconvenience. For a summary of tips on preventing injuries, see the top ten list. If we can't prevent all injuries, it is important to be able to recognize the signs and symptoms of those that exercisers most commonly encounter. This gives you an opportunity to take corrective action in the early stages and limit down time.

and plantar fasciitis. Supination causes excessive wear on the outside of the shoe sole.

Moderate pronation problems can be corrected by wise shoe selection. Most exercise shoes are designed to limit overpronation, not eliminate all inward rotation. A person who overpronates needs motion-control shoes with a straight or semi-curved last and features that limit pronation. The best shoe for a supinator has a curved last to allow normal pronation. Employees in many sports shoe stores are

P.R.I.C.E.

Acute injuries to muscles, joints, and tendons are often accompanied by swelling. Rapid recovery requires keeping the swelling to a minimum. The aim of treatment is to assist the healing process. The recommended treatment for many injuries, whether mild or severe, is protect, rest, ice, compress, and elevate or **P.R.I.C.E.** (see Table 9-3).

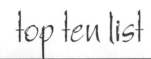

top ten list

Top Ten Tips for Preventing Injuries

1. **Warm up.** Walking, slow jogging, or gentle calisthenics the first 5 to 10 minutes of your workout transition your muscles, heart, and metabolism into a higher gear. You're ready when you feel warmer and begin to break a sweat.

2. **Progress slowly.** Overuse—doing too much, too hard, too soon—is the leading cause of injury. Increase your workload by no more than 10 percent per week. Alternate hard with easy workout days.

3. **Work out regularly.** Sporadic exercise invites injury. Your muscles need several weeks to adjust to the stresses of exercise. Exercise every other day is safer and more effective than weekend workout binges that leave you stiff and sore.

4. **Cool down.** Walk around or continue your exercise at a lower pace a few minutes to give your heart and respiratory rates a chance to transition back toward resting. You will feel better than if you stop suddenly and will avoid a potentially serious drop in blood pressure or even fainting from blood pooling in the extremities.

5. **Stretch for flexibility.** This is most effective during the cool-down when muscles are warm and pliant, stretching is easier and the effects on flexibility are longer lasting (see Chapter 4).

6. **Try cross-training.** Combining aerobic, strength, and flexibility exercises in your weekly program develops balanced fitness and avoids the one-dimensional stresses of doing only one type of workout, in other words, running is a fine aerobic activity, but it tightens hamstrings and calves and doesn't do anything for the abdominals or upper body. Adding stretching and strengthening twice a week keeps the muscles in better shape, can reduce injury risk, and improve the running.

7. **Drink water before, during, and after exercise.** Dehydration leaves you tired and increases susceptibility to heat injury. Drinking 8 oz. of water before, a half-cup every 20 minutes of exercise, and 8 oz. or more afterward is good.

8. **Modify workouts in extreme heat or cold.** In hot spells, shift to early or late workouts, and try noon during cold weather. Pay attention to how you feel and ease back on workout intensity and duration until you acclimatize or until the weather improves.

9. **Pay attention to pain.** Pain is a signal that something is wrong. Trying to work through an injury will prolong or worsen it. If something begins to hurt, or if you're not recovering from one workout to the next, cut back, switch activities, or take a couple days off to give yourself a chance to mend.

10. **Wear good, well-fitted shoes.** They are your first line of defense against impact injuries. Choose those appropriate for the activity and replace them every 400 to 500 miles or before the soles become compressed.

---

table 9-3	Recommended Treatment for Common Injuries

P	=	Protect from further injury
R	=	Rest to allow healing and avoid tissue irritation
I	=	Ice to reduce pain and swelling
C	=	Compress with a wrap to control swelling
E	=	Elevate to reduce swelling

P = Protect

The classic advice of old-time coaches was, "Run it off." On the contrary, it is important to protect the injured area from further tissue damage. A few days rest from the activity in which the problem occurred might be sufficient to protect irritated tissue from re-injury while healing from a minor strain. A medical professional might recommend that a more severely injured limb be protected with crutches, a splint, or sling. The aim is to minimize irritation, tissue

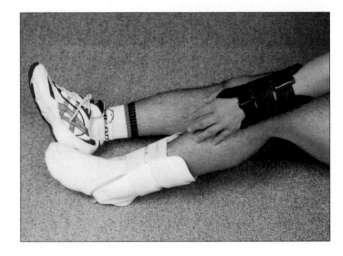

For a serious injury, a medical professional may recommend a splint to protect and rest the area while healing.

bleeding, inflammation, and pain and provide optimal healing conditions.

R = Rest

The injured area should be rested for 24 hours to 72 hours or more depending on the severity of the injury. Switching to a different activity, such as swimming, cycling, or deep water running, can rest a sore area and maintain your conditioning. A minor complaint can become a major problem if you keep aggravating the situation. Healing progresses more rapidly when stress to the area is reduced. Frequently, people will start back into their usual activity before they are ready, and they reinjure themselves. If you are unable to exercise for a week, when you return to your usual workout routine, reduce your duration, frequency, and/or intensity by at least 25 percent. Do not resume your normal workout level until you are free of pain during and after exercise.

I = Ice

Apply ice to the injured part immediately. A convenient way to apply ice is to put ice cubes or crushed ice in a plastic freezer bag and place it on the injured area. Reusable gel ice packs, chemical cold packs, or a pound of frozen peas also work well. Do not apply the ice directly to the skin. A layer of wet towelling or plastic wrap between the ice and skin effectively transmits the cold to the area without risking freezing the skin. Apply the ice for 15 to 20 minutes, stop for 10, ice again if time permits. The ice may make the injured part

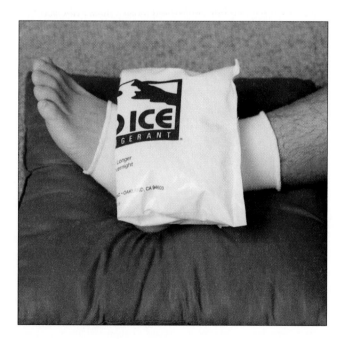

P.R.I.C.E. To transmit cold effectively, wet the elastic wrap prior to applying ice to the injury.

ache for the first 5 to 10 minutes. Keep it on! After 10 minutes, the part will become numb. This will give immediate pain relief and reduce swelling, inflammation, and tissue damage. In deeper blood vessels, circulation increases, bringing blood, nutrients, and healing cells to the injured area. Ice the injured area three times a day for at least the first 48 to 72 hours. Icing should be continued after that time if swelling persists.

If you feel mild discomfort when exercising and suspect an overuse injury, such as tendinitis, you should apply ice to the tender areas right after you work out and reapply it several times a day for the next 48 hours. Remember: You can never go wrong with ice. Sportsmedicine physician Francis G. O'Connor states, "Ice is indicated as long as inflammation persists—from the onset of the injury, through rehabilitation, and into sports return."

C = Compress

When not icing the injury, wrap the part with an elastic wrap to prevent fluid buildup in the injured area. Wrap it snugly but not tightly enough to interfere with circulation. If the part starts throbbing, the wrap may be on too tight. Remove the wrap and reapply it more loosely. Do not sleep with the wrap on.

E = Elevate

Raise the injured area above the level of the heart. This will reduce the swelling by combatting the effect of gravity pulling blood and fluids down to the injured area. Most people with an injured ankle or knee will place it on a pillow for elevation when going to sleep. However, you may move during the night and lose the elevation. Instead, place three or four books under your mattress to raise it approximately 6 to 8 inches.

Heat and Pain Relievers

Many people mistakenly apply heat to an acute injury. Heat applied too early stimulates blood flow and increases swelling and inflammation. Stick with ice for at least the first 48 to 72 hours after an injury and only then, *after swelling has completely subsided*, should heat be applied. At that point, heat may speed healing, relax muscles, and reduce stiffness. Either dry heat (heating pad or lamp) or moist heat (a hot bath, whirlpool, hot-water bottle, damp heat pack) will do. Apply the heat for 10 to 20 minutes, two or three times a day. You can also use it for 5 to 10 minutes before exercising to reduce stiffness.

Over-the-counter liniments and balms are popular methods for producing a warm feeling in muscles. The effect of these products is only superficial—the active ingredients stimulate sensory nerve endings in the skin to produce a sensation of heat. This has no healing effect and may mask the pain.

Aspirin or ibuprofen (such as Motrin or Advil) can reduce the pain and inflammation of minor sprains, strains, and tendinitis. Acetaminophen (such as Tylenol) is less helpful because it has no anti-inflammatory effect. Do not use anti-inflammatories to mask pain so that you can continue to work out—this will worsen an injury. Do not use a therapeutic dose of these pain relievers more than 2 or 3 consecutive days because they increase risk of stomach bleeding. Consult your doctor before using any drugs.

Common Injuries

In pursuit of wellness, you may occasionally push yourself beyond the current capabilities of your structure. Finding your peak and keeping it is a challenge and part of a process of learning about your body's unique strengths and weaknesses. If, in your zeal to experience peak performance, you develop an athletic ailment, it will be minor and you will be able to resume activity within a few days. Here we will discuss the potential causes of, symptoms of, and treatments for the most common injuries listed alphabetically.

Ankle Sprain

A **sprain** is a partial or complete tear of a **ligament,** the fibrous connective tissue that binds bones together to form a joint. A sprain is most often a result of a sudden force, typically a twisting motion that surrounding muscles are not strong enough to control. Both ankles and knees are vulnerable to sprains. An ankle sprain will produce swelling and tenderness on the outside of the ankle. The amount of swelling depends upon the severity of the injury. In severe cases, discoloration or bruising will develop. Range of motion in the ankle may be decreased by swelling and pain. P.R.I.C.E. for the first 72 hours is the best treatment for sprains. It is extremely important to control the amount of swelling in the joint in order to return to activity quickly. Strong, flexible muscles help protect against sprains. For example, to prevent ankle sprain, strengthen ankles with flexion, inversion, and eversion exercises. High-top shoes or a commercial ankle wrap do not reduce risk of re-injury and can provide a false sense of confidence. When you start back into activity, progress gradually. A sprained ankle can take 1 to 2 months to heal.

Blisters

Blisters are a common problem, especially for beginning exercisers. They are an accumulation of fluid under the skin due to excess friction. They are usually only a problem if they become infected or if they cause you to limp. The most common areas for blisters are the bottom of the foot, the sides of the big and little toes, and the back of the heel. Blisters can be prevented by eliminating the friction that causes them. Wear 100 percent acrylic (orlon) socks. Acrylic is best at dissipating moisture and preventing blisters from forming. Cotton socks produce twice as many blisters and even worse is a cotton-acrylic blend. One trick for preventing a blister is to apply a piece of duct tape over an irritated area *before* a blister forms. Never wear new shoes for a workout without first breaking them in by walking around in them at home for a few days. Should a blister be opened? Some say no, let the fluid reabsorb into the system because an open blister invites infection. Others say to pop the blister if it is painful and causes you to limp. The best treatment is to apply a donut pad and lubricant to the blister to reduce friction and pressure. To prevent blisters, some runners wear their socks inside out to avoid the abrasion of the rough interior seam. It may also help to wear two socks on the affected foot—a thin nylon sock inside an acrylic sock. If the blister is lanced, do not remove loose skin, and keep the area clean to prevent infection. Consult your physician if you think it may be infected.

Bursitis

Bursitis is inflammation of a bursa, a fluid-filled sac that lies between tissues and allows tendons, ligaments, muscles, and skin to glide smoothly over one another during activity. There are over 150 bursae, but the most commonly affected lie in the knee, elbow, shoulder, and hip. When a bursa becomes irritated, it begins producing extra fluid and the sac swells, often within 24 hours, causing pain in the affected area. The recommended treatment is to protect the area, rest from activity, ice, compress with an elastic bandage to reduce swelling, and take anti-inflammatory medication. Do not wrap the knee tightly, however, as this could lead to blood clots by compressing the large vein behind the joint.

Chafing

When skin rubs against skin or against clothing, it becomes irritated and can crack and bleed. The most common problem areas are between the thighs, under the armpits, and on the nipples (runner's nipples). While chafing can happen to anyone, frequency increases with greater body fat percentage. Treat chafing by applying petroleum jelly to the affected area. To prevent chafing, select clothing of smooth, nonabrasive material with few or well-covered seams. Synthetics are best. Avoid cotton because it stays wet, causing friction.

Avoid clothing that is tight or that bunches under the arms or between the legs. Wearing tights or knee-length exercise shorts can protect chafed thighs. Nipple chafing can be decreased by going shirtless in warm weather or by applying petroleum jelly and adhesive bandages to the nipples. Women should select a good exercise bra that has flat or covered seams.

Heel Spur

A **heel spur** is a bony growth found on the underside of the calcaneus (heel bone) at the insertion of the plantar fascia. The pull of fascia on the heel can remodel the bone into a spur pointing toward the toes. Heel spurs are common and are not necessarily the sign of a problem. They do not always cause pain, unless there is significant fat pad atrophy or unless they are caused by chronic irritation of the plantar fascia at its insertion. The heel pain of plantar fasciitis is sometimes associated with a heel spur. Treatment involves rest; anti-inflammatory medications; and insertion of a heel pad in the shoe to protect the heel, alleviate inflammation, and to distribute impact during activity.

Iliotibial Band Syndrome

Tightness, burning, and pain on the side of the knee or hip may be related to inflammation of the **iliotibial band,** a long tendon that begins in the buttocks, runs down the side of the thigh, and attaches to the side of the lower leg just below the knee. Common in runners, an overtight iliotibial band may become inflamed from friction of rubbing against the outer knee or hip bone as the knee repetitively flexes and extends. This is primarily an overuse injury and can be treated with decreasing or changing activity, ice, anti-inflammatories, and stretching the IT band, hamstrings, and quadriceps (see stretches in Chapter 4).

Muscle Cramp

A **cramp** is a sharp, involuntary muscle contraction. It may occur during exercise or at rest. The calf is the most common area for a muscle cramp to occur, but cramps may occur anywhere in the body. Muscle cramps may be caused by fatigue. This is a protective mechanism, your body telling you to quit or you will do yourself damage. Cramps may also be related to a strength imbalance, an electrolyte imbalance, or dehydration. Occasionally, low levels of circulating calcium or potassium in the blood can contribute to cramps. Cramps can be treated with fluid intake and with gradual stretching of the muscle. A calf cramp may be treated by extending the foot to a 90-degree angle. Occasionally, gentle massage may help.

Muscle cramps may be prevented by taking precautions when exercising in the heat. Wear light, loose clothing; drink water freely; gradually acclimatize yourself to the heat; and exercise during the cooler hours of the day. Extra salt is not needed. A regular program of stretching may also help prevent muscle cramps.

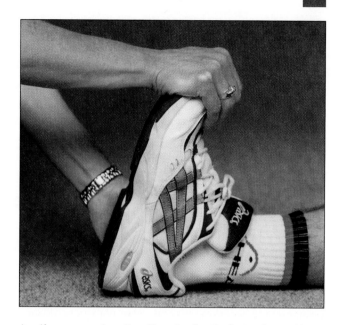

A calf cramp may be relieved by extending the foot and stretching the calf.

Muscle Soreness

Muscle soreness is discomfort or tenderness following an increase in workout level. It may be fairly mild and usually is just a reminder that you had a good workout. There is no real pain but rather a mild achiness when you move the major muscle groups used in the activity. After several sessions of the same activity, soreness will diminish or disappear. Duration of activity and eccentric (lengthening) contractions are highly correlated to muscle soreness. For example, running downhill repeatedly will produce more quadricep soreness than will an equal amount of flat or uphill running. Muscle soreness is thought to be caused by microscopic tears or spasms of the connective tissue. There is no long-term damage from this. Muscle soreness may develop immediately or over a 24- to 36-hour period following unaccustomed exercise and will usually disappear within 1 to 3 days. Other than following a sensible progression, there is no real prevention for muscle soreness. It indicates that some muscles that were out of shape have been stimulated to tone up, usually occurring at the beginning of any new exercise program. For example, a person who has not recently lifted weights will develop muscle soreness following the first workout. There is little that can be done for mild muscle soreness. While stretching is beneficial for flexibility, it has little effect on reducing soreness.

Muscle Strain

A muscle **strain** is a tear of muscle fibers or a tendon and is sometimes referred to as a *pull*. Symptoms include sharp pain, weakness with possible loss of function, spasm or extreme tightness, and tenderness to the touch. There are many different causes, but it most often results from a violent contraction of the muscle. A strain may be caused by fatigue, overexertion, muscle imbalance or weakness, or electrolyte or water imbalance.

A strain may range from mild (more painful than just soreness) to a complete rupture of the muscle. Muscles most likely to be affected are the hamstrings, gastrocnemius, Achilles tendon, erector spinae, groin, and the rotator cuff muscles of the shoulder. Rest, ice, and anti-inflammatories are used to treat muscle strain. Reduce or eliminate activity until the injury starts to heal. The severity of the injury and which muscle is injured will affect the recovery time. The hamstrings usually take the longest to heal and rehabilitate. If the strain is severe, it will heal with a significant amount of scar tissue. Scar tissue is not elastic like muscle, so stretching and strengthening exercises are important to return to normal function. To prevent strains, complete a full warm-up before working out, take care not to overdo, and work toward balancing the strength and flexibility in opposing muscles.

Patellofemoral Syndrome

Pain around and under the kneecap, along with knee stiffness, is characteristic of **patellofemoral syndrome.** Symptoms include pain when walking up and down stairs or after sitting with knees bent for a period of time ("theater sign"), and occasionally mild swelling or a feeling that the knee is "giving way." Patellofemoral syndrome is associated with overuse, always running the same direction on the track, excessive hill running, and rapid ballistic movements such as those done in aerobics. One common cause is structural. Wide hips tend to make the quadriceps pull the kneecap out against the femur, producing inflammation. Loose kneecaps or a quadriceps muscle not strong enough to keep the patella in its groove also may lead to patellofemoral syndrome. The knee will not get better if you continue your activity during the injury.

Rest, ice, and anti-inflammatories are the conventional treatments for this injury. If the knee swells significantly, see a physician. Swelling can indicate a major problem and take much longer to heal.

To prevent recurrence, the knee must be rehabilitated. To stabilize the knee and to assist in correcting the tracking mechanism of the patella, strengthen the quadriceps. Stretching should increase hamstring and iliotibial band flexibility. In severe cases, surgery may be indicated.

Plantar Fasciitis

Plantar Fasciitis causes heel or arch pain. It is most painful when a person takes their first few steps in the morning, but in severe cases, pain may continue throughout the day. It re-

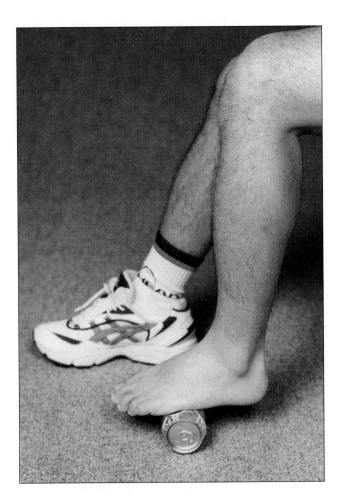

To treat plantar fasciitis, roll a cold can of soda under your arch to ice and stretch the fascia.

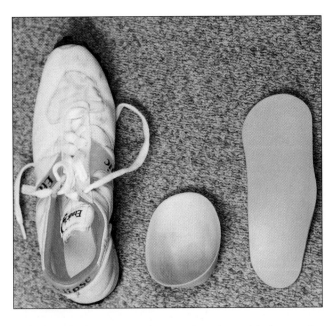

Orthotics or heel cups may reduce symptoms in persistent cases of plantar fasciitis.

sults from inflammation of the plantar fascia, a long thick band of connective tissue on the underside of the foot that attaches the base of the calcaneus to the base of the toes. Inflammation may result from excessive impact, worn shoes, or poor foot mechanics. Anatomical problems frequently cause plantar fasciitis—tight Achilles tendon, high arches, flat feet, or excessive pronation. Also, with age and repeated weight-bearing stress, the fat pad under the heel becomes flattened and less shock absorbent. Rest, anti-inflammatories, calf stretching, ice, and arch supports or heel cups are the recommended treatments. Rolling a can of chilled soda or a frozen plastic bottle of water back and forth under the arch is a good way to apply cold to the area. Orthotics are often recommended to reduce symptoms in persistent/recurrent cases of plantar fasciitis.

Shin Splints

A **shin splint** refers to pain in the front of the lower leg (shin). Early signs are acute burning pain or irritation in the lower third of the anterior tibialis. This may progress to slight swelling, redness, warmth, and inflammation. A variety of factors contribute to shin splints. They often come early in an exercise program and are particularly common in those who are out of shape, overweight, wide hipped, knock-kneed, or duck footed. Working out on very hard or very soft surfaces can bring on shin splints, even if a person is well-conditioned. Switching from a hard to a soft surface or vice versa, excessive mileage, improper footwear, poor foot mechanics, running on a road slope, and running the same direction all the time on an indoor track may cause them. Women, particularly those who wear high heels, are affected nearly three times more often than are men.

Shin splints may be a sign of a long arch problem in the foot. As the long arch begins to sag, it stretches lower leg muscles and causes pain. Another cause is a muscle imbalance between the strong calf muscle and the weak anterior tibialis, which may lead to inflammation of the membrane between the tibia and the fibula. This imbalance can be corrected with exercises to strengthen the anterior tibialis and by stretching the calf. These should be done each workout. If mechanical problems are not corrected, shin splints tend to recur.

To treat shin splints switch to a low-or nonimpact activity and, rub ice on the affected area for 15 to 20 minutes three to four times a day. Aspirin therapy may be indicated for a few days to reduce inflammation. If the pain is persistent, consult a physician to rule out a stress fracture.

Side Stitch

A **side stitch** is a sharp pain just under the ribs, typically on the right side. It may result from participating in vigorous activity before the body has had sufficient warm-up. It may be related to a lack of conditioning, weak abdominals, shallow breathing, consuming a meal too near the time of exercise,

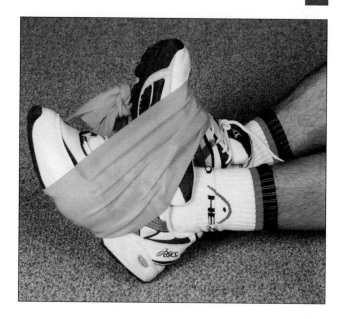

To decrease risk of shin splints, strengthen shins with a set of 15 to 20 toe pulls twice a week using an elastic band.

dehydration, excessive exercise intensity, or **ischemia** (inadequate oxygen) to the diaphragm. Side stitches tend to occur in unfit or new exercisers. Better conditioning brings more efficient blood flow and oxygen delivery to the respiratory muscles. It can be treated by stopping activity and stretching or holding the side. After cessation of the activity for a few minutes, the pain and spasm should subside. Taking a deep breath may also break the spasm. Once the pain has dissipated, activity may resume.

Stress Fracture

A **stress fracture** is a microscopic break in a bone caused by overuse. While it can occur anywhere in the lower legs and feet, it is most common at the end of the tibia near the ankle or in the metatarsals of the feet. Unlike a broken bone, which occurs with a distinct traumatic event, a stress fracture is the result of cumulative overload that occurs over many days or weeks. Overtraining or too-rapid increases in training are the major causes. Bone is living tissue that adjusts to exercise force demands placed on it. As force is applied, bone will remodel itself to better handle the force. If too much force is applied, the bone may fracture before it can successfully remodel. Running excessive mileage, overdoing impact aerobics, wearing worn-out shoes, exercising on hard surfaces such as asphalt or concrete, and having poor foot mechanics may cause a stress fracture. Because they have smaller, lighter bones, women are more susceptible to stress fractures than are men. Especially when combined with hard training, an inadequate intake of calcium and vitamin D can predispose one to the onset—and the recurrence—of stress fractures.

A stress fracture may be confused with a case of severe shin splints but stress fractures are more likely to cause pinpoint pain on the sore bone. Stress fractures are difficult to detect clinically. Frequently, they will not show up on X ray until 3 to 4 weeks after the onset of symptoms. A bone scan can detect a stress fracture much earlier in the injury because it reveals the active bone formation that occurs while the fracture is healing. The pain of a stress fracture will not go away with conventional treatments (ice, ultrasound) or medication. Only rest will decrease the pain.

The best treatment for a stress fracture is rest from the activity that caused it. This does not mean elimination of exercise altogether. Nonimpact activities like riding a bicycle or swimming are good alternatives during the healing phase. Depending on the severity of the stress fracture, activity may be resumed within 2 to 6 weeks of diagnosis. "Running through the injury" is not recommended. This may lead to a nonunion fracture of the bone and a 6- to 8-week recovery period in a cast.

Tendinitis

Anytime you see "-itis," think inflammation. **Tendinitis** is the inflammation of a tendon from repetitive stress. Common signs of inflammation include pain, redness, heat, and swelling. **Tendons** are the fibrous cords that connect muscles to bones. They are vulnerable to inflammation because the force of muscle contractions is transmitted through them. The most commonly affected in runners, walkers, and aerobic dancers is the Achilles tendon, which connects two calf muscles, the gastrocnemius and soleus, to the back of the heel bone. Other areas commonly affected are the knee, shoulder, and elbow ("tennis elbow"). When a tendon is inflamed, normal daily activities, such as opening a door or walking up the stairs, can be painful. Tendinitis is often brought on by muscle tightness or increasing the workload too quickly. Achilles tendon problems are often due to tight calf muscles. When the foot flexes to push off, the powerful Achilles pulls the heel up. If the calf is too tight, it yanks the heel up prematurely, stressing the Achilles tendon. Rest from the activity that caused the injury and stretching to alleviate excessive tightness are recommended. Over-the-counter anti-inflammatory medications (ibuprofen, aspirin) may also help. It may take 2 to 3 weeks to completely heal and rehabilitate. Continuing activity will only delay healing. Meanwhile, you may include alternate activities to maintain fitness. A regular program incorporating stretching and strengthening can help prevent tendinitis.

When to Seek Medical Help

Not all injuries can be self-treated. If symptoms are severe, or if self-treatment is not working, you need professional

---

table 9-3   Injury Specialists

Physical Therapists: These therapists are licensed by the state to administer rehabilitative techniques—from massage to strength and flexibility exercises. Most states require you to obtain a doctor's referral before visiting a registered physical therapist.

Athletic Trainers: Many colleges, universities, and sports medicine clinics have athletic trainers who have extensive knowledge of and experience in dealing with injuries. They are highly trained and must pass rigorous written and practical examinations to become certified.

Sports Medicine Clinics: Because sports medicine is a rapidly growing field, many communities and medical centers have specialized sports medicine clinics. Many clinics have "walk-in" hours and are likely to include some of the specialists already mentioned as part of their staffs.

Orthopedists: These M.D.s with specialized surgical training treat injuries to any part of the musculoskeletal system. Many specialize in athletic injuries.

Podiatrists: These D.P.M.s (doctors of podiatric medicine) treat foot-related problems common to fitness-related injuries. Though not M.D.s, they receive special training and are state licensed. They can prescribe medications, design orthotics, and perform some surgeries.

Chiropractors: These D.C.s (doctors of chiropractic), believing that the alignment of the spine and proper nerve function are essential to body functioning, use manual manipulation and other physical therapy techniques to relieve pain and structural disorders.

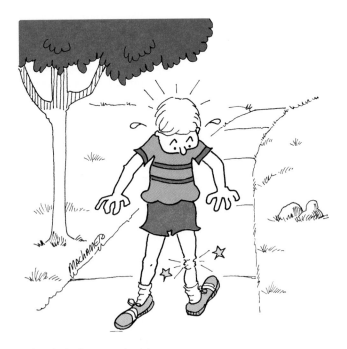

When in doubt, see a physician.

medical treatment. You should seek medical assistance for an injury if you experience any of the following symptoms:

1. The injury is extremely painful or the pain has not decreased in intensity over the course of several days.
2. You heard a distinct "pop" or a "snap" when the injury occurred.
3. You are unable to bear complete weight on the part, or there is a loss of strength and the ability to do normal tasks.
4. The body part is not in its natural anatomical position.

Once injured, whom should you see? Your family doctor will be able to treat common sprains and strains. However, there are other sports injury specialists who can help. Table 9-3 describes some of these specialists.

Communicating with a doctor is an important step in assuming an active role in your health care. Be sure to tell the physician everything that happened leading to the injury: what you felt, signs and symptoms, and any additional information to aid in diagnosing the injury. Do not feel rushed or intimidated by confusing terminology and tests. You are the consumer and are paying for the doctor's time and services. Do not rely on the nurse, receptionist, or friends to explain your injury and treatment. Make sure you completely understand everything you must do to speed your recovery.

Getting Back into Action

There are three steps to getting back into action after injury. First, move the injured part as early as possible, within a pain-free range, to regain flexibility. This motion will increase circulation and reduce stiffness and swelling. As you are able, work all the motions of a joint. For example, in an ankle injury, move the ankle up and down, in and out, 10 to 20 times, three to four times a day. Gradually increase the range of motion. If after moving the part, you feel pain, it should subside within 1 hour. Apply ice and reduce the amount of repetitions in the next session. You may be doing too much too soon.

Second, after obtaining full range of motion, begin to build strength. Gradually increase the strength of a part to equal that of the uninjured side. You can use partner resistance, free weights, rubber tubing, or weight machines. If possible, work under the supervision of a qualified physical therapist or other rehabilitation professional, especially in the early stages of rehabilitation, because this is when you are most susceptible to reinjury.

Third, gradually work your way back to your former activity level. Do not expect to start where you stopped. Frequently, exercisers will try to begin working out at their previous level after merely reducing swelling and pain. Healing

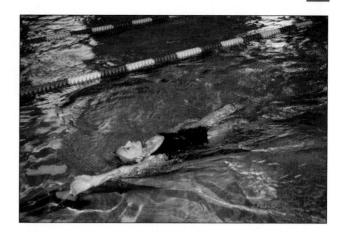

While recovering from an injury, switching to a nonimpact activity such as swimming can maintain your aerobic fitness.

may not yet be complete. The result is often reinjury because the weakened area is unable to withstand the stress. Overload should be gradual with the realization that *more* is not always *better*.

Care of the Lower Back

Without question, back pain is one of the most common conditions affecting Americans—second only to the common cold as a reason for seeing a physician. Eighty percent of Americans will experience back pain sometime in their lives. Back pain affects a largely youthful population, with the first back pain episodes afflicting people in their 20s and 30s. One of the main contributors to this epidemic of poor back health is our sedentary lifestyle. Fortunately, most back pain is preventable with exercise, good posture, and good lifting mechanics.

Ways to Avoid Lower Back Pain

Why does back pain occur? How can risk of back injury be reduced? We often take a healthy back for granted until something goes wrong. Back problems are rarely caused by a single, isolated factor. The 32-year-old computer programmer who hurts his back while pulling the lawnmower chain prefers to blame the lawnmower. His condition may actually be a result of several years of abuse and neglect. The pull on the lawnmower chain merely "triggered" the condition. During high school and college years, our bodies are relatively flexible. As we age, muscles begin to shorten and tighten, decreasing flexibility, especially in the back. Combine this with possible weight gain and declining overall fitness and it becomes evident why back pain afflicts millions. With few exceptions, back problems can be prevented with improved fitness, living and work habits, and posture.

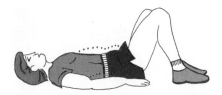

1. Pelvic tilt. Lie on back, knees bent. Press small of back firmly down to floor by tightening the abdominal muscles. Hold for a count of 5.

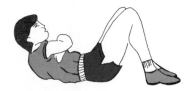

2. Pelvic tilt with curl. Do a pelvic tilt and, while holding this position, curl head and shoulders up until shoulder blades have been lifted from the floor. Hold briefly. Lower slowly.

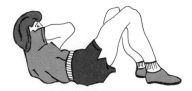

3. Pelvic tilt with twist. Do a pelvic tilt and, while holding this position, curl head and shoulders up, twisting right shoulder toward left knee. Hold briefly. Lower slowly. Repeat other side.

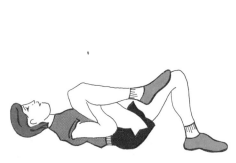

4. Low back stretch. (a) Lie on back. Pull one knee toward chest. Hold for a count of 5. Repeat other leg. (b) Double knee pull. Pull both knees to chest; hold for a count of 5.

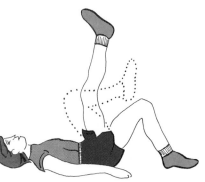

5. Lying hamstring stretch. Lie on back. Bring knee toward chest and extend leg toward ceiling. Flex foot. (You may grasp the back of your thigh with your hands.) Hold 20 seconds. Repeat with other leg.

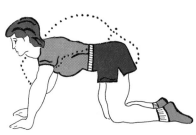

6. Cat stretch. Start on all fours. Round the back upward like a cat. Tighten abdominals Hold for 5 seconds. Relax and return to starting position. Do not let back sag.

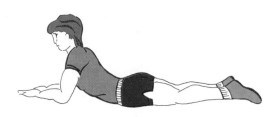

7. Upper back lift. Lie on your stomach with forearms flat on the ground. Tighten abdominals. Lift upper body using back muscles. Do not press with arms. Hold for a count of 5.

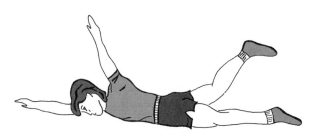

8. Alternate arm/leg lift. Lie on your stomach with arms extended in front. Raise one arm overhead toward ceiling while simultaneously lifting the opposite leg. Hold for a count of 5. Repeat with the other arm and leg.

figure 9-3   Exercises for the lower back.

The most important keys to preventing lower back pain are maintaining strong abdominal muscles and back flexibility. Studies show that people who are physically fit have almost 10 times less back pain. Many of those who suffer back pain are overweight and have weak, sagging abdominals and short, tight back muscles. This puts the back into an overarched position, placing additional stress on the spinal column. Maintaining normal weight and keeping abdominal muscles strong and tight reduces strain on the spine. Strong abdominals keep the pelvis and spinal column stabilized in a normal position. At the same time, it is important to keep the opposing back muscles and hamstrings flexible. People with chronic back problems need to stretch and strengthen regularly using the exercises in Figure 9-3. Exercise, not rest, is recommended for most people with back problems.

Sleeping position plays a role in back health. The one-third of your life you spend sleeping should help, not harm, your back. This makes it important to select a firm but not extremely hard mattress. Sleeping on a mattress that is too hard will leave the back unsupported. Sleeping on a sagging mattress places the back in an unbalanced position. Water beds, properly adjusted, may provide satisfactory back support as an alternative to a traditional mattress.

The fetal position is the best sleeping position for maintaining a healthy back. Lie on your side, pull your knees up to your chest and put a pillow between your knees. This will round the lower back and alleviate back stress. If you must sleep on your back, place a pillow or similar object under your knees to relax the lower back. Sleeping on your stomach increases the arch of the back, shortening the back muscles. Placing a small pillow, or even your arm, under your pelvic bone (abdomen) may help reduce strain on your back.

To decrease back stress when getting out of bed, roll to one side and sit up sideways, using your arms to help. This will eliminate using all of your back and abdominal muscles to get out of bed. This tip is especially helpful if you currently have a back problem.

Good lifting mechanics can reduce the risk of lower back injury. When lifting a heavy weight, bend your knees as if sitting down; keep your head up and looking straight ahead. Your trunk should be held as erect as possible to maintain a neutral spine, and use the large muscles of the buttocks and legs to lift. It is also important not to let the knees pass the toes as you squat in order to avoid excessive knee stress. Combining lifting with a twisting force is one of the most common causes of back injury. Instead, lift the object and pivot with your feet rather than your waist.

Keep your body close to the object. Standing far away from the object will place undue stress on the lower back. Lift with your back straight rather than bent at the waist. When carrying heavy objects such as books, backpacks, and groceries, try to distribute the load equally and close to the body. Do not carry a back pack on one shoulder, as this puts uneven stress on back muscles and is a common cause of back pain.

Finally, obtain help when lifting heavy objects. See the Top 10 list for ways to improve back health.

Workplace Considerations

Many Americans will spend the majority of their work time behind desks or in cars. Sedentary jobs and lifestyle make us vulnerable to back pain. How can you maintain a healthy back if your job entails a lot of sitting? Sit close to your work and keep your hips and knees at a 90-degree angle. This will straighten the lower back and prevent slouching. When you sit in a chair, place both feet on the floor. If the chair is too low, it will increase your back curvature excessively. Use a chair that supports your back in its normal slightly arched position. You can place a small pillow or towel against your lower back to maintain that position. Wearing high-heeled shoes is unhealthy for the lower back. This shortens the Achilles tendon and hamstrings, throws the back into an overarched position, and at the same time overstretches the abdominals. Wear low-heeled shoes to maintain back health.

Maintain good posture while driving, especially when driving long distances. Sitting for extended periods in an automobile is a frequent cause of back pain. To maintain normal spinal curvature, place a small pillow between your lower back and the seat. Sit close enough to reach the accelerator and steering wheel without slumping.

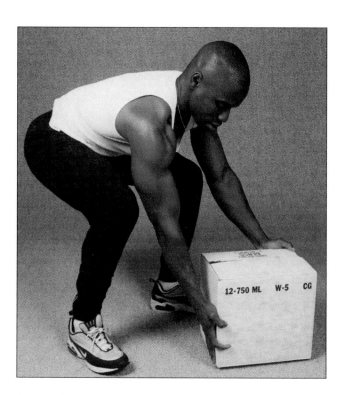

Correct lifting technique.

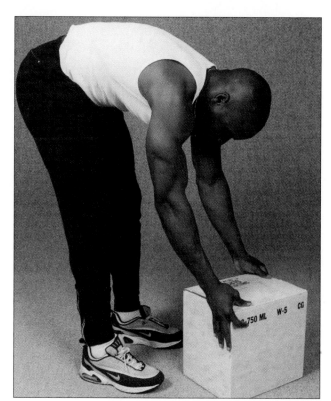

Incorrect lifting technique.

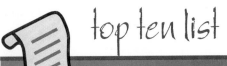

Top Ten Ways to Improve Back Health

1. **Stretch and strengthen.** Weak, tight muscles invite injury. Strengthen the abdominals with abdominal curls and do back stretching/strengthening exercises to maintain a strong, flexible spine (see Figure 9-3).

2. **Use good sitting posture.** Sitting for hours hunched in front of a computer screen can overstress back muscles. Sit erect, knees level with hips, feet flat on the floor. Add a towel roll behind your back to maintain your natural spinal curve.

3. **Use good standing posture.** To decrease back stress, stand with one foot elevated a few inches on a box to relax the back.

4. **Change positions frequently.** When sitting, take frequent breaks—1 to 2 minutes every 30–60 minutes. Stand up, stretch, move around. When standing, vary your body position and shift weight frequently.

5. **Use good sleeping posture.** Sleep on your side with knees bent and a pillow between your knees to relax your back. If you prefer sleeping on your back, put a pillow under your knees to reduce back stress. Avoid sleeping on your stomach.

6. **Use good lifting techniques.** Stand close to the object, bend your knees as if sitting down, keeping the back straight and head up. Tighten your abdominals and lift with your legs, keeping the object close to your body. Avoid bending from the waist and twisting as you lift.

7. **Don't overdo it.** Know your limits. Weekend bouts of yard work, in other words, 2 to 3 hours of gardening and raking the lawn on Saturday or playing 2 hours of basketball when you've been sitting behind a desk all week, overstress the back. Spread out the work and play in shorter bouts over a few days to give your muscles a chance to adjust.

8. **Keep active.** Maintaining a base of fitness throughout the week enables you to go canoeing, play ball, or do that yard work on the weekend with less risk of a stiff, sore back as compared to a couch potato.

9. **Manage your weight.** Carrying extra pounds in front increases the load your back must support. Losing weight decreases back stress 24 hours a day.

10. **Distribute the load.** Habitually carrying a heavy bag, books, or backpack on one side creates uneven spinal stresses. Evenly distribute the load or switch sides to even out the stresses.

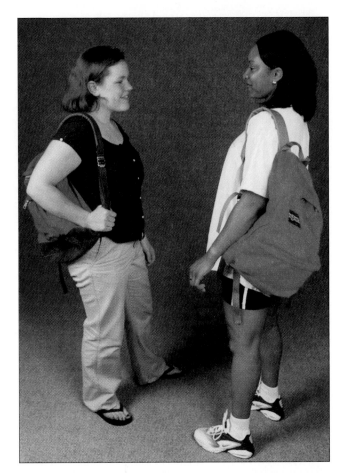

Habitually carrying a heavy backpack on one shoulder may cause back pain.

If your job requires long periods of standing, you can minimize stress on the back by putting one foot on a low stool. Frequently shift your weight from one leg to another. Some occupations put unusual physical stress on the back. Dentists, nurses, and musicians may sit, lift, or move in twisted, awkward positions.

If you must sit, stand, or work in one position for an extended time, get up, stretch, and walk for several minutes. You will feel better, and your back will benefit from the change.

Not to be overlooked is the effect of emotional stress on back health. Stress produces tension, which increases sensitivity to pain, which creates more stress. The stress → tension → pain cycle can exacerbate the symptoms of any injury. Stress reduction and relaxation techniques can play an important role in the treatment of low back problems and other injuries.

Lower Back Injuries

The lower back is made up of many tiny ligaments that hold the vertebrae together from the skull to the tailbone. A sudden twisting force can injure these ligaments. There are also several groups of muscles, called the *erector spinae muscle group*, that parallel the spinal column. These muscles may be injured by lifting a heavy weight, excessively bending and twisting, or sleeping on a sagging mattress.

If your back aches, press the sore area with your fingers. If this does not cause pain, the injury is probably deeper. For sore, achy back muscles, lie on a bag of crushed ice or a cold pack 20 minutes, or alternate 20 minutes of ice with 20 minutes of heat. If you suffer back pain, what symptoms indicate that you should see a physician? If the pain is severe, doesn't decrease with a few days of home treatment, radiates from the back into the buttocks or legs, or is accompanied by numbness or tingling, it may indicate an **intervertebral disc** injury. The intervertebral disc is a cushion that separates the bony vertebrae. Discs are filled with fluid and are flexible through early adulthood but thin and lose their resiliency as we age. A ruptured intervertebral disc may compress nerves, causing pain down the buttocks and legs. Consult a physician who specializes in back pain for these injuries.

Exercises for the Lower Back

Research has shown that 80 percent of patients with back discomfort who visit physicians have no underlying organic disease. Most of these patients are deficient in strength and flexibility of key postural muscles. There are several exercises you can do to maintain a healthy back. We recommend the exercise routine in Figure 9-3. These exercises focus on strengthening the abdominals *and* stretching and strengthening the back. Practice this series daily for best results. The exercises can easily be included as part of your exercise warm-up or cool-down routine. These exercises should not cause any pain, numbness, or tingling in the back and legs. If they do, discontinue them and consult your specialist.

 frequently asked questions

Q. Every time I start a running program, I get shin splints. What can I do to keep this from happening next time?

A. First, check your shoes. Are they less than 6 months (500 miles) old, and are they good running shoes? Well-cushioned shoes designed for the stresses of running are your first line of defense against impact injuries. If your shoes are OK, the problem may be overuse—doing too much too soon. Many beginners, in their zeal to get in shape, try to run a mile their first workout and increase from there. Start with several weeks of walking. Once you can walk two to three miles without discomfort, alternate jogging and walking. Review the progression in Chapter 3 and do not try to progress faster. Try the shin-strengthening exercise in Chapter 5 and stretch calves. Consider alternating days of running with cycling or another nonimpact activity, and do not try to run through the shin splints. If your shins start to ache, switch to a nonimpact activity until they heal. When you start back after a layoff, decrease your workout by 25 to 50 percent, do more walking, and build back slowly.

Q. Which is better for an injury—heat or ice?

A. Ice is the treatment of choice for any acute injury. It decreases pain, limits swelling, and penetrates deep tissues better than heat. Heat applied too early can increase swelling. Once swelling has subsided, heat can be relaxing and can decrease stiffness.

Q. I've been working out for four months and am not doing anything different. Why are my knees starting to bother me?

A. Are you wearing the same shoes you started with? If so, it is time to replace them as the soles compress over time leaving you with less cushioning. Check your workout—are you running on hard surfaces, constantly going the same direction on a track or crowned roads or repeatedly stepping up on curbs with the same leg? Finally, outside of workouts, have you added any new activity such as weekend yard work, or carrying unaccustomed loads? Switch to a nonimpact activity for a few days to give your knees a chance to recover, then modify your workouts to reduce excessive impact or repetitive stresses on your knees.

Q. My joints pop and crack a lot when I move. Is there something wrong with them?

A. Joints can be noisy for a lot of reasons, mostly benign. If there is pain or swelling along with the popping, see your physician. If your joints feel fine, a little noise is common and harmless.

Q. I've read that wearing magnets can relieve back pain. Do they work?

A. Every year a new fad comes along promising results that don't pan out. The body has natural healing ability so if you buy a product and get relief, it is easy to attribute it to that product, when you would have gotten better without it. A randomized, double-blind crossover study of chronic back pain patients found no difference in pain relief between those using real and sham magnets. Don't waste your money.

Q. Does exercise cause arthritis?

A. No. Exercise increases joint lubrication, helps joint range-of-motion, and strengthens muscles that support your joints. Gentle range-of-motion and low-impact aerobic exercises are recommended as a way to decrease the stiffness and pain of arthritis, either rheumatoid or osteoarthritis. Osteoarthritis from joint wear and tear is common in those over 40, may have a hereditary component, and can be brought on by joint injury. So, if arthritis runs in your family or if you have had joint injuries, it is even more important to keep your joints strong and flexible with regular exercise such as walking, swimming, and stretching.

summary

Much soreness and injury can be prevented. Stretching, strengthening, proper warm-up, sensible progressions, and avoiding overuse are the keys. It is better to block injuries at their source than to pay doctors' fees to treat breakdowns. The pursuit of excellence involves learning to balance your strengths and weaknesses and cooperating with your body instead of assaulting it.

You can prevent lower back problems with proper care and treatment. Maintain leg and back flexibility, strengthen abdominals, use correct lifting mechanics, and reduce sources of lower back stress. This is all within your control.

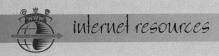 ## internet resources

American College of Sportsmedicine
http://www.acsm.org/sportsmed

The Physician and Sportsmedicine
http://www.physsportsmed.com

lab activity
9–1

Phil A. Case Study

Phil is 20 years old and is a student at State College. He has kept himself in good shape and has been running road races for the past 4 years. This morning, while running on White River Road, he stepped into a chuck hole and sprained his ankle. He was able to limp home. You are one of his best friends, and he has come to you for advice. He asks, "Should I go to a doctor?"

1. List four questions you would ask Phil to determine whether you should recommend a doctor:
   a.

   b.

   c.

   d.

2. Phil answers "No" to your questions. He asks, "What do you think I should do to keep it from swelling?" List and describe five treatments you would prescribe for Phil's injury:

   a.

   b.

   c.

   d.

   e.

3. Phil wants to keep in shape and plans to start running again as soon as possible. He asks, "Do you think I should try to run tomorrow?" List three steps in the progression of getting back into action. Also, tell him how he might keep in shape while his injury heals:

   a.

   b.

   c.

   d.

lab activity

9-2

Action Plan
for the Back

Back Exercises

Complete the series of back exercises that are described in Figure 9-3 in Chapter 9.

1. Describe how your lower back area felt at the completion of the exercise session.

2. Explain how you will fit this exercise regimen into your daily schedule.

Back Care

Explain how you will perform the following tasks using proper body mechanics/alignment:

1. Lifting a garage door to open it:

2. Lifting a heavy box to put in the back of a station wagon:

3. Sitting several hours at a desk studying:

4. Driving a car for 5 hours:

5. Standing/working at a checkout counter for 5 hours:

6. Sleeping:

Name _____

Class/Activity Section _____

Date _____

lab activity 9-3

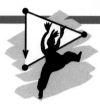

Using HealthQuest

1. Insert HealthQuest CD into your computer.
   In the "Fitness" module, select "Topics", "Specifics on. . . and Exercise-Related Injuries." Read the article for information on how to avoid injury, the most common injuries, and how to care for injuries.

   a. What are three suggestions this article makes for preventing injury?

   b. What are three suggestions this article makes for self-treatment?

   c. Under what circumstances does this article advise you see a doctor?

Eating for Wellness

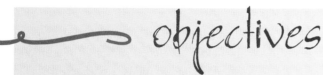

After reading this chapter, you will be able to:

1. Identify the percentages of calories recommended in the diet for carbohydrates, proteins, and fats.
2. List the 10 dietary guidelines for Americans.
3. List the six major nutrients and describe their main function in the body.
4. Identify the health benefits of fiber, and list good food sources of fiber.
5. Differentiate between complex and simple carbohydrates.
6. Identify the correct descriptions of cholesterol, saturated, monounsaturated, and polyunsaturated fats, and state the recommended daily limits of each.
7. Calculate fat gram allowances for specific daily calorie intakes.
8. Describe the role phytochemicals and antioxidants play in nutritional health, and identify foods high in these compounds.
9. Identify four preventive factors relating to osteoporosis.
10. Identify the recommended number of daily servings from the food groups in the Food Guide Pyramid.
11. Give 10 specific examples of small changes that can be incorporated into daily food selections and preparations that could make a significant change in your nutritional wellness.
12. Look at a food label and identify the largest ingredient; calculate the percentage of calories that come from fat, carbohydrate, and protein; identify the sources of fat (including saturated fat); and identify the sources of complex and simple carbohydrates.
13. Identify three ways to eat nutritiously in a fast-food restaurant.

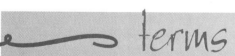

- Antioxidants
- Carbohydrates
- Cholesterol
- Complex carbohydrates
- Fat
- Fat soluble vitamins
- Fiber
- Free radicals
- Glycogen
- Hydrogenation
- Insoluble fiber

- Ketone bodies
- Lactovegetarian
- Macrominerals
- Minerals
- Monounsaturated fat
- Omega-3
- Osteoporosis
- Ovo-lactovegetarian
- Phytochemicals
- Phytoestrogens
- Polyunsaturated fat

- Protein
- Saturated fat
- Semivegetarian
- Simple carbohydrates
- Soluble fiber
- Strict vegetarian (or vegan)
- Trace minerals
- Trans-fatty acids (transfats)
- Triglycerides
- Vitamins
- Water soluble vitamins

I n a world where so many things seem out of our hands, taking control of what you eat is an important personal way that you can impact how you feel. Fundamental knowledge about nutrition can make a tremendous contribution to your level of wellness. It can help you make food choices that will enhance your health and vitality. This knowledge can also help you to decipher the social influences and messages related to eating. This is another step toward assuming self-responsibility for your well-being and health. Learning about nutrition can be exciting. Eating is a daily activity, so you have many opportunities to affect your wellness in a positive way. Food not only sustains life, but has a clear link to *disease prevention.* Scientists are finding that certain foods (especially fruits, vegetables, and grains) are directly associated with the prevention of cardiovascular disease and certain cancers—the leading causes of death in our country. We are fortunate to live in a country where food is plentiful; we have wide and varied choices. We must learn, however, to make healthy choices!

We tend to see diet as affecting only the physical dimension of wellness. Food, however, can be associated with all of the dimensions. Much of our social life revolves

around food. Providing food is an important sign of caring. Eating and being fed are intimately connected with our deepest feelings. Table 10-1 gives examples of how food relates to all seven dimensions of wellness. Perhaps you can think of other connections.

After reading this chapter, you should be able to make responsible food choices in your pursuit of high-level wellness. You have heard it before, but it is remarkably true: You are what you eat.

Changing Times

In the agricultural lifestyle of the past, most people grew and prepared their food. Foods were fresh and simple. Early Americans consumed much greater amounts of fresh fruits, vegetables, and grains and lesser amounts of salt, fats, and refined sugars than Americans do today. In those days, eating out meant eating outdoors—perhaps a picnic or a meal out in the field beside the plow. Today's fast-paced, technological society has contributed to drastic changes in the way we eat. Dual-career and single-parent families are commonplace. As parents juggle careers, child care, social and professional meetings, education, and recreation, meals are often skipped, eaten on the run, or thrown together quickly. More than ever, meals are consumed behind the wheel of a car in what food industry experts call "dashboard dining". Forty percent of the American food budget is spent on food away from home. As a result, the food preparers are often McDonald's or manufacturers of frozen, processed, or snack foods. Food preparation and advertising are big business, so the purpose of mass advertising is to sell products, not necessarily to enhance our nutrition. Supermarket shelves are lined with packaged food products bearing little resemblance to the original farm product. Most are highly processed, often stripped of key nutrients. The result is a new form of malnutrition. Rather than a lack of food, we find ourselves eating too much of the wrong foods. As we have progressed from eating wheat and berries to consuming hot dogs, french fries, and Twinkies, the incidence of heart disease, obesity, Type 2 diabetes, and cancer has increased. This progression has also cost us our vitality and has seriously compromised our immune systems.

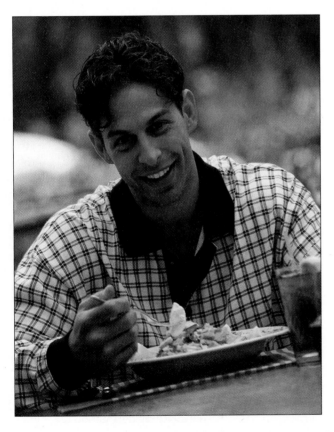

Eating is one of life's pleasures, and the choices we make have a strong impact on our present and future health.

table 10-1	Food Is Associated with Every Dimension of Wellness
Dimension	**How Food is Associated**
Physical	Food is required for physiological nourishment, genetic growth, and survival.
Emotional	Food is often used as a reward, to soothe feelings, and to ease depression or stress.
Social	Food is often at the heart of social events, celebrations, and family interactions.
Intellectual	Having a healthy relationship with food requires informed consumerism, knowledge about the science of nutrition and sound dietary principles, and the ability to read food labels.
Spiritual	Food is used in rituals and is part of spiritual cleansing. Abstention from eating or eating particular foods often accompanies spiritual growth experiences. Food is used in many death rituals throughout the world.
Environmental	The human need for food demands food and crop quality and protection from contamination, protection of the food chain, and strategies for combating world hunger.
Occupational	Food is often a part of business meetings and social gatherings and breaks at work. Also, the income generated by our occupations determines our food choices. Institutional food preparation is big business.

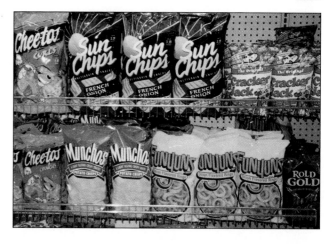

Many of our popular snacks are heavily processed, loaded with fat and sodium, and stripped of key nutrients.

Poor diet is said to contribute to five of the top 10 leading causes of death in our country. Studies repeatedly identify six shortfalls in our eating habits:

1. Too few fruits and vegetables.
2. Too little fiber.
3. Too much fat.
4. Too many refined sugars.
5. Too much food overall.
6. Inadequate water intake.

How many of these habits relate to you?

A survey of American dietary habits revealed some startling facts regarding nutrition knowledge and behavior in our country. Although Americans' concerns about nutrition have increased, only 37 percent rated themselves as "highly careful" about selecting healthy foods. Whereas public awareness of the importance of nutrition continues to grow, action to improve the diet has stalled. A majority of the respondents in the survey felt that changing their dietary habits would mean giving up favorite foods and take too much time. The survey also revealed that most Americans have limited knowledge about dietary guidelines. Only 9 percent of those surveyed could correctly identify the guide-

line for the percentage of fat in our diet, even though 50 percent of the respondents expressed *concern* about fat in their diet! The percentage who knew about sodium and cholesterol was even lower. Despite the low levels of knowledge, 27 percent of those surveyed rated themselves as "very knowledgeable" about dietary guidelines.

Maintaining healthy dietary habits is crucial to lifelong wellness. In college, you are faced with the perhaps new responsibility of buying and preparing your meals or making daily cafeteria selections. Studies indicate that students are especially unaware of or apathetic about the implications of poor dietary habits on the future development of chronic diseases. Television contributes to the problem by presenting mixed messages about diet and nutrition. We are exposed to hundreds of commercials for sugary, high-fat snacks, often featuring enchanting music, jingles, and appealing characters. In prime-time programming, nutrition is anything but balanced—grabbing a snack is the norm. Yet the models used in commercials are extremely thin, attractive, and seemingly healthy.

Healthful eating *can* be enjoyable and is easier to sustain than most people think. The underlying approach for dietary choices should be to combine basic nutrition *knowledge* with positive and practical *action*. Small, gradual changes can collectively produce substantial and sustainable dietary improvements.

The Government Takes Action

As a service to the American people, the U.S. Department of Health and Human Services publishes the *Dietary Guidelines for Americans*. Revised periodically, these guidelines (Table 10-2) help answer the question, "What should we eat to stay healthy and prevent chronic diseases?" The 10 guidelines reflect the newest research on diet and health relationships, with the purpose of giving *practical* suggestions on how to make healthy diet adjustments. It is

table 10-2   The 2000 Dietary Guidelines for Americans*

1. **Aim for a healthy weight.**
   Being overweight or obese increases your risk for many chronic diseases, including cancer. Therefore, choose a lifestyle that combines sensible eating with regular physical activity.

2. **Be physically active each day.**
   Aim to accumulate at least 30 minutes (adults) or 60 minutes (children) of moderate physical activity most days of the week, preferably daily. A moderate physical activity is an activity that requires about as much energy as walking 2 miles in 30 minutes. If you already get 30 minutes of physical activity daily, you can gain even more health benefits by increasing the amount of time that you are physically active or by taking part in more vigorous activities.

3. **Let the pyramid guide your food choices.**
   No single food can supply all the nutrients in the amounts you need. Choose the recommended number of servings from each of the five major food groups in the Food Guide Pyramid. Also select a variety of foods within each group.

4. **Choose a variety of grains daily, especially whole grains.**
   Foods made from whole grains (like wheat, rice, and oats) provide vitamins, minerals, carbohydrates, and fiber necessary for optimal health. The protective substances in whole grains help protect against heart disease and cancer.

5. **Choose a variety of fruits and vegetables daily.**
   Fruits and vegetables are our most concentrated source of vitamins, minerals, and other disease-fighting compounds. The antioxidant nutrients in plant foods have been shown to be protectors from heart disease, cancer, and other chronic diseases. Most fruits and vegetables are also naturally low in fat and calories and high in fiber.

6. **Keep food safe to eat.**
   Safe means that the food poses little risk of foodborne illness. This means storing perishable foods safely; washing hands and foods carefully; and avoiding raw or undercooked meats, poultry, and fish.

7. **Choose a diet that is low in saturated fat and cholesterol and moderate in total fat.**
   Diets high in fat and cholesterol have been linked to heart disease, certain types of cancer, and obesity. Thirty percent or less of calories should come from fat, with less than 10 percent of calories from saturated fat. Dietary cholesterol intake should be less than 300 mg per day. Foods high in trans-fatty acids should also be avoided.

8. **Choose beverages and foods to moderate your intake of sugars.**
   Sugars are added to many processed foods, including many of today's popular low-fat and nonfat foods. Foods containing a lot of sugar provide calories but are often limited in nutrients. They also contribute to tooth decay.

9. **Choose and prepare foods with less salt.**
   Most Americans eat more salt (sodium chloride) than they need. Many people can reduce their chances of developing high blood pressure by consuming less salt. Most of the salt we eat comes from foods that have salt added during food processing or during preparation in a restaurant or at home.

10. **If you drink alcoholic beverages, do so in moderation.**
    Alcoholic beverages supply calories but few or no nutrients. Alcoholic beverages are harmful when consumed in excess. The effects include altered judgment, potential dependency, and many other serious health problems.

*Recommendations for healthy Americans age 2 and over

Source: U.S. Department of Agriculture, U.S. Department of Health and Human Services. "Nutrition and Your Health: Dietary Guidelines for Americans," 5th ed. *Home and Garden Bulletin* no. 232 (2000).

impossible to specify the perfect diet for every individual. However, these guidelines point out positive directions for everyday food selections that can help you maintain optimal health.

In regard to these guidelines, nutritionists concur that the main challenge no longer is simply to determine what eating patterns to recommend. Only issuing and disseminating recommendations is insufficient to produce change in most people's eating behavior. As in making most lifestyle changes, you need:

- *Knowledge* (to identify problem diet behaviors and how to improve them)
- *Motivation* (to make healthy changes)
- A *supportive environment* (to maintain changes in restaurants, supermarkets, worksite and school food services, nutrition labeling, and nutrition education in the schools)

How do you cut salt from your diet? What is a complex carbohydrate? How do you know if your daily diet is under

30 percent fat? What is cholesterol? How do you eat out healthfully? These questions are addressed in the following sections, and we will give practical suggestions as to how to make daily food choices that will enhance your nutritional wellness.

Nutrition Basics

Your body is a priceless machine that needs fuel. This fuel should be composed of six major nutrients: carbohydrates, proteins, fats, vitamins, minerals, and water. These nutrients fulfill three main functions in the body:

1. Provide energy
2. Build and repair body tissues
3. Regulate body processes

Only the carbohydrates, fats, and proteins contribute energy or calories (kcal) to your diet. To function at optimal efficiency, you need a balance of each of the six essential nutrient groups.

Carbohydrates

Carbohydrates are the major source of energy for the body. They are the body's preferred form of energy. They provide 4 calories per gram. Carbohydrates are stored in the liver and in muscles in the form of **glycogen.** Most dietitians recommend that our daily caloric intake be 55 to 60 percent carbohydrate. Carbohydrates have mistakenly earned the reputation of being fattening. If we analyze the two types of carbohydrates, this unearned reputation can be understood. Carbohydrates, with the exception of milk sugar, come from plants. The two types are **simple carbohydrates** (sugars) and **complex carbohydrates** (starches).

Simple Carbohydrates (Sugars)

When you see the suffix *-ose* as an ingredient on a package label (as in sucrose, fructose, dextrose, maltose) or see *corn sweetener, corn syrup, molasses, sorbitol,* or *honey,* think *sugar.* The presence of these refined and processed sugars in our diet accounts for carbohydrates' "fattening" reputation. Instead of consuming the natural simple sugars found in fruits and vegetables, we consume too much of these hidden processed sugars.

The major sources of added sugars in Americans' diets are:

1. soft drinks
2. cakes, cookies, pies
3. fruit ades and drinks such as fruit punch and lemonade
4. dairy desserts such as ice cream
5. candy

These refined sugars have been extracted from their natural sources and have little nutritional value other than the calories they contain—hence the name "empty calories." Americans consumed an average of 154 pounds of sugar per person in 1999, up 25 pounds from 1986. Excess sugar throws the entire body chemistry off balance, causes fatigue, and dramatically weakens the immune system for up to 6 hours after ingestion. Even if you profess not to eat sweets, you probably consume more sugar than you realize because it is hidden in so many processed foods such as chocolate milk, ketchup, barbecue sauce, cereals, and juice drinks. For example, one average 12-ounce cola drink contains 9 teaspoons of sugar. Eight ounces of low-fat fruit yogurt contain 7 teaspoons of sugar. Jell-O is 83 percent sugar. Check your breakfast cereal. Some are nothing more than "candy" fortified with vitamins. Look for cereals with no more than 5 or 6 grams of added sugar per serving.

Complex Carbohydrates (Starches)

The starches are potatoes, rice, whole grains, beans, fruits, and vegetables. These foods are low in calories. They are nutritionally dense, a rich source of vitamins and minerals that provide a steady amount of energy for many hours. What *is* fattening are the calorie-rich additives we often add to these foods (butter, sour cream, jams, gravies, sauces). Complex carbohydrates should comprise 45 to 50 percent of our total caloric intake, while simple sugars should be limited to only 10 percent. Carbohydrates supply many vital nutrients such as vitamins, minerals, and water. In addition, they supply an important nonnutrient: dietary fiber. **Fiber** is the part of plant food that is not digested in the small intestine, where most other foods are digested and absorbed into the bloodstream.

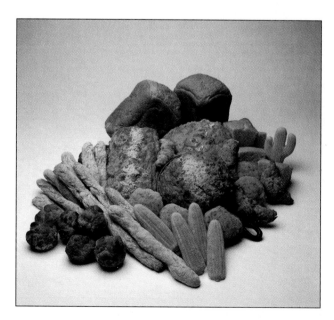

Whole-grain products are better for your health than refined flours.

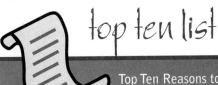

Top Ten Reasons to Eat More Fiber

1. It curbs overeating. Because fiber-filled foods take up more room in your stomach than other foods, you feel full faster.
2. It decreases your hunger. Fiber is slower to digest, so it keeps hunger at bay longer.
3. It whisks away calories. Because most fiber leaves the body undigested, the calories in fiber-rich foods are less accessible to the body. For each gram of fiber you consume, you absorb about seven fewer calories from food.
4. It lowers the "bad" cholesterol. Soluble fiber lowers harmful LDL cholesterol, possibly reducing heart disease risk.
5. It cuts the fat. Fiber-rich foods are naturally low in fat.
6. It may reduce diabetes risk. Eating fiber while reducing sugar in the diet has been linked to reduced risk of diabetes.
7. It keeps you regular. Fiber is called your body's "broom" because the insoluble fiber binds with water to usher waste out of the body.
8. Its sources are nutrient-dense. Fruits, vegetables, and fortified high-fiber breads and cereals are filled with tons of vitamins, minerals, and antioxidants.
9. It may protect against breast cancer. Fiber binds to estrogen—an important breast-cancer risk factor—reducing blood levels of this hormone.
10. It may protect against colon cancer. Fiber binds with and removes carcinogens from the body.

wellness flash

How much is 30 grams of fiber?

If you were to eat 1 cup of bran cereal, 1/2 cup of carrots, 1/2 cup of beans, a medium-sized apple, and a medium-sized pear in one day, you would get 30 grams of fiber.

To many people, *fiber* is synonymous with *oat bran*. Fiber is not a single substance but a large group of widely different compounds with varied effects on the body. Formerly called *roughage* or *bulk,* fiber was once thought of primarily as a filler—it takes up room, leaving less space for high-fat, high-calorie items. That is still one of fiber's potential benefits, and it is in foods rich in vitamins and minerals. But researchers recognize that fiber plays a role in reducing the risk of heart disease, cancer, and diabetes. Look at the Top Ten reasons we should eat more fiber. As you can see, a high-fiber diet contributes to health in a multitude of ways. There are two types of fiber: insoluble and soluble. Both play important roles in your nutritional health.

Insoluble fiber is from the cell walls of plants and is not digested by the body. Insoluble fiber absorbs water as it passes through the digestive tract, increasing fecal bulk. It quickens the passage of food through the system, helping to prevent constipation. This type of fiber acts as a deterrent to digestive disorders, including cancer of the colon and rectum, because it decreases the time in which your system is exposed to toxic substances in waste materials. Whole wheat bran is the richest source of insoluble fiber. This valuable bran is lost when whole wheat flour is refined to produce

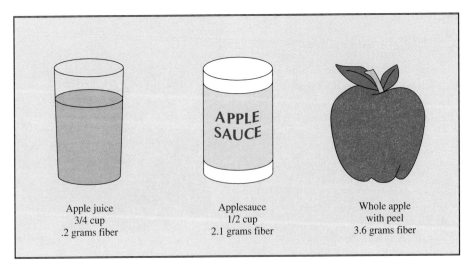

A fiber profile.

table 10-3 Dietary Fiber in Foods

Almost all fruits, vegetables, and whole-grain products contain some of both types of fiber. Realize, however, that "wheat flour" and "enriched flour" are *not* whole grains. Most pizza crusts, breads, crackers, pastas, and pancakes are made of enriched or refined flours, low in fiber because in the processing, the valuable bran has been removed. Try to get your fiber from a variety of the following sources.

Good Sources of Insoluble Fiber More Than 5 Grams Total Fiber	Good Sources of Soluble Fiber More Than 5 Grams Total Fiber
• High-fiber wheat bran cereal (1 oz) • Lentils (dried, cooked, 1/2 cup)	• Pinto, kidney, navy beans (dried, cooked, 1/2 cup)
3 to 5 Grams Total Fiber	**3 to 5 Grams Total Fiber**
• Whole-wheat crackers (6) • Potato (medium, with skin) • Popped corn (4 cups) • Shredded-wheat cereal (1 oz) • Brown rice (cooked, 1/2 cup) • Brussels sprouts, broccoli, spinach (cooked, 1/2 cup) • Wheat germ (3 Tbsp) • Whole-wheat flour (1 oz)	• Oat bran, oatmeal (dry, 1 oz) • Barley (dry, 1 oz) • Berries (1/2 cup) • Apple, pear (medium, with skin) • Orange, grapefruit (medium) • Raisins (1/2 cup) • Okra, cabbage, peas, turnips, sweet potato (cooked, 1/2 cup) • Chickpeas, split peas, lima beans (cooked, 1/2 cup) • Carrots (cooked, 1/2 cup)
1 to 2 Grams Total Fiber	**1 to 2 Grams Total Fiber**
• Whole-wheat bread (1 slice) • Pasta (cooked, 1 cup) • Rye bread (1 slice) • Corn (1/2 cup) • Low-fiber wheat cereal (1 oz) • Banana (medium)	• Cauliflower (cooked, 1/2 cup) • Peach, nectarine (medium) • Apricots (2) • Pineapple (1/2 cup)

white flour (used in most breads, crackers, and cereals). Lentils, skins of fruits and root vegetables, and leafy greens are other good sources of insoluble fiber.

Soluble fiber travels through the digestive tract in a gel-like form, pacing the absorption of carbohydrates. This prevents dramatic shifts in blood sugar levels and can help control diabetes. A diet rich in soluble fiber has also been shown to reduce blood cholesterol levels, especially LDL, thus reducing the risk of cardiovascular diseases. However, this effect primarily occurs when coupled with a diet low in saturated fats. Oat bran, beans, vegetables, and fruits are rich sources of soluble fiber, though most plant foods contain both types of fiber. Animal foods never contain fiber.

According to the National Cancer Institute (NCI), one-third of cancer deaths may be related to what we eat. Eating between 25 and 35 grams of fiber daily is recommended (about double the amount of the current American diet). Not enough is known about how each kind of fiber (soluble and insoluble) works, so the NCI does not recommend any set dietary ratio for either type. Table 10-3 shows the fiber content of some common foods.

For busy students and adults, breakfast is one of the best meals to get a jump start on fiber consumption for the day. Look at Table 10-4 for comparisons of various popular breakfast foods. As you can see, careful selection of a breakfast cereal plus adding some fresh fruit gives you a great start toward those 25 to 35 grams.

Proteins

Hundreds of different kinds of proteins make up the cells of your body. **Protein** is the major substance used to build and repair tissue, maintain chemical balance, and regulate the formation of hormones, antibodies, and enzymes. Protein can also be used as a source of energy, but only if there are not enough carbohydrates or fats available. It is not an efficient source of energy, however. When protein is broken down, the nitrogen part of the protein molecule is left. The kidneys are overworked trying to excrete this excess nitrogen. Also, if your body must rely on protein for energy, the protein is not available for building and repairing tissue—its real function.

Each gram of protein provides 4 calories of energy. We need protein daily, and most of us consume more than enough. The recommended dietary allowance of protein for adults is 45 to 65 grams a day, depending on body weight.

table 10-4   Fiber in Breakfast Foods

There is a wide variance in fiber content in breakfast selections. The amount that constitutes one serving is in parentheses. HINTS: An addition of fruit can add 2 to 5 more grams of fiber; sprinkle on 2 tablespoons of wheat germ for an additional 2 grams.

Kellogg's All-Bran (1/2 c) = 10 grams	Raisin Bran (1 c) = 8 grams
Multi-Bran Chex (1 c) = 7 grams	Shredded Wheat (1 c) = 6 grams
Frosted Mini-Wheats (24 bite size) = 6 grams	Grape-Nuts (1/2 c) = 5 grams
Bran Flakes (3/4 c) = 5 grams	Wheat Chex (1 c) = 5 grams
Total (3/4 c) = 3 grams	Whole wheat toast (1 slice) = 3 grams
Wheaties (1 c) = 3 grams	Instant oatmeal (1 packet) = 3 grams
Honey Nut Cheerios (1 c) = 2 grams	Blueberry bagel (1) = 2 grams

The following foods have only 1 gram of fiber:

Froot Loops (1 c)	Pop Tart (1)	Special K (1 c)
Frosted Flakes (3/4 c)	Wheat toast (1 slice)	English muffin (1)
Cap'n Crunch (3/4 c)	Nutri-Grain bar (1)	Granola bar (1)
Lucky Charms (1 c)	Eggo waffle (1)	Banana nut muffin (1)
Egg McMuffin (1)	Biscuit sandwich (1)	Croissant sandwich (1)

The following foods have 0 grams of fiber:

Cocoa Pebbles (3/4 c)	Corn Pops (1 c)	Donut (1)
Eggs (any amount)	Corn Chex (1 c)	Rice Krispies (1¼ c)
White bread toast (1 slice)	Danish (1)	Yogurt (8 oz)

This is only 180 to 260 calories. Protein needs vary throughout the life cycle, due to different growth stages. Growing children need more protein per body weight than adults. Pregnant or lactating women, and people over age 55, may need a little extra protein. Persons age 19 and older can approximate their daily protein need in grams by multiplying their weight (in pounds) by 0.36.

Example: 130 lb. person × 0.36 = 46.8 or 47 grams of protein daily
To give you an idea of how little food this is,
47 grams of protein would be:
4 oz. of meat (a piece roughly the size of your palm)
2 cups skim milk

Example: 180 lb. person × 0.36 = 64.8 or 65 grams of protein daily
Sixty-five grams of protein could be fulfilled with:
1 cup oatmeal
1½ cups macaroni and cheese
1½ cups skim milk
1 large bowl of chili with beans

Most Americans consume too much protein. (Average consumption is about 100 grams per day.)

Good sources of protein are found in animal and plant foods. Meat, poultry, fish, eggs, and milk products are good sources of animal protein. Many of these sources also contain high amounts of fat and cholesterol, so you are wise to select some plant sources of protein: legumes (beans and peas), whole grains, pastas, rice, and seeds. These plant proteins are also a great source of fiber.

Fats

Fat is the most concentrated form of food energy, providing 9 calories per gram, more than twice the energy provided by carbohydrates and proteins. Fat adds texture and flavor to food. It helps satisfy the appetite because it is digested more slowly. Also known as *lipids,* fats are necessary for growth and healthy skin and for transporting fat soluble vitamins in the body. Fats are also linked to hormone regulation. Because of their concentrated form, fats are an efficient way to store energy. Like protein, however, fats are not a good *single* source of energy. Fats burned for energy in the absence of carbohydrates produce a toxic waste product called *ketone bodies. Ketosis,* a buildup of poisonous **ketone bodies,** causes fatigue and nausea and overtaxes the kidneys, resulting in nerve and brain damage. Fat is burned more completely in the presence of carbohydrates, another reason to have a diet high in complex carbohydrates (and to avoid weight-loss diets that promote very low carbohydrate and calorie intakes).

An important distinction should be made among the three types of fatty acids. Ninety-five percent of dietary fat consists of molecules called **triglycerides,** which are made up of fatty acids. The three types of fatty acids are classified

table 10-5   Comparison of the Three Types of Fats

	Characteristics	Examples	
Saturated	• No more room for hydrogen atoms • In animal products and some vegetable products • Raises cholesterol levels in the blood • Solid at room temperature	Coconut oil Palm oil Cheese Hot dogs Chocolate Cocoa butter Poultry skin Luncheon meats Regular ice cream Sour Cream	Butter Milk Beef Bacon Lard Pork Lamb Veal Cream
Polyunsaturated	• Can accept four more hydrogen atoms • Lowers total cholesterol and LDLs without affecting HDLs	Corn oil Cottonseed oil Soybean oil Safflower oil Sesame oil Sunflower oil Mayonnaise Almonds Most margarines	Fish Pecans Walnuts Flaxseed
Monounsaturated	• Can accept two more hydrogen atoms • Lowers total cholesterol and LDLs, and raises HDLs.	Peanut oil Olive oil Avocados Canola (rapeseed) oil	Olives Peanuts Cashews

Fat Comparison

	Saturated Fat	Monounsaturated Fat	Polyunsaturated Fat	Cholesterol mg/Tbsp
Canola Oil	6%	62%	32%	0
Safflower Oil	10%	13%	77%	0
Sunflower Oil	11%	20%	69%	0
Corn Oil	13%	25%	62%	0
Olive Oil	14%	77%	9%	0
Soybean Oil	15%	24%	61%	0
Cottonseed Oil	27%	19%	54%	0
Chicken Fat	30%	48%	22%	11
Lard	41%	47%	12%	12
Palm Oil	51%	39%	10%	0
Butter	54%	30%	16%	33
Coconut Oil	77%	6%	17%	0

according to their chemical structures. Table 10-5 identifies and compares the three types of fats.

An easy observation shows that, with a few exceptions, **saturated fats** are primarily in foods of animal origin, whereas most vegetable fats are unsaturated. Additionally, all animal fats contain cholesterol. (Vegetable foods have no natural presence of cholesterol.) Diets high in fat, especially saturated fat, have a strong link to heart disease and stroke. They elevate blood cholesterol levels that, in turn, can lead to clogged arteries (atherosclerosis). **Polyunsaturated fats** come mostly from plant foods and are a healthier fat to consume. **Monounsaturated fats** also come from plant foods. When "mono" fats replace saturated fats in the diet, they not

only decrease total and LDL cholesterol, but also appear to raise HDLs—an added benefit.

Regardless of the types of fats, we need to limit their consumption. We eat too much total fat. Americans consume approximately 37 to 40 percent of their daily calories in fats—much of which is saturated. It is recommended that our diet consist of no more than 30 percent fat (10 percent of each of the three types). Some nutritionists emphasize an even more prudent recommendation of only 10 to 20 percent of daily calories from fat. The excessive fat in our diet is the main reason Americans suffer so many heart disease deaths. Thirty to 40 percent of cancers in men and 60 percent of cancers in women have been attributed to diet, with

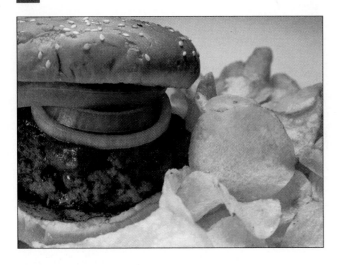

Our love for fats contributes to heart attacks, strokes, and some cancers.

excess fat being linked to cancer more frequently than any other dietary factor. Excess dietary fat is linked to cancer of the colon, breast, and prostate. The amount and type of dietary fat eaten—not the amount of cholesterol consumed—have the greatest impact on the blood cholesterol level. Dietary cholesterol also affects the level of blood cholesterol but to a lesser and more variable extent than does the fat content of the diet.

Monounsaturated fat and polyunsaturated oils can be turned into solid unhealthy saturated fats by a manufacturing process called **hydrogenation.** This technique adds hydrogen atoms to these fats as a way to prolong the shelf life of a product. Avoid completely and partially hydrogenated oils! Like saturated fats, they elevate your blood cholesterol level. During the process of hydrogenation, some fatty acid molecules become rearranged and convert to a **trans-fatty acid** (sometimes called **transfats**). Transfats are linked to coronary artery disease because they raise the bad LDL and decrease the good HDL in the blood. Some scientists believe transfats are more harmful than saturated fats on artery health. Transfats have most recently been linked to lymphoma (cancer of the lymph glands). Foods typically high in transfats include: margarine, crackers, cookies, doughnuts, pies, french fries, chips, cakes, taco shells, frostings, and candy. Transfats are not listed on food labels. And, because foods can still be called "cholesterol-free", implying a certain healthfulness, this is misleading if it contains hydrogenated oils and trans-fatty acids.

We need to be careful of these "hidden" fats in commercially prepared foods. Whereas it is obvious that butter, oils, and the visible fat on meats have a high fat content, the fat in crackers, peanut butter, pastries, and dairy products is less obvious. It is important to be able to decipher food labels and understand where the fats are in our heavily processed food supply. Remember . . . completely or partially hydrogenated oils equals trans-fatty acids.

Newly developed fat substitutes (like Olestra) have emerged in many commercially prepared foods. These substitutes are made from soybeans or various milk and egg proteins with the purpose of duplicating the taste and texture of fat—without the caloric fat content. Read the food labels for any side effects or contraindications from these substitutes. Some can cause abdominal distress.

Regardless of the source, all fats should be limited in our diet. Table 10-6 shows you how to figure your daily fat allowance to adhere to the 30 percent fat-calorie guidelines recommended in the *Dietary Guidelines for Americans.*

With so much emphasis on low-fat eating, some may try to cut their fat grams to almost zero. A little dietary fat is necessary for basic metabolic functions, especially for the absorption of fat-soluble vitamins. A minimum of 15 to 25 grams per day should satisfy these requirements.

Cholesterol

Cholesterol is not a true fat. It is a fatlike waxy substance found in animal tissue. It plays a vital role in the body's functioning. Your liver manufactures all of the cholesterol that you physically need. However, most of us consume more cholesterol by eating animal products (meat, egg yolks, cheese, dairy products, liver). A diet high in fats and cholesterol has been linked to atherosclerosis, therefore you are prudent to limit animal products in your diet. It is recommended that you restrict cholesterol consumption to 300 milligrams per day. (One egg yolk equals approximately 213 mg cholesterol; a hamburger patty or chicken breast has approximately 80 mgs.) Remember, vegetable foods contain no cholesterol, unless it is added in processing or food preparation.

Fish Oils

Studies of the diets of Eskimos and Asian fishermen have revealed interesting information about fats. Their diets provide 40 percent of daily calories from fats. Yet Eskimos are listed

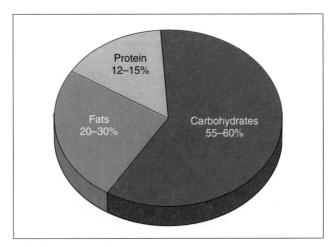

Daily diet recommendations.

table 10-6 — Determining Your Fat Gram Allowance

The American Heart Association and the *Dietary Guidelines for Americans* recommend that we consume no more than 30 percent of our daily calories from fat. For better artery health and weight loss, 20 to 25 percent consumption is recommended. If you know your approximate daily caloric intake, it is easy to calculate your desired fat grams.

Example: Terry consumes 2,000 calories per day. He wishes to stay at the recommended 30 percent fat-calorie guideline.

30% × 2,000 calories = 600 fat calories
600 calories ÷ 9 (calories per gram of fat) = 66.6 or 67 grams of fat

An easy way to estimate your fat gram limit per day is to divide your ideal weight in half. Keep your number of fat grams per day under this number. (If your ideal weight is 140 lbs., your fat gram limit should be 70 g per day.)

Fat Grams per Day for Specific Calorie Intakes and Percentages

Daily Calories	10%	20%	25%	30%
1200	13g	27g	33g	40g
1400	16g	31g	39g	47g
1600	18g	36g	44g	53g
1800	20g	40g	50g	60g
2000	22g	44g	56g	67g
2200	24g	49g	61g	73g
2500	28g	56g	69g	83g
2800	31g	62g	78g	93g

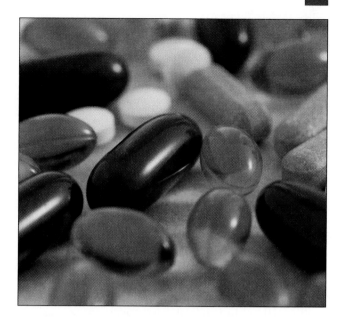

Taking vitamin/mineral supplements cannot replace a balanced diet, but can fill some specific nutritional gaps for some.

among people with the lowest rates of heart disease in the world. Why? They eat lots of fish, and fish are rich in polyunsaturated fats called **omega-3.** A diet rich in omega-3 fatty acids inhibits atherosclerosis in coronary arteries and can reduce the blood cholesterol level. The American Heart Association recommends eating fish twice a week to get heart-healthy omega-3 fatty acids. The best omega-3 sources are salmon, mackerel, herring, tuna, and sardines. Omega-3s are also available from plant sources such as flaxseed and walnuts.

Vitamins

Vitamins are the organic catalysts necessary to initiate the body's complex metabolic functions. Although these chemical substances are vital to life, they are required in minute amounts. Because of our adequate food supply, symptoms of vitamin deficiencies are rare. However, some factors may alter one's requirements (aging, illness, stress, pregnancy, smoking, dieting). Vitamins fall into two categories: fat soluble and water soluble. Vitamins A, D, E, and K are **fat soluble vitamins,** which means they are transported and stored by the body's fat cells and liver. They are stored in the body for relatively long periods (many months). Vitamin C and the B-complexes are **water soluble vitamins.** They remain in various body tissues for a short time (usually only a few weeks). Excesses are excreted.

Are vitamin supplements necessary? Vitamins do not contain energy or calories. Therefore, extra vitamins will not provide more energy or power. Eating a variety of foods is a preferred way to maintain an adequate intake of vitamins. However, in today's lifestyle, most people are not consuming a varied and balanced diet. Manufacturer's processing and preserving, food irradiation and chemical pollution, nutrient-depleted soil, and shipping and storage practices have significantly reduced the nutritional value of our foods. Other lifestyle factors, such as smoking; consuming alcohol; stress, and using drugs, such as aspirin and oral contraceptives, may increase the need for vitamin or mineral supplementation. Most medical authorities have been reluctant to recommend supplements on a broad scale for healthy people eating healthy diets. However, the accumulation of research in recent years has shown that extra amounts of certain vitamins (especially the antioxidants) may play a significant role in preventing chronic diseases like heart disease and cancer. Also, because most Americans aren't eating enough fruits, vegetables, and whole grains, supplementing with vitamin B_{12}, vitamin D, folic acid, vitamin E, and calcium are most common. Anyone with irregular diet patterns, on a weight-reduction regimen, pregnant or lactating women, strict vegetarians, or elderly people should consider a nutritional supplement or multivitamin. This could offer nutritional insurance. Consult your health professional to assess your personal needs.

Minerals

Minerals are inorganic substances critical to many enzyme functions in the body. Two groups of minerals are necessary to the diet: macrominerals and trace minerals. **Macrominerals** are needed in large doses (more than 100 mg daily). Examples are calcium, phosphorus, magnesium, potassium, and sodium. **Trace minerals** are needed in much smaller amounts. Examples are iron, zinc, copper, iodine, and fluoride, and selenium. Table 10–7 lists vitamins and minerals, their functions, good food sources of each, and adult recommendations.

Three minerals deserve special attention: calcium, iron, and sodium.

Calcium

Calcium is the body's most abundant mineral and is critical to many body functions. If the calcium supply in the blood is too low, the body withdraws calcium from the bones. This inadequate supply of calcium is a major factor contributing to **osteoporosis,** an age-related condition of insufficient bone mass. Healthy bone is living tissue that is continuously being replenished. An adult body replaces about 20 percent of its bone each year. In osteoporosis, the formation of bone fails to keep pace with lost bone tissue. The result is porous, brittle bones susceptible to fracture. Women are more susceptible to osteoporosis because they have smaller, less dense bones. However, men are also at risk. Men are more likely to suffer a hip fracture from osteoporosis than to develop prostate cancer.

In the United States, osteoporosis affects more than 25 million people (80 percent of whom are women) and causes more than 1.5 million fractures to vertebrae, wrists, and hips each year. It is the major underlying cause of bone fractures in postmenopausal women and men over 65. Some bone loss is normal with aging in both males and females, so it is important that you build strong bones now. Consumption of adequate dietary calcium from preadolescence through young adulthood is critical for building bone mass. Current calcium consumption is dangerously low among teenagers, adult women, and the elderly. It's estimated that most Americans consume only 500 milligrams of calcium daily.

Your present habits determine your bone density later in life. Up to about age 25, as calcium is added to the diet, the rate at which bone is replaced is greater than the rate at which it breaks down. By age 25–30, you've reached your peak bone mass—the point at which your bones are as dense and strong as they'll ever be. Forty to sixty percent of this peak bone mass is built during the teenage years. By age 40, bone mass begins to slowly decline in both men and women. After menopause, women lose bone mass rapidly due to a drop in estrogen level. Osteoporosis cannot be cured—it can only be prevented or its progression delayed. That is why it is essential that teens and young adults take action to build as much bone mass as possible while they are young to slow the rate of bone loss later in life. See Table 10–8 for the recommended calcium intake for various age groups.

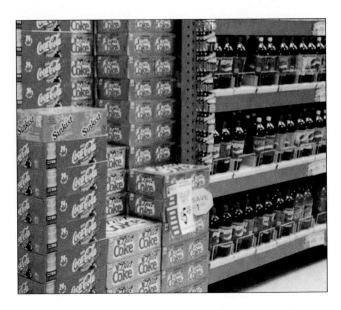

The average teenager consumes three cans of carbonated soft drinks every day. Twice as much soda as milk is consumed today; 20 years ago the reverse was true. The result? Fat teens and brittle bones.

Recent studies show that calcium isn't only for strong bones. A high daily intake of calcium (1200 to 1500 mg) has been shown to help protect against heart disease and colorectal cancer as well. (Note: The safe upper limit for calcium intake has been set at 2,500 mg a day. Experts think going above that on a regular basis may invite kidney stone formation.) To keep your bone "banks" filled, check out the top ten list.

Iron

Iron deficiency is a nutritional problem for some, particularly women, teenagers, and endurance athletes. Due to menstruation, women need to ingest more iron than men (women need 15 mgs daily; men need only 10 mgs). Iron deficiency may cause chronic fatigue and listlessness. To increase your iron intake, take the following steps:

1. Eat foods rich in iron (lean meats, poultry, fish, fortified cereals and grains, green vegetables, beans, peas, and nuts).
2. Consume iron-rich foods with foods high in vitamin C to triple iron absorption (a hamburger and tomato; cereal and orange juice).
3. Keep consumption of tea and coffee under 3 cups per day (caffeine reduces the absorption of iron).
4. Use cast-iron cookware (iron is absorbed into the food in a form readily assimilated into the body).

Iron supplementation should not be done indiscriminately. Prolonged consumption of large amounts can cause a disturbance in iron metabolism for some, contributing to atherosclerosis and heart attacks. This excessive iron buildup is more prevalent in men than women, because women lose

table 10-7 Vitamins and Minerals

Vitamins	Functions	Sources	Adult Recommendations
Fat Soluble			
A	Promotes growth and repair of body tissues; keeps skin cells moist; builds resistance to infection; promotes bone and tooth development; aids in vision	Green leafy vegetables, yellow fruits and vegetables, eggs, butter, margarine, cheese, milk, liver	800–1,000 mcg* RE**
D	Regulates absorption of calcium and phosphorus; promotes normal growth of bone and teeth	Vitamin D fortified dairy products, fish, eggs, fortified margarines, sunlight (absorbed through the skin)	400 IU ** (age 51 and over); 200 IU (ages 9–50)
E	Essential in preventing oxidation of other vitamins and fatty acids; maintains cell structure	Vegetable oil, green and leafy vegetables, whole grains, egg yolks, nuts, wheat germ	15 mg**** (22 IU)
K	Aids in blood clotting	Cabbage, cauliflower, spinach, green vegetables, liver, cereals	60–80 mcg
Water Soluble			
C (Ascorbic acid)	Builds resistance to infection; aids in tissue repair and healing; involved in tooth and bone formation	Citrus fruits, strawberries, tomatoes, potatoes, melons, broccoli, peppers, cabbage	women = 75 mg men = 90 mg
B_1 (Thiamin)	Needed to convert carbohydrates into energy; promotes normal function of nervous system	Whole grains, fortified grain products, milk, pork, legumes, nuts, meats	1.0–1.5 mg
B_2 (Riboflavin)	Combines with proteins to make enzymes that affect function of eyes, skin, nervous system, and stomach	Meat, dairy products, whole grains, green leafy vegetables	1.2–1.7 mg
B_3 (Niacin)	Aids in energy production from fats and carbohydrates	Meat, poultry, fish, liver, nuts, whole grains, legumes	13–19 mg
B_6	Aids in protein metabolism and red blood cell formation	Whole grains, meat, fish, poultry, legumes, milk, green leaf vegetables	1.6–2.0 mg
Folic acid (Folacin)	Aids in red blood cell formation; aids in synthesizing genetic material	Meat, poultry, fish, eggs, broccoli, asparagus, legumes	400 mcg
B_{12}	Aids in function of body cells and nervous tissue	Animal foods only; meat, poultry, fish, eggs, dairy products	2 mg

Minerals	Functions	Sources	Adult Recommendations
Macrominerals			
Calcium	Aids in bone and tooth formation, aids in use of phosphorus helps muscle contraction and heart function	Dairy products, green leafy vegetables, broccoli, fish	1300 mg (age 9–18); 1,000 mg (age 19–50); 1200 mg men (age 51 and over); 1500 mg women (age 51 and over)
Phosphorus	Aids in metabolism and energy production	Dairy products, eggs, meat, fish, poultry, legumes, whole grains	700 mg
Magnesium	Activates important enzyme reactions	Whole grains, nuts, legumes, green vegetables	320–420 mg
Potassium	Regulates body fluids and the transfer of nutrients across cell walls	Citrus fruits, juices, bananas, potatoes	2,000–5,000 mg
Sodium	Regulates body fluids cells; aids in muscle contraction	Table salt, milk, seafood (abundant in most foods except fruits)	1,100–3,300 mg
Trace			
Iron	Essential for oxygen transport in the blood	Liver, meat, poultry, fish, dried fruit, whole grains, legumes, green vegetables	10–15 mg
Zinc	Aids in metabolism and growth of tissue	Seafood, poultry, eggs, whole grains vegetables	12–15 mg
Copper	Involved with iron in the formation of red blood affecting overall metabolism	Liver, nuts, shellfish, meat, poultry vegetables	1.5–3.0 mg
Iodine	Forms thyroid hormone	Iodized salt, seafood	150 mcg
Fluoride	Involved in formation of bones and teeth	Fluoridated water, seafood, green vegetables	3.1–3.8 mg
Selenium	Necessary for normal growth and development, and for use of iodine in thyroid function; has antioxidant properties	Seafood, meat, liver, grains	55 mcg

*mcg = micrograms.

**RE = retinol equivalents, a measurement of vitamin A activity

***IU = International Units

****mg = milligrams

table 10-8	Optimal Calcium Requirements (Recommendations of the National Institutes of Health)

Age	Calcium mg/day
1–3	500
4–8	800
9–18	1,300
19–50	1,000
51 and older (men)	1,200
51 and older (women)	1,500

For your information:

1 cup yogurt = 300 mg	1 cup cottage cheese = 150 mg
1 cup milk = 300 mg	1½ oz cheese = 350 mg
1 cup cooked broccoli = 50 mg	3 oz sardines = 370 mg
½ cup ice cream / frozen yogurt = 100 mg	4 oz tofu = 145 mg
1/2 cup spinach = 100 mg	1 slice whole wheat bread = 25 mg
8 oz orange juice with calcium = 350 mg	1 packet instant oatmeal = 150 mg
1/3 cup nonfat dry milk = 300 mg	

Note: Food labels list calcium content as "% Daily Value." To convert to milligrams (mg) of calcium add a zero. For example, if one serving has 15% DV for calcium, it has 150 mg.

blood through menstruation each month. Individuals concerned about their iron level should consult a physician.

Sodium

Many people can reduce their chances of developing high blood pressure by consuming less salt. The American Heart Association and National Academy of Science recommend no more than 2,400 milligrams of sodium per day for healthy adults. (One teaspoon of table salt contains 2,400 milligrams of sodium.) Many Americans consume much more than that daily: 5,000 to 10,000 milligrams! We consume sodium most commonly in the form of table salt and in the processed foods we eat. Even if you never salt your food, 90 percent of processed foods contain sodium—even milk does. In this way, sodium becomes "hidden" in our diet. Sodium is also present in other popular condiments, such as monosodium glutamate (MSG), meat tenderizer, ketchup, salsa, soy sauce, mustard, barbecue sauce, and baking soda. It is even present in many medications—antacids, for instance. Fast-food restaurants often add sodium to their products. Eating a McDonald's Quarter Pounder with Cheese, large fries, and a chocolate shake will give 1,590 milligrams of sodium. "Hidden" salt is a problem in this age of processed foods. Excess sodium consumption has been one factor linked to hypertension in some sodium sensitive individuals. Excesses of sodium also increase calcium loss in urine, which is detrimental to bone density. Therefore, be

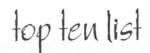

top ten list

Top Ten Ways To Keep Your Bone "Banks" Filled

1. Eat calcium-rich foods every day—low-fat dairy products, spinach, broccoli, fish with edible bones (salmon, sardines). Sprinkle nonfat dry milk into casseroles, soups, meat loaf, and so on.
2. Get regular vigorous exercise (exercises that create muscular contraction and gravitational pull on the long bones, such as walking, jogging, aerobics and weight training).
3. Do not smoke. Smoking reduces the production of estrogen and negatively affects calcium absorption.
4. Avoid excesses of alcohol and sodium. Both increase urinary loss of calcium.
5. Avoid excessive protein intake. Eating a lot of extra protein increases the rate of calcium loss from the body. The currently popular high-protein, low-carbohydrate diets contribute to the dissolution of bone.
6. Cut back on soft drinks. The phosphoric acid in colas interferes with the skeleton's ability to absorb calcium. Today's teens have tripled their consumption of soft drinks and cut their consumption of milk by more than 40 percent, robbing them of bone-building calcium during this critical stage of bone formation. The risk? More bone fractures and a future of osteoporosis.
7. Be sure to consume foods rich in vitamins A and D to enhance absorption of calcium.
8. If you have a lactose intolerance (have trouble digesting dairy products), lactose-free products are available at some stores. Or experiment with dairy foods lowest in lactose: ricotta, mozzarella, parmesan, American, and cheddar cheeses; tofu; some yogurts; sherbet; 1 percent low-fat cottage cheese.
9. Look for calcium-fortified foods such as orange juice and cereals.
10. If a high calcium intake through foods is impossible, consider a calcium supplement—ideally in the form of calcium citrate, the most readily absorbed form.

conscious of your sodium intake, and try to keep it within the recommended range.

Water

Water is often called the forgotten nutrient. However, it is *the most important* nutrient because it serves as the medium in which the other nutrients are transported. Almost all of the body's metabolic reactions occur in this medium. Water also helps rid the body of wastes, aids in metabolizing stored fat, and helps control body temperature. Water composes approximately two-thirds of your body weight. Your exact percentage of water weight varies depending on your body composition. Lean tissue contains more water than does fat tissue. Lean muscle tissue is about 73 percent water; fat tissue is only 20 percent water. Some nutritionists claim that the average American is in a constant state of dehydration. Dehydration can result in feelings of fatigue, stress, headaches, constipation, and hunger. You should drink before you feel thirsty, because thirst is a sign that you're already dehydrated. The minimum amount of water a healthy person should drink is eight to ten 8-ounce glasses a day. Some experts have suggested dividing your weight in half and using that number in ounces as a target for your daily water intake. For example, a 140-pound person should drink about 70 ounces of water daily. More is recommended if you are overweight, exercise a lot, or live in a hot climate. Alcohol and caffeinated beverages such as coffee, tea, and colas don't count because they act as diuretics and increase your need for water. Water is also a component of many foods (i.e., apples, lettuce, melons, potatoes, tomatoes, green beans, fruit juices). Are you getting enough water? If so, your urine is clear, almost colorless.

Phytochemicals and Antioxidants: Disease Fighters

Research is exploding in a new area of dietary study: examining the power of specific food components to ward off chronic diseases. These food components, known as **phytochemicals** (meaning "plant chemicals") are present in foods such as fruits, vegetables, grains, legumes, and seeds. Phytochemicals are also in garlic, licorice, soy, and green tea. Phytochemicals have been associated with the prevention and treatment of at least four of the leading causes of death in the United States: cancer, cardiovascular diseases, diabetes, and hypertension.

There are hundreds of helpful phytochemicals. These plant pigments and enzymes interact with hormone receptors, suppress malignant changes in cells, enhance immune function, and reduce cholesterol levels. Excitement is building in this new area of nutrition research as scientists continue to uncover the relationship between these plant chemicals and disease prevention. Phytochemicals, with peculiar names like carotenoids, pectins, lignins, flavonoids, indoles, lycopene, quercetin, and lutein, translate into a cornucopia of fruits and vegetables. Eating a wide variety of colorful fruits and vegetables gives you a full range of these powerful internal bodyguards that help fight off everything from cataracts to cancer to arthritis.

One particular group of phytochemicals, called **phytoestrogens** (plant estrogens), have a structure similar to the body's own hormones. Found particularly in soy products (soy milk, soy nuts, tofu, etc.), they may reduce the long-term harmful effects of the body's own hormones, commonly associated with breast, colon, and prostate cancers. Soy products may also be linked to the reduction of blood cholesterol.

Phytochemicals, along with certain vitamins (C, E, and selenium), are known as antioxidants. **Antioxidants** are compounds that come to the aid of every cell in the body that faces an ongoing barrage of damage because of the normal aging and oxygenation process (living and breathing), environmental pollution, chemicals and pesticides, additives in our processed foods, stress, and sun radiation. As aging and exposure occurs, our body creates **free radicals,** singlet oxygen molecules that damage our cells and tissues. This free radical assault on our body contributes to a number of chronic diseases such as atherosclerosis, arthritis, cancer, cataracts, heart disease, stroke, and an array of other degenerative diseases. Free radicals cause us to "rust out". Antioxidants (phytochemicals, carotenoids, vitamins C and E, etc.) that are plentiful in fruits and vegetables neutralize these free radical chemical reactions, thereby suppressing cell deterioration and slowing the aging process.

Realizing the power of these substances, Americans need to take action by eating a wide variety of fruits and vegetables—at least five servings per day.

Why not just take a supplement? Millions of Americans do, believing that they cannot get all the antioxidants and phytochemicals into their diets. We face a daily challenge to try to eat a healthy diet. In our "grab-and-go, microwave, drive-through" world, we rarely see broccoli burgers, cabbage tacos, or spinach nuggets! If you are considering taking dietary supplements, consult a knowledgeable health professional, because megadoses of some nutrients can cause side effects.

Antioxidant All-Stars

- broccoli
- green and red peppers
- cantaloupe
- spinach
- carrots
- tomatoes
- raspberries

- strawberries
- kale
- brussels sprouts
- blueberries
- sweet potatoes
- cabbage
- raisins and grapes

The Well-Balanced Diet

Eating healthy is exciting. Nutritious eating does not doom you to "nutrition martyrdom"—eating flavorless foods, counting grams, measuring portions, or passing up favorite desserts. Eating right means having a wide variety of foods, some in moderation, throughout the week. There are no "forbidden" or "bad" foods—only bad eating habits. If you have a high-fat snack one day, make sure you balance it with low-fat foods at other meals. Eating should remain one of life's pleasures. Americans are fortunate to have food choices that are varied, plentiful, and safe to eat. Nutritionists often refer to three words when attempting to simplify the principles of good nutrition: *variety*, *moderation*, and *balance*. Do you eat the same thing for breakfast every day? For lunch? For snacks? Despite our access to diverse foods, we have a tendency to consume relatively few types of foods and often become locked into standard meals that many times are culturally influenced. Why not have spaghetti, rice, chili, or pizza for breakfast rather than eggs, bacon, and donuts? The ten dietary guidelines provide a sound framework for helping us make food choices.

The Food Guide Pyramid

In 1956, the U.S. Department of Agriculture (USDA) introduced the "basic four food groups" to graphically convey healthy nutrition to Americans. For almost four decades, the "basic four" (dairy products, meats, fruits and vegetables, breads and grains) were drawn on school chalkboards and printed in nutrition booklets. As the science of nutrition grew more sophisticated, and the roles of fats and carbohydrates became better understood, the "basic four" design came under fire. Nutritionists argued that giving dairy products and meats equal emphasis with fruits, vegetables, and grains has caused heart disease and some cancers. In 1992, the USDA introduced the Food Guide Pyramid (Fig. 10-1), with grains taking up the largest space on the bottom, as the foundation of our diet. Fruits and vegetables are the next largest component. Meat, dairy, and fats occupy smaller spaces near the top. Eating according to this pyramid, with the greatest emphasis on grains, fruits, and vegetables, is the key to sound nutrition and is in harmony with the *Dietary Guidelines*. Fats and sugars can be added to grains, fruits, and

vegetables (with sauces, toppings, and preparation methods), making them less healthy choices. It is up to you to make wise choices. How well do you conform to the pyramid and *Dietary Guidelines*? Look at Table 10-9 to see how you compare to the typical American.

To further promote healthy eating, the National Cancer Institute initiated a national "Five a Day for Better Health" program to encourage Americans to eat five or more fruits and vegetables every day. You have probably seen examples of this massive campaign—television and magazine ads, billboards, and grocery bag notices. Think about your dietary intake during the past 3 days. Did you consume "five a day"? See the top ten list on how to add more fruits and veggies to your day. Start a five-a-day campaign, and remember . . . the darker, richer colors usually have more nutritional value.

Making Positive Changes

All of this information about nutrition can seem confusing and sometimes appear contradictory; for example, how do you consume enough meat for iron, yet reduce saturated fat? If you make sure you get plenty of calcium, how do you watch out for those high-fat dairy products? Eggs are a good source of protein, but how do you make sure daily cholesterol milligrams don't exceed 300? You certainly hear

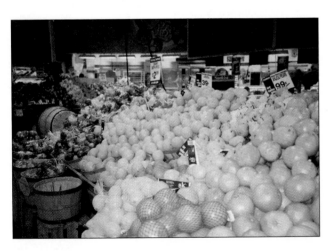

Fruits and vegetables are true "disease fighters". Eat a variety of each every day.

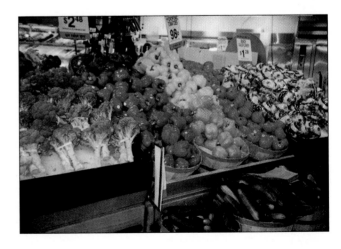

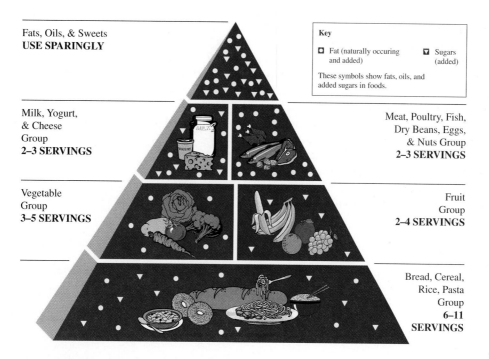

Fats, Oils, & Sweets
USE SPARINGLY

Key

☐ Fat (naturally occuring and added)   ▽ Sugars (added)

These symbols show fats, oils, and added sugars in foods.

Milk, Yogurt, & Cheese Group
2–3 SERVINGS

Meat, Poultry, Fish, Dry Beans, Eggs, & Nuts Group
2–3 SERVINGS

Vegetable Group
3–5 SERVINGS

Fruit Group
2–4 SERVINGS

Bread, Cereal, Rice, Pasta Group
6–11 SERVINGS

What is the Food Guide Pyramid?

The Pyramid is an outline of what to eat each day. It's not a rigid prescription but a general guide that lets you choose a healthful diet that's right for you. The Pyramid calls for eating a variety of foods to get the nutrients you need and at the same time the right amount of calories to maintain a healthy weight. The Pyramid also focuses on fat because most American diets are too high in fat, especially saturated fat.

Fat

● In general, foods that come from animals (milk and meat groups) are naturally higher in fat than foods that come from plants. But there are many low-fat dairy and lean meat choices available, and these foods can be prepared in ways that lower fat.

Fruits, vegetables, and grain products are naturally low in fat. But many popular items are prepared with fat, such as french-fried potatoes or croissants, making them higher-fat choices.

The number of servings you need depends on how many calories you need. This depends on your age, sex, height and weight, and activity level.

Added sugars

▼ These symbols represent sugars added to foods in processing or at the table, not the sugars found naturally in fruits and milk. It's the added sugars that provide calories with few vitamins and minerals.

Most of the added sugars in the typical American diet come from foods in the Pyramid tip—soft drinks, candy, jams, jellies, syrups, and table sugar we add to foods such as coffee or cereal.

Added sugars in the food groups come from foods such as ice cream, sweetened yogurt, chocolate milk, canned or frozen fruits with heavy syrup, and sweetened bakery products such as cakes and cookies.

What counts as a serving?

Milk, yogurt, and cheese group (2–3 servings)	Meat, poultry, fish, dry beans, eggs, and nuts, group (2–3 servings)	Vegetable group (3–5 servings)	Fruits group (2–4 servings)	Bread, cereal, rice, and pasta group (6–11 servings)
1 c. milk or yogurt 1 1/2 oz. natural cheese 2 oz. processed cheese 1 1/2 c. ice cream, frozen yogurt 1 c. cottage cheese 1/2 c. ricotta cheese	2–3 oz. cooked lean meat, poultry, or fish 1/3 c. nuts 4 T. peanut butter 1/2 c. tofu 2 eggs 1 c. cooked dried beans	1 c. raw leafy greens 1/2 c. other kinds of vegetables (raw or cooked) 3/4 c. vegetable juice 1/2 med. potato or 1/2 c. potatoes 1/2 c. salsa	1 medium apple, banana, orange 1/2 c. chopped, cooked, canned, fruit 6 oz. juice 7 med. strawberries 12 grapes 1/4 c. dried fruit	1 slice bread 1/2 bun or bagel 3/4–1 c. dry cereal 1/2 c. cooked cereal, rice, or pasta 3–4 small, plain crackers 1 small tortilla 1 4 in. pancake 2 c. light microwave popcorn

figure 10-1   Sizing up portions. By using common references, you can estimate serving sizes. For example, a closed fist takes up about as much space as a cup of food. The palm of your hand, minus the fingers, or a deck of cards is about the size of a 3-ounce serving of meat. A slice of hard cheese the size of your thumb or 2 dominoes is roughly equivalent to 1 ounce. One medium potato is the size of a computer mouse. Two tablespoons peanut butter is the size of one golf ball.

Source: U.S. Department of Agriculture, Human Nutrition Information Service; USDA's Food Guide Pyramid, *Home and Garden Bulletin* No. 249 (1992).

enough about what *not* to eat. We believe in a positive approach to a wellness lifestyle, and Table 10-10 gives many tips to help you eat more nutritiously in today's fast-paced world. These suggestions are ways to incorporate the dietary guidelines into sensible and simple practices. Significant changes in your nutritional health can be accomplished with *simple* changes, without excluding commercially prepared foods or drastically reducing the amount of food you eat. For example, using Prochaska's transtheoretical model for behavior change (see Chapter 2), clients have been successful in lowering and maintaining their dietary fat intake to below 30 percent of their calories by using five specific action-based techniques:

1. Switching to low-fat or nonfat cheeses and dairy products
2. Eating bread, rolls, pancakes, and muffins without butter or margarine
3. Taking the skin off chicken
4. Using low-cal or nonfat salad dressings
5. Regularly eating fruit or veggies as snacks (grapes, raisins, carrots, bananas, etc.)

You may want to go back and review Prochaska's behavior change theory to help identify your current stage of change. Look at the specific behavior change strategies that could help you make a healthy dietary change. See Table 10-11 for one example.

People eat food, not numbers. So rather than focusing on constant measuring, counting, and weighing, dietary

top ten list

Top Ten Answers to How Am I Supposed to Eat All Those Fruits and Vegetables?

We are supposed to eat five servings of some combination of fruits and vegetables every day. Many nutrition experts believe we should consume at least nine servings to get the phytonutrients and fiber necessary for disease prevention and optimal health. Yet, only 24 percent of Americans eat five daily servings, and a mere 5 percent consume seven. Contrary to what most say, it is surprisingly easy to eat five or more servings of fruits and vegetables every day. Here are some suggestions for adding produce to your life:

1. Start your day with a glass of 100% fruit juice (not fruit "drink"). Six ounces is a serving.
2. Top your cereal or pancakes with sliced bananas, berries, apples, or raisins.
3. Create a veggie omelette, pizza, pita sandwich, or burrito.
4. Iceberg lettuce is the least nutritious of vegetable greens. Try romaine, spinach, red leaf, chicory—add other veggies.
5. Add chopped fruits to yogurt, pudding, and as an ice cream topping.
6. Add tomatoes, carrots, zucchini, peppers, broccoli to pasta and rice salads and pasta sauces. Frozen or canned veggies work fine.
7. Top baked potatoes with assorted cooked veggies or salsa.
8. Fortify stews, soups, and casseroles with extra veggies (e.g., add broccoli, peppers, or peas to your standard macaroni and cheese).
9. Replace chips with raw veggies for dipping.
10. Keep dried fruits, raw veggies, and fresh fruits ready for quick snacks.

table 10-9   We're Not Watching What We Eat

Americans are doing fairly well at watching cholesterol intake. But we're not eating nearly enough fruit, and only a third of us are taking it easy on the salt, government data show:

	Daily Recommended Amounts	Percentage of People Meeting Daily Recommendations[1]
Grain	6-11 servings	22%
Vegetables	3-5 servings	32%
Fruits	2-4 servings	17%
Milk	2-3 servings	26%
Meat	2-3 servings	26%
Total fats	30% of calories	38%
Saturated fats	Less than 10% or calories	40%
Cholesterol	300 milligrams of less	72%
Sodium	2,400 mg or less	35%

[1] — 1996, latest year available

Source: The Healthy Eating Index. Department of Agriculture

change should involve practical changes that can become lifetime habits. It is not advisable or possible to do a complete overhaul of your diet. It is easier, and usually more lasting, to make small and gradual changes. Realize that no one is perfect or eats perfectly all of the time. You do have choices, though. As you pursue wellness, try to do the best you can with the knowledge that you now have about nutrition.

A good way to assess your nutritional habits is to record everything you eat for 3 to 7 days in a log. By observing types and quantities of food consumed, you can best judge if your diet is nutritionally sound—that is, if it con-

table 10-10   Thirty Tips for Nutritional Wellness

1. Use fresh, unprocessed foods whenever possible.
2. Remove the skin from poultry (the source of most of the fat).
3. Eat low-fat dairy products. There are plenty of reduced fat cheeses available. Switch to skim or 1 percent milk.
4. Try salsa on baked potatoes for a nonfat topping.
5. Trim all excess fat from meats; eat leaner cuts of red meats (i.e., "loin" or "round"). "Select" is lower in fat than "choice" or "prime."
6. Eat fish once or twice a week (baked or broiled, *not* fried or breaded).
7. Instead of focusing a meal around a meat, use a small amount of meat (diced, shaved, chopped, sliced) to mix in with vegetables and rice or pasta.
8. Steam, bake, broil, or roast foods using a cooking rack to allow fat to drain from the food.
9. Select salad oils, cooking oils, and margarines made with unsaturated fats. Soft, tub margarines with liquid oil listed as the first ingredient are good choices.
10. Try bagels, muffins, or whole wheat toast with jam or apple butter (without butter or margarine), rather than croissants, donuts, sweet rolls, or biscuits.
11. Use a nonstick vegetable oil spray for sautéing.
12. Use deli luncheon meats such as shaved chicken breast and turkey instead of high-fat bologna, salami, beef, or hot dogs.
13. Remove the salt shaker from the table; experiment with recipes by substituting herbs and other seasoning for salt.
14. Use applesauce in place of the oil in brownie, cookie, and cake recipes.
15. Replace snack items such as potato chips, salted nuts, and crackers with fresh fruit; raw vegetables; unsalted, unbuttered popcorn; pretzels; or rice cakes.
16. Use plain, low-fat yogurt as a substitute for sour cream in dips and on baked potatoes. Fat-free sour cream and cream cheese are also available. Evaporated skim milk can substitute for cream in recipes.
17. Eat a meatless dinner several nights a week.
18. Use ground turkey in casseroles, chili, spaghetti sauce, and skillet dinners that normally require ground beef.
19. When making scrambled eggs, separate the eggs, eliminating half of the yolks. If a recipe calls for one egg, substitute two egg whites to reduce the cholesterol.
20. After making soups, broths, or chili, scrape off the congealed fat.
21. Substitute fruit juices or plain water for soft drinks.
22. Top off your meals with fresh fruit for a nutritionally "sweet" dessert. Try frozen yogurt, juice bars, graham crackers, vanilla wafers, fig newtons, or angel food cake to satisfy your sweet tooth.
23. Decrease, at least by half, the margarine or butter called for in preparing packaged rice and pasta mixes (with minimal effect on taste).
24. Take advantage of nonfat chips, dips, snacks, cereals, cookies, and crackers that are appearing on grocery shelves almost daily. (Remember, however, that "no fat" doesn't necessarily mean "no calories.")
25. Try canned fruit with natural juices as a tasty topping for pancakes and french toast, rather than butter and syrup.
26. Top pizzas and baked potatoes with broccoli, mushrooms, zucchini, peppers, and onions rather than meats.
27. Try powdered "nonbutter" sprinkles or "butterlike" sprays as toppings for vegetables.
28. Make burritoes and tacos with beans, peas, rice, or lentils as fillers.
29. Use breads and cereals that list 100% whole wheat or "whole grain" as the first ingredient.
30. Select cereals with at least 2 grams of fiber but no more than 2 grams of fat per serving.

forms to the *Dietary Guidelines* and mimics the Food Guide Pyramid. Keeping a food log can help you set goals for making positive dietary changes. (There is a sample Food Log form in the Lab Activities section at the end of this chapter.) An appendix with the nutritive values of popular fast foods is provided at the end of the book. You may prefer to use one of the many computer programs or websites available for dietary assessment. At www.cyberdiet.com you can find a complete nutritional breakdown of thousands of foods. It may be tedious to keep records for several days, but this experience creates an awareness of food choices and quantities as well as of where improvements can be made.

Nutrition Labeling

Now that you understand the basics of nutrition, how do you find out the nutritional content of the foods you are eating? You do this by reading labels. Read about what you are eating. Part of self-responsibility is becoming a nutritionwise consumer. The federal government regulates food labeling and requires processed and packaged foods to have uniform labels. This uniformity can help consumers make healthy choices. Study the sample label in Figure 10-2 to learn how to read a label.

Points to remember when reading labels follow:

1. Check serving size. If not careful, you may eat two to three servings if the stated serving size is skimpy.
2. Watch for hidden sugars added to a product: syrup, sucrose, molasses, corn sweetener, dextrose, maltose, honey, and so on.
3. Check fat content. Avoid hydrogenated fats.
4. Some crackers, pastries, cookies, candies, and instant cocoas are made with coconut and palm oil, more saturated than beef fat.

table 10-11 — Tips for Behavior Change: Eating Five Servings of Fruits/Vegetables Every Day

Stages of Change: In what stage are you?

1. Precontemplation: "I don't like fruits and vegetables, and I'm in good health. So why would I want to eat them?"
2. Contemplation: "I realize fruits and vegetables have a lot of nutritional value and could probably cut my risk of future chronic diseases."
3. Preparation: "I've been spending more time in the produce section of the grocery store, learning more about different fruits. I have even started buying and trying some new kinds."
4. Action: "I have been eating five servings everyday for about 2 months."
5. Maintenance: "I eat at least five servings (sometimes more!) everyday and have done so for over 6 months. I can't imagine not eating them everyday!"

Processes of Change

After identifying your current stage, try using some of the following selected processes and behavior strategies appropriate for your particular stage—to facilitate your transition into the next stage (refer to Fig. 2-2).

- Consciousness-raising: read about health benefits of eating fruits and vegetables.
- Social liberation: investigate new fruits and vegetables at the grocery and new recipes.
- Self-reevaluation: write down pros and cons of making this major dietary change.
- Self-liberation: map out a plan (i.e., drink a glass of juice and slice a banana onto cereal at breakfast; carry an apple in backpack for a snack; have a green vegetable at dinner every night; snack on grapes, carrot sticks, or other fruits/veggies while studying).
- Reward: treat yourself to a rich fruit dessert once a week (cobbler, pie, etc.).
- Environment control: have plenty of fruits/vegetables available in room/apartment.

table 10-12 — Label Descriptions

Free. The product contains no amount of, or only "physiologically inconsequential" amounts of one or more of these components: fat, saturated fat, cholesterol, sodium, sugars, and calories. For instance, "calorie free" means that there are fewer than 5 calories per serving, and "sugar free" and "fat free" indicate that there are less than 0.5 grams per serving.

Low. This food could be eaten frequently without exceeding dietary guidelines for one or more of the following components: fat, saturated fat, cholesterol, sodium, and calories. Thus, the following terms are used:

Low fat. 3 grams or less per serving.

Low saturated fat. 1 gram or less per serving.

Low sodium. Less than 140 mgs per serving.

Very low sodium. Less than 35 mgs per serving.

Low cholesterol. Less than 20 mgs per serving.

Low calorie. 40 calories or less per serving.

Lean and extra lean. The following terms can be used to describe the fat content of meat, poultry, seafood, and game meats:

Lean. Less than 10 grams of fat, less than 4 grams of saturated fat, and less than 95 mgs of cholesterol per serving and per 100 grams.

Extra lean. Less than 5 grams of fat, less than 2 grams of saturated fat, and less than 95 mgs of cholesterol per serving and per 100 grams.

High. One serving of the food contains 20 percent or more of the Daily Value for a particular nutrient.

Good source. One serving of the food contains 10 to 19 percent of the Daily Value for a particular nutrient.

Reduced. A nutritionally altered product contains 25 percent less of a nutrient or of calories than the regular, or reference, product.

Less. A food, whether altered or not, contains 25 percent less of a nutrient or of calories than the reference food.

Light. A nutritionally altered product contains one-third fewer calories or half the fat of the reference food; or the sodium content of a low-calorie, low-fat food has been reduced by 50 percent.

---

5. Select *whole* wheat bread ("wheat flour" means refined *white* flour—the bran and wheat germ have been removed). All whole wheat bread is brown, but not all brown bread is whole wheat.

6. Fortified foods contain added vitamins and minerals not originally in the food or were present in lower amounts. Breakfast cereals are commonly fortified. Can you name the vitamin milk is commonly fortified with?

7. Enriched foods have lost nutrients during processing and then had them replaced by the manufacturers. For instance, when wheat is turned into white flour, it loses at least 50 to 80 percent of many nutrients. Of these, iron, niacin, thiamin, and riboflavin are replaced; but other nutrients lost in the milling process, such as fiber, zinc, and copper, are not restored.

One of the problems in food labeling has been the confusing descriptors that manufacturers put on food products, for which there have previously been no definitions (for example, *lite* or *light* could have meant light in calories, color, texture, or weight). Under law, specific, uniform definitions have been assigned to descriptors used on the label of any product. Table 10-12 defines these label descriptors. Consistency in these terms will help shoppers who do not scrutinize the numbers on food labels but who want to pick up a "low-sodium" or "fat-free" version of foods as they walk through the supermarket. Now, shoppers cannot be misled.

Serving sizes are standardized to reflect the amounts of foods people actually eat. They are also expressed in common household and metric measures. (You should note whether you are consuming more than one serving.)

This mandatory list of nutrients includes those most important to today's consumers. In the past, the concern was vitamin and mineral deficiencies. Now the worries pertain to fat, cholesterol, sodium, types of carbohydrates, and protein amounts.

This means that in a 2,000 calorie diet 65 grams is equal to 30 percent fat.

This information can help you calculate what percentage of calories of this food comes from fat, carbohydrates, and protein.
e.g.:
TOTAL FAT = 13g
13g × 9 = 117 calories
117 ÷ 261 = .45
This macaroni and cheese is 45 percent fat.
TOTAL CARBOHYDRATE = 31g
31g × 4 = 124 calories
124 ÷ 261 = .47
This macaroni and cheese is 47 percent carbohydrate.
TOTAL PROTEIN = 5g
5g × 4 = 20 calories
20 ÷ 261 = .08
This macaroni and cheese is 8 percent protein.

MACARONI AND CHEESE

Nutrition Facts

Serving Size 1/2 cup (114g)
Servings Per Container 4

Amount Per Serving

Calories 261   Calories from Fat 117

	% Daily Value*
Total Fat 13g	**20%**
Saturated Fat 5g	**25%**
Cholesterol 30mg	**10%**
Sodium 660mg	**28%**
Total Carbohydrate 31g	**11%**
Sugar 5g	**
Dietary Fiber 1g	**4%**
Protein 5g	**

Vitamin A 4% • Vitamin C 2% • Calcium 15% • Iron 4%

* Percents (%) of a Daily Value are based on a 2,000 calorie diet. Your Daily Values may vary higher or lower depending on your calorie needs:

	Calories	2,000	2,500
Total Fat	Less than	65g	80g
Sat Fat	Less than	20g	25g
Cholesterol	Less than	300mg	300mg
Sodium	Less than	2,400mg	2,400mg
Total Carbohydrate		300g	375g
Fiber		25g	30g

1g Fat = 9 calories
1g Carbohydrates = 4 calories
1g Protein = 4 calories

** No daily values have been determined for sugars and protein intake.

Ingredients: Enriched wheat flour (contains niacin, reduced iron, vitamin B$_1$, vitamin B$_2$, folic acid), cheddar cheese cultures, partially hydrogenated soybean and/or cottonseed oil, non-fat milk, salt, corn syrup, monosodium glutamate, citric acid, natural and artificial flavors, yellow 5 and 6

% Daily Value shows how a food fits into the overall daily diet. For each item, it shows the percentage or recommended daily consumption for a person eating 2,000 calories a day (e.g., 5 grams of saturated fat is 25 percent of the *recommended* daily value of 20 grams).

Percentage of daily requirements for selected vitamins and minerals

Recommended daily amounts of each item for two average diets. (If you eat less than 2,000 calories, you will have to adjust the Daily Values.)

Based on 10 percent consumption

Based on 60 percent consumption

Voluntary components that will be allowed on labels are calories from saturated fat, polyunsaturated fat, monounsaturated fat, potassium, soluble and insoluble fiber, sugar, alcohol, other carbohydrates, and other essential vitamins and minerals.

Ingredients are listed in descending order by weight. The ingredient in the largest quantity is always listed first.

figure 10-2   How to read a food label.

wellness flash

The costs of eating out. Frequent restaurant dining can ruin more than your budget. Those who eat out 6 to 13 times per week take in nearly 300 more calories, nearly 20 more grams of fat, and 400 more milligrams of sodium daily than those who dine out 5 or fewer times per week.

Eating Out

One out of every five Americans eats at a fast-food restaurant daily. Eating out has become routine for many of us. Meal preparation time at home has decreased due to changing lifestyles, and it is evident this trend will not reverse. In this fast-paced world, people want food fast. Many fast-food restaurants pride themselves in the ability to have a meal in your hands 90 seconds after you place your order. Most fast-food chains supply nutrient information on their food products. What has this information revealed about the nutrient value of fast food? Are fast foods junk foods? Nutritionists have found that fast-food items do have significant amounts of some nutrients (especially protein), but many tend to be low in fiber and high in calories, sodium, and fat. How often do you rely on these foods? What other foods are you eating during the day? Occasional visits to fast-food restaurants will have little effect on the nutritive value of your total diet. In response to consumer demand, many chains have become diversified and have added many more items to their menus. Many offer lower-fat items. However, it is difficult to get ample amounts of fruits and vegetables by eating consistently at fast-food establishments. Check out the top ten list of suggestions for healthy eating at fast-food restaurants.

Restaurant-eating in general (not only fast foods) has become a way of life for many. Many restaurants offer low-fat, low-calorie offerings, often identified on the menu in a separate "healthy fare" category. Some list fat grams and other nutritional information. Having nutritional knowledge can help you make healthy selections. Ask the server how foods are prepared. Are they baked or fried? Can lower fat sauces or condiments be substituted? Can the vegetable of the day be substituted for french fries? Salads are not always healthy if loaded with bacon, high-fat cheeses, and full-fat dressings. Check out the à la carte menu. Baked potatoes, salads, vegetables, and soups can often be ordered to make up a meal. When looking at your overall diet, keep your entire day's and week's intakes in perspective. No foods should be totally forbidden. Everyone enjoys an occasional burger and fries or pepperoni pizza. Try to live by the "80-20 rule": 80 percent of the time eat nutritionally-dense, healthy foods; 20 percent of the time . . . indulge! Remember: *variety*, *moderation*, and *balance*.

top ten list

Top Ten Fast Tips for Fast Foods

1. Think about what else you have eaten or will eat in the day. Fit this meal into your total fat, sodium, and calorie intake.
2. Salad bars are a wise choice for vitamins A and C and fiber; go easy on the dressings, high-fat cheeses, bacon, olives, sour cream, and refried beans. If the bar has pita bread, tacos, or tortillas, why not stuff these with veggies?
3. Potato bars are another good choice if you avoid the heavy cheese and butter-type sauces, bacon, and sour cream.
4. Chicken and fish sound healthy, but many are coated with fat. Select the baked or grilled without breading or skin.
5. Pizza is a great choice, especially if the toppings are vegetables; avoid the pepperoni, sausage, bacon, and olives.
6. Hamburgers—order the small one instead of the "jumbo" burger.
7. Drink skim milk or juices instead of a shake or soda.
8. If eating Mexican food, emphasize soft corn tortillas, beans, chicken, and vegetables (easy on the cheese).
9. For breakfast, avoid croissants, biscuits, sausage, bacon, butter, and the danish. Better choices are pancakes, English muffins, bagels, bran muffins, and whole grain cereals.
10. Ask for salad dressings "on the side" and use sparingly. Select nonfat or low-fat dressings.

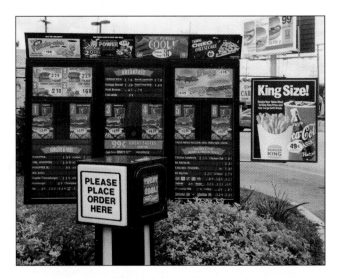

We spend 40 percent of our food dollars taking-out, driving-thru, or sitting down for a restaurant meal. In comparison, in 1980 it was only one-fourth of our budgets.

diversity issues

America loves more than burgers and fries. Ethnic foods are popular. Check out these suggestions. (Remember . . . any foods in huge portions can contribute extra fat, calories, and salt.)

	TRY	AVOID
MEXICAN	rice and beans, salsa, soft tacos, chicken or bean burritos, chicken or vegetable fajitas, corn tortillas, grilled chicken or seafood, nonfat or low-fat refried beans	refried beans made with lard, taco chips and shells, cheese sauces, sour cream, guacamole, fried appetizers, chimichangas
CHINESE	soups, steamed rice, soft noodles, chicken, shrimp, stir fries, vegetables, Hunan or Szechuan dishes	breaded and fried meats, fried rice, fried noodles, egg rolls, wontons, General Tso's chicken
ITALIAN	marinara and tomato-based sauces, grilled fish and chicken, minestrone soup, pasta primavera, pasta with red or white clam sauces, vegetable pizza	alfredo, carbonara or other cream sauces, parmigiana dishes, cannelloni, ravioli, manicotti, garlic bread, fried calamari, pepperoni pizza, and sausage pizza
INDIAN	baked breads (chapati), Tandoori chicken or fish, yogurt-based curry dishes, dal (lentils)	fried breads (bhatura, poori, paratha), ghee (clarified butter), fried appetizers (pakoras), samosa, korma
THAI	chicken and seafood dishes (larb, po tak), broiled beef with onions (yum neua)	fried fish, chicken or duck, curries, peanut sauces, yum koon chaing (sausage with peppers)

Special Nutritional Concerns

High-level wellness means adjusting to life changes and seeking information for special situations. This section discusses dietary considerations for vegetarians; pregnant mothers; the elderly; and those persons engaging in regular, vigorous exercise.

Vegetarian Diet

For a variety of health and moral reasons, many people prefer a vegetarian diet. A vegetarian diet can be nutritious and healthy. From not eating animal foods, vegetarians normally have lower body fat, blood cholesterol, blood pressure, and rates of coronary heart disease than do meat eaters. Studies show that mortality rates are lower for vegetarians than for nonvegetarians and that they have a lower-than-average risk of various cancers and Type 2 diabetes. There are different vegetarian diets, however. Careful planning and food selection is important to avoid nutritional deficiencies. All vegetarian diets emphasize the use of vegetables, fruits, and grains as main staples. Some diets exclude all animal products, while some include dairy products and eggs.

Here are the types of vegetarian diets:

1. **Strict vegetarian** (or **vegan**) consumes only plant foods. (Vitamin B_{12} supplementation is recommended because it is not in any plant foods.)
2. **Lactovegetarian** will consume plant foods and dairy products. (No meat or eggs.)
3. **Ovo-lactovegetarian** will consume plant foods, dairy products, and eggs.
4. **Semivegetarian** only excludes red meat.

Meat is not essential to your diet, but protein is. Therefore, following a vegetarian diet requires careful planning and food selection to consume sufficient vitamins and minerals (especially the vitamin Bs, vitamin D, calcium, zinc, and iron). Search for good quality protein sources such as legumes (beans), nuts, grains, seeds, and soybean products. A thorough knowledge of nutrition is essential. For example, combining a good source of vitamin C with whole grains and legumes will greatly enhance iron absorption from grain and legumes. Drinking fortified soybean milk will help you obtain calcium and vitamin B_{12}.

Pregnancy

Many women become more nutritionally aware and eat more wisely during pregnancy. This makes sense. It is an enormous responsibility to be in control of the nutritional well-being of another human. Good nutritional habits before conception give the baby an even healthier start. Good nutrition can improve infant birth weight and reduce infant mortality. It has become recognized that a deficiency in folic acid (a B vitamin) is linked to neural tube birth defects. Therefore, the U.S. Public Health Service has issued a public health recommendation that all women of childbearing age should consume 0.4 milligrams (or 400 mcg) of folic acid per day. The evidence is so clear and the concern so great that the FDA has mandated that folic acid be added to "enriched" grain products.

Pregnancy is not a time to diet. Weight gain and some increased fat deposition are necessary and healthy. Be sure to increase calcium, iron, and protein. Your physician may recommend a vitamin supplement, because many vitamin needs are increased. Although some additional vitamins and minerals are needed, only about 300 extra calories per day are necessary for fetal growth and metabolic expenditure. A woman may be "eating for two," but normal energy expenditure is not double. Therefore, it is important to eat nutritionally dense foods. Twinkies, chocolate chip cookies, and potato chips offer few nutrients to that growing baby. Alcohol and caffeine should be limited, because they increase nutrient excretion and adversely affect fetal development.

Aging

Many factors may interfere with good nutrition in older adults: economics, isolation, dentures, chronic health disorders, loss of taste, and medications. Nutrient absorption may decrease, especially for calcium and zinc. The widow or widower whose partner had always prepared the meals might start eating fast foods or frozen dinners. The depressed and lonely surviving partner may eat very little. Proper nutrition throughout life and into later life can minimize degenerative changes and help you maintain productivity and wellness. However, your 65-year-old body will not be the same one you fed at 25. If you decrease activity and your body composition changes (increase in fat, decrease in lean), then caloric intake should be decreased. Maintaining an active lifestyle can keep energy requirements from decreasing drastically. Although energy needs may drop as you age, nutrient needs do not diminish significantly. You must make your calories count. Be sure to eat adequate fiber and calcium and fewer fats and refined sugars. In many ways good nutrition (along with proper exercise) can help slow the aging process.

Sports and Fitness

Do you play competitive basketball? Are you training for a half-marathon? Is lap swimming every morning your fitness routine? Nutrition complements physical activity as you pursue a wellness lifestyle. However, the basic nutritional needs of an active person vary little from those of the more sedentary. *Everyone* needs a wide variety of healthy foods. If you are physically active, you burn more calories and have less chance of gaining weight (while eating more). Nevertheless, you do not need a special diet. There are many myths surrounding athletic performance and nutrition. An athlete (even a body builder) does not benefit from consuming a lot more protein. The typical American diet contains adequate amounts of protein—even to support an athletic lifestyle. The usual recommendation for athletes is to consume 15 percent of daily calories from protein. Athletes who train heavily may need a little more. These increased protein needs can be satisfied easily by small adjustments in the normal diet—skim milk, yogurt, skinless chicken breast, and beans can provide excellent high-quality protein.

The main fuel for exercising muscles, glycogen, comes from carbohydrates. The best are complex (breads, pastas, cereals, potatoes, rice, fruit), which provide plenty of vitamins and minerals. Persons engaged in fitness activities should consistently follow the 55 to 60 percent carbohydrate diet-proportion guidelines. For those engaging in heavy exercise training, a diet with 60 to 70 percent of its calories from carbohydrates may be necessary to refuel glycogen stores. High-sugar snacks consumed before exercising can decrease performance. Carbohydrate loading (that is, manipulating diet and training to increase glycogen stores in the muscles) has not been shown to be effective for athletes participating in events requiring less than 1½ to 2 hours of continuous, noninterrupted effort.

The benefits of vitamin and mineral supplementation is a current area of study in regard to nutrition for competitive athletes. Large doses of the antioxidants vitamins C, E, and beta-carotene have shown promise in minimizing muscle damage and soreness in hard-working athletes. Research is exploding in this area.

Dehydration is a major contributor to poor athletic performance. Athletes, like everyone else, should drink eight to ten glasses of water every day. They should also drink a cup or more of water immediately before exercise and another ½ to 1 cup every 15 minutes during exercise. Do not wait until you are thirsty. Thirst is not a reliable indicator of dehydration because it usually does not occur until after 2 to 4 pints of body water are lost. The inclusion of electrolytes in sports drinks has been shown to be beneficial for rehydrating athletes. Sports drinks with 4 to 8 percent carbohydrate concentrations work best. (See Chapter 6 for more information on sports drinks.) In regard to nutrition, the key to sports and fitness performance is the same key to general wellness and vitality: a balanced diet.

frequently asked questions

Q. I work out quite a bit, endurance biking and weight training. Don't I need a lot more protein than a casual exerciser?

A. Many athletes overestimate the amount of protein they need, thinking that more is better. Some studies indicate that more grams of protein than the normal recommendation (i.e., weight in pounds multiplied by 0.36) may help some, while other studies show no improvement in workload capacity or strength. The studies that recommend more protein, weight in pounds multiplied by 0.54 to 0.64 is the additional amount sufficient for strength and endurance athletes. If you are typical, you probably eat more than enough protein. For example, if you weigh 180 pounds, your recommended protein intake is approximately 65 grams (180 lbs × 0.36). If you increase to: 180 lbs × 0.54 or 180 lbs × 0.64, the result is 97 to 115 total grams of protein. To put this in food perspective, 70 grams of protein would be: 8 oz of skinless chicken breast and 2 cups of skim milk. An addition of 1 cup oatmeal, 1 cup cottage cheese, and 2 tablespoons peanut butter brings the total to 115 grams of protein. As you can see, the typical American diet contains a sufficient amount of protein to support even the most active lifestyle. Remember, more carbohydrates, *not* protein, are needed for energy fuel; and excessive protein does not build muscle faster. Excessive protein intake causes the body to excrete calcium (weakening bones), and puts extra strain on the kidneys.

Q. I hate milk and know I don't get enough calcium. Can't I take a calcium supplement? If so, what kind?

A. It is best to get enough calcium in the diet, but like you, many people struggle at this. There are many types of calcium supplements, some more absorbable than others. The most absorbable form of calcium is calcium citrate, and it can be taken without food. Avoid oyster shell calcium, dolomite, and bone meal products due to possible lead contamination. Calcium carbonate (the type found in antacids) is less absorbable than calcium citrate. Also, you absorb more from divided doses (500 mg or less) than taking a high dose of calcium all at once. In addition to calcium, it is important to get the recommended levels of magnesium, zinc, and vitamin D to enhance the absorption of calcium. Remember, you can also obtain calcium from nondairy

foods: calcium-fortified orange juice, sardines, oatmeal, whole grains, broccoli, tofu, and so on.

Q. I keep seeing more foods labeled "organic" in my grocery store. What does that mean?

A. In the past, "organic" had never been officially defined. Growers and manufacturers could slap the word "organic" on any food they wanted and not be breaking any regulations. This has changed. Under the new federal regulations, "organic" indicates that a food has been made with ingredients grown without chemical fertilizers, genetic engineering (scientific tinkering with a plant's DNA), and irradiation (a process that uses low levels of radiation to kill bacteria). "Organic" meat denotes that the animals have not been administered antibiotics, have access to outdoor land, and have been fed organically grown feed.

Q. Which is better to eat—butter or margarine?

A. It is best to limit consumption of *all* fats, including butter and margarine. Butter is high in saturated fat, which raises "bad" LDL cholesterol. Regular margarine is high in trans fatty acids (hydrogenated oils), known to increase the "bad" LDL cholesterol *and* decrease the "good" HDL cholesterol. Therefore, if you must use a spread, look for lower fat or lighter kinds of margarines that say "trans-free" on the label. These would be better for you. Both margarine and butter have the same number of calories, approximately 100 calories per tablespoon. You may want to try some of the butter sprinkles, butter flavored mixes, and butter sprays, which are fat free.

Q. I don't like many vegetables. Is it okay to get my five-a-day strictly from fruit?

A. Fruits and vegetable contain about the same vitamins and minerals, but vegetables offer a wider array of phytochemicals and carotenoids that help fight cancer, heart disease, and more. How about trying to add some new sauces or spices to vegetables to make them more flavorful? Or, add shredded carrots, zucchini, or spinach to pasta sauces or meat loaf. Add some steamed broccoli or peas to your macaroni and cheese. Throw a handful of veggies into your soup. They make great pizza toppings. There are many creative ways to add vegetables to your diet. And you may find you like them!

summary

Although diet is not singled out as a specific risk factor for coronary heart disease, dietary factors are often interrelated with patterns of physical activity as major contributors to heart disease, stroke, obesity, atherosclerosis, osteoporosis, and some types of cancer. While many dietary components are involved in diet and health relationships, a primary factor is our high consumption of fats (especially saturated fats). These are often consumed at the expense of fruits,

vegetables, and complex carbohydrates that may be more conducive to health.

Like many, you may admit to having some poor nutritional habits. You may rationalize this with some of the following:

- I'll do better after I get out of school and have more time. (Frankly, you will probably be busier after graduation.)

- But I feel fine! (Like smoking, poor eating habits may not noticeably affect your health for years.)
- I don't have any control over what the cafeteria serves. (However, you do have *choices* in the cafeteria and between meals.)
- I don't have enough money to buy the right foods. (On the contrary, milk is cheaper than soft drinks; a bunch of bananas costs less than a bag of potato chips.)
- I'm going to die anyway, so I might as well eat what I like. (Yes, we are all going to die. However, lifetime dietary habits significantly affect the *quality* of the last 10 to 20 years of your life.)

Wellness involves making informed choices rather than rationalizing. Improved eating habits can positively affect your health—now and later in life. Therefore, learn about the foods you are eating. Read food labels. The heart of good nutrition is ten *dietary principles*, a *pyramid of choices*, and *three simple words*. A diet that emphasizes *variety*, *moderation*, and *balance* is a big step toward achieving high-level wellness. A variety of foods is available to you, and it is up to you to make responsible choices: complex carbohydrates high in fiber and foods low in fat, cholesterol, sodium, and refined sugars.

 internet resources

Organizations

American Dietetic Association
www.eatright.org

American Heart Association
1-800-AHA-USA1
www.americanheart.org/dietaryguidelines
www.deliciousdecisions.org

American Institute for Cancer Prevention (AICR)
www.aicr.org

Center for Science in the Public Interest
www.cspinet.org

Cooking Light Magazine
www.cookinglight.com

National Osteoporosis Foundation
www.nof.org

USDA Food and Nutrition Information Center
www.nal.usda.gov/fnic

Vegetarian Resource Group
www.vrg.org

Vegetarian Times Magazine
www.vegetariantimes.com

Websites

www.cyberdiet.com

www.dietitian.com

www.dietsite.com

www.5day.com

www.healthyfridge.org

www.healthyideas.com

www.meals.com

www.navigator.tufts.edu

www.nutrition.gov

www.purefood.org

www.weightdirectory.com

Name _____

Class/Activity Section _____

Date _____

Food Log

Write down everything you eat and drink for three to five full days. Make copies of the log as needed. Be sure to note the approximate quantity of food and assess combination foods (e.g., pizza, casseroles, tacos, salads) to list the foods in them. Keep track of the number of servings in each food group. Use the columns at the right to record calories, sodium milligrams, fat grams, cholesterol milligrams, and so on, as desired.

Date _____
(12:01 A.M. to 12:00 midnight)
Other categories: calories, calcium,
cholesterol, fat, etc.

Major Food Groups—Servings

Time	Food	Amount	Bread, cereal, rice, pasta	Vegetable	Fruit	Meat, poultry, fish, beans, eggs, nuts	Milk, yogurt, cheese	Fats, oils, sweets				
	Totals =											
	Recommendations		6–11	3–5	2–4	2–3	2–3	Sparingly				

Vitamin supplements:

Date _____
(12:01 A.M. to 12:00 midnight)
Other categories: calories, calcium,
cholesterol, fat, etc.

Major Food Groups—Servings

Time	Food	Amount	Bread, cereal, rice, pasta	Vegetable	Fruit	Meat, poultry, fish, beans, eggs, nuts	Milk, yogurt, cheese	Fats, oils, sweets				
	Totals =											
	Recommendations		6–11	3–5	2–4	2–3	2–3	Sparingly				

Vitamin supplements:

Analyze Your Diet

After completing the *Food Log*, analyze your diet as follows.

1. Looking at the ten *Dietary Guidelines for Americans*, how does your diet measure up with *each* guideline?

    1.   6.

    2.   7.

    3.   8.

    4.   9.

    5.   10.

2. Look at the Food Guide Pyramid. Do you meet the daily criteria for recommended servings in each food group?

Compare your daily servings to what is recommended. Comment.

   a. Bread, cereal, rice, and pasta group: d. Milk, yogurt, and cheese group:
      My servings =____   My servings =____

   b. Vegetable group: e. Meat, poultry, fish, dry beans, eggs, and nuts group:
      My servings =____   My servings =____

   c. Fruit group:
      My servings =____

3. Identify three positive dietary changes that you could implement that would enhance your nutritional wellness. Include *what* you would do and a *specific strategy* for how you would do it.

   a.

   b.

   c.

How Much Fat?

1. Lisa consumes 1,800 calories per day. To keep her percentage of fat right at 30 percent of her calories, figure how many *grams* of fat she can consume per day. _____ (Show your work.)

   If Lisa wants to eat even *healthier* and limit her fat percentage to 20 percent of her daily calories, how many fat grams per day can she consume? _____ (Show your work.)

2. Robert consumes 2,700 calories per day. To keep his percentage of fat right at 30 percent of his calories, how many *grams* of fat can he consume per day? _____ (Show your work.)

   If Robert wants to eat even *healthier* and limit his fat percentage to 20 percent of his daily calories, how many fat grams per day can he consume? _____ (Show your work.)

What About You?

(Multiply your body weight by 15 to approximate your caloric intake for a day.)

_____ lbs. × 15 = _____ calories

Number of daily fat grams at 30 percent of calories = _____ (Show your work.)

Number of daily fat grams at 20 percent of calories = _____ (Show your work.)

Label Reading Assignment

Honey Wheat Muffin Mix

Directions	**Nutrition Facts**
Combine mix with: 　1/3 c. milk 　1 T. oil 　1 egg Stir and pour into prepared muffin tin. Bake 15 minutes at 400°.	Serving Size 1 muffin (from 31g mix) Servings Per Container 6

Amount Per Serving	Mix	Prepared
Calories	123	162
Calories from Fat	27	54

	% Daily Value**	
Total Fat 3g*	4%	10%
Saturated Fat 0.5g	3%	7%
Cholesterol 0mg	0%	12%
Sodium 210mg	9%	9%
Potassium 15mg	<1%	1%
Total Carbohydrate 23g	8%	8%
Dietary Fiber <1g	2%	2%
Sugars 12g		
Other Carbohydrate 11g		
Protein 1g		
Calcium	0%	2%
Iron	2%	2%

Not a significant source of vitamin A and vitamin C.

*Amount in mix. As prepared, one serving provides 6g fat (1.5g saturated fat), 35mg cholesterol, 220mg sodium, 45mg potassium, 24g total carbohydrate (12g sugars) and 3g protein.

**Percent Daily Values are based on a 2,000 calorie diet. Your daily values may be higher or lower depending on your calorie needs:

	Calories:	2,000	2,500
Total Fat	Less than	65g	80g
Sat Fat	Less than	20g	25g
Cholesterol	Less than	300mg	300mg
Sodium	Less than	2,400mg	2,400mg
Potassium		3,500mg	3,500mg
Total Carbohydrate		300g	375g
Dietary Fiber		25g	30g

Calories per gram:
Fat 9　•　Carbohydrate 4　•　Protein 4

Ingredients: Enriched Wheat Flour, Sugar, Hydrogenated Vegetable Oil (Coconut and/or Palm Kernel), Corn Syrup, Salt, Cellulose Gum, Dextrose, Rice Flour, Artificial Flavor

Look at the muffin mix label and complete the following:

1. What constitutes one serving?

2. Why are there two columns (mix, prepared)?

3. How many grams of fat are there in two prepared muffins? _____

4. In one prepared muffin, figure the
   a. percent of calories from fat: _____

   b. percent of calories from carbohydrates: _____

   c. percent of calories from protein: _____

5. Give one source of complex carbohydrate:

6. Give one source of simple carbohydrate:

7. Name the source of cholesterol in this prepared product:

8. Name and comment on the sources of fat in this prepared product:

9. What is your overall assessment of this food (i.e., nutritional density; sodium, fat, cholesterol content; types of carbohydrates; fiber content)?

Using HealthQuest

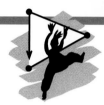

1. Insert HealthQuest CD into your computer.

2. Click on "Nutrition and Weight Control" from the menu. Click on "Introduction" and read.

3. Click on "Introduction" again and go to "Wellness Activities." Click on the "How's Your Diet?" activity.

4. Read the instructions, then go through the assessment (14 questions). When you have finished, click on "Show Score" and then on each of the histogram bars for feedback on your fats, carbohydrates, proteins, fruits and vegetables.

   What was your score in each category? (These percentages are like a test score—i.e., 100 percent is perfect)

   Fats _____   Proteins _____

   Carbohydrates _____   Fruits and Vegetables _____

   List four *specific* dietary changes you could implement that would enhance your dietary profile.

   1.   3.

   2.   4.

Close this out (bottom left corner) and click on "Wellness Activities" again, then on "Topics."

Click on either: "Specifics On," "Our Changing World," or "Key Articles."

Peruse the topics under these three categories. Select three topics and read the information. Summarize what you learned.

1. Topic = _____

2. Topic = _____

3. Topic = _____

lab activity
10–7

Changing Behavior Using the Transtheoretical Model

Using a highlighter, trace a path on the algorithm as you answer each question. Highlight your stage of change.

Do you consume at least five servings of fruits and/or vegetables every day?

Yes → Have you done this consistently over the last 6 months?

    Yes → Maintenance

    No → Action

No → Do you plan to adopt this practice within the next 6 months?

    Yes → Within the next month?

        Yes → Preparation

        No → Contemplation

    No → Precontemplation

lab activity @ chapter ten

Once you've identified which stage of change you are in, it is important to use the processes most useful in progressing to the next stage—*or* remaining in maintenance. In the box, write your stage of change. Then, list the processes that are most useful in that stage (see Fig. 2-2 in Chapter 2). Use only the number of processes that apply to your stage of behavior change. You may not need to use all six. Under each process, give two specific behavior strategies (see Table 2-1 in Chapter 2) that could help you progress to the next stage—*or* maintain, if you're in the maintenance stage.

The stage I am in = _____ .

Process 1.   _____

        Behavior strategy – a.

        Behavior strategy – b.

Process 2.   _____

        Behavior strategy – a.

        Behavior strategy – b.

Process 3.   _____

        Behavior strategy – a.

        Behavior strategy – b.

Process 4.   _____

        Behavior strategy – a.

        Behavior strategy – b.

Process 5.   _____

        Behavior strategy – a.

        Behavior strategy – b.

Process 6.   _____

        Behavior strategy – a.

        Behavior strategy – b.

11

Aiming for a Healthy Weight

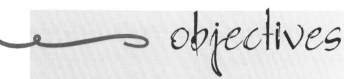 objectives

After reading this chapter, you will be able to:
1. Differentiate between overweight and obesity.
2. Explain the purpose of the body mass index (BMI) and identify a BMI associated with health problems.
3. List seven health conditions associated with obesity.
4. Explain how the location of fat on the body is linked to health risks and calculate waist-to-hip ratios.
5. Describe how each of the following factors contributes to obesity: energy balance, fat cells, set point, heredity, metabolism, and nutrient composition of food.

6. Define basal metabolic rate (BMR), and identify five factors that affect it.
7. Distinguish a healthy weight loss program from a fad/diet program.
8. Identify and explain the three major components of effective lifetime weight management.
9. List five ways exercise helps in weight management.
10. Compare and contrast the eating disorders: bulimia nervosa, anorexia nervosa, and binge eating disorder.

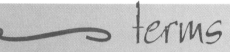 terms

- Anorexia nervosa
- Basal metabolic rate (BMR)
- Behavior modification
- Binge eating disorder
- Body fat
- Body mass index (BMI)
- Bulimia nervosa

- Calorie (kcal)
- Cellulite
- Eating disorder
- Essential fat
- Fat cells (adipose cells)
- Fat-free mass
- Glycogen

- Lean-body mass (muscle mass)
- Liposuction
- Obesity
- Overweight
- Set point
- Storage fat
- Weight cycling (yo-yo syndrome)

chapter eleven

Americans are preoccupied with weight. It is likely that you know your weight within 5 pounds. Every birth announcement gives the baby's weight to the exact ounce. Weight scales are commonplace in American bathrooms. This preoccupation has made weight control a multibillion-dollar business. Americans spend approximately $33 billion yearly on weight-reduction products (including diet foods and drinks) and services.

The craze to lose weight (whether needed or not) is reflected by the millions of Americans who report that they are dieting. Approximately half of women and one-third of men in the United States are trying to lose weight at any moment. Bookstore shelves and magazine racks are crammed with diet plans guaranteed to help you lose those extra inches. Television, radio, and newspapers further advertise a multitude of weight-loss options. Advertisements nailed to telephone poles promise: "lose 30 pounds in 30 days." With all of this attention and effort, one would predict that the American population would be lean. Actually, obesity is a major health problem in our country. Overweight and obesity account for 300,000 U.S. deaths per year, second only to tobacco as the most preventable cause of death. The prevalence of obesity increased from 15 percent in 1979 to 27 percent in 1999 (almost doubling in only 20 years). This unprecedented epidemic is consistent in all states; in both sexes; and across all age groups, races, and educational levels. The greatest magnitude of increase was found in the following groups:

- 18- to 29-year olds (7.1 to 12.1 percent)
- college-educated (10.6 to 17.8 percent)
- Hispanic ethnicity (11.6 to 20.8 percent)

Because the obesity trend is increasing so rapidly, many health professionals feel that obesity is the most common and serious health threat to Americans. "At the rate we're going now, every American will be overweight in 20 years," maintains Barbara Rolls, Ph.D., a professor of nutrition at Penn State University who has studied obesity for more than two decades.

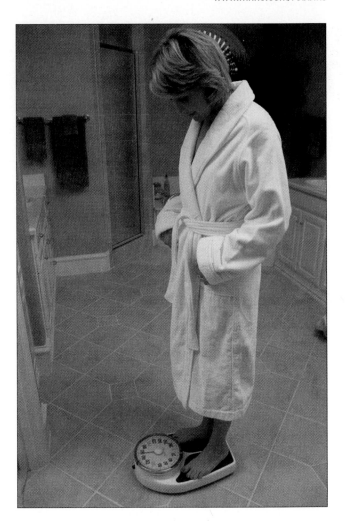

Although people are concerned about their weight, obesity is on the rise.

Although there appears to be an increased interest in diets and dieting, decreasing fat consumption, and overall "healthy" eating, few dieters achieve their weight goals. Most of those who do lose weight are unable to keep the weight off. On the other extreme, the incidence of anorexia nervosa and bulimia nervosa is at an epidemic level. The paradoxes of these facts reveal how complex America's weight problem is.

Maintaining a reasonable body weight is a definite wellness issue. Your body is the vehicle by which you function in society. Being overfat can affect you physically, emotionally, socially, and occupationally. The purpose of wellness is to strive toward full potential, so maintaining a reasonable body composition is one step toward achieving wellness. Knowledge gives you the tools to plan your lifetime weight-management scheme. It is important that you understand body composition facts, effective weight-loss principles, weight-management guidelines, and the influence of heredity and environment on weight control.

wellness flash

Sorry Walt Disney, but it isn't such a small world after all (at least in the United States) . . . 61 percent of adults are overweight or obese; with a whopping 27 percent considered to be obese.

Understanding Body Composition

Your body is composed of body fat and fat-free mass. **Fat-free mass** includes muscle, bone, body fluids, and organs. Muscles, part of your fat-free mass, are often specifically referred to as **lean-body mass** or **muscle mass.** Body fat is classified as either essential fat or storage fat. **Essential fat,** required for normal body functioning, is stored in major body organs and tissues such as the heart, muscles, intestines, bones, lungs, liver, spleen, and kidneys and throughout the central nervous system. Females have additional essential fat in the breasts and pelvic region for child bearing and other hormone-related functions. **Storage fat** is the extra fat that accumulates in adipose cells (or fat cells) around internal organs and beneath the skin surface to insulate, pad, and protect the body from trauma and extreme cold. As you learned in Chapter 3, there are different ways of assessing body composition. Knowing your body composition (especially your percentage of body fat) can help you set realistic weight goals.

Overweight Versus Obesity

Too often, the terms *overweight* and *obesity* are used interchangeably. **Overweight** refers to an excess of body weight compared to a set standard (in this case, a body mass index of 25 to 29.9). **Obesity** refers specifically to having an abnormally high proportion of body fat (a body mass index ≥ 30). You may at one time have seen height-weight charts published by the Metropolitan Life Insurance Company. These charts, based on mortality rates of persons who purchased life insurance policies, have been widely distributed since the 1940s. Metropolitan regularly updates these charts. You have probably seen one of these charts in a physician's office or magazine and looked to see where you rank. There has been considerable controversy and criticism over the appropriateness of these charts. They list desirable weight ranges for three specific frame sizes. The frame sizes give too much latitude of choice, and non-Caucasians are underreported in these tables. Also, the mortality data for life insurance purposes does not necessarily correlate to a desirable weight for wellness, vitality, and quality of life.

A more suitable measure for assessing the relationship between weight and health risk is the body mass index (BMI). **Body Mass Index (BMI)** is a direct calculation based on your height and weight and is a guideline for determining healthy weights and risky weights. BMI has been universally adopted by scientists and health professionals. BMI is computed from the following equation:

$$BMI = \frac{\text{weight in kilograms}}{(\text{height in meters})^2}$$

A second (and somewhat simpler) method of calculating your BMI is:

BMI = [(weight in lbs × 705) ÷ height in inches] ÷ height in inches

Table 11-1 allows you to quickly determine your BMI. Note the classifications below the chart. These standards have been adopted worldwide and are referred to in many articles and reports on obesity and weight management. In this way, overweight and obesity are clearly defined. BMI is not gender specific. For example, a 5'6" woman who weighs 155 pounds is considered overweight. If she weighs 186 pounds, she is classified as obese. A 6'0" man weighing 184 pounds is overweight. At 221 pounds, he is considered obese. Table 11-2 distinguishes the current BMI classifications for American adults. Also look at Figure 11-1 to see comparisons of ethnic groups in regards to percentages of overweight.

One disadvantage of using the BMI is that it remains a measure of weight and height, not fatness (i.e., it doesn't distinguish between body fat and muscle mass). Therefore it may not be appropriate for an athlete or body builder. Also, for the elderly who have lost a lot of muscle mass, their BMI may reflect a "healthy weight," when in actuality they have reduced nutritional reserves. Therefore, an analysis of your body fat percentage using the skinfold calipers gives a more accurate body composition assessment (i.e., body fat versus lean body mass). A woman over 30 percent body fat or a man over 25 percent are considered obese. (See Chapter 3 for more on skinfold measuring and body composition.)

Risks Associated with Obesity

The health implications of excess weight are becoming more clear. Obesity is identified as a risk factor in 5 of the 10 leading causes of death. The major killers associated with obesity are heart disease, some types of cancer, stroke, type 2 diabetes,

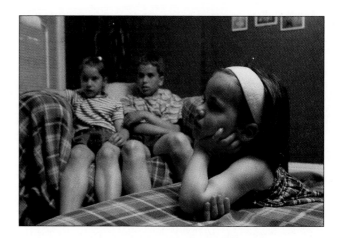

The prevalence of overweight in children in the United States has more than doubled in the past 3 decades. The 20-plus hours per week the average child spends watching TV and videos is a major contributing factor.

table 11-1   Find Your Body Mass Index (BMI)

Find your height, then look across that row. Your BMI is at the top of the column that contains your weight.

Body Mass Index (BMI)

Height	19	20	21	22	23	24	25	26	27	28	29	30	35	40
							Weight (pounds)							
4'10"	91	96	100	105	110	115	119	124	129	134	138	143	167	191
4'11"	94	99	104	109	114	119	124	128	133	138	143	148	173	198
5'0"	97	102	107	112	118	123	128	133	138	143	148	153	179	204
5'1"	100	106	111	116	122	127	132	137	143	148	153	158	185	211
5'2"	104	109	115	120	126	131	136	142	147	153	158	164	191	218
5'3"	107	113	118	124	130	135	141	146	152	158	163	169	197	225
5'4"	110	116	122	128	134	140	145	151	157	163	169	174	204	232
5'5"	114	120	126	132	138	144	150	156	162	168	174	180	210	240
5'6"	118	124	130	136	142	148	155	161	167	173	179	186	216	247
5'7"	121	127	134	140	146	153	159	166	172	178	185	191	223	255
5'8"	125	131	138	144	151	158	164	171	177	184	190	197	230	262
5'9"	128	135	142	149	155	162	169	176	182	189	196	203	236	270
5'10"	132	139	146	153	160	167	174	181	188	195	202	207	243	278
5'11"	136	143	150	157	165	172	179	186	193	200	208	215	250	286
6'0"	140	147	154	162	169	177	184	191	199	206	213	221	258	294
6'1"	144	151	159	166	174	182	189	197	204	212	219	227	265	302
6'2"	148	155	163	171	179	186	194	202	210	218	225	233	272	311
6'3"	152	160	168	176	184	192	200	208	216	224	232	240	279	319
6'4"	156	164	172	180	189	197	205	213	221	230	238	246	287	328
			NORMAL					OVERWEIGHT				OBESE		

Interpreting Your BMI

- ≤18.9 Underweight
- 19–24.9 Healthy Weight (little health risk)
- 25–29.9 Overweight (increased health risk)
- ≥30 Obesity (greatest health risk)

Source: National Institutes of Health; National Heart, Lung and Blood Institute

table 11-2   BMIs and Current Classifications of American Adults (Ages 20 years and older)

Healthy Weight (BMI ≥ 19 to < 25	36%
Overweight (BMI ≥ 25)	61%
Obese (BMI ≥ 30)	27%

Source: Centers for Disease Control and Prevention, National Center for Health Statistics, December 2000.

and atherosclerosis. Obesity can aggravate high blood pressure, cardiovascular problems, liver disorders, and arthritis. Obesity is often found in conjunction with diabetes and gallbladder disease. Recent statistics show an alarming rise in the number of cases of type 2 diabetes due to the increasing obesity rates in the United States.

Obesity complicates surgery and pregnancy. Pulmonary problems, heat intolerance, and reduced fertility are more prevalent in the obese. Among obese women there is an increased risk of endometrial uterine, and breast cancers. Obese men face an increased chance of colon, rectum, and prostate cancer. Obesity restricts mobility, increases fatigue, and decreases overall body efficiency. Figure 11-2 shows the percent increase in risk of various conditions related to specific BMIs.

The high prevalence of obesity in the United States is not only linked to numerous chronic diseases, but is responsible for a substantial portion of total health-care costs. Obesity health-care costs exceed $100 billion per year. This figure does not include the psychosocial costs of obesity—from lowered self-esteem to eating disorders to severe clinical depression. The psychological and social consequences of obesity are often overlooked. Obese people also face a tremendous amount of prejudice and discrimination. Their educational and professional opportunities often suffer.

Until recently, modest weight gains throughout adulthood of initially lean individuals were overlooked and even culturally expected. Results from the ongoing Nurses' Health Study (a 14-year tracking of 115,818 nurses) have revealed that even *modest* (11 to 17 lbs) weight gains after 18 years of age increase one's cardiovascular disease risk. The researchers concluded that there is a large fraction of the population falsely reassured that their weight is not a health concern because they are not "overweight." The study found that a person's weight at midlife (30 to 55 years) has the greatest influence on heart disease risk. Those with a BMI of 23 to 27 had a 31 percent increased risk; those with the lowest risk had a BMI below 21. Those with a BMI ≥ 30 have a 50 to 100 percent increased risk of death from *all* causes, compared to those with healthy BMIs (19 to 24.9).

Location of Fat

Studies suggest that it is not only body fat percentage and BMI related to health, but the location of excess fat is a strong risk factor also. Fat distributed primarily in the abdominal area (called *apple-shape obesity*) is characteristic of many men (but also present in some women). This apple-shape obesity is linked to increased risk for coronary heart disease, hypertension, high cholesterol, type 2 diabetes, and some forms of cancer. Fat distributed in the lower extremities, around the hips, buttocks, and thighs (called *pear-shape obesity*) does not present as great a risk. Pear-shape obesity is more common in women. The two types of fat have bio-

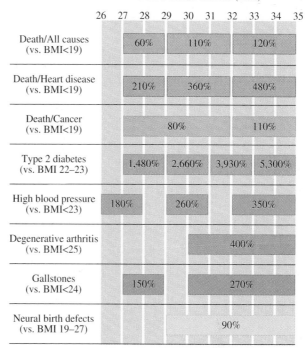

figure 11-2   Weighing the risks. Percent increase in risk by level of obesity. At BMIs of 27 and higher, one's risk for various disorders increases significantly.

Source: New England Journal of Medicine, Annals of Internal Medicine, American Journal of Clinical Nutrition, Journal of the American Medical Association, Circulation

Diversity Issues: Overweight Statistics of Selected Ethnic Groups in the U.S. (ages 20 years and older) Represents BMI ≥25

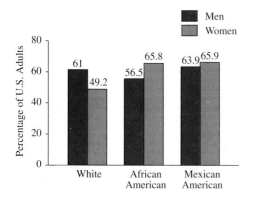

figure 11-1   No specific percentages are available for Native Americans or Asian-Americans. However, Native Americans have higher percentages, and Asian-Americans have lower percentages than the three groups listed in the graph.

Source: National Institutes of Health

chemical differences. Abdominal fat experiences much more enzyme activity, dumping more fatty acids into the bloodstream. Hip-thigh fat activity is more stagnant. Unfortunately, this hip-thigh fat is more difficult to lose than is abdominal fat. Some obesity experts feel that one's waist-to-hip ratio is as important as the BMI in predicting potential weight-related health problems because abdominal fat is so heavily linked to diseases. Waist-to-hip ratio can be calculated by dividing the number of inches around the waistline by the circumference of the hips. See Table 11-3 for examples of waist-to-hip ratios. For example, someone who has a 30-inch waist and 40-inch hips has a ratio of 0.75. A woman whose ratio is 0.80 or higher is at risk, as is a man whose ratio is 0.95 or above.

Some feel that the waist circumference *alone* can be a predictor of risk. Men with a waist circumference over 40 inches and women with a waist circumference over 35 inches are classified as high risk no matter what their BMI. An excess of abdominal fat in women has been linked to breast cancer. Whereas the distribution of fat has some genetic link, a comprehensive program of a low-fat, reduced-calorie diet and regular exercise can help reduce body fat stores, regardless of where they are located.

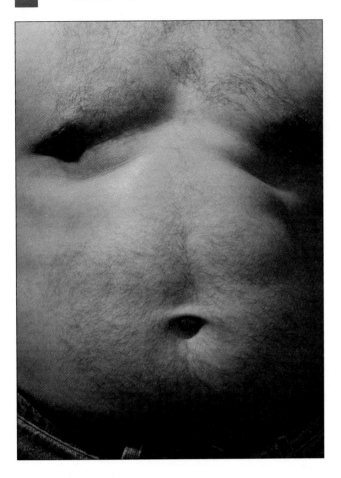

A man or woman having a large amount of abdominal fat increases the risk of heart disease, stroke, Type 2 diabetes, and cancer.

What Causes Obesity?

For years, the popular explanation for obesity was that people became obese because they ate too much. Obesity was viewed as a condition resulting from a lack of self-control around food. In scientific terms, obesity occurs when a person's caloric intake exceeds the amount of energy he or she burns. What causes this imbalance between consuming and burning calories is unclear. Evidence suggests that obesity is a complex puzzle of metabolic, genetic, psychological, behavioral, social, and environmental factors—not solely a result of a lack of individual willpower. It is clear that no single factor results in obesity. In an attempt to explain the causes of obesity, several factors have to be examined. These include energy balance, fat cells, set point, heredity, metabolism, and the nutrient composition of food.

The Energy Balance Equation

The energy balance equation states that energy input (calories consumed) must be equal to energy output (calories ex-

pended) for body weight to remain constant. Any imbalance in energy input or energy output will result in a change in body weight. If you eat more calories daily than your body expends in activity, you will store the excesses as fat. If you eat fewer calories than you burn, you will lose weight. It is unrealistic to assume that the equation must be exactly equal every day to maintain your weight. Some days you eat more; some days less. Some days you are more active than you are other days. Several days of imbalance in one direction will produce a change in body weight.

This explanation assumes that a calorie is a calorie, whether it is calories from candy or from a vegetable. A **calorie** (actually a **kcal**) is a measure of energy. One pound of body fat equals 3,500 calories of stored energy. Therefore, consuming an extra 3,500 calories will cause you to gain 1 pound of fat. If you burn an extra 3,500 calories with activity, you will lose 1 pound. To cause a reduction in body weight, you (1) reduce calorie intake below the energy requirement; (2) increase the calorie output through additional physical activity above energy requirements; or (3) combine the two methods by reducing calorie intake and increasing calorie output. So how do you lose 10 pounds? By creating a calorie deficit of 500 calories daily (by either increasing exercise or decreasing food intake) for 7 days, you will lose 1 pound (3,500 calories). By maintaining this deficit, you will be 10 pounds lighter in 10 weeks.

However, weight loss is not necessarily this simple. For some, cutting calories causes feelings of fatigue, resulting in a decrease of energy expenditure. As body weight is reduced, the energy costs of movement go down proportionately, thus reducing caloric output. Also, individual differences in resting metabolic rates, cellular makeup, and lean tissue need to be considered. That is why knowledge about other factors is necessary to fully understand the complexities of weight loss.

Regardless of the problems that come with relying solely on the energy balance equation as the only way to understand weight loss and weight gain, this equation is the best way of explaining why, in this age of modernization and decreased physical demands, so many Americans are too fat. Most are not active enough to use the calories consumed. Food in America is plentiful, available, and relatively inexpensive. It is also high in sugar, calories, and fat. More frequent eating is encouraged by numerous societal changes: the growth of the fast-food industry, 24-hour supermarkets, "pop-in" pantries, the increased marketing of snack foods, the number of "all you can eat" buffets, and the growing tendency to socialize with food and drink have all added calo-

table 11-3 — Sample Waist-to-Hip Ratios

$$\text{Waist-to-Hip Ratio} = \frac{\text{Waist circumference}}{\text{Hip circumference}}$$

(see Chapter 3 for specific measuring instructions)

$$\frac{\text{waist}}{\text{hip}} = \frac{26"}{35"} = 0.74 \qquad \frac{\text{waist}}{\text{hip}} = \frac{40"}{42"} = 0.95$$

$$\frac{\text{waist}}{\text{hip}} = \frac{32"}{40"} = 0.80 \qquad \frac{\text{waist}}{\text{hip}} = \frac{40"}{37"} = 1.08$$

$$\frac{\text{waist}}{\text{hip}} = \frac{38"}{42"} = 0.90 \qquad \frac{\text{waist}}{\text{hip}} = \frac{45"}{39"} = 1.15$$

Higher risk is associated with a ratio >0.8 for women and >0.95 for men.

recommended 30 minutes of exercise five times per week at *any* intensity! Twenty-five percent are completely sedentary.

How many calories do you need to maintain a desirable body weight? Table 11-4 helps you estimate your daily caloric need based on your activity level. Remember, this is only an approximation and may vary between individuals. To lose or gain weight, the calorie intake must be adjusted upward or downward.

Fat-Cell Theory

The size and number of fat cells in the body determine degrees of fatness. **Fat cells** (also known as **adipose cells**) are storage sites for energy. The body increases fat storage in two ways: by increasing the *number* of fat cells and by increasing the *size* of the fat cells. As might be expected, the body increases its number of fat cells during childhood and teenage growth spurts. Fat cells also expand and contract as energy is stored or burned. They can expand to two to three times their normal size, but they cannot enlarge endlessly. At some point, new fat cells are created in response to the body's need to store more excess energy. It is well-accepted that, contrary to earlier theories, increases in fat cell number can occur throughout adult life. This capacity to increase cell numbers when a maximum cell size is reached depends on the age and sex of the person and on the site of the fat tissue. Unfortunately, once a fat cell has been created, it exists for life. Fat cells do not seem to be destructible. There are about 25 billion fat cells in a normal-weight individual versus 60 to 80 billion in the extremely obese.

Therefore, the fat-cell theory proposes that weight reduction in adults is a result of decreasing the size of the fat cells, shrinking them by using the energy stored in them or not filling them at all. This theory also explains why people who grow a large number of fat cells during childhood have a predisposition to obesity as adults. They can reduce the amount of fat stored in the cells, but the excess number of fat cells is still there, waiting to be filled again.

ries to our day. Although many people are consuming lower-fat food items, *low fat* doesn't necessarily mean *low calorie*. Surveys indicate that our daily caloric intake is increasing, while our caloric expenditure is decreasing. Countless labor-saving devices at home and work and our passive leisure-time activities (television, Internet, computer games, videos) have contributed to creeping obesity. Phoning, faxing, e-mailing, and express mail don't burn many calories (unless you're the express mail delivery person!). Many neighborhoods lack sidewalks for safe walking, and the automobile is used to travel even the shortest distances. There are fewer opportunities in daily life to burn calories. We live increasingly sedentary lives. The average American watches 16 hours of television per week and only 22 percent get the

table 11-4 — Determining Your Daily Caloric Needs

The following is a method for estimating the caloric needs for healthy, nonpregnant adults. Older individuals (over age 50) should further reduce calories by 10 to 20 percent. These are only estimates. Individual activity factors and body frames vary from person to person.
Formula: Weight × Activity level = Calories needed daily

Activity Level	Calories Needed Per Pound Per Day	
	Female	Male
Inactive (little or no regular exercise; desk job; light work)	× 12	× 14
Moderately Active (20–30 minutes of exercise at least 3–4 times per week)	× 14	× 16
Very Active (30–45 minutes of vigorous, sustained exercise 5–7 times per week)	× 16	× 18

Example: female = 140 lbs (desirable weight) × 14 (moderately active) = 1,960 calories per day
male = 180 lbs (desirable weight) × 14 (inactive) = 2,520 calories per day

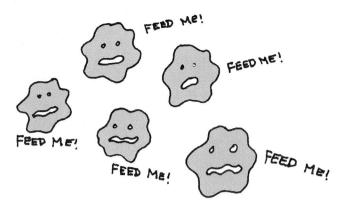

Fat cells are with you forever.

Knowing that obese children often become obese adults, it is easy to see one way to prevent obesity. Control the development of new fat cells during childhood and teenage years with regular exercise and sensible eating. This makes more sense than letting children become obese in the first place. This fact makes us question why daily physical education is being cut from most school programs. In this day and age, children need more daily exercise, not less.

When going on a low calorie diet, the adult with an excessive number of fat cells gets caught in a trap. A large number of empty fat cells is a biologically abnormal state. The body's natural tendency is to defend its fat cell size. As a result, the appetite control center in the brain is stimulated, causing the dieter to eat more calories. This condition of "starved fat cells" is the reason most dieters (especially in the obese category) eventually regain their lost weight. This is also the reason obese people on treatment programs tend to stop losing weight when their fat cells shrink to normal size. In this way, obesity can become a lifelong condition. *Prevention* is the key.

Set-Point Theory

The set-point theory maintains that every individual is programmed to be a certain weight and that the body regulates itself to maintain that "set" weight. Studies of people in alternating states of semistarvation and gorging have shown that, once intervention ceases, they return to their former weights. What determines your **set point?** The hypothalamus in the brain may act as a body weight thermostat, lowering body metabolism and increasing hunger if fat levels fall below the set point. Here is where the set-point theory and fat-cell theory merge. The set-point mechanism is thought to respond to signals sent out by the fat cells as to the amount of fat in storage. The weight at which this occurs may depend on the number of fat cells. Consider two 180-pound women. Sara has a normal number of fat cells, which are enlarged. Mary has an excessive number of fat cells of normal size. Sara has a greater chance of weight loss, because

she can reduce her cell size and still sustain adequate fat volume. Mary faces a harder battle, because her body will work to maintain her cell size. This theory also helps explain why attempts at permanent weight loss by crash dieting are not successful. The body naturally fights against this starvation state.

The set-point theory is based on survival. How else could populations endure famine or our ancestors survive periods of food shortages? Heredity influences the set point, too. Some people have naturally higher set points, causing maintenance of higher levels of body fat. Whereas some individuals have naturally low set points.

Can you change your set point? Some studies show that sustained consumption of a high-fat diet (the typical American diet?) raises the set point and that regular, vigorous exercise can lower the set point. Exercise stimulates changes in metabolism, thus causing the body to use fat rather than protect against its losses. Knowing this it is easy to see how our growing sedentary lifestyles and dietary habits are more likely connected to America's obesity problem than are brain thermostat alterations. We've gone from lean to fat because we eat more and exert ourselves less.

Heredity

"I can't lose weight; it's in my genes!" Many would view this exclamation made by many obese persons as an excuse for their physical state. Research about genetic influences of obesity lends some (but not *total*) credibility to this exclamation. Children with obese parents do have a greater tendency to become obese adults. Is this an inherited tendency or a result of inappropriate behaviors learned and reinforced at home? Studies of families (especially twins) have provided insights to this question. A classic study conducted by Claude Bouchard showed that adult identical twins were similar in *total* fat gain and *distribution* of fat gain when consistently overfed for 100 days. There were huge differences between pairs of twins as to body weight gains, body composition changes, and waist/hip circumference changes. Between twins, however, there were striking similarities. Similar research shows that adult twins tend to be similar in body weight and body mass index regardless of whether they were raised together in the same home or separated in early childhood and raised in different environments. Heredity seems to influence the number of fat cells in the body, how much fat is stored, where it is stored, and metabolic rates. However, scientists have concluded that genetics are responsible for only 33 percent of these factors. Scientists are actively investigating the possible existence of a "fat gene" that may influence levels of fatness.

Although these facts address a role heredity has in obesity, heredity is only a *tendency* or predisposing factor that can be influenced by environmental components and behaviors. Those people predisposed to be overweight or obese will have more difficulty controlling their weight, but it is certainly not impossible for them to attain and maintain a healthy weight with healthy eating habits and regular exercise.

Metabolism

Every individual expends a certain amount of energy, even at rest, to sustain the vital functions of the body such as brain activities, organ function, and temperature regulation. This energy requirement is called the **basal metabolic rate (BMR)** and accounts for approximately 60 to 75 percent of calories burned in 1 day. A true measure of basal (resting) metabolism is taken when you have been lying quietly but awake and without food for 12 to 15 hours. Most men have a BMR requirement of 1,600 to 1,800 calories daily; most women need 1,200 to 1,450 calories daily. Lab Activity 11-3 provides you an opportunity to determine your BMR. BMR is the largest component of your daily energy expenditure, so it can significantly affect body weight over time. It is an important yet highly individual factor in the development of obesity.

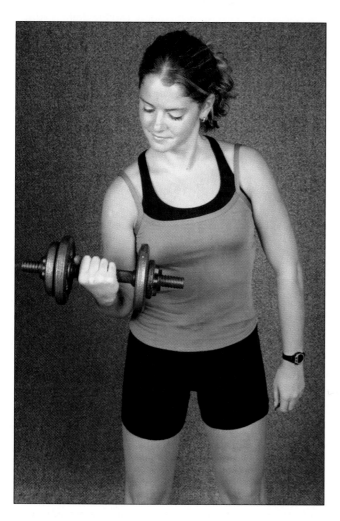

Doing resistance training exercises increases lean-body mass, which in turn increases metabolism.

Your BMR is a result of several interrelated factors, including age, gender, body size, nutritional status, musculature, activity level, and genetics. Pay particular attention to Table 11-5. It depicts how BMR is affected by each of these factors.

Although some of your BMR is genetically inherited, you can affect it with exercise. An aerobic workout that includes resistance training (free weights, machines, or exercise band) can increase muscle mass. The more muscle mass you have, the higher your BMR. Fat, being storage tissue, is inactive and has low metabolism; whereas muscle tissue is active and has a high metabolism. Women especially can counteract a slow metabolism by participating in exercise programs that include resistance training. In this way, they can increase their muscle mass. Middle-aged women often experience a dramatic slowdown of their metabolisms due to hormonal changes. They too can keep their "energy burners" fired up with regular exercise. The actual workout burns calories too! Your total daily caloric expenditure is influenced by:

1. Basal Metabolism = 60 to 75 percent
2. Digestion = 10 percent (e.g., if you consume 2,000 calories a day, you burn 200 of them by digesting the food)
3. Physical Activity and Exercise = anywhere from 15 to 40 percent (*you* control this!) Remember . . . *all* physical activity burns calories.

table 11-5 Factors That Affect Basal Metabolic Rate

Gender	Women generally have lower BMRs than do men (about 5 to 10 percent lower) due to smaller size, greater body fat, and less muscle mass.
Musculature	Increased muscle mass or tone increases BMR. Muscle tissue is more metabolically active than is fat. As muscles atrophy from inactivity, BMR declines.
Age	For both men and women, BMR declines by about 2 to 3 percent per decade after age 25. Loss of lean muscle mass typically occurs with aging as well. Maintaining a regular exercise program (including resistance training) can help prevent a decline of lean muscle mass and BMR as you age.
Body size	Smaller body surface area results in lower BMR.
Nutritional status	Fasting, very low calorie diets, or long-term undernutrition lower BMR.
Activity level	BMR increases during exercise and may remain elevated somewhat after exercising.
Genetics	We inherit physiological tendencies, and, as a result, BMR is inherently higher in some people and lower in others.

Nutrient Composition

The energy balance equation approach to weight loss/gain is based on the premise that all calories are created equal. That is, for weight loss, the *source* of calories is not important as long as the total calorie deficit is greater than the caloric intake. Studies report that total caloric intake is not correlated to obesity as much as dietary fat is. The premise is that a calorie is *not* a calorie. Fat is converted into body fat with greater ease than are carbohydrates and proteins. For example, for every 100 carbohydrate calories consumed, 23 calories are burned metabolizing it (converting it to a storable form), and about 77 calories are stored. In contrast, for every 100 fat calories consumed, only about 3 calories are used to metabolize it, leaving a whopping 97 calories available for storage in the fat cells. (There *is* one predominantly carbohydrate substance that has been found to easily convert to body fat—alcohol. This confirms the direct correlation between alcohol consumption and weight gain.) Some studies have shown that normal-weight and overweight persons may consume approximately the same number of calories, but the overweight persons derive a greater proportion of their calories from fat.

What About "Dieting"?

Most people who want to lose weight think immediately of going on a diet. This notion is reinforced by the number of new fad diets advertised each year. In this connotation, the word "diet" implies a distinctive way of eating that involves special foods or food combinations; caloric or food restrictions; or special powders, pills, or shakes. Whereas in reality, the word diet should imply a way of eating for a lifetime. Popular weight-loss diets are viewed by the user as a temporary inconvenience that will be discontinued as soon as the weight goal has been reached. "Going on" a diet implies "going off" it. Dieters assume that weight will be lost quickly and immediately. Chances are, however, that the excess pounds have accumulated gradually over a period of years. These pounds are maintained by ingrained habits. Most fad diets rely on rigid food choices. Food becomes the enemy and mealtime a battle to be fought. Practicing restraint can result in food cravings, binges, guilt, and self-deprecation. Many popular diets do not emphasize physical exercise. More than half of the overweight adults trying to lose weight are doing so by eating fewer calories. Yet, less than one-third are increasing physical activity. This is a reflection of our sedentary lifestyle and the emphasis on dieting as a means to control weight. Diets have special appeal and sound easy. Most of them, however, are nutritionally inadequate, too low in calories, potentially dangerous, and fail to teach lifelong eating habits. Table 11-6 lists some of the most common diet plans.

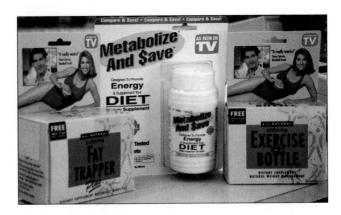

Be wary of diet aids that focus on a "quick fix."

If you choose to go on a very low-calorie diet, up to 70 percent of the weight loss during the first 3 days is water. This is predictable because your body needs carbohydrates for energy. Being starved of carbohydrates, it uses **glycogen** (stored carbohydrates) for energy. As you use this glycogen, you lose water, because each gram of carbohydrate is stored with 3 grams of water. Your body also uses protein for energy, resulting in a loss of muscle tissue. Crash dieting can cause headaches, ketosis, and loss of bone mineralization. If you go on a very-low-calorie diet (less than 800 calories per day), your body slows its metabolism (BMR) significantly. After all, your body doesn't know that there is a grocery store a block away. It reacts as if you were dying from starvation. Therefore, your body saves energy by burning fewer calories. This conservation of energy causes the diet to be even less effective. Depression, irritability, fatigue, and feelings of deprivation often follow. The survival urge to eat eventually wins out and weight is regained. When this happens, the crash dieter may become fatter for five reasons:

1. If old eating habits are resumed, the regained weight is fat; some of the weight loss was most likely lean tissue.
2. Metabolism can stay depressed.
3. Overeating (especially a preference for dietary fat) may occur in response to the past deprivation.
4. More fat cells can develop if the existing cells fill to capacity and divide.
5. Metabolic alterations can occur (i.e., fat can be stored more efficiently; the body conserves fat stores as a protective phenomenon against future losses).

Weight Cycling

Fad dieting does not produce lasting results, and repeated bouts of dieting result in improved efficiency in the body's adaptive response to semistarvation. The body interprets drastic dieting as a mortal threat, so basal metabolic rate slows in an effort to maintain life. This metabolic response

table 11-6 Diet Plans: Claims and Reality

Diet Plan	Claims	Reality
Commercial weight loss company (Weight Watchers, etc.)	Promotes a high-carbohydrate, low-fat diet. Provides advice on portions, food choices, calorie intake. Moderate loss of 1–2 lbs per week. Individual counseling and group support. (Note: Some commercial companies require purchase of their prepackaged foods, which can be expensive.)	Can be safe and effective if healthy lifelong eating habits and portion control are learned.
Meal-replacement drinks (Slim-Fast, Sweet Success, etc.)	A liquid shake replaces one or two meals a day. Shakes contain sugar, protein, and vitamins and are low in calories.	May be hungry; less satisfying. Calorie intake may be too low. Lacks fiber. Weight often regained when stopped because food selection has not been learned.
"Fat-Burning" diets (cabbage soup diet, grapefruit diet, etc.)	Certain foods can accelerate the body's ability to burn fat. Eating large quantities of these foods results in fast weight loss.	No foods exclusively burn fat. Low in calories (which causes the weight loss). Boring and not nutritionally balanced. Weight is regained easily.
Low carbohydrate/High protein diets (Adkins, Protein Power, etc.)	Severely restricts carbohydrates such as bread, cereals, starchy vegetables. Claims that carbs increase insulin, which promotes fat accumulation. Eat a lot of protein and fat.	Not supported by scientific evidence. Low calories. Loss of water and muscle causes the weight loss. High fat, low calcium, and lack of antioxidants contributes to future diseases. May cause bad breath, fatigue, dizziness, head-aches, constipation. Weight is regained when eating returns to normal.
Ornish diet ("Eat More, Weigh Less")	Fat-free foods and a lot of fruits, vegetables, whole grains, beans; limited dairy. Weight loss occurs despite eating ample amounts of food.	Healthy for heart and cancer prevention. Effective for weight loss, but hard for some to adhere to due to lack of fats. May be low in calcium and iron if not careful.
Diet pills	Claims to burn fat, absorb extra fat, increase metabolism, and/or suppress appetite.	Promoted as a "quick fix." May contain amphetamine-like substances (ephedra, ma huang), which may cause heart irregularities and jitters. Some herbs may help with appetite in some, but safety is an issue. Lifelong eating habits not learned.
Glycemic index ("The Glucose Revolution")	Carbohydrates that break down quickly (i.e., have a high glycemic index—G.I.) cause a quick blood sugar and insulin rise, resulting in fat storage. Slow-release carbohydrates (low G.I.), fill you up, cause a slower release of glucose, decrease blood sugar fluxuations, and burn body fat.	Is a balanced approach of consuming adequate protein, low fat (under 30%), and 60% carbohydrate (of low G.I.: whole grains, legumes, vegetables, some fruits) and reducing refined breads, cereals, rices, potatoes, and snacks). Is sensible and healthy, but requires learning high G.I. from low G.I. foods.
Insulin-Resistance diets ("The Zone," etc.)	Meals/foods must be eaten in proper carb-to-protein-to-fat ratio (40:30:30) to combat the insulin production that may prompt fat storage.	No scientific evidence that a diet of complex carbs causes the body to store fat or increase appetite. Nor does food combining make a difference. Is low in calories, which causes the weight loss.

causes greater difficulty in losing weight and greater efficiency in gaining weight. As a result, many obese people have repetitive bouts of weight loss and weight gain. This cycle is known as **weight cycling** (or the **yo-yo syndrome**). In this cycle, fat is often lost slower and regained faster with each repeated dieting bout. Therefore, yo-yo dieting affords the body repeated opportunities to enhance its efficiency at storing energy—a function of fat cells. Incessant dieting may be one reason many Americans are fatter today than ever.

Much attention has been focused by the lay press and professional journals on possible physiological and psychological dangers of weight cycling—even suggesting that stay-ing overweight may be safer in terms of heart disease or premature death than riding the diet roller coaster. Experts on a National Institutes of Health task force reviewed 43 human studies on yo-yo dieting, finding that the evidence for the claimed adverse health effects is not convincing or consistent (i.e., yo-yo dieting by itself does not increase the risk of dying from heart disease). The scientists admitted, however, that repeatedly regaining hard-lost pounds *may* result in depression and a loss of self-esteem. Millions of overweight people stand to benefit from loss of fat, and worries about weight cycling should not be a deterrent. Although health problems associated with weight cycling have not been proven, the health-related problems of obesity are well known. As with any attempt at changing a habit, you may experience cycles of success and relapse before succeeding. This information accentuates even more dramatically the need to learn *skills* for maintaining weight loss and to *prevent* obesity from occurring altogether. Losing weight—and maintaining a healthy weight—is a lifelong commitment.

Reliable Weight-Loss Programs

Are there any reliable weight-loss programs? Yes. There are some good programs available, as long as the dieter understands the purpose and limitations of commercial-based plans. Enrolling in a weight-control program is an investment of time, energy, and money. Ask yourself if you are ready to lose the weight *and* do what it takes to keep it off. Losing the weight is only half the battle. Keeping it off demands lifestyle changes that are lifelong. It is especially important for the morbidly obese to seek professional help in losing weight. These persons would be wise to consult one of the hospital-based programs available in many communities or meet with a registered dietitian. New fad diets appear almost weekly and disappear almost as quickly, so it is unrealistic to assess every particular diet for strengths and weaknesses. Instead, look at the top ten guidelines in evaluating any weight-loss program.

The goal of weight loss is fat loss, which takes time and long-term lifestyle change. Many diets are variations on the food restriction theme, are unpleasant, and fail to teach modification of eating behavior. Scarcity and deprivation often lead to bingeing and subsequent feelings of guilt and despair. Just about any type of food restriction will result in weight loss. The key is keeping the weight off by learning to live with food–forever!

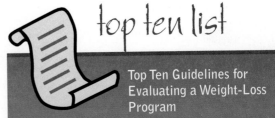

top ten list

Top Ten Guidelines for Evaluating a Weight-Loss Program

1. It should use real, regular food available in supermarkets.
2. It should provide an energy deficit to allow slow, safe weight loss of 1 to 2 pounds per week.
3. It should encourage the reduction of fat in the diet.
4. It should encourage a safe, personalized exercise program.
5. It should not promise a quick fix or advertise claims that sound too good to be true.
6. It should teach lifelong changes that allow freedom and flexibility for individual lifestyles and not list "good" and "forbidden" foods.
7. It should make possible the enjoyment of social situations such as eating out, holidays, and special occasions.
8. It should allow for basic energy needs (never under 1,200 calories daily) and be nutritionally balanced (the Food Guide Pyramid, U.S. dietary guidelines, etc.).
9. It should not be too costly.
10. It should teach techniques and strategies for *maintaining* positive behavior change.

A final question to ask yourself when considering a diet plan should be, "Can I live on this diet for the rest of my life?"

Lifetime Weight Management: Strategies for Success

The factors that contribute to obesity are so numerous and complex that it is impossible to pinpoint one cause. Having knowledge of the theories of obesity should help you understand some of these complexities. Fat cells, metabolism, set points, genetics, and energy expenditure all play a role. Behaviors that have developed over time are also intricately involved. One unrefuted truth emerges in nearly all weight-control studies: *Permanent weight control involves a lifelong commitment to good eating habits and regular exercise*. There is evidence that young adults in their early 20s gain a disproportionate amount of weight by the time they are 30, making them an important population segment for obesity pre-

vention efforts. If you are in this age group, this should help motivate you to commit to a lifetime weight-management plan. Weight management is a lifestyle. Maintaining a reasonable body composition is, rather than isolated bouts of crash dieting or sporadic exercise, a result of lifelong integration of three management components:

1. Food management
2. Emotional management
3. Exercise management

Food Management

We must eat everyday to sustain life. And, eating is one of life's pleasures. To lose or maintain weight, it is essential to have a good framework for making sensible, well-balanced food choices. Basic weight-management principles are not different from general good nutritional recommendations (low fat, sugar, and salt and high complex carbohydrates and fiber). Cutting the fat from your diet reduces a tremendous number of calories. "I lost weight without eating less!" is often the exclamation of persons who substitute fiber-rich grains, fruits, and vegetables for fat in their diets. Fiber fills you up and slows the absorption of food, which regulates blood sugar and insulin levels. You may want to conduct an experiment by trying some of the foods on the top ten list of "filling foods." Do they fill you up?

The eating plan for weight control on which most experts agree is one that is relatively low in fat and sugar and high in fruits, vegetables, and grains. This diet does not only help with weight, but it helps prevent disease while ensuring adequate intake of all essential nutrients. The *2000 Dietary Guidelines for Americans* and the Food Guide Pyramid (see Chapter 10) describe such an eating plan.

It appears that the main causes of obesity are eating too many fats, sugars, and calories *and* participating in only low levels of physical activity. Carbohydrates and the new fat-free foods have calories, too. Some people think that they can eat as much of a fat-free food as they want without gaining weight! Overall calorie consumption cannot completely be ignored. Although many Americans are consuming less fat as a percentage of total calories, average daily calorie consumption has increased (up an average of 150 calories per day). That's a weight gain of 15 extra pounds a year! One culprit is that portion and serving sizes have increased tremendously. The words "biggie," "supersize," and "double stuff" commonly describe ordinary servings. For example, a standard one-serving bran muffin should be the size of a cupcake. Some oversized deli muffins pack a whopping 550 calories and 26 grams of fat!

Restaurants are especially guilty of over feeding us. Plates overfilled with pasta, nachos, french fries, and steak are common. Parking lots at all-you-can-eat buffets are packed. Surprisingly, one survey revealed that most Americans (78 percent) believe that the *kind* of food they eat is more important for managing weight than the *amount* of

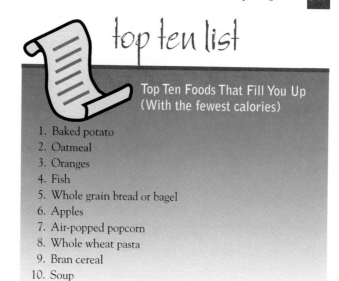

top ten list

Top Ten Foods That Fill You Up
(With the fewest calories)

1. Baked potato
2. Oatmeal
3. Oranges
4. Fish
5. Whole grain bread or bagel
6. Apples
7. Air-popped popcorn
8. Whole wheat pasta
9. Bran cereal
10. Soup

food they eat. Many foreigners who visit the United States often express amazement at the amount of food served in American homes and restaurants. Being aware of portion sizes and calorie amounts is as important as understanding fat content in foods. Use the serving sizes on the Food Guide Pyramid (in Chapter 10) as a guideline, and learn to "eye ball" the servings you are consuming. Also be sure to look at food labels to determine what is considered "a serving."

What is considered a low-fat diet? Most dietitians recommend that the diet be composed of a *minimum* of 20 percent fat of total caloric intake. Some fat is necessary, especially for fat-soluble vitamins to be used. Therefore, a fat intake of 20 to 25 percent of daily calories is a reasonable low-fat diet. (This is slightly below the American Heart Association's recommendation of 30 percent for heart health.) Table 10-6 in Chapter 10 translates fat intakes of 10 to 30 percent into daily fat grams for various caloric levels. Being aware of caloric values of foods, the food groups, portion sizes, sources of "hidden" fats, and energy needs can help you make sensible food choices. Figure 11-3 gives examples of how the Food Guide Pyramid can be personalized for sensible and healthy caloric intakes depending on your weight management agenda. Learning to read food labels and alter recipes to lower the fat content is where nutritional knowledge plays a major role in lifetime weight management. See Chapter 10 for fat-lowering tips.

Traditional weight-loss diets often feature a lot of "can" and "cannot have" foods. Sensibility in food choices does not mean that you will never again eat chocolate cake. There should never be guilt or forbidden foods. Instead, lifetime weight management means seeing how much or where chocolate cake fits into your total diet. Reduce, don't eliminate, certain foods. Balance your food choices over time. Gradual rather than drastic changes in dietary patterns lead

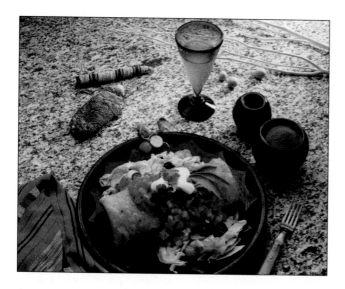

As restaurant serving portions become larger, Americans are "supersizing" their way to obesity.

For weight management (losing, maintaining, or gaining), counting servings from the food guide pyramid is an easy way to adjust your food intake for specific calorie requirements. In this way, balance and variety can be assured.

1200 CALORIES	1500 CALORIES		1800 CALORIES	2400 CALORIES
2	2	MEAT	2	3
2	2	MILK	3	3
2	3	FRUIT	3	4
3	3	VEGETABLES	4	5
6	7	GRAINS	8	10

Example: an 1800-calorie day (in parentheses after each food item: calories/fat grams/number of servings)

BREAKFAST	SNACK	LUNCH	SNACK	DINNER	SNACK
2 oz. cereal (220/5/2) 1 c. skim milk (80/0/1) 6 oz. orange juice (90/0/1)	1/2 bagel (100/1/1)	2 slices whole wheat bread (140/4/2) 3 oz. deli-style turkey (120/4/1) 1/2 c. green beans (25/0/1) banana (100/0/1)	apple (85/0/1)	2 burritos: 2 sm. tortillas (180/4/2) 3 oz. chicken, diced (240/6/1) 1/2 c. chopped, cooked broccoli (30/0/1) 1 1/2 oz. mozzarella cheese (120/8/1) 1 c. lettuce (10/0/1) 1/2 c. salsa (40/0/1) 1 c. frozen yogurt (160/4/1)	2 c. microwave popcorn (60/4/1)

TOTALS: 1800 calories
40 grams fat (20% of calories)
meat = 2 servings
milk = 3 servings
fruit = 3 servings
vegetables = 4 servings
grains = 8 servings

figure 11-3   Food Guide Pyramid weight management plan.

wellness flash

Food industry messages often drown out health messages . . . for example, more than $33 billion per year is spent on advertising sugary soft drinks, candy, and fatty snacks. In contrast, the National Cancer Institute's maximum annual advertising budget to promote the "5-A-Day" (fruit and vegetable) campaign is $1 million.

to successful maintenance. Healthful eating does not happen by accident, and it is not always easy. The 10,000 food advertisements we watch per year on television are not for broccoli and cantaloupe. The commercials say, "Eat, eat, eat" but show a woman who is so thin that it appears she never eats! For lifetime weight management it is essential to learn about the nutritive value of foods and devise strategies for making good choices over the course of each day.

Emotional Management

Why do you eat? "Because I am hungry!" you answer. If everyone ate only when they were in the physiological state of hunger, few would have a weight problem. We are surrounded with opportunities to eat more than we need to. Food is inexpensive and everywhere. Eating behavior is strongly influenced by psychological, social, and emotional factors. We eat out of emotional needs. We eat when we're happy; we eat when we're sad. Food becomes a substitute for other things. We confuse physical hunger with emotional hunger.

Controlling eating habits begins with having an understanding of why you eat and what cues trigger eating. Do you eat when you are bored? Lonely? Angry? Stressed? Do you eat when you turn on the television? Read? Do you eat when something smells good? When others are eating? Even positive feelings can trigger eating—earning an A on a term paper, celebrating the end of final exams, looking forward to a fun party. For emotional eaters, food serves as a comfort. Their "fix" is food, a means of self-nurturing.

For emotional management, spend time observing your eating behavior. Keep a journal or diary, recording the food you are eating and the feelings that accompany that moment. (There is an eating diary in Lab Activity 11-1 at the end of this chapter.) Learn to recognize the cues and connections between your thoughts, feelings and behaviors. Before you eat, ask yourself: "Why am I reaching for food at this time?" After you've spent some time observing your eating patterns, think of replacement activities to cope with the situation. Go for a walk; chew a stick of gum; drink a glass of water; call a friend; surf the Internet; suck on a mint; play a CD; work on a crossword puzzle. If you are one of those people who experiences occasional food cravings, try using the 4 D's:

- *Delay* at least 10 minutes before you eat so that your action is conscious, not impulsive.
- *Distract* yourself by engaging in an activity that requires concentration.
- *Distance* yourself from the food.
- *Determine* how important it is for you to eat the craved food.

Using behavior modification strategies can help emotional eaters. **Behavior modification** is the use of techniques to enhance awareness or consciousness about a behavior and to subsequently alter the behavior. Behavior modification is based on the premise that all behaviors are learned responses to environmental cues or antecedents. In using these techniques, people make eating a more conscious act, and healthier behavior patterns are integrated into the day-to-day routine. These include slowing the act of eating, altering susceptibility to the cues (separating eating from other activities, such as watching TV), and breaking behavior chains. Table 11-7 gives examples of some behavior modification techniques.

Changing eating behavior demands commitment and perseverance (unlike the magic potion or easy pitches delivered in many popular magazines). Too often, commercial weight-loss programs reward persons for the total number of pounds lost, creating undesirable behaviors such as going on crash diets, skipping meals, and using drugs and diuretics. According to some weight-management researchers, the use of rewards for weight loss is inappropriate because weight loss is not a behavior. It is the outcome of a complex interaction of emotions and behaviors over time. As discussed in Chapter 2, behavior change is a complex process that involves stages and coping techniques within each stage. You may want to go back to Chapter 2 and review Prochaska's behavior-change theory to see which techniques can be incorporated into managing emotional eating. Table 11-8 may help you identify your stage of change in terms of weight loss. Some example techniques are listed with selected processes, as well. To continue with or maintain a weight loss, you must be able to identify your high-risk situations in which difficulties with feelings or social situations threaten a relapse. Developing

table 11-7 Behavior Modification Techniques

1. Keep an eating diary to maximize awareness of eating.
2. Eat in one room only; sit at a table—don't stand.
3. Prepackage healthy snacks or meals and take them with you.
4. Keep a weight, fat gram, or calorie graph.
5. Never read or watch TV while eating.
6. Use smaller plates.
7. Always leave some food on your plate.
8. Drink a lot of water throughout the day and during meals.
9. Prepare, serve, and eat one portion at a time.
10. Do not place serving dishes on the table.
11. Grocery shop from a list and never on an empty stomach.
12. Leave the table after eating and clear dishes directly into the compost pile or garbage; brush your teeth immediately or chew gum.
13. Keep problem food out of sight or not in the house.
14. Keep healthy food accessible and visible.
15. Eat slowly; chew each bite thoroughly; put utensils down between bites; eat with your nondominant hand; cut food into smaller pieces.
16. Rehearse strategies in advance for eating out, special occasions, and high-risk situations.
17. Substitute alternative activities for eating (write a letter; go for a walk; jog; pay bills; sew; play tennis; etc.).
18. Don't do nonfood-related activities in the kitchen; stay out of the kitchen as much as possible; close the kitchen down after a meal.
19. When eating out, plan to share large portions with a companion. Or take extras home for another meal.
20. Snack from a plate, not the package, so you don't absentmindedly eat more than you realize.

and practicing coping strategies for dealing with these situations is an essential part of emotional management. Find more constructive ways to vent your feelings without food. Remove yourself from former patterns of behavior and develop new rituals that will ensure your success. Food stops taking on the role of nurturer when people learn to nurture themselves. Emotional management works best when you are reinforced by social support—family, friends, dietitians, community, and weight-loss support groups. And, finally, don't forget to acknowledge and reward your accomplishments and successes. This builds confidence!

Exercise Management

Americans have become fatter because calorie output has declined drastically. Our diet hasn't changed as much as our exercise habits. Television viewing, which substantially decreases activity levels and may influence diet, is a strong factor in obesity, especially among children and adolescents. In adults there is a direct relationship between the number of hours spent watching television and a person's level of obesity. The Internet, computers, video games, and VCRs have decreased overall activity levels. American technology has

table 11-8 Tips for Behavior Change: Losing Weight

Stages of Change: In What Stage Are You?

1. Precontemplation: "As far as I'm concerned I'm not too heavy."
2. Contemplation: "I think I should probably lose some weight; maybe after Christmas I'll try."
3. Preparation: "I am currently planning my weight-loss program."
4. Action: "I have been doing the things I need to do to lose weight (dietary change and exercise) for 3 months, and it is working."
5. Maintenance: "I have been successful at losing weight and maintaining that loss for over 6 months."

Processes of Change:

After identifying your current stage, try using some of the following selected processes and behavior strategies that are appropriate for your particular stage—to facilitate your transition into the next stage [refer to Figure 2-2]

- Consciousness-raising: read about people who have successfully lost weight.
- Social liberation: check out low-fat and low-calorie options at your favorite lunch/dinner spots.
- Self-reevaluation: assess and write down your feelings and disappointments due to your dependence on food.
- Reward: treat yourself to a low-fat yogurt every Saturday after a week of healthy food choices.
- Environment control: throw out junk-food snacks stored in desk drawer/shelves.
- Helping relationships: ask roommate to refrain from storing/eating snacks in your room.

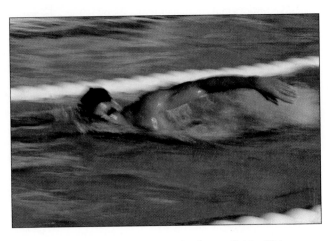

Participating in regular aerobic exercise is essential for lifelong weight management.

been ingenious in discovering ways for us to save energy, thus throwing off our energy balance. Electric garage door openers, riding lawn mowers, electric toothbrushes, and drive-up banks are a few examples of activity-robbing conveniences.

The secret to lifelong weight management is exercise, not dieting. While exercise is an important part of an initial weight-loss program, it is the single best predictor of long-term weight *maintenance.* A year-long study of overweight men and women compared body weight losses between two groups: those who dieted only and those who combined diet with exercise (brisk walking/jogging three times per week for 25 to 45 minutes). The diet-plus-exercise group increased loss of body fat, especially in the dangerous abdominal fat area. In another study using three behavioral weight loss treatment groups (diet only, exercise only, and diet plus exercise), at the end of 1 year, the combination diet plus exercise group lost the most weight. However, by the end of 2 years, the *exercise only* group maintained their weight loss much better than the other two groups. During the second year, the participants were without professional contact or guidance made available to them during the first year. The researchers discovered that exercise was easier for participants to adhere to than a restrictive diet. The exercise became a self-reinforcing behavior that the participants truly enjoyed and planned to continue. Regular exercise contributes to fat loss in several ways.

It Burns Calories

Table 11-9 shows how many calories you burn per minute in various activities. Note that the larger person burns more energy than does the lighter person engaged in the same activity. Also notice how aerobic activities burn considerably more calories per minute than do light, day-to-day tasks. Most people burn approximately 100 calories per mile whether walking or jogging. If this does not seem like a lot, look at it this way: You only burn about 1 calorie per minute while sitting. Remember that weight gain does not occur overnight; nor does weight loss. A pound of fat is lost by burning 3,500 calories. No one ever said it must all be done at once and only by jogging. Liberating large amounts of energy from our body reservoirs requires time—typically measured in months, if not years. Whereas the Centers for Disease Control and Prevention recommends 30 minutes of exercise per day for heart and overall health, research reveals that to lose and maintain weight loss, much more caloric expenditure from exercise is necessary. Studies indicate that burning approximately 2,800 calories a week with exercise (about 400 calories daily) should be the goal if weight is an issue. This would equate to about one hour of moderate intensity activity per day or walking 4 miles. If more vigorous exercise is preferred (e.g., jogging, aerobic dance, lap swimming, etc.), about 40 minutes per day is recommended. This may sound like a lot, but it doesn't all have to be done at one time. Doing intermittent activity (i.e., in 10 minute bouts) throughout the day is as effective as continuous exercise. Therefore, find ways to weave increased energy expenditure into day-to-day living: Walk to work or during breaks, take stairs instead of elevators, ride a bike on errands.

There is some question as to whether exercise increases postexercise basal metabolic rate. If there is some slight increase in metabolism after exercise, the total effect on energy balance is minimal. The greatest benefits of exercise in weight control are in the calories burned in the ac-

table 11-9   Caloric Expenditure per Minute for Various Activities

The figures in this table are only for the *time* you are performing the activity (not standing, waiting, resting). Variances may occur if you are running uphill, walking with hand weights, biking into a strong head wind, and so on. There may be small differences between males and females, but not enough to make a significant difference. You can approximate your expenditure if you are between the body weights listed.

Body Weight	120	150	180	210
Sitting and writing	1.5	1.9	2.3	2.7
Standing with light work, cleaning, etc.	3.3	4.1	4.9	5.7
Aerobic dance	7.3	9.1	10.9	12.7
Basketball (recreational)	6.0	7.5	9.0	10.5
Bicycling (10 mph; 6 min/mile)	5.1	6.4	7.6	8.9
Bicycling (15 mph; 4 min/mile)	8.7	10.9	13.1	15.3
Dancing (active; square; disco)	5.4	6.8	8.2	9.5
Golf (foursome, carrying clubs)	3.3	4.1	4.9	5.7
Racquetball	7.8	9.8	11.7	13.7
Roller skating (9 mph)	5.1	6.4	7.6	8.9
Running (6 mph; 10 min/mile)	8.7	10.9	13.1	15.4
Running (7 mph; 8:35 min/mile)	10.2	12.8	15.4	17.9
Running (8 mph; 7:30 min/mile)	11.6	14.6	17.6	20.5
Skiing, downhill; cross country (4 mph; 15 min/mile)	7.8	9.9	11.9	13.8
Soccer	7.2	9.0	10.8	12.6
Stair step machine	5.7	7.0	8.7	10.2
Swimming (crawl, 35 yds/min)	5.9	7.3	8.8	10.2
Swimming (crawl, 45 yds/min)	6.9	8.7	10.4	12.2
Tennis (recreational singles)	6.0	7.5	9.0	10.6
Walking (3 mph; 20 min/mile)	3.3	4.1	4.9	5.7
Walking (4 mph; 15 min/mile)	5.1	6.4	7.6	8.9
Walking (5 mph; 12 min/mile)	6.5	8.2	9.8	11.5
Weight training	6.2	7.8	9.4	11.2

tual exercise and in the positive effects it has on developing and maintaining lean body mass.

It Prevents Loss of Lean Muscle Mass

Exercise builds muscle tissue. And, since muscle cells are metabolically active, they burn more calories in basal metabolism (at rest) than do fat cells. As a result, someone with a lot of muscle mass burns more calories throughout the day *outside* of the exercise session. This is a key factor especially for women of all ages (who typically have less muscle mass and more fat than men), and for *both* men and women during middle age when metabolism can slow down due to loss of muscle tissue. Doing resistance training exercises 2 to 3 days per week using free weights, machines, or an exercise band, along with daily aerobic exercise is the perfect plan for maintaining lean muscle mass.

It Decreases Abdominal Fat

Excessive fat located in the abdominal area (apple-shape obesity) is linked to increased risk of heart disease and type 2 diabetes. Studies show that most of the positive effects of physical activity on heart disease risk factors (especially blood pressure and cholesterol) have to do with reductions in this intra-abdominal fat. This is true for both men and women. So, regular physical activity attacks abdominal fat.

It Is a Natural Appetite Suppressor

Moderate exercise has a tendency to decrease the appetite for a time after the workout because blood is diverted from digestive organs to skeletal muscles. You may feel thirsty but not usually hungry. This is why exercising during a lunch break helps you control weight. After exercising, you feel satisfied with a light lunch. Extremely intense exercise tends to lower blood sugar, which may stimulate appetite. To burn fat, keep your exercise at a moderate intensity and work to increase the duration. (Be sure not to view exercise as an excuse for eating more.)

wellness flash

At rest, muscle tissue burns approximately 40 calories per day per pound. At rest, fat tissue burns approximately 2 calories per day per pound.

It May Lower Your Set Point

The set-point theorists believe that regular, vigorous exercise is the one sure way to lower your body's fat level. Maintaining an active lifestyle stabilizes the set point at this lower level.

It Helps Maintain Weight Loss

Most health professionals agree that losing weight is easy; keeping it off is more difficult. To avoid the negative consequences of weight cycling, more attention is being given to *maintenance* of weight loss. Exercise has been shown to be one of the few factors correlated with long-term weight maintenance. A change in lifestyle that includes a consistent exercise regimen across the life span is the fundamental key to successful weight-loss maintenance.

It Improves Self-Esteem

For overweight, sedentary individuals, exercise may not be a richly reinforcing experience at first. It may be difficult for them to get out and exercise in public. They may feel self-conscious about their bodies. They may have negative feelings about exercise because of past embarrassing experiences. As exercise becomes a satisfying habit, the individual begins to experience a new sense of well-being and power. Anxiety and depression are reduced. As weight comes off, self-image is enhanced. Self-esteem and self-confidence are improved. These psychological benefits received from regular participation in physical activity are often the additional impetus necessary for adhering to a weight-loss/maintenance program. This positive self-concept helps reinforce all other areas of weight management, including food selection, feelings of anxiety, and feelings of control.

As you incorporate food management, emotional management, and exercise management into your life, you'll never see a need to "go on a diet." Look at the top ten tips from successful losers and maintainers for final insight into lifetime weight management.

Gaining Weight: A Healthy Plan for Adding Pounds

While many overweight people face the challenge of shedding extra pounds, those who are underweight face the challenge of trying to hold on to each pound and perhaps add more. The key to gaining weight is shifting the body weight equation so that you take in more calories than you burn. Add 2 to 3 substantial snacks between three moderate-size meals. Rather than eating high-fat and sugary foods, choose "calorie-dense" foods packed with nutrients. Increase your caloric intake to compensate for the energy burned while exercising. Here are some suggestions:

- Mix beans, nuts, cheese, peas, or lean meats into casseroles, side dishes, and pasta.

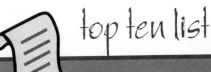

top ten list

Top Ten Tips from Successful Losers and Maintainers

Most people declare that losing weight is easier than keeping it off, especially if they followed some restrictive, unrealistic "diet" to achieve their initial weight loss. These tips from successful losers and maintainers address *lifetime* weight management—how to lose it *and* keep it off forever!

1. Focus on a *healthy* eating style, not "dieting."
2. Choose low-fat over higher-fat foods when available (e.g., dairy, salad dressing, sauces, sour cream, cream cheese, cooking spray, etc.)
3. Control portions. Everything has calories, even fat-free foods. Take half of that huge restaurant portion home with you.
4. Plan for exercise every day (include both aerobic and resistance training exercises). Make movement a part of your life.
5. Allow favorite foods—in moderation.
6. Fill up on fiber (fruits, vegetables, whole grains).
7. Don't skip meals. "Grazing" or eating smaller, but more frequent meals or snacks improves metabolism and reduces cravings and binging.
8. Set realistic goals. Working on losing 5 pounds at a time is easier than focusing on losing all 50 pounds.
9. Evaluate your relationship with food. Are you truly physiologically hungry or are you eating because of stress, boredom, anxiety, or habit? Develop coping and problem-solving strategies.
10. Drink at least eight 8-oz. glasses of water a day.

Finally, if you've eaten one too many chocolate chip cookies or haven't made it to the gym for a few days, don't give up. Take lapses in stride. Try to ascertain why the lapse occurred, learn from it, and move on. Weight management is a lifelong process, not an all-or-nothing contest. Remember . . . small changes can bring big results.

- Combine yogurt, fruit, wheat germ, and ice in a blender to make a shake.
- Spread peanut butter on bananas, apples, toast, or bagels.
- Replace sodas with fruit juices or skim milk.
- Replace cookies and doughnuts with nuts, raisins, dried fruits, bran muffins, yogurt, puddings, and fruit.
- Replace hamburgers and fries with thick-crust vegetable-topped pizza.

- Prepare hot cereals with milk instead of water; add nuts, peanut butter, fruit, and wheat germ.
- Top cold cereal with bananas or raisins.
- Eat hearty soups.
- Add garbanzo beans, seeds, tuna, croutons, cottage cheese, and lean meat to salads.

wellness flash

Twenty years ago fashion models weighed 8 percent less than the average women; today they weigh 23 percent less.

Culture and Weight

Why people diet and other weight-related issues are shaped by cultural environments. In the 1880s, full-figured actress Lillian Russell was the epitome of beauty. During these times, a surplus of fat was equated with wealth and success. The twentieth century brought about a decline in fatness as a social asset. Insurance companies began observing the increased death rate among those extremely overweight. The socially elite began diminishing the enormity of banquet menus. President William Howard Taft, weighing in at 355 pounds in 1909, began facing ridicule for his size. Corsets gave way to exercise, massage, raised hemlines, and penny scales. Hollywood stars, such as Jean Harlow and Gloria Swanson, gave diet and beauty advice that focused on reducing food intake. Thinness became equated with glamour, success, and desirability. After the Depression, the knowledge that excessive fat was linked to heart disease became a publicized issue. Weight reduction became a national pastime—a craze. Mail-order companies began making large profits with their weight-loss gimmicks. The market eventually gave way to new low-calorie foods and drugs designed to fool the body's hunger sensations. At the same time, labor-saving machines reduced the energy output necessary in daily life. The message that emerged by the 1960s was, "Thin is in." The desire for an unrealistic slimness, particularly among women, has caused many to be preoccupied with their bodies and with dieting. Diet books become instant best-sellers.

There She is . . . Miss Unrealistic America

This thin standard is perpetuated in all channels of social influence: families, peers, and the media. The message is pounded home over and over: "You can never be thin enough." This notion has been documented in studies of *Playboy* centerfolds and Miss America Pageant contestants from 1959 to the present, indicating a shift toward a thinner ideal shape for women in our culture. At the same time there has been a significant increase in diet articles in popular women's magazines. The cultural ideal for women's body size keeps getting thinner, though the average woman weighs 144 pounds and wears between a size 12 and 14. This cultural index of the "ideal" woman's body is 13 to 19 percent below the expected weight for age and height. A body

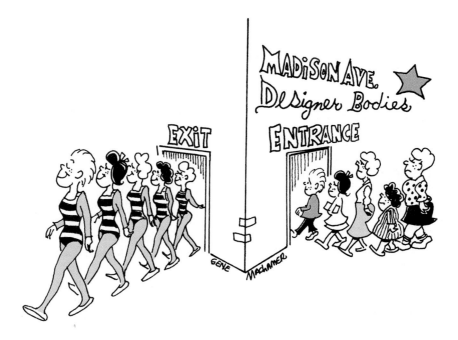

Many feel pressured to pursue the development of a model-like body.

weight below 15 percent of expected weight is one of the criteria for diagnosing anorexia nervosa, so what does this say about our cultural ideals?

With extreme slimness as a cultural norm, it becomes clear why fear of fat, fad dieting, surgical fat removal, and eating disorders abound. The overweight, obese, and even normal-weight individuals evaluate themselves in society's mirror, defining themselves as unattractive and as failures. Such harsh evaluations are a result of an acceptance of society's distorted concept of the ideal body. Every day we see pictures of models in magazines that are air brushed and electronically altered—a "manufactured ideal!" One study found that 3 minutes spent looking at models in a fashion magazine caused 70 percent of women to feel depressed, guilty, and shameful. Advertisements suggest that we invest money, time, and hope into trying to reach this ideal. Unfortunately, the results are often feelings of despair and inferiority.

The media and fashion industry need to take responsibility for using models who depict fitness and health rather than emaciation. Some already have. With the popularity of fitness and wellness programs in our country, we hope the image is changing. The "one size fits all" standard *must* change.

Men Are Joining In

A growing number of teenage boys and men are worried that their muscles aren't big enough or their bodies aren't lean enough. Bombarded with images of muscular, half-naked men on the covers of the emerging men's magazines and in advertisements, men are facing the cultural pressures that women have felt for decades. An increasing number of men are dieting, compulsively weight training, and abusing supplements and steroids as they strive for this ideal. This obsession for some goes beyond working out for health. It can affect school work, jobs, personal relationships, and self-esteem.

Eating Disorders

Obsession with weight and the desire to be thin begins early in life. Even third-graders are dieting and fretting about their weight. Our culture, especially, socializes girls to be concerned about their physical appearance. For them, thinness equates with attractiveness and social approval. The message is, "Work hard in school, but be popular and pretty." On the other hand, a male's self-concept is linked to physical dominance and sports competence. Most adolescent boys desire to be bigger and stronger. Studies have shown that females consistently desire to weigh less than their ideal body weight, whereas males do not.

Few measure up to the fashion industry's ideal, so dieting is commonplace. At the same time, obesity is dramatically rising among children in our country. The dilemma of

preventing obesity yet avoiding a fostering of "thin mania" presents a tremendous challenge.

The frequency of dieting among teenage girls is alarming. It is estimated that two-thirds of teenage girls in the United States have dysfunctional or abnormal eating behavior, one-half are undernourished, and one-third feel negative about their bodies. One in five take diet pills. One survey of teenage girls revealed that most were more afraid of becoming fat than they were of cancer, nuclear war, or losing their parents! Fear of fat, obsessive dieting, and a distorted body image can lead to a psychological eating disorder. An **eating disorder** is defined as a disturbance in eating behavior that jeopardizes a person's physical or psychosocial health. Bear in mind that preoccupation with weight and dieting are not synonymous with an eating disorder. An eating disorder is an extremely serious psychopathological state. Most professionals agree, however, that dieting precedes the onset of an eating disorder. Eating disorders are viewed as multidimensional in cause and nature. Factors that increase vulnerability can be genetic, biological, psychological, personality, sociocultural, and familial. Thus, the treatment must include all components. The general causes for disordered eating include:

1. Society's definition of the "perfect body" as unrealistically thin and lean.
2. Family characteristics such as over-involvement and high expectations.
3. Personality traits like "perfectionism," the desire to achieve, and competitive drive.
4. A genetic propensity to being overweight.
5. Pressure from others to lose weight.

It is estimated that 8 million Americans struggle with eating disorders. One million are men. Certain populations are especially at risk. These include gymnasts, dancers (especially ballet), cheerleaders, pom-pom performers, distance runners, and models. Although more women than men suffer from eating disorders, there is a higher than normal incidence of eating disorders in certain subgroups of males where slenderness is encouraged: models, dancers, wrestlers, and long-distance runners.

High school and college-age students are also vulnerable due to academic and social stresses and peer pressure to conform. Most social events take place around eating and drinking: parties, dates, late-night snacks. Physical attractiveness is important, and the stresses of growing up and

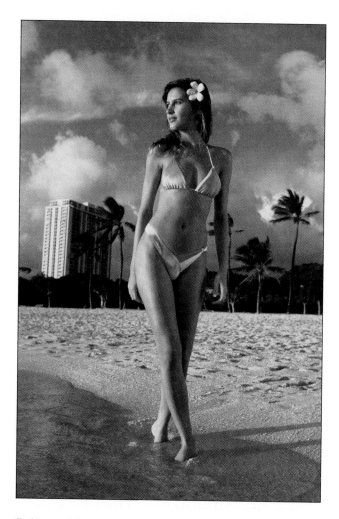

Fashion models perpetuate the unrealistic ideal of extreme thinness, especially to young women.

leaving home intensify these pressures. Rather than a strict addiction, eating disorders are a response to our societal influences, dieting culture, fat discrimination, overachieving perfectionism, and media images. Two of the most common eating disorders are bulimia nervosa and anorexia nervosa. They may occur separately or together. A third eating disorder is called binge eating disorder.

Bulimia Nervosa

Bulimia is a Greek word meaning *ox* and *hunger*. The disorder was so named because the sufferer eats like a hungry ox. That is, **bulimia nervosa** is characterized by a compulsive need to eat large quantities of food (bingeing) to the point of gorging, followed by purging through vomiting, use of laxatives, or fasting. Often, the binge is a response to an intense emotional experience, such as stress, loneliness, or depression, rather than the result of a strong appetite. Nevertheless, most bulimics are not aware of what precipitates these

uncontrollable binges, nor are they able to stop them. The diagnostic criteria for bulimia are as follows:

1. Recurrent episodes of binge eating (rapid consumption of a large amount of food in a discrete time).
2. A feeling of lack of control over eating behavior during the eating binges.
3. Self-induced vomiting, use of laxatives or diuretics, strict dieting or fasting, or excessive exercise to prevent a weight gain.
4. Persistent overconcern with body shape and weight.
5. Two binge episodes a week for at least 3 months.

Bulimia is the most common eating disorder. Some surveys suggest the prevalence of bulimia to be as high as 19 percent in college-age women and 5 percent in college-age men.

Bulimia frequently starts as normal, voluntary dieting behavior but later becomes compulsive, uncontrollable, and pathological. The bulimic's eating binge involves a rapid gulping of enormous quantities of food. Preferred foods are high in calories and sweet tasting and can be eaten rapidly without preparation: ice cream, cookies, candy, bread, cheese, chips, doughnuts. The consumption of this food is not a pleasurable pastime but a compulsion. Up to 10,000 calories can be consumed in one sitting, followed by abdominal pain and discomfort. The binge generates guilt, depression, and anxiety. Purging follows, reducing the anxiety and fear. Then the cycle begins again.

The bulimic is aware of his or her abnormal behavior and has great fear of not being able to stop. He or she has feelings of guilt and shame about the behavior. Bulimia is a secret habit and can continue for many years undetected. The weight of most bulimics is normal or fluctuates within 10 pounds as a result of the binge-purge cycle.

The physical effects of bulimia include electrolyte imbalance (especially potassium), low blood sugar, esophageal lacerations, dehydration, and nerve and liver damage from low potassium. Tooth enamel is eroded by the stomach acid brought up with vomiting. Severe abdominal pain is common. In rare cases, actual rupture of the stomach has occurred. Bone density is lost if the disorder continues for many years.

People with bulimia need professional help and are often tearful and desperate when they finally seek help. Psychotherapy is necessary to understand the underlying cause of the disorder and to help reshape the bulimic's feelings of self-worth and self-confidence. Bulimics tend to be extroverted perfectionists—high achievers—and are often academically or vocationally successful. Yet bulimics have troubled interpersonal relationships, low self-esteem, poor impulse control, and high levels of anxiety and depression and are self-critical and sensitive to rejection. It is not uncommon to see other impulsive behaviors among bulimics, including kleptomania, alcohol and drug use, and sexual promiscuity. The treatment goal is to get the bulimic to cope with his or her stresses and body image insecurities through less destructive ways and to feel more comfortable with who they are. Bulimia is difficult to cure, and some struggle with this disorder for life.

Anorexia Nervosa

Far less common than bulimia, **anorexia nervosa** is a psychological disorder in which self-inflicted starvation leads to a drastic loss of weight. Although anorexia is less prevalent than bulimia, it is associated with more frequent physical problems and greater mortality. The mortality rate from anorexia—estimated between 10 and 20 percent—is the highest of any mental disorder. Whereas the bulimic has a general dissatisfaction with his or her body weight, the anorexic is obsessed with achieving thinness. Individuals with anorexia nervosa have an iron determination to become thin and an intense, irrational fear of becoming fat. They vehemently deny their impulse to eat, their appetite, and their enjoyment of food. The term *anorexia* is a misnomer, because loss of appetite is usually rare until late in the illness. While bulimics feel shameful about their abnormal behavior, anorexics justify their weight-loss efforts.

Found primarily in early and middle adolescent females, anorexia may result in physical deterioration to the point of hospitalization or even death. Anorexia carries a 19:1 female-to-male ratio, with a prevalence estimated at 1 percent among adolescent girls. The diagnostic criteria for anorexia are as follows:

1. Refusal to maintain body weight at or above a minimal normal weight for age and height (i.e., a body weight that is 15 percent below normal).
2. Intense fear of weight gain or becoming fat, despite being significantly underweight.
3. A disturbed perception of body weight, size, or shape (i.e., feeling "fat" although emaciated).
4. In females, amenorrhea for at least three consecutive menstrual cycles.
5. Rigid dieting.
6. Food rituals and excessive exercise.

Anorexia often starts as innocent dieting that turns into irrational behavior characterized by severe caloric restriction; fasting; relentless exercising; diuretic and laxative use; and, in some cases, self-induced vomiting. The anorexic pursues and maintains thinness despite an emaciated appearance that is so apparent to others.

Anorexics display an extraordinary amount of energy for exercise and schoolwork in spite of their starvation state. However, they avoid social relationships, have low self-esteem, and are fearful of change. Despite an aversion for eating, anorexics are preoccupied with food. They may prepare elaborate meals for others, collect recipes, carry or hide snacks, and memorize the caloric content of various foods. Bizarre eating habits are commonplace. Anorexics have been known to cut a raisin in two and chew each half for several minutes. In many situations, they may pretend to be eating while putting food into their napkin or feeding the dog under the table.

Family stress and social pressure contribute to this disorder. Most anorexics come from middle- to upper-class families that place a high premium on achievement, perfection, and physical appearance. Their families are often overcontrolling and overprotective. Anorexics exhibit extreme perfectionism accompanied by a profound sense of ineffectiveness. Only by restricting food intake do they feel a sense of control and capable of coping with life's stresses.

Anorexia causes the physiological complications that accompany any malnutritive state: chronic fatigue, dry and scaly skin, hair falling out, lack of menstruation, drops in blood pressure, and cardiac complications. Constipation is commonplace. Bone growth is retarded, increasing the risk of fractures and osteoporosis. Anorexics have an unusual sensitivity to cold due to their low body-fat percentage.

Treatment for anorexia nervosa involves medical, psychological, and nutritional help. The major obstacle to treatment is the patient's denial that any problem exists. The entire family must be involved, because the anorexic's behavior has deep psychological origin: low self-esteem, struggle for control and independence, and fear of physical sexual development.

Binge Eating Disorder

Classified separately from anorexia or bulimia, binge eating disorder (sometimes called compulsive overeating) has become a serious problem. **Binge eating disorder** (BED) is defined as recurrent episodes of eating characterized by eating, in a discrete time, an amount of food much larger than most people would eat in a similar period, and accompanied by a sense of lack of control or a feeling that one cannot stop. At least three of the following must be part of the binge episode:

1. Eating much more rapidly than normal.
2. Eating until uncomfortably full.
3. Eating large amounts of food when not hungry.
4. Eating alone because of embarrassment about how much is eaten.
5. Feeling disgusted with oneself, depressed, or guilty about eating.

Most people overeat from time to time, and many feel that they eat more than they should. Compulsive overeaters, however, experience marked distress regarding their binging behavior, and engage in binge eating on average at least 2 days a week for 6 months. They tend to overeat when home alone, while normal eaters tend to overeat in restaurants and social situations that are associated with positive feelings.

In some ways, people with binge eating disorder are similar to bulimics. Both engage in frequent binges, are preoccupied with food and body weight, experience intense feelings of body dissatisfaction, and set unrealistically high dieting standards. Both use food to fill an emotional void.

However, some important differences distinguish bulimics from people with BED. People with BED do not regularly compensate for their behavior by dieting or purging. Whereas bulimics dwell on the importance of thinness, serious binge eaters would be happy to be an average body weight. Individuals with BED are usually very overweight and most seek treatment for obesity. Compulsive overeaters make up 25 to 45 percent of Americans who seek treatment for obesity and 5 to 8 percent of obese people in general. They eat even if they aren't hungry. Whereas bulimics engage in the extremes of severe dieting and eventual binging, people with BED rarely restrict food. Table 11-10 will help you assess whether you have a problem with compulsive overeating.

The goal in treating binge eaters is to normalize eating—to help them say "no" to overeating. They need help in adopting a plan of healthy eating and overall moderation *without* rigid rules. Binge eaters need help in learning to cope with the underlying emotions that perpetuate this eating problem—anxiety, loneliness, depression, shame, inferiority, and fear of criticism. Finally, binge eaters need to learn to accept that which cannot be changed about their bodies.

What Can Be Done?

Eating disorders appear to be increasing in incidence, so implementation of prevention programs is desperately needed. The most obvious and effective site for prevention is the schools. However, all segments of society need to absorb some of the responsibility, including parents, coaches, advertising executives, the media, and the entertainment business. Society needs to send the message of healthy acceptance of self and body. Not everyone is meant to be a size 6.

If you suspect a friend, roommate, or relative of having an eating disorder, you probably wonder what you can do to help. Eating disorders are not solely about food and eating but are manifestations of emotional distress. Therefore, just begging someone to start eating or put on some weight is futile. Nor will ignoring the situation or waiting to see what happens solve the problem.

table 11-10	Are You a Compulsive Overeater?

1. Do you eat when you're not hungry, but don't know why?
2. Do you constantly think about food throughout the day?
3. Do you go on eating binges for no apparent reason and find yourself unable to stop?
4. Do you have feelings of guilt and remorse after overeating?
5. Do you look forward with pleasure and anticipation to the time when you can eat alone?
6. Do you eat sensibly in front of others, and then binge when you're alone?
7. Is your weight affecting the way you live your life?
8. Do you eat to escape from worries or trouble?
9. Does your eating behavior make you or others unhappy?
10. Have you tried "dieting," only to fall short of your goal?

If you answered "yes" to over half of these questions, you may want to seriously think about your relationship with food and consult a professional.

The first step to recovery is indisputable: Locate professional help as soon as possible. Congress has mandated that every state establish a system of community mental health centers to assist people with a variety of psychological problems. These centers are a good source for providing treatment or helping you locate professionals who specialize in treating eating disorders. Even though psychotherapy has become more prevalent and accepted in the last 25 years, some still avoid it. For whatever reason, psychotherapy still carries a stigma with some people.

Your anorexic or bulimic acquaintance may deny the condition or balk at your suggestion to seek help, therefore it may be difficult to persuade her or him to seek help. However, both physical and psychological evaluation are crucial at the onset of treatment. You cannot force someone to get help. It is important, however, to be direct and honest while showing sincere concern and support. You may have to be tough, even make the appointment, and insist on accompanying the anorexic or bulimic to see the specialist.

 frequently asked questions

Q. *I have cellulite on my thighs. Is there any special way to remove it?*

A. There is no such thing as **cellulite.** It is a slang term used to describe the dimpled fat found primarily on the buttocks and thighs of women. Concentrated areas of fat tend to bulge in some women because, with age, their connective fibers become taut and their skin thin. This fat is like any other fat in that only a comprehensive program of exercise and calorie reduction will remove it. No miracle creams, saunas, diets, or devices specifically break up cellulite.

Buying a product that claims to do this only reduces your wallet.

Q. *The only place I feel I have too much fat is on my abdomen. Is there any way to just lose fat there?*

A. The concept of *spot reduction* (that is, selectively burning off fat from a particular body area) is a myth. No one can dictate where body fat will accumulate or from where it will be removed. Genetics determine your body build and preferred fat storage sites. Exercising a specific body area

frequently asked questions

does not burn fat in just that area. Fat stores from throughout the body are mobilized during exercise. So your abdomen will lose fat only after a combined program of total-body aerobic exercise and calorie management, not solely by doing 100 curl-ups a day. It is possible to "spot tone," however. Those 100 curl-ups create strong abdominals.

Q. *My friend had his stomach stapled and lost a considerable amount of weight. What about this and other surgical treatments of obesity?*

A. Surgery for obesity should not be taken lightly and should be considered only as a last resort for the morbidly obese (those at least 100 pounds above ideal weight). Even the nonsurgical means of jaw wiring and inserting balloons in the stomach are drastic measures in tackling obesity. As with any major medical procedure, these methods have inherent risks and medical complications. Also, their long-term effectiveness is questionable, unless a drastic lifestyle change accompanies the procedure. **Liposuction** (suctioning fat from under the skin) has become popular as a method of removing body fat from selected body parts. This surgical procedure, performed by physicians who specialize in cosmetic surgery, is another questionable approach to permanent weight loss.

Q. *I have seen a lot of advertisements from health salons promoting effortless exercise machines for weight loss. Do they work?*

A. Because many people do not understand the basic principles of fat metabolism, they fall prey to the appeal of these ads. After all, they say you don't have to sweat or even change clothes. It takes only minutes. Roller machines, oscillating tables, electrical muscle stimulators, and power-driven vibrators are promoted as equipment that removes fat or breaks up fatty deposits. These devices are worthless gimmicks. They have no value in reducing fat because of the lack of effort on the part of the participant. Remember, fat loss is a result of burning more calories than you consume. These machines are doing the work, so few calories are burned. Using active machines such as stationary bicycles, rowing machines, stair climbers, and cross-country skiing machines are effective ways to burn calories, because they require *you* to exert energy.

Q. *What about body wraps, rubberized suits, and other special weight-reducing apparel? I've worn some of these and they seem to work.*

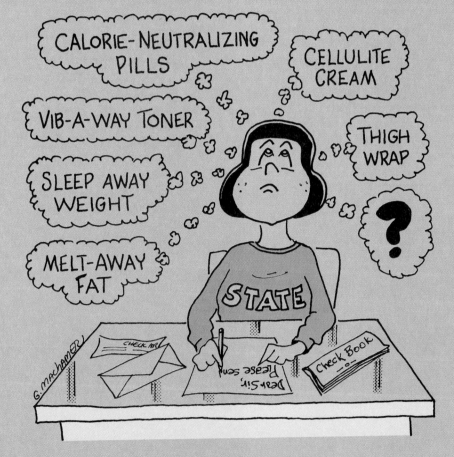

Weight-loss gimmicks reduce your wallet not your waist.

A. Waist belts or body wraps do nothing more than squeeze water out of one tissue area into another. Think about the indentation that occurs on your wrist after wearing a rubber band there for several minutes. This circumference loss is only temporary until rehydration occurs. Rubberized or vinyl suits can be dangerous, especially if worn while exercising. These suits trap the heat and perspiration given off by the body, not allowing the natural process of evaporation—the body's normal cooling process. These suits make you like a turkey basting in its juices. Water, not fat, is lost by the body, and the danger of life-threatening overheating is possible. Again, as soon as the body is rehydrated, weight is regained.

Q. *I am heavily involved in competitive sports. As a result, I am very muscular. When I stop competing, how do I avoid having all of that muscle turn into fat?*

A. Your concern is fueled by a common misconception. Muscle can no more turn into fat than a cat can turn into a dog. Neither can fat become muscle. The cellular makeup of each is different. If you stop activity altogether, your muscles will atrophy and lose tone. Calories not needed to fuel your body will be stored as fat. To avoid this, continue some regular exercise and modify your calorie consumption, being sure your energy input and output are relatively equal.

Q. *I have heard that I will burn more fat if I work out at the lower end of my target heart rate range rather than at a high intensity. Is this true?*

A. This low-intensity fat-burning idea is a misunderstanding based on an oversimplification. It is true that the higher the exercise intensity, the more the body prefers to use glycogen rather than fat for fuel. Some have interpreted this to mean that to burn fat, low-intensity exercise is best. However, the type of fuel used during exercise does not make a great deal of difference. The most important exercise variable is *total* caloric expenditure. Because you don't fatigue as quickly when exercising at a low intensity, you may be able to work out for a longer time and feel more comfortable while doing it. The result is more total calories expended due to the longer workout time.

Q. *I am concerned because my sister is very much overweight. She doesn't act like it bothers her, but I think it does. What can I do to motivate her to lose weight?*

A. Often, we have relatives or friends who have health-robbing habits (smoking, being overweight, not exercising). Because we care about them, it is natural to want to help. In the case of your sister, do not nag or criticize her. Instead, set a good example and talk about why you do the things you do (select certain foods, behavior modification tricks, etc.). Try to include her in your practices. Invite her to go on a walk, bike riding, or to an aerobics class. Grocery shop or eat out together. Share recipes and food preparation ideas. Show that you care. Make a pact with her (you will try to stop biting your fingernails, while she tries to lose weight). Be there for her. However, realize that she is ultimately responsible for herself. Nevertheless, be her friend, confidante, and number one cheerleader. A strong support system is essential in any weight management program.

Summary

Obesity is acknowledged as this country's most important nutrition-related disease. It is a complex disorder, no longer considered only a problem of overeating or lack of willpower. It is caused by multiple factors—some within your control and some beyond. Genetics, environment, and culture combine to complicate the act of nourishing our bodies. It is important to understand body composition and be able to differentiate between overweight and obesity. Many health problems are associated with obesity, so concern with weight control should begin sufficiently early in life to reduce the risk of developing obesity. Prevention is the treatment of choice. The factors affecting obesity give insight into the complexities of losing excess body fat.

"Monday I start my diet" is far too often the battle cry for losing weight. This diet mentality has contributed to the obesity problem. Dieting and concerns about appearance have also contributed to the increasing incidence of eating disorders. Because successful weight management has been elusive for many obese individuals, the marketplace has provided many legitimate as well as unfounded claims about products and services. Therefore, consumer education is essential. Effective weight management involves food management, emotional management, and exercise management. Whereas dieting is temporary, restrictive, and negative, lifestyle weight management is a positive, flexible means of dealing with food for life and health. It is a lifestyle of low-fat eating and regular exercise, amidst established cultural patterns and social and economic forces. No gimmick or gadget can replace this lifestyle approach.

Regular exercise is the key ingredient in maintaining a healthy body composition. Technological advances have increased the quality of our lives in many ways but have eliminated much daily physical exertion. It is a challenge to find ways to fit activity into your life. However, lifelong weight management and total wellness depend on it. Only when we start considering food as fuel and accepting a range of healthy body weights will obesity begin to be eradicated.

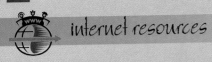
internet resources

Organizations

American Anorexia/Bulimia Association
165 W. 46th Street, Suite 1108, New York, NY 10036
(212) 575-6200
   www.aabainc.org

American Dietetic Association
   www.eatright.org

Anorexia Nervosa and Related Eating Disorders
P.O. Box 5102, Eugene, OR 97405
(503) 344-1144
   www.anred.com

Cooking Light Magazine
   www.cookinglight.com

Eating Disorders Awareness and Prevention
603 Stewart Street, Suite 803, Seattle, WA 98101
(206) 382-3587
   www.edap.org

National Association of Anorexia Nervosa and Associated
Disorders P.O. Box 7, Highland Park, IL 60035
(847) 831-3438
   www.anad.org

National Eating Disorders Information Centre
   www.nedic.on.ca

Overeaters Anonymous
P.O. Box 44020, Rio Rancho, NM 87174
(505) 891-2664
   www.overeatersanonymous.org

Partnership for Healthy Weight Management
   www.consumer.gov/weightloss

The Center for Eating Disorders
   www.eatingdisorders.org

Web Sites

   www.about-face.org
   www.cyberdiet.com
   www.dietitian.com
   www.ediets.com
   www.healthyweight.net
   www.nourishnet.com
   www.shapeup.org
   www.weight.com
   www.weightdirectory.com
   www.weightfocus.com

Name _____

Class/Activity Section _____

Date _____

Why Do You Eat?
(An Eating Diary)

Use the following eating diary to analyze the reasons you eat. Knowing the cues and factors that affect eating can help you manage your eating behavior. (Make copies of this diary as needed to record multiple days.)

Date: ____

Time of day	Location	Companion(s) (if any)	Food	Portion Size/ Quantity	Hunger Level (0–5) 0 = not hungry 5 = very hungry	Feelings/Mood (before eating)	Feelings/Mood (after eating)

Observations:

Strategies for change:

How Active Are You?

Finding the time to exercise can be a challenge. However, there are several times during a day that you can weave activity into your life (i.e., walking rather than driving; riding a stationary bike while watching TV; taking the stairs rather than the elevator; getting up 45 minutes earlier in the morning to jog). Use the following log to keep track of your activity during the day. Then, analyze *when* and *how* you could adapt your lifestyle to include more activity. (Make copies of this log as needed to record multiple days.)

Date: _____

Activity	Time of Day	Location	Duration	Positive Outcomes	Negative Outcomes (if any)

Assess your activity level today (If you did any of the activities listed in Table 11-9, how many calories did you burn?).

Describe ways you could fit more activity into your day:

What obstacles do you face in trying to be active?

What are your strategies for combatting these obstacles and for adhering to a lifetime of activity/exercise?

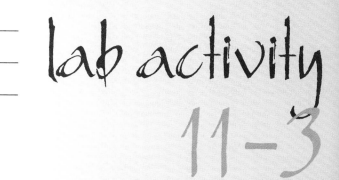
Estimating Your Basal Metabolic Rate (BMR)

Precise measurement of your BMR can be achieved only in a laboratory. However, you can compute an estimate of your BMR by using the following equations:

Males: BMR = 1.0 cal/hr/kg × body weight (kg) × 24 hr/day

Females: BMR = 0.9 cal/hr/kg × body weight (kg) × 24 hr/day

Compute yours:

Step one: Convert your body weight in pounds to kilograms (kg): _____ (your weight in lbs) ÷ 2.2 = _____ (weight in kg)

Step two: Multiply weight in kilograms by 0.9 (females) or 1.0 (males) to get calories per hour: _____ (wt in kg) × 0.9 or 1.0 = _____ (cal/hr)

Step three: Multiply calories per hour by 24 hours: _____ (cal/hr) × 24 hours = _____ YOUR BMR (calories per day)

Note: For both men and women, BMR can decline by about 2 to 3 percent per decade after age 25 due to the loss of lean muscle mass.

Example:	The estimated BMR of a female who weighs 135 pounds
	Step one: 135 lbs ÷ 2.2 = 61.4 weight in kg
	Step two: 61.4 kg × 0.9 = 55.26 cal/hr
	Step three: 55.26 cal/hr × 24 hours = 1326 BMR (cal/day)

Remember . . . the BMR does not include any calorie expenditure from activity or exercise that you do throughout the day.

Comment on the day's intake:

Do you have any areas to improve? What are your strategies for improvement?

SAMPLE

CALORIES ≈ 2100

BREAKFAST	SNACK	LUNCH	SNACK	DINNER	SNACK
2 oz. cereal	apple	chef's salad:	bagel with	stir fry:	popcorn
1 c. milk		lettuce	2 T. peanut	chicken breast	Coke
6 oz. orange juice		tomato	butter	Chinese vegetables	
banana		carrots		1 c. rice	
		ham/egg		1 c. yogurt	
		breadstick		1 c. milk	
		Jell-o			

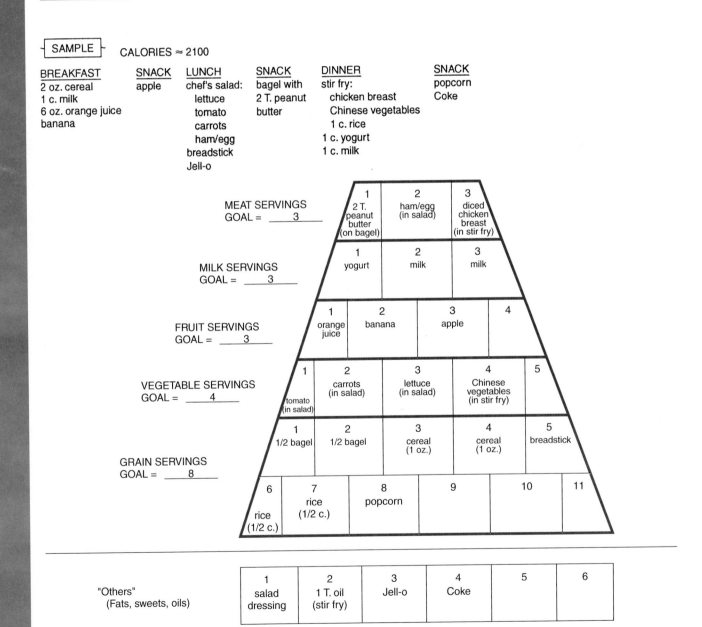

MEAT SERVINGS
GOAL = ___3___

| 1 2 T. peanut butter (on bagel) | 2 ham/egg (in salad) | 3 diced chicken breast (in stir fry) |

MILK SERVINGS
GOAL = ___3___

| 1 yogurt | 2 milk | 3 milk |

FRUIT SERVINGS
GOAL = ___3___

| 1 orange juice | 2 banana | 3 apple | 4 |

VEGETABLE SERVINGS
GOAL = ___4___

| 1 tomato (in salad) | 2 carrots (in salad) | 3 lettuce (in salad) | 4 Chinese vegetables (in stir fry) | 5 |

GRAIN SERVINGS
GOAL = ___8___

| 1 1/2 bagel | 2 1/2 bagel | 3 cereal (1 oz.) | 4 cereal (1 oz.) | 5 breadstick |
| 6 rice (1/2 c.) | 7 rice (1/2 c.) | 8 popcorn | 9 | 10 | 11 |

"Others"
(Fats, sweets, oils)

| 1 salad dressing | 2 1 T. oil (stir fry) | 3 Jell-o | 4 Coke | 5 | 6 |

Weight Management Plan

Date: _____

Current weight: _____

　Goal weight: _____

Current body fat percentage: _____

　Goal body fat percentage: _____

Current body mass index (BMI): _____

　Goal body mass index (BMI): _____

Waist: _____ Hip: _____

　　　Current waist-to-hip ratio: _____

　　Goal waist-to-hip ratio: _____

　　　　(waist ÷ hip)

I. Food Management

- Calories per day: _____ (goal)

- Fat grams per day: _____ (goal)

- Food Guide Pyramid compliance and strategies for improvement:

- Snack strategy:

- Food preparation adjustments:

II. Emotional Management

Behavior modification and coping strategies:

1.   4.

2.   5.

3.   6.

III. Exercise Management

Physical activity strategies:

Sunday	Monday	Tuesday	Wednesday	Thursday	Friday	Saturday

Using HealthQuest

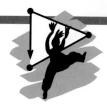

1. Insert HealthQuest CD into your computer.

2. Click on "Nutrition and Weight Control" from the menu. Click on "Introduction" and read.

3. Click on "Introduction" again and go to "Wellness Activities." Click on the "Energy Balance" activity.

4. Click on "Introduction" and read. Go back and click on "Energy Balance."

    Enter your personal information (press "Enter" after feet, inches, pounds)
    Click on "Body Mass Index." Record your BMI _____

        Record your recommended caloric intake _____

    Click on "More About BMI" and read.

    Your body composition classification is: _____

5. Proceed and complete the "Energy In" (daily food intake) and "Energy Out" (daily Energy output) for a typical day. Don't forget to record all of the sedentary activities in the "Energy Out." (Use the "Help" button as needed.)

    What was your "Energy In" for the day? _____

    What was your "Energy Out" for the day? _____

    Comment on this activity:

12

Preventing Cancer

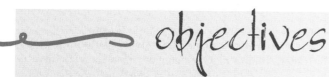

After reading this chapter, you will be able to:

1. Identify how cancer deaths rank in overall death statistics.
2. List four primary and four secondary risk factors for cancer.
3. Give four guidelines for preventing sun overexposure.
4. Give four guidelines for selecting foods that reduce cancer risk, and apply the guidelines to a menu.
5. List three early detection factors for cancer.
6. Recognize the proper procedure and schedule for conducting a breast or testicular self-exam.
7. Identify cancer's seven warning signals.
8. Identify the most common cancers and their risk factors.

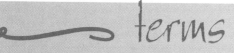

- Antioxidants
- Benign
- Beta-carotene
- Cancer
- Carcinogens
- Crucifera
- Free radicals
- Human papilloma virus (HPV)
- Malignant
- Melanoma
- Metastasis
- Phytochemicals
- Precancerous
- Tumor

A wellness lifestyle implies taking responsibility for your health and making wise choices. The purpose of this chapter is to discuss how to decrease cancer risk, which is strongly affected by personal lifestyle choices. Adult cancer is largely a preventable disease. While no one would choose to have cancer, a person might choose to use tobacco, tan excessively, or eat a high-fat diet, factors that can initiate and promote cancer. You will learn which behaviors increase health risks and how to decrease these risks to enhance your state of wellness.

Cancer Incidence

Cancer is the second most common cause of death in the United States, after heart disease. See Figure 12-1 for cancer death rates by site and gender. According to present rates, about one in three Americans will eventually have cancer. Although gains have been made in cancer treatment and survival, the total number of cancer deaths has increased. Changes in diet and lifestyles coupled with a longer life expectancy has resulted in more time for carcinogens to affect cells. While cancer is most common in people over 55, it can strike at any age. The earlier a cancer is detected, the simpler the treatment and the higher the survival rate. We know that simple lifestyle changes can cut your risk of cancer. For this reason, it is important to understand cancer risk factors and warning signals and to practice self-exams.

What is Cancer?

Cancer is not a single disease, but a group of over 100 different diseases characterized by abnormal cell growth and replication. Normally, cells grow and are replaced in an orderly manner. Enough new cells grow to replace those that are worn out and injured. Cancer cells lack controls to stop the growth process and continue to grow and multiply without restraint. This loss of control of cell growth may be due to a variety of factors. Ultraviolet radiation from sunlight, tobacco smoke, viral infections, diet, and chemicals in food and in the environment all have been implicated.

It is possible that all of us at some time experience potentially cancerous changes in our cells. These **precancerous** cells usually die or are destroyed by the immune system. Few live long enough to cause harm. If one abnormal cell survives, it can replicate into billions of cells, forming a lump or **tumor.** Tumors may be benign or malignant. **Benign** tumors are usually nonthreatening. Although they can grow large enough to interfere with organs and bodily functions, they seldom cause death. They usually resemble surrounding tissue, remain localized, and spread by expansion, like a wart or mole. They do not spread to other parts of the body. They can be removed completely by surgery and are not likely to recur. **Malignant** tumors are cancerous. They differ from surrounding tissue and tend to spread through **metastasis.** In metastasis, cells break away from the primary tumor and migrate to other tissues through the lymph or blood systems where they continue to grow. They have lethal potential because they invade and destroy normal tissues and spread to other parts of the body.

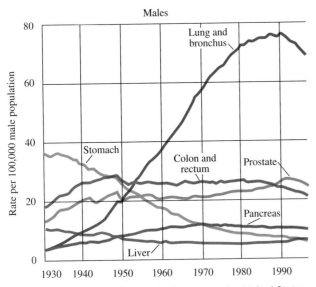

Age-adjusted cancer death rates,* males by site, United States, 1930–1996.

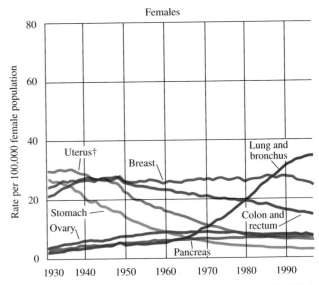

Age-adjusted cancer death rates,* females by site, United States, 1930–1996.

figure 12-1   United States, 1930–1996.

*Per 100,000, age-adjusted to the 1970 U.S. standard population. **Note:** Due to changes in ICD coding, numerator information has changed over time. Rates for cancers of the liver, lungs, and bronchus and colon and rectum are affected by these coding changes.

Source: US Mortality Public Use Data Tapes 1960–1996, US Mortality Volumes 1930–1959, National Center for Health Statistics, Centers for Disease Control and Prevention, 1999.

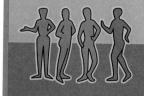

diversity issues

Rates of incidence of certain types of cancers differ among countries, races, and socioeconomic groups. Some differences occur because of cultural habits practiced for a lifetime. For example, in Japan and China, where soy foods are eaten almost every meal, deaths from prostate and breast cancers are one-fourth of what they are in the United States. In the United States, a diet rich in high-fat meat and processed and refined food results in high rates of colorectal cancer, rare in countries where the diet consists largely of unrefined grains, fruits, and vegetables.

Likewise, cultural influences affect rates of certain types of cancer among socioeconomic groups. Smoking is an example. At one time, smoking symbolized sophistication, affluence, and maturity, and over half the population smoked, but this has changed. Nevertheless, while smoking has declined to less than a quarter of the population, 50 million Americans, mainly the less educated, still smoke. Also an unacceptably high number of teenagers are using tobacco, which foreshadows grim health problems for that group in the future.

Not only cultural influences, but racial background or genetics can affect cancer rates. People with brown, olive, or black skin have a measure of protection against skin cancer provided by melanin, a natural skin pigment. Darkly pigmented blacks can have up to 30 times more melanin than people with pale white skin and are less likely to suffer skin damage due to sun exposure. However, blacks are more prone to a type of melanoma that most often appears on the palms, soles, nail beds, and mucous membranes and is often detected at a later, less treatable stage.

While genetics is a factor in cancer risk, behavioral choices are a much more powerful determinant. Following a healthy diet, avoiding tobacco and sun overexposure, and being physically active decrease cancer risk for all populations.

How to Cut Your Risk of Cancer: Primary Risk Factors

People hear so much about cancer, they often get the feeling that everything causes cancer. If everything causes cancer, then there seems to be no use in trying to avoid it. They feel that there is little they can do to make a difference in their cancer risk or that it is not worth the effort. They are wrong. Cancer, like heart disease, is largely preventable. Up to 85 percent of cancers may be related to lifestyle factors over which you have control. Only 2 percent can be blamed on environmental factors. These cancers occur as a result of cumulative exposure to **carcinogens,** substances that cause cancer, and/or a weakened immune system that does not effectively scavenge precancerous cells. There are four major risk factors for cancer that are within your control.

Primary risk factors for cancer are:

- Tobacco use
- Sun overexposure
- Diet
- Inactivity

Several other factors contribute to increased risk of cancer. Secondary risk factors for cancer, some of which are controllable, include:

- Obesity
- Excessive alcohol consumption
- Exposure to some viral infections, for example, hepatitis B
- Exposure to radiation, workplace hazards, and certain chemicals

Choices you make daily can greatly cut your cancer risk. It is a matter of education and habit change. What follows is a discussion of what you can do.

wellness flash

Sunscreen loses its potency within 1 year. Check the expiration date or write the purchase date on yours so you will know if it is still effective.

Tobacco Use

This includes cigarettes, pipes, cigars, snuff, and chewing tobacco. Tobacco contains many carcinogens that increase the risk of developing several types of cancers. (See Chapter 13 for additional information on the effects of tobacco.) Frequent exposure to toxins ingested from tobacco products weakens the immune system and decreases the body's ability to cleanse itself of precancerous cells. In addition, when a smoker is exposed to other carcinogens, there seems to be a synergistic effect that multiplies cancer rates beyond what would be expected from the effect of each alone. For example, smoking, combined with the use of alcohol, greatly increases the risk of cancer. The number of smokers is decreasing in the United States. However, the use of smokeless tobacco, especially "dipping snuff," has increased. Whereas tobacco use is most often implicated in lung cancer, tobacco products can produce a variety of oral cancers, including cancer of the lip, tongue, mouth, and throat.

The good news is that cancers caused by tobacco are 100 percent preventable. If you don't use tobacco, don't start. If you are a tobacco user, quit. People who quit, no matter what age, live longer, healthier lives than those who keep using tobacco. For the majority of Americans who don't use tobacco, reducing sun exposure and eating healthfully are the most powerful tools for decreasing cancer risk.

Sun Overexposure

Overexposure to the sun is the main cause of skin cancer. It is estimated to strike one of every six Americans, making it the most common cancer. We have been a nation of sun worshipers and are seeing the consequences. How ironic that the price of a "healthy" tan can be premature skin aging and wrinkling and skin cancer. It is never good to lie in the sun to tan, but you can still enjoy outdoor activities and minimize negative effects by following the guidelines in Table 12-1.

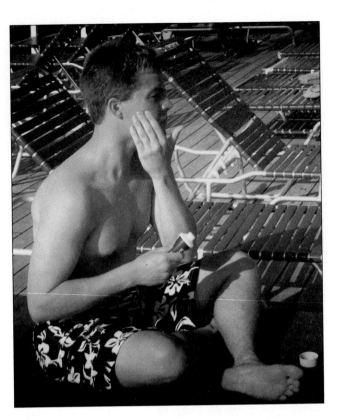

Use SPF 15 sunscreen if you are going to be out in the sun even 15 to 30 minutes.

table 12-1	How to Reduce Sun Exposure

1. Avoid prolonged exposure to the sun when ultraviolet (UV) radiation is strongest, between 10:00 A.M. and 3:00 P.M., even on overcast days.
2. Plan activities for early morning or late evening.
3. When you will be working or playing outside for even 15 to 20 minutes, *apply a sunscreen rated SPF 15 or higher.* Use at least 1 ounce (about 2 tablespoons). Newer formulations protect from both UVB and UVA radiation. Reapply every 2 hours or after swimming or perspiring.
4. Avoid tanning, even in tanning parlors or with sunlamps. There is no such thing as a safe tan. Tanned skin is damaged skin. The UVA light emitted by tanning booths still can cause sunburn, premature skin aging, and increased risk of skin cancer.
5. Protect children from too much sun. Skin damage occurs with each unprotected sun exposure and accumulates over a lifetime. Perhaps most of the damage is done in childhood and adolescence. Even one bad burn in childhood can double the risk of skin cancer.
6. Know what skin cancer looks like and examine your skin at least once a month. If you find unusual moles or skin spots, have them examined by your physician.

Diet

About one-third of cancers can be prevented by a healthful diet. Certain foods seem to be related to an increase or decrease in some kinds of cancers; for instance, a high-fat diet seems to play a role in the development of breast, colon, and prostate cancers. A multitude of studies show that by eating whole-grain foods, fruits, and vegetables and by avoiding high-fat red meat, bacon, and processed meats, we could significantly reduce our overall cancer risk as shown in Table 12-2. The food pyramid in Chapter 10 and the ten dietary guidelines are excellent models to follow. However, many Americans are not making these simple dietary adjustments. Only 24 percent of Americans eat the recommended five servings of fruits and vegetables a day. Eating a variety of fruits, grains, and vegetables is not only more healthful, but less expensive than buying a lot of high-fat meat and highly processed foods such as hot dogs, fries, chips, doughnuts, and junk cereals.

Concerns have been voiced about pesticide and chemical residues in fruits and vegetables, as well as about irradiation of fresh produce and poultry. There is no doubt that the production, processing, and transportation of food in our mass-market world raises concerns that necessitate further research. Nevertheless, we do know that sun exposure, a fatty diet, and tobacco products are three highly controllable areas

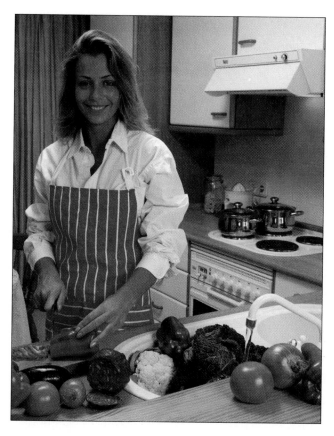

Eating five servings of fruits and vegetables a day can reduce cancer risk.

where your behavior has a major impact. Taking positive steps in these three areas makes more sense than worrying about food products over which you have little control.

By making positive choices in your daily diet and following the guidelines listed here, you can promote good health now and can reduce your cancer risk in the future. Healthy dietary changes you can make can be found in Table 12-3, and a sample 1-day dietary plan incorporating many of these suggestions is given in Table 12-4.

1. *Decrease fat intake, particularly from animal sources.* Eat low-fat meats and dairy products, as well as vegetarian meals. Cut way back on fried foods (average one serving or less a day) and fatty sweets (pastry, cookies). Decrease consumption of foods high in saturated fat and trans fat. Limit consumption of red meat, particularly high-fat meat. High-fat diets are related to increased risk of cancer of the colon, rectum, prostate, and endometrium. Some studies have also linked a high-fat diet with increased risk of breast cancer. Whether this risk is related to the amount of fat, type of fat, calories in fat, or some other factor in dietary fats is not yet clear. Information on dietary fat is found in Chapter 10.

2. *Choose most of the foods you eat from plant sources.* Eat five or more servings of fruits and vegetables a day, as well as six or more servings of whole-grain breads and cereals, brown rice, pasta, or beans. Diets rich in fruits and vegetables (french fries don't count) protect against many cancers, particularly those occurring in the gastrointestinal and respiratory tracts such as cancers of the colon, lung, stomach, esophagus, mouth, and throat. Grains are important sources of many nutrients such as selenium and folic acid, which some studies have associated with lower risk of colon cancer. It is not yet known exactly what factors in plant foods provide protective benefits. Fiber has long been thought to be protective against colon cancer, but recent studies leave this open to question. Certainly, consuming more plant foods leaves less room for high-fat, empty-calorie foods, and plant foods are rich in essential vitamins, minerals, and protective **phytochemicals** (plant chemicals). Scientists are studying many substances in plants in an effort to learn specifically what substance or combination of substances are protective against cancer.

3. *Eat cruciferous vegetables:* Broccoli, cauliflower, brussels sprouts, cabbage, turnip greens, and other members of the mustard family help prevent certain cancers from developing. Phytochemicals unique to **crucifera** (cabbage, turnip, and mustard family) stimulate liver enzymes responsible for inactivating toxic chemicals.

4. *Include foods rich in vitamins C and E, folic acid, and beta-carotene in your diet each day:* Citrus fruits, tomatoes, green peppers, baked potatoes, broccoli, and strawberries are high in vitamin C. Dark-green and deep-yellow fresh vegetables and fruits such as carrots, corn, spinach, winter squash, peaches, and

table 12-2 **Cancer Deaths Preventable by Healthy Diet**

What you eat every day *can* make a difference! Eating more plant foods, less fat and meat can greatly cut your risk of cancer. The National Cancer Institute estimates that a healthier diet can reduce your risk of cancer by these amounts:

Colon/rectal	75%
Prostate	75%
Breast, pancreas	70%
Endometrium, gall bladder	50%
Stomach	35%
Lung, mouth, larynx, cervix, bladder, esophagus	20%
Other types	10%
Overall estimate	32%

Source: National Cancer Institute

table 12-3   Healthy Changes

Improving your nutritional well-being to reduce cancer risk due to diet can be as simple as making healthier substitutions for foods that you often eat. Here are some suggestions.

Eat Less Often	Eat More Often
Meats	
High-fat meat, ribs	Loin, flank steak, roasts, round steak, tempeh
Fried chicken	Chicken with skin removed
Fried fish	Broiled fish
Hamburger	Soy burger, ground turkey, tofu in stir-frys
Regular hot dogs, bologna	Low-fat hot dogs or bologna
Bacon, ham, pepperoni	Canadian bacon
Other fried meats	Meats baked, grilled, roasted, steamed
Dairy	
Full-fat or 2% milk	1% or skim milk
Regular sour cream	Lite or fat-free sour cream or plain yogurt
Full-fat cheese	Fat-free or low-fat cheese
Full-fat cream cheese	Fat-free cream cheese
Fats	
Butter, margarine	Lite or whipped butter or none
Regular salad dressing	Lite or fat-free salad dressing and mayonnaise
Snacks	
Potato chips, corn chips	Low-fat popcorn, pretzels, soy nuts, baked corn chips
Cookies	Low-fat cookies, graham crackers, fruit, carmel or chocolate rice cakes
Ice cream	Frozen yogurt, pudding pops, popsicles, frozen bananas or grapes
Donuts, croissants	Whole-grain bagels with low-fat spread
Candy bar	Fruit, Lifesavers, gum, breath mints
Cocoa, cappucino	Low-fat cocoa, low-fat cappucino

table 12-4   One-Day Sample Menu

Breakfast	Whole- grain cereal, toast, or low-fat muffin; skim or soy milk; and fruit.
Lunch	Tuna or chicken sandwich made with whole grain bread; low-fat dressing; soup, salad, or vegetables; and skim milk.
Dinner	Pasta or rice dish with small amount of meat or tofu; beans; two vegetables; whole-grain bread; and skim milk.
Snacks	Low-fat popcorn; fruit; frozen yogurt; soy nuts, or raw vegetables with a low-fat dip.

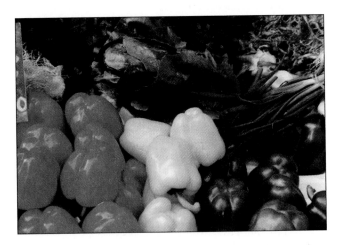

Brightly colored vegetables are rich in phytochemicals, which bolster the body's cancer defenses.

apricots contain up to 500 or more natural carotenoids. While much research has focused on **beta-carotene,** many other carotenoids are stronger **antioxidants,** and it may be that a combination of these and other phytochemicals make them cancer-protective. Green and leafy vegetables, whole grains, egg yolks, nuts, and wheat germ contain folic acid

and vitamin E. Folic acid is a B vitamin that guards against cell mutations and chromosome abnormalities that may be involved in initiation of cancer. Folic acid works synergistically with other antioxidant vitamins and phytochemicals to neutralize **free radicals,** potentially dangerous

top ten list

Top Ten Cancer-Fighting Foods

Five servings of fruits and vegetables a day is a good start in preventing cancer, but some plant foods are more powerful than others in reducing cancer risk. Here are the best—include them in your weekly shopping list and enjoy them often.

1. Cruciferous vegetables: cabbage, cauliflower, kale, broccoli, collards, brussels sprouts. Contain sulphaphorone, indoles, isothyocianates, which reduce the risk of lung, breast, and stomach cancer.
2. Dark green leafy vegetables: spinach; orange plant foods: carrots, sweet potato, apricots; yellow vegetables: corn, squash. Contain carotenoids, the plant form of vitamin A; antioxidants; and phytochemicals, which neutralize free radicals and bolster the body's cancer defenses.
3. Tomatoes, tomato sauce. Contain lycopene, which defends against prostate, lung, stomach, and endometrial cancers.
4. Soy foods (soy burger, soybeans, tofu), flaxseed. Contain phytoestrogens, which lower the risk of breast and prostate cancer.
5. Red grapes, purple grape juice. Contain grapes, which have flavonoids, phenols, and resveratrol, which inhibit cancer cell growth.
6. Garlic, onions, leeks. Contain allyl sulfides, which lower the risk of colon and stomach cancers.
7. Citrus fruits. Contain terpenes such as limonene and flavonoids, which inhibit cancer cell growth.
8. Prunes, berries (blueberries, strawberries). Contain antioxidant powerhouses, which neutralize damaging free radicals.
9. Whole-grain breads, cereals. Contain folate, fiber, and phytonutrients, which lower the risk of breast, colon, and endometrial cancers.
10. Green tea. Contains polyphenols, which inhibit growth of cancer cells. Black tea may provide some benefit.

substances that produce precancerous cellular damage. These foods also help strengthen the body's immune system. More information on food sources of these vitamins and minerals is given in Chapter 10.

5. *Consume charcoal-grilled, salted and nitrite-cured, smoked, and pickled foods in moderation:* Charring and cooking meats at high temperatures for long periods produces carcinogens. The preservative nitrate in processed meats such as hot dogs, luncheon meats, bacon, beef sticks, and beef jerky forms cancer-causing substances when broken down by the body.

wellness flash

Number of U.S. states in which at last half of the adult population eats five or more servings of fruits and vegetables a day: Zero!

6. *Consume low-fat dairy products and other calcium-rich foods daily:* Calcium appears to neutralize potentially carcinogenic substances in the digestive tract, reducing the risk of colorectal cancer. Also, processed cheese contains a cancer inhibitor, a form of linoleic acid, which may be incorporated into body cells of people who consume it, locking in a defense against cancer.
7. *Include soy foods in your diet.* If you are not eating soy foods now, it's a good time to start. Soy not only has heart-healthy benefits, but may protect against breast and prostate cancer. Breast and prostate cancer rates are far lower in some Asian countries where soy foods are consumed daily. While American and Asian diets differ in many ways, when scientists compared 1,200 Japanese women who had breast cancer with 23,000 who did not, the cancer-free women ate much more soy foods than those with cancer. Another study in Singapore found that premenopausal women who consumed the most soy had over 60 percent less risk of breast cancer than those who ate the least. Researchers state that soy appears to work by increasing production of enzymes that detoxify free radicals. Researchers also believe

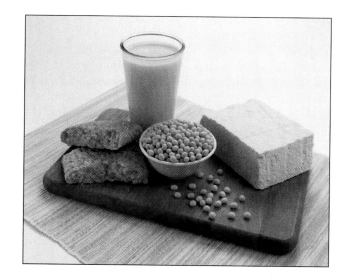

A variety of soy foods.

that phytochemicals in soy called phytoestrogens may occupy estrogen receptors and prevent the growth and proliferation of certain cancers that feed on estrogen. However, it is possible to get too much of a good thing. Breast cancer patients or those at high risk for breast cancer should not load up on soy or take isoflavone pills extracted from soy. While one to two servings a day are fine, there is concern that too much soy could cause estrogen imbalances that stimulate breast cancer growth. Soybeans and products such as tofu, soy milk, and tempeh are good sources of protective phytochemicals. While many Americans are unfamiliar with soy-based foods, dubious about the taste, or unfamiliar with how to prepare them, soy dishes can be tasty, and soy is easy to work into your daily diet. Try soy burgers, soy corn dogs, or soy chicken nuggets or try soy milk on breakfast cereal. Soy burger crumbles work well in spaghetti sauce and chili. Soy nuts make a good snack. Even one serving of soy a day decreases cancer rates.

wellness flash

Twenty-two percent of U.S. adults are physically active for at least 30 minutes, five times a week. Twenty-eight percent of U.S. adults don't participate in any leisure-time physical activity.

Inactivity

Thirty minutes of physical activity 4 to 5 days a week pays big dividends. Experts speculate that exercise enhances overall health and well-being and stimulates the immune system, which may then scavenge abnormal cells more effectively. Having a strong immune system is a key factor in preventing cancer because we are exposed to carcinogens every day. Researchers also speculate that exercise decreases the production of some reproductive hormones in both men and women, decreasing the risk of cancers that depend on these hormones to develop, such as breast and prostate cancers. Many studies have found an association between physical activity and reduced risk of breast cancer. In one study, women who exercised at least four times a week had a 37 percent lower risk of breast cancer than sedentary peers. A study of Harvard alumni found that men who burned at least 1,000 calories a week in physical activity had half the risk for colon cancer of inactive men. (One thousand calories is the approximate equivalent of walking 2 miles a day, 5 days a week.) This is true for women as well. A Harvard study of women found that for every day a woman walks a half-hour,

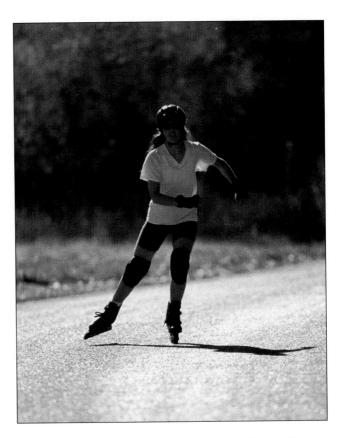

Thirty minutes of exercise a day pays big dividends in preventing cancer.

her risk of colon cancer is decreased by 10 percent. Other studies show that the more you exercise, the more protection you get. Exercise appears to prevent colon cancer by helping to speed food through the digestive system, leaving less time for carcinogens to remain in contact with the colon.

Inactivity may be a greater risk than obesity in the cancer equation. Studies done at the Cooper Institute in Dallas have shown that exercise is beneficial in reducing cancer risk even for those who are overweight. Thousands of people were treadmill tested for cardiorespiratory fitness then tracked for long-term health. Studies based on that data indicated that physically active individuals who are overweight have a lower risk of cancer than people who are overweight and sedentary, though they still have a higher risk than those who are thinner and fit. Whatever your weight, good health habits can pay off.

Secondary Risk Factors for Cancer

While the primary factors are the strongest contributors to increased cancer risk, several other preventable factors also affect risk of having cancer. These include obesity; excessive alcohol consumption; exposure to some viral infections; and exposure to radiation, workplace hazards, and certain chemicals.

Obesity

Body size matters in cancer risk. Obese individuals particularly those who are obese and sedentary, increase their risk of cancer of the breast, colon, and reproductive organs. The more overweight a person is, the greater the risk. Whether increased risk is due to sedentary lifestyle, greater caloric intake, greater fat intake, body fat mediated hormonal factors, or a combination of these is uncertain. People who carry extra weight in the abdomen are at higher risk for breast and endometrial cancer. The good news is that those who are apple-shaped (as opposed to pear-shaped, having bigger thighs and hips) can reduce their risk by losing weight. It appears to be fairly easy for apple-shaped people to lose weight where it counts because fat leaves the abdomen first. While the explanation for the reduced risk is uncertain, researchers believe that weight loss reduces the amount of sex hormones available to stimulate possible precancerous cell growth in the reproductive organs. To reach and maintain a healthy body weight, see Chapter 11 for information on how to balance caloric intake with physical activity.

Excessive Alcohol Consumption

Avoid alcohol or limit alcohol intake to two drinks a day or less. Excessive alcohol consumption increases the risk of several cancers. Esophageal and liver cancers occur more frequently among heavy drinkers of alcohol especially when the drinking is accompanied by cigarette smoking or chewing of tobacco. Coupled with poor diet, alcohol increases the risk of developing colon cancer because it interferes with folic acid metabolism. Studies have also shown an increased risk of breast cancer in women who regularly consume more than three alcoholic drinks per week. Factors that cause this effect are not yet known, but researchers speculate that the association may be due to the carcinogenic effect of alcohol, it's breakdown products in the body, or alcohol-mediated changes in hormonal levels such as estrogens. Whatever the cause, for those who drink regularly, reducing alcohol consumption is a good way to decrease risk of cancer.

Exposure to Some Viral Infections

Some viral infections can initiate cellular damage that leads to cancer. For example, the hepatitis B virus is linked to liver cancer, human papilloma virus (HPV) is linked to cervical cancer, and human immunodeficiency virus (HIV) is linked to Kaposi's sarcoma. Risk of exposure to these can be reduced by behavioral changes. For example, condom use during sex can prevent sexual exposure to hepatitis B, HPV, and HIV. This is particularly important for young adults, because the highest risk age group for STDs is in the late teens to early 20s.

Exposure to Radiation Workplace Hazards, and Certain Chemicals

Avoid excessive exposure to ionizing radiation. Ionizing radiation includes X rays, radon, and UV radiation. While most medical X rays emit low-dose radiation, it is still wise to use protective shields to cover body areas not being X rayed. There is also a potential problem of radioactive radon gas in the home in certain areas of the country. You can buy an inexpensive radon detector to test for radon, which increases the risk for lung cancer, especially in cigarette smokers. If you detect radon, professionals can advise you regarding steps to take to increase ventilation and seal the home against radon infiltration.

Be aware of hazards in the workplace. Exposure to asbestos and other industrial materials increases risk, especially when combined with smoking. Minimize exposure to these products by wearing protective clothing and equipment and by following standard safety procedures.

Limit your exposure to pesticides and insecticides. Not all chemicals are carcinogenic, but a few that are proven carcinogens include benzene, PCBs, DDT, vinyl chloride, arsenic, aflatoxin, chloroform, and formaldehyde. Read and follow label instructions with household and garden chemicals and use natural products when possible (e.g., soap spray to kill aphids).

Early Detection

Early detection is taking action to diagnose cancer in its earliest, most treatable stage. This includes three parts:

- knowing cancer's warning signals
- practicing self-exams
- having regular cancer-related checkups by a physician

Once metastases spread from the primary site, cancer becomes much more difficult to cure. Although not all cancers can be detected through self-exams, such exams, along with awareness of cancer's seven warning signals (Table 12-5) can alert a person to the need to consult a physician.

| table 12-5 | Cancer's Seven Warning Signals (CAUTION) |

1. Change in bowel or bladder habits
2. A sore that does not heal
3. Unusual bleeding or discharge
4. Thickening or lump in breast or elsewhere
5. Indigestion or difficulty in swallowing
6. Obvious change in wart or mole
7. Nagging cough or hoarseness

If you have a warning signal, see your doctor!

Source: Courtesy of American Cancer Society.

table 12-6	Cancer Checkups
Breast	Do a monthly self-exam; clinical examination of the breast every 3 years from age 20 to 40 and then every year; a screening mammography by age 40, one every 1 to 2 years from age 40 to 49, and yearly from age 50.
Colorectal	Have a digital rectal examination by a physician during an office visit yearly after age 40; the stool blood test every year after age 50; the proctosigmoidoscopy examination every 3 to 5 years after age 50.
Cervical	Get an annual Pap test and pelvic exam if you are a woman who is or has been sexually active or are age 18 or over. After three or more consecutive satisfactory annual exams, the Pap test may be performed less frequently at the physician's discretion.
Testicular	Do a monthly self-exam.
Skin	Perform a monthly self-exam.
Prostate	Have an annual rectal/prostate examination as part of your regular annual checkup if you are a man over age 40.

See your physician for cancer-related checkups. Even if you have no symptoms, it is important for early detection of cancer to have periodic cancer-related checkups (Table 12-6). Until all cancers can be prevented, protect yourself with knowledge about cancer signs, self-exams, early detection, regular checkups, and prompt treatment.

For most people without symptoms, cancer-related checkups are recommended every 3 years from ages 20 to 39 and annually for those over age 40. People who are at high risk for certain cancers may need tests more often.

Common Cancers

While many types of cancers exist, some are much more common than others. The most common cancers in order of occurrence are:

Men	Women
• Prostate	• Breast
• Lung	• Lung
• Colon/Rectal	• Colon/Rectal

For men in the 15- to 34-year-old age group, testicular cancer is the most common. While it is second in occurrence for both men and women, lung cancer is the leading cause of cancer deaths because of its low survival rate. Although they are the most frequently occurring cancers, affecting nearly one in six Americans, skin cancers are not usually included in cancer statistics because almost all nonmelanoma skin cancers are easily cured if detected early. Even so, there are over 9,000 skin cancer deaths yearly. See Figure 12-2 for leading sites of new cancer cases and deaths.

Skin Cancer

Skin cancer accounts for 40 percent of cancers. Sun overexposure during childhood and teen years accounts for over three-fourths of your lifetime exposure to the sun's ultraviolet radiation. Well-browned skin is a sign of injury to the skin, not a sign of health. While anyone can get skin cancer, people are most susceptible if they work out in the sun, live in sunny climates, or have blonde or red hair, light-colored eyes, or fair skin that doesn't tan easily (Table 12-7).

There are three types of skin cancer that may be caused by UV radiation: basal cell, squamous cell, and malignant melanoma. Basal cell cancers, the most common, are

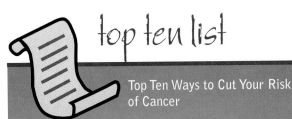

top ten list

Top Ten Ways to Cut Your Risk of Cancer

1. Avoid tobacco of any kind
2. Reduce sun exposure
3. Eat more fruits, vegetables, and grains; decrease red meat and dietary fat
4. Exercise 20 to 30 minutes most days of the week
5. Maintain a healthy weight
6. Drink little or no alcohol
7. Use protective measures against STDs
8. Minimize exposure to radiation, workplace hazards, and chemicals
9. Know cancer's seven warning signals
10. Practice self-exams, and see your physician for cancer-related checkups

Cancer Cases by Site and Sex

Male	Female
Prostate 180,400	Breast 182,800
Lung and bronchus 89,500	Lung and bronchus 74,600
Colon and rectum 63,600	Colon and rectum 66,600
Urinary bladder 38,300	Uterine corpus 36,100
Non-Hodgkin's lymphoma 31,700	Non-Hodgkin's lymphoma 23,200
Melanoma of the skin 27,300	Ovary 23,100
Oral cavity 20,200	Melanoma of the skin 20,400
Kidney 18,800	Urinary bladder 14,900
Leukemia 16,900	Pancreas 14,600
Pancreas 13,700	Thyroid 13,700
All sites 619,700	All sites 600,400

Cancer Deaths by Site and Sex

Male	Female
Lung and bronchus 89,300	Lung and bronchus 67,600
Prostate 31,900	Breast 40,800
Colon and rectum 27,800	Colon and rectum 28,500
Pancreas 13,700	Pancreas 14,500
Non-Hodgkin's lymphoma 13,700	Ovary 14,000
Leukemia 12,100	Non-Hodgkin's lymphoma 12,400
Esophagus 9,200	Leukemia 9,600
Liver 8,500	Uterine corpus 6,500
Urinary bladder 8,100	Brain 5,900
Stomach 7,600	Stomach 5,400
All sites 284,100	All sites 268,100

figure 12-2   Leading sites of new cancer cases and deaths—2000 Estimates*

*Excludes basal and squamous cell skin cancer and in situ carcinomas except urinary bladder.

© 2000, American Cancer Society, Inc., Surveillance Research

---

table 12-7   What Is Your Skin Type?

Skin Type	Sunburn and Tanning History	SPF
I	Always burns, never tans*	20–30
II	Burns easily, tans minimally	15–20
III	Burns moderately, tans gradually to light brown	15
IV	Burns minimally, tans well to medium brown	15
V	Rarely burns, tans profusely to dark	10–15
VI	Never burns, deeply pigmented	10–15

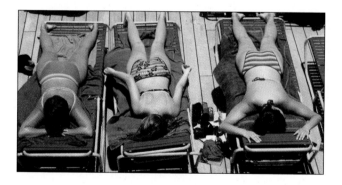

Sun overexposure causes most skin cancers.

---

raised pearly nodules that involve the outer layers of skin. Squamous cell cancers are either wartlike growths that ulcerate in the center or pinkish, raised, opaque nodules. These cancers are rarely fatal, do not tend to metastasize, and can be removed by a physician.

Malignant **melanoma,** which usually starts as a dark wart or mole, is the most rapidly increasing type of skin cancer in the United States. It has a deadly tendency to metastasize and accounts for over 75 percent of skin cancer deaths. The problem is particularly severe for men and whites. Men die of melanoma at twice the rate of women. People with naturally dark skin, type VI, have a built-in measure of protection. About 98 percent of malignant melanoma occurs in whites, though African Americans tend to be diagnosed at a later stage. Malignant melanoma diagnosed at an early stage can be treated, but when it penetrates even one-tenth of an inch into the skin, the survival rate decreases by 50 percent. Contributing to increasing rates of skin cancer is that, in the upper atmosphere, the thinning ozone layer allows more of the sun's damaging ultraviolet radiation to reach the skin. As a result, skin cancer rates are increasing by about 4 percent per year, faster than any other cancer. Approximately 90 percent of skin cancers can be prevented by protecting the skin from the sun's rays.

While young people often think of themselves as immune to skin cancer, nearly one-third of melanomas occur in people under age 45. The most common sites are the upper back and back of the legs, but it can occur anywhere from the scalp to the soles of the feet. You don't have to be a dermatologist to recognize a potential melanoma. Know what skin cancer looks like and examine your skin at least once a year using the skin self-exam in Figure 12-3. Learn where your moles are and what they look like, and then you will notice if there are any changes. If you find unusual moles or skin spots, the American Academy of Dermatology suggests using the ABCD test for early detection of malignant melanoma (Figure 12-4). Besides moles, watch for sores that do not heal; unusual bumps; and chronically scaly, red, or pinkish patches of skin. If detected early, skin cancer has an 85 to 99 percent cure rate. Table 12-8 summarizes the risk factors for skin cancer.

Breast Cancer

Breast cancer is the most common cancer in women, but it is more curable than lung cancer, so it ranks as the second leading cancer killer. It is estimated that the lifetime risk of breast cancer is one out of nine. Getting older is the most important risk factor for breast cancer. However, young

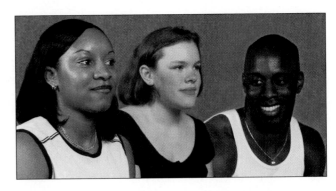

Skin cancer risk is greater with fair skin. Melanin in darker skin provides a measure of protection from damaging UV rays.

table 12-8   Risk Factors for Skin Cancer

While anyone can get skin cancer, these characteristics indicate higher risk:

- Light skin color
- Family history of skin cancer
- Personal history of skin cancer
- A typical mole or a large number of moles
- Freckles (indicating sun sensitivity and sun damage)
- Severe sunburn in childhood
- Chronic sun overexposure

Your skin self–exam

The best time to do this simple monthly exam is after a bath or shower. Use a full-length and a hand mirror so you can check any moles, blemishes, or birthmarks from the top of your head to your toes, noting anything new– a change in size, shape, or color or a sore that does not heal.

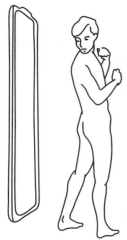

1. Examine your body front and back in the mirror, then right and left sides, arms raised.

2. Bend elbows and look carefully at forearms and upper underarms *and* palms.

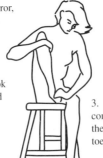

3. Sit, if that is more comfortable, to look at backs of the legs, feet—spaces between toes *and* soles.

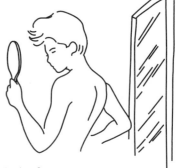

4. Examine back of neck and scalp with the help of a hand mirror, part hair (or use blow dryer) to lift it and give you a close look.

If you do the exam regularly, you will know what is normal for you and can feel confident in your examination. Remember the ABCDs, and check with your physician or clinic if you find something.

figure 12-3   Skin self-exam.

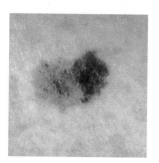

A—Asymmetry: Is one half unlike the other?

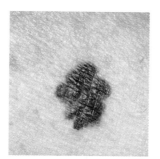

B—Border irregularity: Does it have an uneven, scalloped edge rather than a clearly defined border?

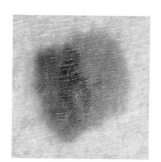

C—Color variation: Is the color uniform, or does it vary from one area to another– from tan to brown to black, or from white to red to blue?

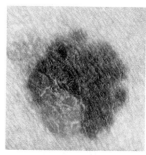

D—Diameter larger than one-fourth inch: At its widest point, is the growth as large as or larger than a pencil eraser?

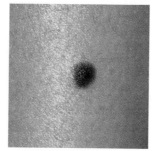

Normal mole

figure 12-4 ABCD test for malignant melanoma.

Breast Self-Examination

1. In the shower:
Examine your breasts during bath or shower; hands glide easier over wet skin. Fingers flat, move gently over every part of each breast. Use the right hand to examine the left breast, left hand for the right breast. Check for any lump, hard knot, or thickening.

2. Before a mirror:
Inspect your breasts with arms at your sides. Next, raise your arms high overhead. Look for any changes in the contour of each breast: a swelling, dimpling of skin, or changes in the nipple.

Then rest palms on hips and press down firmly to flex your chest muscles. Left and right breast will not exactly match; few women's breasts do.

Regular inspection shows what is normal for you and will give you confidence in your examination.

3. Lying down:
To examine your right breast, put a pillow or folded towel under your right shoulder. Place right hand behind your head—this distributes breast tissue more evenly on the chest. With left hand, fingers flat, press gently in small circular motions around an imaginary clock face. Begin at outermost top of your right breast for 12 o'clock, then move to 1 o'clock, and so on around the circle back to 12. A ridge of firm tissue in the lower curve of each breast is normal. Then move in an inch, toward the nipple, keep circling to examine *every part of your breast*, including nipple. This requires at least three more circles. Now slowly repeat procedure on your left breast with a pillow under your left shoulder and left hand behind head. Notice how your breast structure feels.

Finally, squeeze the nipple of each breast gently between thumb and index finger. Any discharge, clear or bloody, should be reported to your doctor immediately.

figure 12-5 Breast self-examination.
Source: Courtesy of American Cancer Society.

women should not feel complacent because breast cancer can occur at any age. Although rare, about 2 percent of breast cancers are in men. Other risk factors for breast cancer include the following:

- A sister or mother who has had breast cancer, especially if it occurred before menopause; early onset of menstruation (before age 12)
- Experiencing menopause after age 50 (both situations increase the lifelong exposure to high estrogen levels)
- Obesity (fat cells produce estrogen)
- Never having given birth

These factors together account for only 25 percent of breast cancer. White women have a somewhat higher risk than African American or Hispanic women or those of Asian origin.

The incidence of breast cancer is slowly rising, but no one knows why. It could be partly because more women are being diagnosed at earlier ages, thanks to mammography. It might be partly attributed to some as yet unidentified dietary or environmental factor (e.g., PCBs or DDT). High fat intake and sedentary lifestyle are currently suspects. The good news is obesity and sedentary lifestyle are two risk factors that you *can* control. A breast self-exam can detect cancer in its early, curable stage and should be practiced monthly (Figure 12-5).

Prostate Cancer

This is the most common cancer (excluding skin cancer) and the second leading cause of cancer deaths in men. It affects about one in six men over a lifetime. The warning signs of prostate cancer are weak or interrupted urine flow; inability to urinate or difficulty starting and stopping urine flow; the need to urinate frequently, especially at night; blood in the urine; pain or burning on urination; and continuing pain in the lower back, pelvis, or upper thighs. Most of these symptoms are nonspecific and may be similar to benign conditions such as infection or prostate enlargement.

Prostate cancer generally occurs in men over 50; risk increases with age. Studies link dietary fat, and consumption of red meat to increased risk of this cancer.

Lung Cancer

Lung cancer is a rare disease except among smokers. Exposure to sidestream cigarette smoke increases the risk for nonsmokers. Lung tissue damage and cellular changes that precede lung cancer have been observed in 93 percent of active smokers but in only 6 percent of exsmokers and 1 percent of nonsmokers. If a smoker quits, these early precancerous cellular changes are reversible, and the damaged bronchial lining often returns to normal. If the smoker continues, the abnormal cell growth may progress to cancer.

wellness flash

On average, smokers die nearly 7 years earlier than nonsmokers and have an added 2 years of disability.

Between 1960 and 1990, lung cancer deaths increased in women by over 400 percent and surpassed breast cancer deaths by 50 percent. Lung cancer, the leading cancer killer for both men and women, has a low survival rate because it is seldom discovered in its earliest stages. By the time it has grown large enough to produce noticeable symptoms or to be visible on X ray, it is already well advanced. It metastasizes readily through the bloodstream to the brain and other organs and is difficult to treat. The 5-year rate for lung cancer survival is 13 percent and has not changed, despite advances in cancer treatment, in 40 years.

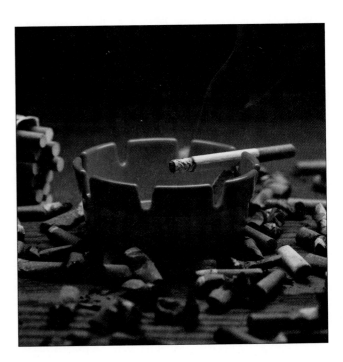

Cancers caused by tobacco use are 100 percent preventable.

Colon and Rectal Cancer

In populations where fruits and vegetables are consumed in abundance and animal foods are scarce, colon cancer is a rare disease. In the United States, however, it is the third leading cancer killer. A genetic tendency to develop

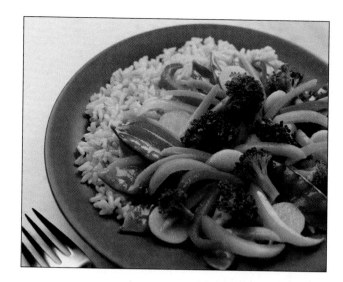

Eating more plant foods and less meat and high-fat foods can reduce the risk of colon cancer as much as 75 percent.

testicle, a dull ache in the lower abdomen and groin, a sensation of heaviness, and pain in the testes. Your risk of getting testicular cancer is 40 times higher if you have a testicle that never descended into the scrotum or descended after age 6.

Lives could be saved if more testicular cancers were detected and treated early. The 5-year survival rate of testicular cancer is 91 percent. Treatment does not mean losing your "manhood" or your ability to have normal sex, and it doesn't mean you can't have children.

Men discover most testicular cancers by learning how to examine their testicles. In doing this once a month, you can greatly increase the chances of finding a testicular cancer early if it does occur. All young men should learn and practice the monthly testicular self-examination, detailed in Figure 12-6, from adolescence on. The technique is simple.

noncancerous polyps in the colon, combined with a diet high in animal fat and low in fruits and vegetables may cause half, perhaps all, colon cancer. Dietary habits and preferences are formed young and practiced over a lifetime. Chronic exposure to carcinogens in high-fat and highly refined and processed foods can eventually stimulate precancerous changes in cells. While high-fiber dietary supplements have not proven beneficial, in thousands of studies, components within plant foods have shown the ability to protect against cancer. Studies of adults whose childhood diets were low in salads and cruciferous vegetables or high in processed meats found that they were more likely to get colon cancer as compared to adults who ate healthier diets. This does not mean that you are doomed by poor childhood eating habits, but many studies consistently indicate that eating a diet rich in fruits, vegetables, whole grains, and beans can protect against many forms of cancer. A lifetime commitment to healthy eating is more effective than a short-term dietary change because cancer can take many years to develop. High levels of physical activity also are associated with lower risk of colon cancer—by increasing intestinal motility and limiting exposure of colon cells to potentially carcinogenic compounds.

Testicular Cancer

Most people think that cancer is a disease old people get. Cancer of the testicle is different. It is not one of the most common types of cancer in this country, but it is the most common cancer in young men between the ages of 15 and 34. Warning signs include a swelling or hard lump in the

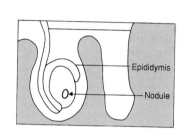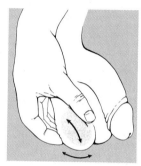

figure 12-6 Testicular self-examination.
Source: Courtesy of American Cancer Society.

Uterine and Cervical Cancer

With the widespread use of Pap smears for early detection, the death rate from uterine cancer has declined. Cervical cancer, often seen in young women, has been linked to the **human papilloma virus** (HPV), which can be spread through sexual contact. Risk factors for cervical cancer include:

- becoming sexually active at an early age
- having had several different sex partners
- genital infections such as herpes and HIV
- smoking (it weakens the immune system)

A Pap test, in which cells from the cervix and uterine lining are examined under a microscope, is a simple procedure that can be done at intervals by physicians as a part of each pelvic examination. If cervical cancer is detected at an early stage, it can easily be removed. Use of the Pap test, along with timely treatment can prevent nearly all deaths from cervical cancer. Use of condoms can prevent sexual infections that initiate the disease.

Coping with Cancer

What can you do when someone you care about is diagnosed with cancer? Many of us will face this at some time in our lives because cancer affects one in three people. You may have mixed emotions: anger and grief that this could happen to someone close to you, fear of the future, or compassion and sympathy for what that person is facing. You might feel uncomfortable around that person, not knowing what to say or do, and tend to avoid him or her or avoid discussing the illness. What can you do? Plenty. First, you should realize that cancers overall have a 50 percent cure rate. Second, loving support of friends and family increases the quality of life and survival rate to such an extent that it is a powerful adjunct to medical treatment. A study at Stanford University found that women with advanced breast cancer who participated in weekly support groups doubled their predicted life expectancy and lived an average of 18 months longer than those who were not in support groups. Here are several things you can do to help a friend or loved one deal with cancer:

1. Share your thoughts and feelings and encourage your friend to do so. Allow your friend to express hopes, fears, and sadness; accept those feelings without trying to change them. Showing your love and concern and discussing mutual fears can bring you closer and provide great comfort. There is no right way to feel about cancer, no right way to react. Being honest and open strengthens relationships.

2. Offer to accompany your friend on a visit to the doctor or hospital. You can provide transportation to and from treatments, take notes while the doctor gives instructions, and provide support.

3. Instead of saying "Call me if you need anything," offer specific help: cook a meal, do the dishes, do laundry, walk the dog, take the kids to the park, pick up medicine from the pharmacy.

4. Encourage your friend to join you in some enjoyable activities . . . go to a movie or rent some comedy videos, go for a walk together, go on a picnic, or have a potluck dinner with friends.

5. Contact a cancer survivor who can talk to your friend, answer questions, and share insights of someone who has successfully walked down the same road.

6. Help your friend contact a cancer support group. While you can't know what your friend is going through, other cancer patients do and can provide the kind of open discussion and empathy that reduces distress and strengthens coping skills. Provide transportation to meetings. Some resources that may help you locate support groups: The American Cancer Society (800-227-2345) and The National Cancer Institute's Cancer Information Service (800-422-6237). Also check with your friend's physician, church, hospital, or on the Internet.

What if *you* are diagnosed with cancer? How can you cope? Here are some suggestions:

1. Take an active role: learn everything you can about the cancer and treatments.

2. Ask lots of questions so you understand what is happening to you and what your options are. Think of what you can do to enhance your recovery and discuss it with your doctor.

3. Take care of yourself. Exercise, eat healthfully, get enough sleep, manage stress. Your immune system needs every advantage you can give it. If you don't feel like going for a walk, try stretching or yoga. Ask your doctor how long you need to wait after a chemotherapy treatment to exercise.

4. Build a support system. Many studies point to the positive effect of a good support system on health and the immune system. Some friends won't feel comfortable knowing that you have cancer because of their fear of the disease or the fear that you will die. They may not know what to say or do, and as a result you could become socially isolated. Have friends and relatives join you in a walk, a meal, shopping, or going to a movie. Ask friends for help with research, transportation to medical appointments, cooking meals, home maintenance, and so on. Learn to graciously accept help.

5. Talk about your feelings. Sharing your concerns openly and honestly with a friend or family member may bring you closer and help you cope better.

6. Find a cancer support group. Talk to a cancer survivor. We don't know why, but there is something about sharing experiences that helps people in support groups live longer than those who go it alone.

7. Maintain your sense of humor. Do something that makes you laugh everyday. Watch a funny video, have a good laugh with a friend. A sense of humor helps you cope with cancer and treatments. Cultivate positive feelings to mobilize your body's healing energies and to make yourself feel better.

frequently asked questions

Q. My grandfather and father had skin cancer. Does cancer run in families?

A. All cancers are caused by a malfunctioning gene that controls cell growth and replication. The American Cancer Society estimates that about 5 to 10 percent of cancers are related to an inherited gene that predisposes a person to a certain type of cancer, such as certain types of breast cancer. Having an inherited copy of a damaged gene doesn't mean that cancer is inevitable, rather that the risk is higher and it is more important than ever that a person practice preventive behaviors. Gene malfunctions in most other cancers are initiated by external factors such as sunlight and chemical exposure (e.g., tobacco use) or internal factors such as hormones. Most skin cancers are related to sun overexposure, although if you inherited fair skin that burns easily, you are more susceptible to UV damage than someone who inherited a darker skin tone.

Q. I sunburned nearly every summer during childhood. Am I doomed to have skin cancer?

A. While sunburns and sun overexposure during childhood increase your lifetime risk of skin cancer, the skin does have a capacity to heal. While it isn't inevitable, if you are at higher risk, it is especially important to know what skin cancer looks like, to examine your skin monthly, and to use sunscreen when you are outside. What are you doing now to take care of your skin?

Q. I smoked two packs of cigarettes a day for 3 years but quit and haven't had one in 5 years. What is my risk of cancer?

A. After five smoke-free years, your risk is about half that of a smoker. After 10 smoke-free years, it will be the same as if you never smoked.

Q. I heard blueberries are high in antioxidants. Should I eat them instead of other fruits?

A. No. There is no one perfect food. Eating a lot of one food at the expense of others can shortchange you on a balance of nutrients. Your best bet is to eat a variety of fruits and vegetables rather than concentrating on a few.

Q. The only vegetable I like is corn. Can't I just take a vitamin pill or a few supplements instead of eating fruits and vegetables to reduce cancer risk?

A. While some experts recommend vitamin supplements, others feel that this causes us to get more vitamins than our bodies can use, and the excess are excreted in the form of expensive urine. Both groups agree on this: pills cannot make up for a bad diet. There is good evidence that a diet rich in certain fruits, vegetables, and whole-grain products lowers the risk of some types of cancer, but it is not yet clear whether it is the antioxidants, folic acid, or another of the dozens of phytochemicals in these foods that makes them cancer-protective. A plant may be more than the sum of its nutrients. While taking a pill probably won't hurt, no one compound, or even a small group of compounds, will replace hundreds of nutrients, many of which we are only beginning to learn about. Don't count on a vitamin to replace a diet abundant in fruits and vegetables.

Q. Do tanning beds provide a safe tan?

A. Tanning beds used to emit only UVA ("tanning") rays, but now many approximate natural sunlight, emitting a mix of UVA and UVB ("burning") radiation. UVA rays penetrate deeper into the skin than UVB and can cause serious damage. Both kinds injure the skin, collagen, and immune response and encourage wrinkling and skin cancer. It is a myth that tanning beds will provide a safe "base" tan before a midwinter vacation. The protection is minimal, and you will still burn unless you apply sunscreen.

Q. Are self-tanning lotions safe?

A. While many previous products turned the skin orange, some newer products contain an FDA-approved dye, dihydroxyacetone (DHA). It stains skin a light brown and is safe to use because it appears to work only on the outermost skin layer. Best results are obtained for people with skin types II and III who have applied the product two to four times within 1 day. Skin darkened with a dye does not provide UV protection, and you still need to wear sunscreen to guard against burns.

summary

You can significantly increase your chances of living a healthy, active life, free of disabling disease, by making wise daily personal choices. Your risk of cancer can be greatly decreased with awareness of primary and secondary risk factors and appropriate lifestyle changes. These involve avoiding tobacco; reducing sun overexposure; eating more plant foods and fewer high-fat animal products; regular exercise; maintaining a healthy weight; using little or no alcohol; using protective measures against viral infections, and minimizing exposure to radiation, workplace hazards, and some chemicals. Early detection is also important. This includes knowing cancer's seven warning signals, performing regular self-exams, and having regular cancer-related checkups. Cancer is not inevitable. Acting to control risks in your immediate environment is a powerful way to enhance your total wellness.

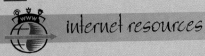 *internet resources*

American Cancer Society, Inc.

   http://www.cancer.org
   1 (800) ACS-2345

American Institute for Cancer Research

   http://www.AICR.org
   1-800-843-8114

Breast cancer

   http://www.susanlovemd.com
   http://www.breastcancer.com

Centers for Disease Control and Prevention

   http://www.cdc.com

National Cancer Institute

   http://www.cancernet.nci.nih.gov
   1(800)4-CANCER

OncoLink

   http://www.oncolink.org

Y-Me Breast Cancer Support

   Program, 1 (800) 221-2141.

Web MD

   http://www.mywebmd.com

What is Your Cancer Risk?

Cancer isn't always something that "just happens." Behaviors that you practice regularly over a lifetime can increase or decrease your risk of a serious illness, including cancer. Take this test to check your risk related to personal behaviors, then assess what changes you can make to reduce your risk. Scores below 40 indicate increased risk of cancer due to personal behavior.

Yes

1. I do not smoke.

      6

2. I do not use smokeless tobacco

      4

3. I am rarely exposed to sidestream smoke

      2

A. Tobacco avoidance score _____

4. I avoid tanning, even in tanning booths

      4

5. I use at least SPF 15 sunscreen when outside for 15 minutes or longer

      3

6. I use a hat, long sleeved shirt, and protective clothing if I must be outside for several hours in the sun

      3

B. Sun protection score _____

7. I seldom eat fried foods

      1

8. I eat meat only a couple times a week

      1

9. I usually consume low-fat dairy products

      1

10. I eat five or more servings of fruits and vegetables daily

      1

11. I eat whole-grain products regularly

      1

12. I eat cruciferous vegetables two or more times weekly

      1

13. I often eat deeply colored or leafy green vegetables

      1

14. I consume fruits and vegetables high in vitamin C five or more times a week

      1

15. I rarely eat charcoal-grilled or smoked meats

      1

16. I rarely eat heavily salted or pickled meats

      1

17. I seldom eat nitrate-processed meats such as hot dogs, beef jerky, or bacon

C. Dietary habits score _____

lab activity @ chapter twelve

18. I am physically active 20 to 30 minutes 3 to 5 days a week   4

19. My physical activity includes 3 or more days of aerobic activity following the F.I.T.T. formula   4

D. Exercise habits score   _____

20. I am or within 5 pounds of my ideal weight   4

21. I use little or no alcohol   3

22. I use protective measures to avoid STDs   3

23. I limit my exposure to insecticides, X rays, and known carcinogens in the workplace (e.g., asbestos, PCBs)   3

E. Secondary factors score   _____

24. I know cancer's seven warning signals   3

25. I do a monthly breast or testicular self-exam   3

26. I do a regular skin self-exam   3

27. I follow the regular cancer checkup schedule   3

F. Early detection score   _____

Grand Total (A+B+C+D+E+F) = _____

On what three behaviors did you score the highest points? (Tobacco avoidance, sun protection, exercise habits, early detection, etc.) These are behaviors that you will want to maintain.

Behavior   **Points**

1.

2.

3.

1. Over the next 3 weeks, 3 to 6 months, 1 year or more, what changes can you make to reduce your cancer risk?
   a. 3 weeks—

   b. 3 to 6 months—

   c. 1 year or more—

Cancer Type and Risk Factors

Cancer is a group of over 100 different diseases, each with different risk factors. Listed are the most common cancers and their risk factors. If several of your relatives have had the same type of cancer, family history may also increase your risk.

The white boxes indicate risk factors for a particular type of cancer. If a box is black, it is not a risk factor for that cancer (e.g., tanning is a risk factor for skin cancer, but not lung cancer). Place an X in each white box that applies to you to see if your habits place you at risk, then assess if there are any changes you can make to reduce your risk.

Type of Cancer

Risk Factor	Skin	Lung	Colon/Rectal	Breast	Prostate
Smoking					
High-fat diet					
Eat few fruits and vegetables					
Tan or sunburn					
Obesity					
Inactive					
Alcohol					
Family history					

lab activity @ chapter twelve

1. For what cancers do you have two or more risk factors?

2. Give three strategies that you can practice to reduce your risk of cancer.
   a.

   b.

   c.

Name _____

Class/Activity Section _____

Date _____

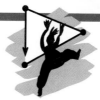

lab activity 12-3

Using HealthQuest

1. Insert the HealthQuest CD into your computer.

2. Click on "Cancer" from the menu. Click on "Introduction" and read.

3. Click on "Introduction" again and go to "Wellness Activities." Click on the "Cancer: What is Your Risk?" activity. This activity gives your risk levels and how to decrease risk for the most common cancers. Complete the 15 questions.

4. For which cancers do you have an increased risk? Why?

5. What are three specific actions that you can take to decrease your cancer risk?
   a.

   b.

   c.

6. For which cancers is your risk low? Why?

7. What are three specific cancer protective behaviors that you currently practice?
   a.

   b.

   c.

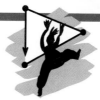

lab activity @ chapter twelve

8. Close this out (bottom left corner) and click on "Wellness Activities" again, then on "Topics."

9. Click on either: "Specifics On," "Our Changing World," or "Key Articles." Peruse the topics under these three categories. Select three topics and read the information. Summarize what you learned.

   a. Topic = _____

   b. Topic = _____

   c. Topic = _____

Cancer Prevention and Your Diet

An estimated 35 percent of cancers are related to dietary habits, which you can control. Food selection and food preparation habits can greatly increase or decrease your lifetime risk of certain kinds of cancers. To evaluate your eating habits, record everything you eat or drink for 3 days. See Lab 10-1 and check Figure 10-1 for serving sizes. Then, total the servings of foods that fall within the categories and assess how you can adapt your diet to decrease your risk.

Foods That Decrease Cancer Risk:

Over three days, how many servings did you consume of the following foods?

Servings:

1. Cruciferous vegetables (broccoli, cauliflower, brussels sprouts, bok choy, cabbage) _____
2. Dark green leafy vegetables, orange or yellow plant foods _____
3. Tomatoes, including tomato paste, tomato sauce _____
4. Soy foods (tofu, soy burgers, soybeans, soy milk, soy cheese) _____
5. Red grapes, purple grape juice, prunes, berries _____
6. Onions/garlic _____
7. Citrus fruits (oranges, grapefruit) _____
8. Skim milk/low fat cheese _____
9. Whole grains (oatmeal, brown rice, whole-grain bread) _____
10. Green or black tea _____

Cancer prevention score _____

Foods That Increase Cancer Risk:

Over three days, how many servings did you consume of the following foods?

Servings:

1. Fried foods (fried potatoes, donuts, fried fish) _____
2. Other high-fat foods (chips, cookies, crackers, Twinkies, cake, pie, candy bars) _____
3. Butter, margarine, mayonnaise, oil, regular salad dressing _____

4. High-fat meats or poultry with skin   _____

5. Pickled or salt-cured foods   _____

6. Nitrite-cured or smoked meats (bacon, hot dogs, sausage, pepperoni, jerky, bologna)   _____

7. Whole milk, ice cream, sour cream, cheese and other full-fat dairy products   _____

8. Charcoal-grilled or BBQ meats   _____

9. Alcoholic drinks   _____

Cancer promotion score   _____

Risk Assessment

Subtract your servings of cancer promoters from cancer risk reducing foods. A score of 15 or above is excellent, 10 is average, below 5 indicates increased risk related to dietary habits

1. My score is: _____. This is: excellent—average—increased risk (circle one).

2. Three things that I can do to reduce my cancer risk due to diet are:
    a.

    b.

    c.

Planning a Dietary Defense Against Cancer

Dietary defense against cancer is as close as your next meal. Complete Lab 12-4, *Cancer Prevention and Your Diet*. Consult Table 12-3, "Healthy Changes," then list cancer-preventing foods that you can add to your diet over the next week. Also note cancer-promoting foods that you can eliminate or reduce consumption of and healthier substitutes.

Over the next week, I will add the following foods to my diet:

Breakfast
1.
2.
Lunch
1.
2.
Supper
1.
2.

Over the next week, I will reduce consumption of the following foods and/or substitute healthier choices

Eliminate/Reduce	**Healthier Substitute**
Breakfast	
1.	
2.	
Lunch	
1.	
2.	
Supper	
1.	
2.	

lab activity

12-6

Lunch Box Guidelines

Cancer-risk reduction is as simple as choosing your next meal. Use the dietary guidelines in Chapter 12 to complete the following items:

1. Give four *different* dietary guidelines for reducing cancer risk and, using the following menu, select a food that exemplifies each guideline.

2. List two dietary habits that increase cancer risk and use the following menu to select a specific food example for each.

Residence Hall Dining Service Menus

Lunch

Cream of Chicken Soup, Lentil Soup, Toasted Bacon Sandwich, Tuna in Lettuce Cup, Veggie Burger, Yogurt, Sliced American Cheese, Luncheon Meats and Cheeses on Deli Line, Dill Pickles, Potato Chips, Buttered Whole Kernel Corn, Bread and Butter
Salad Bar includes: Shredded Lettuce, Chopped Broccoli and Cauliflower, Fresh Spinach, Soy Nuts, Apple Sauce, Canned Onion Rings, Bacon Bits, Tomato Slices, Cottage Cheese, Shredded Cheddar Cheese, Shredded Carrots
For dessert: Strawberries, Soft Serve Frozen Yogurt, Ice Cream Cone

Dinner

Baked Lasagna, Turkey Breast Fillet, Tofu Stir-Fry, Beans and Corn Bread, Cooked Spinach, Corn on the Cob, Mashed Potatoes, Turkey Gravy, Parsley Buttered Potatoes, Broccoli Spears, Honey Glazed Baby Carrots, Whole-Grain Roll and Butter
Salad Bar includes: Combination Salad, Alfalfa Sprouts, Fresh Spinach, Pea Peanut and Cheese Salad, Croutons, Tomato Slices, Cauliflower Buds, Bacon Bits, Shredded Cheddar Cheese, Cubed Ham, Cottage Cheese, Parmesan Cheese
For dessert: Peaches, Soft Serve Frozen Yogurt, Ice Cream Cone

lab activity @ chapter twelve

Changing Behavior Using the Transtheoretical Model

Using a highlighter, trace a path on the algorithm as you answer each question. Highlight your stage of change.

Do you practice a monthly breast or testicular cancer self-exam?

Yes   No

Have you done this consistently   Do you plan to start doing this
over the last 6 months?   within the next 6 months?

Yes   No   Yes   No

                                    Within the next month?

                                    Yes   No

| Maintenance | Action | Preparation | Contemplation | Precontemplation |

lab activity @ chapter twelve

Once you have identified which stage of change you are in, it is important to use the processes most useful in progressing to the next stage—or remaining in maintenance.

   In the box, write your stage of change. Then, list the processes that are most useful in that stage (see Fig. 2-2 in Chapter 2). Use only the processes that apply to your stage of behavior change. You may not need to use all six. Under each process, give two specific behavior strategies (see Table 2-1 in Chapter 2) that could help you progress to the next stage—or maintain, if you're in the maintenance stage.

The stage I am in = [   ] .

Process 1. _____

        Behavior strategy – a.

        Behavior strategy – b.

Process 2. _____

        Behavior strategy – a.

        Behavior strategy – b.

Process 3. _____

        Behavior strategy – a.

        Behavior strategy – b.

Process 4. _____

        Behavior strategy – a.

        Behavior strategy – b.

Process 5. _____

        Behavior strategy – a.

        Behavior strategy – b.

Process 6. _____

        Behavior strategy – a.

        Behavior strategy – b.

13

Understanding Substance Abuse and Addictive Behavior

objectives

After reading this chapter, you will be able to:

1. Give three out of five reasons alcohol/drug dependence is considered a disease.
2. Define the following terms: drug, addiction, alcoholism, tolerance, passive smoking, 'roid rage, and synergy.
3. List five factors that affect alcohol absorption.
4. Describe the effects of alcohol on the central nervous system and personal behavior.
5. Differentiate between alcohol use, abuse, and alcoholism.
6. Identify family behaviors that reduce one's risk of alcohol-related problems.
7. Identify the blood alcohol concentration (BAC) at which a person is regarded legally drunk.
8. Describe the "Zero . . . One . . . Three Rule for Lower-Risk Drinking."
9. Explain why a person may not feel intoxicated but have a BAC of 0.10 percent or more.
10. List the harmful effects of alcohol on the body.
11. Choose a correct guideline to follow if you overindulge in alcohol or a friend passes out from alcohol overindulgence.
12. List five tips/strategies for drinking less or not at all.
13. Differentiate between fetal alcohol syndrome (FAS) and fetal alcohol effect (FAE).
14. Identify the number one cause of preventable death and health problems in this country.
15. Identify the health hazards related to passive smoking.
16. Identify the two most common illegal drugs used in the United States.
17. Describe which psychoactive drugs are classified as depressants, narcotics (opioids), stimulants, psychedelics, and inhalants.
18. Identify the side effects of marijuana, cocaine, anabolic steroids, caffeine abuse, LSD, heroin, MDMA (Ecstacy), and GHB and Rohypnol "Roofies."
19. Describe the relationships between cocaine and crack and between crank and ice.
20. List four drugs that affect physical performance and describe how they do so.
21. List three of four common kinds of nonprescription drugs that can lead to physical dependence if overused and describe how prescribed drugs can be abused.

terms

- Addiction
- Alcohol (ethyl alcohol, ethanol)
- Alcoholism
- Amotivational syndrome
- Amphetamines
- Anabolic steroids
- Binge drinking
- Blackout
- Blood alcohol concentration (BAC)
- Caffeine

- Cocaine
- Crack
- Crank
- Delta-9-tetrahydrocannabinol (THC)
- Depressants
- Diuretics
- Drug
- Fetal alcohol effect (FAE)
- Fetal alcohol syndrome (FAS)
- Flashbacks

- Gamma-Hydroxybutyrate (GHB)
- Heroin
- Ice
- Inhalants
- LSD (Lysergic acid diethylamide)
- Marijuana
- MDMA (Ecstacy)
- Methamphetamine
- Narcolepsy

- Narcotics
- Nitrosamines
- Passive smoking
- Psychedelic drugs
- Psychoactive drugs
- Rohypnol ("Roofies")
- 'Roid rage
- Stimulants
- Synergistic reaction
- Testosterone
- Tolerance

We live in a drug saturated environment. We have drugs for everything—anxiety, depression, infection, and pain. A **drug** is a chemical that alters a person's physical or mental condition. The question is not whether to use drugs, because most people do, but, rather, when, where, why, and how much to use them. Most of us use over-the-counter drugs, such as aspirin. Others of us use prescribed drugs for a medical condition. Still others misuse and abuse legal and illegal drugs at the cost of our bankbooks, our relationships, and our lives (Table 13-1). Alcohol is addressed first because it is the most abused legal drug in our society. This chapter includes alcohol use assessments, responsible drinking guidelines, and strategies for drinking less to help you make decisions and take action about your alcohol use. Other drugs addressed are tobacco, illegal psychoactive recreational drugs, (depressants, narcotics, marijuana, stimulants, and psychedelics) drugs affecting physical performance, and over-the-counter and prescription drugs. Before we discuss specific drugs, let's examine addiction in general.

Addiction

Addiction is a pathological or abnormal relationship with an object or event. It is characterized by using a substance or behavior repeatedly. Addiction is an illness that progresses from a definite, though often unclear, beginning toward an end point. Beginning as a voluntary, pleasurable act, it becomes a reflective and compulsive behavior. The most insidious of addictions is alcoholism, recognized as a disease by the American Medical Association since 1956. This recognition eliminates notions that the alcoholic is a weak-willed person, who could quit drinking if he or she wanted. Recognizing alcoholism and other drug dependence as a disease implies five points:

1. *The disease can be described.* The compulsion to drink (or to use other drugs) is manifested in habits that are inappropriate, unpredictable, excessive, and constant.
2. *The course of the disease is predictable and progressive.* It will get worse; it is as simple as that. Sometimes, there will be plateaus when the drinking and/or drug behavior seems to remain constant for months or even years. But over time the course of the disease will move inevitably toward greater and more serious deterioration. This deterioration can be physical, mental, and spiritual.
3. *The disease is primary.* Alcoholism/drug dependency is a primary disease. Other problems the victim may have cannot be treated until the dependency is treated.
4. *The disease is permanent.* Once you have it, you have it. Trying to learn to use drugs/drink moderately will not work. The chances for successful treatment are much better in the earlier stages of the disease.
5. *The disease is terminal.* If you have a chemical addiction and do not successfully arrest it, you will die from it. Whether the chemical complicates a heart condition, high blood pressure, liver problems, or a bleeding ulcer or precipitates a stroke or suicide, it is still the agent that causes the death.

A useful assessment for recognizing any chemical dependency is to ask, "Is the alcohol or other drug causing *any* continuing disruption in my life—or the lives of those close to me?" (i.e., physically, mentally, emotionally, socially, or economically). If the answer is "yes" and you do not stop drug use, despite damage to home life, school performance, or career, then your chemical usage constitutes harmful dependence. This question is useful in assessing any type of compulsive behavior, including gambling, shopping, and having sex.

Addictive Behaviors Other Than Alcohol or Other Drug Use

In the past, the focus of the term *addiction* has been centered exclusively around the use of alcohol and other drugs. Recently, a more neutral term, *dependence*, has been substituted for addiction. *Dependencies* or *addictionlike* behaviors may include objects or events such as food, gambling, sex, shoplifting, work, spending, exercise, and television. Although these addictive objects or events are different, they produce the desired and pleasurable mood change the addict seeks:

- The gambler feels excited when studying a racing form.
- The alcoholic feels relaxed and happy when drinking at the neighborhood bar.
- The food addict feels rewarded and comforted when eating or shopping for food.
- The shoplifter senses a thrill when stealing a magazine from the drugstore.
- The sex addict gets aroused when browsing in a pornographic bookstore or when searching for a new sex partner.
- The addictive spender feels exhilarated during a shopping spree.
- The workaholic feels an extreme sense of accomplishment while working all day on Sunday.

These objects and events have a normal, socially acceptable function. Food is to nourish, gambling is for fun and excitement, sex is for intimacy, and drugs are to help overcome illness. Most people have a normal, healthy relationship with these things, but dependent behavior results in an abnormal relationship. Dependent individuals seek a

table 13-1 Substance Use Is Not Just a College Problem—It Begins Much Earlier

Drugs used today are more potent, more dangerous, and more addictive than ever. Initial drug use occurs at an increasingly early age. It erodes the self-discipline and motivation necessary for learning and is closely tied to dropping out of school. Fifty-seven percent of high school seniors in the United States have used an illicit drug at least once before they finish high school. Thirty-six percent have used an illicit drug other than marijuana.

Tobacco acts as a "gateway drug." It is generally the first drug used by young people who enter a sequence of drug use that can include tobacco, alcohol, marijuana and harder drugs. The surgeon general's report revealed that for the 12-to 17-year-olds who reported having smoked in the past 30 days were three times more likely to use alcohol, eight times more likely to smoke marijuana, and 22 times more likely to use cocaine, within those past 30 days than those 12-to 17-year-olds who had not smoked during that time. Further, teen smoking is linked to other high risk behaviors: fighting; carrying weapons; attempting suicide; and engaging in early, frequent, and unprotected sexual intercourse. Facts on high school tobacco use:
- 35 percent of high school girls smoke.
- 36 percent of high school seniors smoke.
- At least 4.5 million adolescents are current smokers.
- 22 percent of high school students smoke cigars; 27 percent of 14- to 19-year-olds report having smoked a cigar in the previous year.
- 9.3 percent of high school students use smokeless tobacco.

Report from the commission on Substance Abuse Among America's Adolescents, (ages 12 to 17) found:
- 23.5 percent of 12-year-olds said they knew someone who used hard drugs such as cocaine or heroin.
- Support for the theory that teenagers who use cigarettes, alcohol, or marijuana—so called gateway drugs—run a greater risk of moving to harder, more addictive substances. (Teens who drink and smoke are 30 times more likely to use marijuana; and teens who drink and use marijuana are 17 times more likely to use heroin, cocaine, and LSD later.)
- The percentage of eighth-graders using marijuana during or before seventh grade climbed from 7.7 to 12.7 percent.
- More than half of eighth-graders had tried alcohol last year, three-fourths found it easy to get, and one-fourth admitted getting drunk.
- Binge drinking among eighth-graders increased from 12.9 to 15.6 percent.

Small-town Rural Teens and Drug Use:
A study by the national Center on Addiction and Substance Abuse reported that rural eighth-grade students were more likely to use drugs than their peers in large metro cities. A population of 50,000 or less put a town in the rural classification.

The study revealed that they are:
- 100 percent likelier than those in urban centers to use amphetamines, including methamphetamines.
- 50 percent likelier to use cocaine.
- 83 percent likelier to use crack cocaine.
- 34 percent likelier to smoke marijuana.
- 70 percent likelier to have gotten drunk and 29 percent likelier to drink alcohol.
- Twice as likely to smoke cigarettes and nearly five times likelier to use smokeless tobacco.

Among tenth-graders, use rates in rural areas exceeded those in large urban areas for every drug except marijuana and the drug known as ecstasy.

Among twelfth-graders, use rates in rural America exceeded those in large urban areas for cocaine, crack, amphetamines, inhalants, alcohol, tobacco, cigarettes, and smokeless tobacco.

Adult drug use was about equal across communities of all sizes.

Youth Drug Use: (R=rural) (U-urban)

Marijuana
| R | 11.6% |
| U | 8.6% |

Amphetamines
| R | 5.1% |
| U | 1.4% |

Crack
| R | 1.1% |
| U | 0.6% |

Heroin
| R | 0.7% |
| U | 0.6% |

table 13-2   How Addictions Affect the Wellness Dimensions

Physical	Addicts don't take good care of their bodies. Addictions over time affect various parts of the body—an alcoholics liver, a bulimic's throat. The added stress of addiction takes its toll on the heart and every other organ of the body; malnourishment is common; the body's immune system breaks down. A body is more accident prone. Suicidal thoughts may become actions.
Social	Addicts become withdrawn and isolated from others, become loners, and interact only with the object or event of addiction. Their responsibility to family, school, job, and so on, diminishes.
Emotional	Feelings of guilt and shame increase; depression is common; unresolved issues increase; mood swings increase; anxiety increases; fits of rage for no reason occur; and paranoia develops (the addict starts to question everyone and everything).
Intellectual	Logic breaks down; the addicts behavior doesn't make sense to him/her; schoolwork falters; he/she loses touch with world events; judgment is impaired.
Spiritual	Addicts are not "connected" in a meaningful way to the world around them; they lose feelings of belonging and being an important part of the world; they lose the sense of knowing themselves; the importance of self drifts farther away; values and priorities shift; addicts begin to rationalize.
Environmental	Addicts show little concern for the health and well-being of the environment, such as conserving natural resources and energy. The addiction (compulsive behavior) consumes his/her energies.

pleasurable mood change to fulfill personal needs. The addict turns to the addiction just as someone else may turn to a spouse or best friend for support, nurturing, and intimacy. As the addiction progresses, the addict becomes more preoccupied, withdrawn, and isolated. Table 13-2 illustrates how this type of behavior affects all dimensions of wellness.

We know that chemical addictions produce physiological dependence resulting in withdrawal symptoms when the substance is denied. When the object of other dependencies (i.e., food or gambling) is withdrawn, withdrawal symptoms also result (i.e., anxiety, irritability, or moodiness).

A person can switch an addictive relationship from object to object and event to event. For example, former alcoholics can become chain smokers. Switching from object to object helps create the illusion that the problem has been taken care of, when in reality one dangerous relationship has replaced another.

Many experts predict that compulsive gambling will soon become a serious national problem. There may be good cause for this concern: Consider the millions of dollars spent in the legal and illegal gambling industry every day. Commercial bingo, dog and horse racing, state and interstate lotteries, and video gambling are on the increase. Gambling casinos are no longer confined to Nevada and New Jersey; they can be found on Native American reservations and floating up and down our rivers, and they are being built in more states every year. Sports gambling is also booming. As gambling becomes legal in more states, the number of problem gamblers rises proportionally. Current figures estimate that between 3 and 11 percent of the entire adult U.S. population are compulsive gamblers. Gambling is meant for

wellness flash

Worldwide online gambling revenue in 1999 was 2.4 billion. It was 651 million in 1998. There are over 300 gambling sites on the Internet.

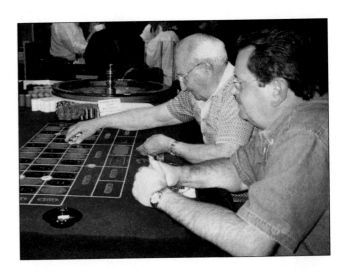

Gambling is meant for fun but can turn into a devastating compulsion in some people.

table 13-3 — Do You Have a Gambling Problem?

Yes	No	
____	____	1. Do you frequently gamble with more money than you can afford?
____	____	2. Do you bet on something whenever you can or gamble more than you intended?
____	____	3. Have you ever lost time from school or work because of gambling?
____	____	4. Is gambling making your home life unhappy or is it having a negative effect on your relationships with others?
____	____	5. After losing, do you go back as soon as possible to recoup your losses?
____	____	6. Have you ever lied about your gambling or stolen or borrowed money to gamble or to pay a gambling debt?
____	____	7. Have you ever felt guilty about how much you gamble or about what happens when you gamble?
____	____	8. Have you ever been criticized for your gambling or is it affecting your reputation?
____	____	9. Are you reluctant to use gambling money for "normal" expenditures?
____	____	10. Do you ever gamble to escape worry or trouble?
____	____	11. Have you ever considered suicide as a result of your gambling?
____	____	12. Does gambling make you careless about the welfare of your family or friends??

Scoring: One "Yes" answer indicates you may have a problem. Two or more "Yes" answers indicate that you could be addicted or heading that way.

table 13-4 — Do You Have a Shopping or Spending Problem?

The most prominent symptom of a shopping or spending problem is obvious: *Debt!*

Yes	No	
____	____	1. Do you shop or spend money when you're disappointed, angry, or scared?
____	____	2. Are your shopping/spending habits causing emotional distress or chaos in your life?
____	____	3. Do you find yourself arguing with others about your shopping/spending habits?
____	____	4. Do you feel lost without your credit cards?
____	____	5. Do you buy items on credit that you wouldn't buy with cash?
____	____	6. Do you experience a rush of euphoria and anxiety at the same time when you spend money?
____	____	7. Does spending or shopping feel like a reckless or forbidden act?
____	____	8. Do you feel guilty, ashamed, embarrassed, or confused after you shop or spend money?
____	____	9. Do you lie to others about what you bought or how much money you spend?
____	____	10. Do you think excessively about money?
____	____	11. Do you spend a lot of time juggling accounts and bills to accommodate your spending?

Scoring: If you said "Yes" to four of the questions, you might have a shopping or spending problem.

amusement, recreation, and excitement, but it can turn into a devastating compulsion in some individuals. Take the self-assessment in Table 13-3 to determine if you have or someone you know has a gambling problem.

The glut of credit cards bombarding our mail boxes, as well as online shopping available around-the-clock and non-stop TV shopping networks, is assisting in the expansion of shopping or spending compulsions. Take the self-assessment in Table 13-4 to determine if shopping or spending is becoming a problem for you.

Individuals with addictions or who exhibit addictive-like behaviors to substances, objects, or events need professional help. A partial listing of organizations, agencies, and resource centers that give information and assistance with addictions can be found at the end of this chapter.

Addictive Personality

Is there such a thing as an addictive personality? Do some individuals possess such a personality? This controversial topic continues to produce heated debate among psychologists. Although the addictive personality type has not been confirmed by research, some experts feel that this personality type does exist. They believe the addictive personality may be found in persons who don't know how to have healthy relationships, have been taught not to trust people, and have never learned to "connect" with others, community, their emotions, and spiritual powers greater than themselves.

These experts believe that early life experiences determine whether a person will live in a state of dependency. They argue that the family environment is the most important determinant because the family is where we learn about relationships. For example, in abusive families, the children are often treated as objects, thus developing low self-esteem and mistrust in people. Also, in neglectful families, children may learn to be passive, to feel dead inside, and they will seek out someone or something that makes them feel alive. This theory reflects the idea that people often form addictions because of the positive feelings (mood change) they experience when using a particular substance or repeating a behavior.

Experts claim there is no single characteristic or constellation of traits inevitably associated with addiction. So who is vulnerable? Possibly the individual who

- has a low sense of self-esteem;
- has a sense of alienation;
- is unable to turn to others for comfort;
- possesses a need for instant gratification;
- is impulsive;
- displays antisocial behavior (is willing to go outside the boundaries of what is normally accepted);
- cannot control strong feelings;
- rebels against authority;
- likes to try exciting and dangerous things;
- lies easily;
- is a perfectionist—a high achiever;
- seeks approval from others;
- fears personal criticism;
- is overly concerned with how others perceive him or her; or
- tends to be submissive and dependent.

Many people display these characteristics without becoming addicts. This leads some experts to believe that the personality disorders and antisocial behavior that accompany chemical abuse are the result of this abuse, not the cause of it. They claim there is no way to predict who will become an addict.

Alcohol

Alcohol is the most misunderstood drug in America. Some say alcohol is a beverage, and others say that it is a drug. They say it is a mood-altering chemical in liquid form or that it is sinful and dangerous. Others say it is a rite of adulthood and is safe. What a conflicting set of statements. What is alcohol and what does it do? **Alcohol** (technically known as **ethyl alcohol** or **ethanol**) is a central nervous system depressant. The central nervous system (CNS) is composed of the brain and the spinal cord. A CNS depressant is a chemical that slows brain functions. Alcohol slows reaction time, dulls alertness, and impairs body coordination. It intensifies emotions, lowers inhibitions, and increases risk-taking behaviors. It also disrupts judgment and reasoning power. On the positive side, alcohol is a good social lubricant; on the negative, it can be unhealthy and unsafe if abused.

Alcohol Absorption

Most healthy bodies process alcohol in the same manner. Alcohol is water soluble and is transported throughout the body by the blood, which is mostly water. The amount of alcohol in the blood is expressed as a percentage; for example, 0.10 percent **blood alcohol concentration (BAC)** or blood

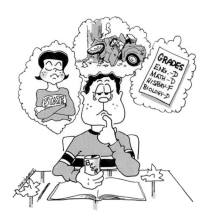

There are many consequences of abusive drinking.

alcohol level (BAL). With the first sip, alcohol briefly irritates tissues of the mouth and esophagus. Alcohol rapidly enters the bloodstream through the small intestine and, to a small degree, through the stomach. A fraction exits in breath, sweat, and urine. Alcohol is chiefly metabolized (i.e., chemically broken down) in the liver, through which the entire blood supply circulates every 4 minutes. Enzymes in the liver metabolize alcohol into acetaldehyde, a highly toxic chemical. This is converted into acetate and, finally, into carbon dioxide and water. The process is slow, taking roughly an hour for each ounce of pure alcohol. Despite vigorous folklore, nothing will speed up liver function or sober up the intoxicated. A person who is drunk and drinks coffee does not become sober, only wide awake.

The mind-altering effects of alcohol begin soon after it hits the bloodstream. Within minutes, alcohol enters the brain, numbing nerve cells and slowing their messages to the body. In the heart, cardiac muscles strain to cope with alcohol's depressive action, and the pulse quickens. If drinking continues, alcohol builds in the bloodstream and disrupts the centers in the brain that govern speech, vision, balance, and judgment. As more alcohol is ingested, the drinker may lose consciousness. Alcohol is a hazardous anesthetic, with a narrow range between deadness and dead. At a BAC of 0.4 to 0.6 percent, the drinker is comatose and in danger of dying from respiratory failure.

Speed of Alcohol Absorption

How quickly alcohol is absorbed into your bloodstream depends on five factors: body weight, gender, speed of consumption, food intake, and beverage imbibed. How is alcohol absorption affected by body weight and gender? It is not a myth that a man can drink the same amount of alcohol as a woman of equal weight and have a lower BAC. This means a woman can get drunk faster than a man does. There are several explanations for this:

- Women generally weigh less than men do, so the same amount of alcohol is concentrated in a smaller body mass

- Even at the same weight, women typically have a higher percentage of body fat and less body water than men do (alcohol is diluted in body water)
- When alcohol enters a woman's body, it becomes more concentrated and therefore has a more potent effect than the same amount of alcohol would in a man's body
- The enzyme found in the gastric system (small intestine and stomach) that metabolizes alcohol before it is absorbed into the bloodstream is less active in women. So, even if a man and a woman weigh the same, have the same proportion of body fat, and drink the same amounts, more alcohol is likely to reach a woman's blood, brain, and liver than a man's. This phenomenon has more serious long-term consequences for women. They are more likely to develop damage to the liver, heart muscle, and brain at lower levels of alcohol intake. Alcohol may also put them at increased risk for osteoporosis and breast cancer
- Studies reveal that alcohol has a greater effect on driving skills in women so they are at increased risk of having a fatal car accident.

Speed of consumption and food intake also affect the rate of alcohol absorption. A 12-ounce can of beer sipped over an hour's time is not absorbed into the bloodstream as fast as a beer that is gulped quickly. Food in the stomach inhibits alcohol absorption. Without inhibitors in the stomach, alcohol is absorbed extremely fast through the stomach walls and small intestine. The type of beverage also affects absorption. Carbonated drinks, such as champagne, rum and coke, and whisky and soda, are absorbed even faster than water-diluted drinks.

There are three major types of alcoholic beverages: beer, wine, and distilled spirits (i.e., hard liquor such as whiskey, vodka, gin, and brandy). A standard serving of any one beverage contains approximately the same amount of alcohol. Thus, one 4-ounce glass of wine, one 12-ounce beer, one 12-ounce wine cooler, and one shot glass of liquor provide approximately the same amount of alcohol. One person's wine glass is another person's beer mug, so always measure your drinks. See the photo of the three servings of alcohol.

Often, wine coolers are not perceived as alcoholic beverages because of their fruit juice base and sweet taste. Beware. They contain the same amount of alcohol as beer or any other alcoholic beverage (about 4 percent to 7 percent). These drinks may provide the bridge from soft drinks to other alcoholic beverages for many young people.

Your alcohol history determines how quickly you feel the effects of this drug. It is based on your lifetime alcohol consumption, the frequency of your drinking, and the tolerance you have acquired. The number of drinks it takes for you to feel a "buzz" increases as your tolerance to alcohol increases. **Tolerance** is the body's physical adjustment to the habitual use of a chemical. Due to alcohol tolerance, an ex-

perienced drinker with a BAC of 0.10 percent may not feel drunk. On the other hand, an inexperienced drinker may feel intoxicated at that same BAC because a tolerance has not developed (Table 13-5).

If you are in a "chugging" contest, many of the previously mentioned factors come into consideration. Chugging is not proof of maturity or a route to social acceptance. Chugging will only make you drunk, incoherent, and accident prone. It is dangerous and may cause convulsions, blackouts (loss of memory during a period of drinking), passing out (unconsciousness), vomiting, nausea, and death. There are between 200 and 400 alcohol poisoning deaths annually in the United States. Nearly all are due to chugging contests.

Considering all the factors that affect alcohol absorption rate, is your level of alcohol use a low- or high-risk behavior?

Impact of Alcohol

Alcohol is by far the most devastating drug—wrecking families and friendships, impairing health, jeopardizing careers, and filling jails, hospitals, and morgues. Alcohol accounts for 50 percent of deaths from motor vehicle crashes, one-third of drownings, and about half of deaths caused by fire. Alcohol is linked to half of homicides, a third of suicides, and two-thirds of assaults. Social workers report that alcohol is a factor in

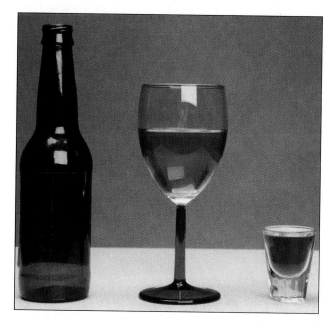

All standard-size drinks provide the same amount of alcohol.

table 13-5 Percentage of Blood Alcohol Concentration (BAC)

Number of Drinks*	Body Weight (pounds)				
	120	140	160	180	200
2	0.06	0.05	0.05	0.04	0.04
4	0.12	0.11	0.09	0.08	0.08
6	0.19	0.16	0.14	0.13	0.11
8	0.25	0.21	0.19	0.17	0.15
10	0.31	0.27	0.23	0.21	0.19

Effects Related to Blood Alcohol Concentration (BAC)

BAC%	Effect
0.03	Relaxation, mood change
0.04	Reduced visual acuity (as much as wearing dark glasses), slight euphoria, and loss of shyness
0.05	Decrease in motor skills, judgment impaired, caution reduced
0.08	Inhibitions lowered; unexpected behavior
0.10	Legally intoxicated; movements and speech impaired
0.18	Difficulty staying awake
0.20	Very drunk; loud and difficult to understand; emotions unstable, staggering/muscular coordination reduced; has the appearance of a "sloppy" drunk
0.30	Loss of consciousness
0.40+	Onset of coma; possible death due to respiratory arrest

*One drink equals 1 1/2 oz. of 80-proof alcohol, 12 oz. beer, or 4 oz. wine
Source: Mothers Against Drunk Driving and PRIDE.

nearly 50 percent of their domestic violence cases. Over 36 percent of the male population in prison report that they were under the influence of alcohol at the time of their crimes. The greatest tragedy is that the *number one killer* of teenagers is *drinking and driving*. The majority of these drinkers started early, before they had turned 13. As you can see in Table 13-6, over 80 percent of college students report some drinking, ranging from occasional to heavy. Alcohol consumption is one of the major reasons for absenteeism among college students. It is involved in 90 percent of campus rapes, 25 percent of student deaths, and 40 percent of academic problems, and it is the major contributor to campus violence, property damage, and the disruption of sleep and study time. Alcohol is implicated in thousands of unwanted pregnancies and cases of sexually transmitted diseases, including AIDS. Thousands of college students drop out because of drinking. See Table 13-5 to learn how nondrinking college students are affected by the drinking of their classmates. The single most dangerous consequence of alcohol use may be that it produces a false sense of confidence, even invulnerability that often leads to disregard for the health, safety, and welfare of self and others.

Health and Long-Term Effects of Alcohol

Alcohol is a toxin, and its harmful effects on the body are great. A few drinks may make you drowsy and can interrupt

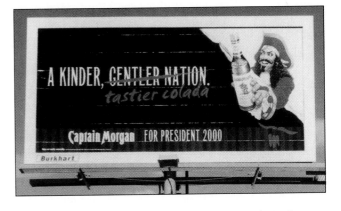

Drinking and driving killed a human being every 31 minutes in 1999. Some say billboards advertising alcohol should be banned.

patterns of sleep. Over time, heavy drinking can cause brain damage (it speeds the death of brain cells); damage nerve endings; and increase the risk of heart disease, high blood pressure, hemorrhagic stroke, and cancer (mouth, throat, stomach, intestines, pancreas, and liver). It can depress the immune system and cause gastritis, pancreatitis, anxiety, delirium tremens (DTs), and malnutrition. Alcohol is a primary cause of liver failure. When alcohol is present in the liver, it preempts the breakdown of fats, which then accumulate within the liver cells. As fatty cells enlarge, they can rupture or grow into cysts that replace normal cells. After

table 13-6   College Binge Drinking and Problems Drunks Cause Sober Students

What is the extent of alcohol consumption on campus?
- 81 percent drank alcoholic beverages
- 43 percent (2 out of 5 students) binged in the 2-week period (**Binge drinking** is defined as *five* drinks at one setting for men and *four* at one setting for women.)
- 23 percent were frequent bingers (at least three times in the last 2-week period (increased since 1993)
- 21 percent were occasional binge drinkers
- 37 percent were nonbinge drinkers
- 19 percent were abstainers (increased since 1993)
- 13 percent thought they were problem drinkers
  (Binge drinking *decreased* among dormitory residents and *increased* among students living off campus.)

Frequent binge drinkers describe their alcohol-related problems. Because of drinking:
- 63 percent missed class
- 46 percent got behind in schoolwork
- 62 percent did something they regretted
- 54 percent forgot where they were/what they did
- 42 percent engaged in unplanned sexual activities
- 20 percent did not use protection during sex
- 23 damaged property
- 13 percent got into trouble with campus/local police
- 27 percent got hurt or injured
- 57 percent drove after drinking
- 48 percent had five or more alcohol-related problems

Binge drinking was most common at:
- Colleges in Northeast and North Central states
- Residential colleges
- Coed colleges
- (2 out of 3 students who live in a fraternity or sorority houses are binge drinkers.)

Binge drinking was least common at:
- Colleges in the West and South
- Traditional African American colleges
- Commuter colleges
- Women's colleges

Sober students are affected in a number of ways: at the big drinking schools, sober students were twice as likely as those at the lowest drinking level schools to be insulted or humiliated; to be pushed, hit, or assaulted; and to experience unwanted sexual advances from drinking students. They were two and one-half times as likely to sustain property damage, to end up taking care of a drunken student, and to have their study or sleep time interrupted by classmates drinking.

Source: Henry Wechler, et al. "College Binge Drinking in the 1990's: A Continuing Problem. Results of the Harvard School of Public Health 1999 College Alcohol Study." The study surveyed colleges that participated in the 1993 and 1997 surveys. Over 14,000 students at 119 colleges in 39 states participated.

years of heavy drinking, fibrous scar tissue, or cirrhosis, impedes the normal flow of arterial and venous blood through the organ, resulting in liver failure and death.

Does drinking alcoholic beverages guard against heart disease? Recent studies of men suggest *light-to-moderate* alcohol intake (*one drink per day*) is the amount associated with a reduction in mortality. This is due to a reduced risk of coronary artery disease because of increased HDL level. Alcohol also protects the heart by reducing the tendency of the blood to form clots. *But so does aspirin.* However, among women with similar levels of alcohol consumption, an increased risk of breast cancer was noted that complicates the balance of risks and benefits. Light-to-moderate intake of alcohol appears only to reduce mortality risk in some women who are at high risk for coronary heart disease in the first place. Also, while light alcohol consumption may reduce coronary artery disease, it has destructive effects on the heart muscle. This is especially true in women who appear to be more susceptible to cardiomyopathy (or heart muscle destruction)—even when they drink less than men.

So this one bit of HDL information about the "protective" relationship of alcohol consumption and heart disease should not be perceived as a "green light" to drink. Keep in mind the cons overwhelmingly outweigh the pros of drinking alcoholic beverages. For coronary heart disease protection, not smoking, following a proper diet, and staying physically active are far superior methods to the consumption of alcohol.

Use, Moderate Use, and Abuse

About two-thirds of Americans use alcohol. These individuals enjoy an occasional alcoholic beverage (no more than one to two drinks per week). Others, however, drink in moderation or abuse alcohol. *Moderate* drinking means no more than *two* drinks a day for most men, no more than *one* drink a day for most women, and no more than *five* drinks per week. Who is the alcohol abuser? It is the individual who drinks more than *three per day* or more than *five drinks per week*. The alcohol abuser is also guilty of **binge drinking** (i.e., five or more at one setting for men and four or more at one setting for women). Any time a person consumes this amount of alcohol at one setting it is considered to be binging—regardless of if it is only once per week or even once per year. The alcohol abuser is the drinker who considers alcohol to be something other than a beverage to be consumed with meals or to celebrate special occasions. Alcohol abusers "use" alcohol as a medication to kill pain, to alter emotions (when mad or depressed), to help them sleep, or to cope with life. If you drink when pregnant or drink and drive, you are an alcohol abuser. See Table 13-7.

The morning after a night of abusive drinking, you may experience the following conditions: oversensitivity to light and sound; a hangover; dehydration; nausea; bloodshot eyes; "bags" under the eyes; and **blackout** (cannot remember all or parts of the night before). To avoid abusing alcohol follow the Zero . . . One . . . Three Rule for Lower-Risk Drinking in Table 13-8.

College Binge Drinking/Positive Norming and Harm Reduction

Studies such as the Harvard School of Public Health College Alcohol Study indicate that students who drink at the binge level create enormous problems for themselves and for other students at their college (Table 13-6). As Table 13-9 reveals, frequent binge drinkers consumed two-thirds of the alcohol students drank. They also accounted for more than three-fifths of the more serious alcohol-related problems on campus. But, only 23 percent of college students are frequent binge drinkers—a minority on our campuses. No doubt about it, there is a great deal of alcohol being consumed on our college campuses. However, most students who consume alcohol are not causing a lot of problems. It's the minority, the frequent bingers, that are visible and the ones creating most of the havoc. See Figure 13-1.

The perception on most campuses is that everyone is consuming vasts amounts of alcohol and causing numerous problems for themselves and everyone else. Studies indicate that this is not the true picture (Table 13-9 and Fig. 13-1). These studies suggest that students tend to overestimate the acceptability and the actual drinking behavior of their peers. This creates a *false perception* and cements beliefs that such extreme norms exist and may serve to justify and explain extreme behavior. This in turn, may influence students to engage in heavy drinking. The "Everyone is doing it, so I'm a nerd if I don't, too!" mentality. The reality is, as the Harvard data revealed, that nondrinkers or nonbinge drinkers are the majority. The study further revealed that the median number of drinks consumed per week by all students, regardless of drinking status, was 1.5. When students were divided by

---

table 13-7 — Use, Moderate Use, and Abuse of Alcohol

Use
- No more than one to two drinks per week

Moderate Use
- Two per day for men; one per day for women; no more than five per week
- Use of alcohol to celebrate special occasions
- Use of alcohol as a beverage with meals

Abuse
- More than three per day or more than five per week
- Binge drinking (i.e., five or more at one setting for men and four or more for women)
- Use of alcohol
  — to medicate or kill pain
  — to alter emotions
  — to get drunk
  — to induce sleep
  — to cope with life's problems
  — when pregnant

Source: Anna Lamb, Alcohol Education, Coordinator. Ball State University, Muncie, IN 47306, (317) 285-8437.

---

table 13-8 — The Zero . . . One . . . Three Rule for Lower-Risk Drinking

0 = No level of drinking is recommended. Never drink and drive—even one block.

1 = Drink only one alcoholic beverage per hour if you do drink.

3 = Never drink more than three alcoholic beverages per day (or more than five per week).

Source: Concept partially developed by Enjoy Michigan Safety Coalition. Fur by Michigan Office of Highway Safety Planning.

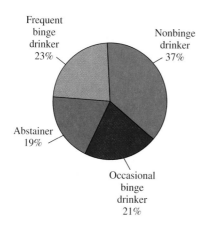

figure 13-1 When it comes to college alcohol use, nonbinge drinkers and abstainers (when totaled together) are the majority.

table 13-9	Share of the Alcohol Consumed by College Students	
		Mean Number of Drinks Per Week
• Frequent Binge Drinkers (Binged 3 or more times in past 2 weeks)	68%	14.5
• Occasional Bingers	23%	4.8
• Other	9%	0.8

As this table illustrates, frequent binge drinkers account for 68 percent of the alcohol consumed on our college campuses even though they represent just 23 percent of the student population. This minority of college drinkers makes a big impact on our campuses, though.

drinking pattern, the median number of drinks per week was 0.8 for those who did not binge drink. This is the reality on most campuses. So not everyone is getting into trouble with alcohol. It's the highly visible minority. How many drinks per week do frequent bingers consume? See Table 13-9.

So what can be done to bring reality to the forefront and diminish false perceptions? One alcohol intervention technique achieving high success rates is to challenge and attempt to correct these inaccurate perceptions. It is frequently called "positive norming" and is coupled with "harm reduction." This technique uses a variety of strategies to help students internalize accurate norming information. The accurate norms help the student deal with peer pressure and not succumb to that pressure to drink when they may not wish to or not consume more than they want. Read "Strategies for Dealing with Alcohol" and "Harm Reduction" ideas in "Commonly Asked Questions" later in this chapter for more information.

Alcoholism

No one plans on becoming an alcoholic, yet alcoholism is on the rise. Even newborn infants may be addicted if the mother abused alcohol during pregnancy. Most alcoholism is a result of abusive drinking. The difference between the alcohol abuser and the alcoholic is control over drinking. The abusive drinker can stop. The addict cannot. Ask yourself, "Do you *want* it, or do you *need* it?"

Alcoholism is a drug (chemical) dependence. It involves progressive preoccupation with drinking, leading to physical, mental, or social dysfunction. Approximately one of ten Americans is an alcoholic. The point where heavy drinking merges into alcohol dependence is blurry. The behaviors may appear to be the same. For example, both the abuser and addict may suffer from blackouts, passing out, arrests, hangovers, absenteeism, accidents, violence, poor job or school performance, and poor relationships.

table 13-10	Social Self-Assessment

You are least likely to have problems with alcohol if
1. You were exposed to alcohol in relatively small quantities early in life by your family or within the context of a religious or cultural group;
2. Your family members viewed alcohol as a food and consumed small quantities, primarily at mealtime;
3. Your parents set a good example by practicing lower-risk drinking behaviors;
4. Your family did not view drinking alcoholic beverages as a means of demonstrating maturity, adulthood, or masculinity/femininity;
5. Abstinence with respect to the consumption of alcoholic beverages was accepted as a legitimate choice;
6. Drunkenness was not an acceptable form of behavior;
7. Alcohol was viewed as a beverage and not as the central focus of a group activity;
8. Rules and rituals associated with drinking were known and understood by all group members and they were reasonable and agreeable to those members.

Source: National Institute on Alcohol Abuse and Alcoholism.

Heredity explains some alcoholism because a history of alcoholism in the family puts you at higher risk. The rate of alcoholism is 40 to 50 percent in children of alcoholics and 7 to 10 percent in the general population. What you inherit is not the disease but a predisposition to the disease. Scientists are looking for biological markers (i.e., variations in neurotransmitters, certain blood enzymes, and brain waves) to eventually identify influential genes. One researcher reports that there are different types of alcoholics, just as there are different types of diabetics and schizophrenics. He claims that a cluster of symptoms is needed to lead to dependence. Abusive drinking and craving are pivotal.

wellness flash

Young people who begin drinking before age 15 are four times more likely to develop alcoholism than those who begin drinking at 21.

The way in which you were introduced to alcohol as a child strongly influences your attitudes and drinking behavior as an adult. Table 13-10 lists factors indicative of those who would experience the fewest problems with alcohol in adulthood. How do you stack up with these factors?

The *alcohol abuser* needs to change his or her drinking behavior by quitting or following the Zero . . . One . . . Three Rule for Lower-Risk Drinking. The *alcoholic* must quit. No alcoholic should quit "cold turkey" (abruptly) without proper supervision, however, as the body has become dependent upon alcohol. When you abruptly stop using alcohol, you will probably experience some withdrawal symptoms, which can be dangerous. Some of these symptoms are profuse sweating, coldness, tremors or shakes, nausea, headaches, and hallucinations (auditory or visual).

Anyone who drinks should ask the following questions: Does anyone in my family (even one member) have a history of alcoholism or drug abuse? Am I drinking too much? When am I drinking? Where am I drinking? What am I drinking? Why am I drinking? Are most of my friends heavy drinkers? Do I seek out events at which alcohol will be served? Do I have to have a drink? Do I make up excuses to drink? Do I intend to control my alcohol intake but never do?

If you are not satisfied with your answers, consider getting a professional assessment. Take the quiz in Table 13-11 to find out if you have a drinking problem. See Table 13-12 for tips on how to make behavior changes in relation to controlling your consumption of alcohol.

For those with an alcohol problem, help is available. There is hope. Many people have gone to treatment centers, hospitals, clinics, and self-help groups for assistance in dealing with drinking problems.

One popular group that offers assistance to alcoholics of all ages is Alcoholics Anonymous (AA). AA was founded in 1935 by two alcoholics: a stockbroker and a surgeon who met in Akron, Ohio. They discovered that leaning on each other for emotional support was crucial to keeping them on the wagon. The group they started had only 100 members during the first 4 years. It now has a worldwide membership

table 13-11   Do You Have a Drinking Problem?

Yes	No		
___	___	1.	Do you occasionally drink heavily after a disappointment, a quarrel, or someone gives you a hard time?
___	___	2.	When you have trouble or feel under pressure, do you drink more than usual?
___	___	3.	Have you noticed that you are able to handle more alcohol than you did when you first started drinking?
___	___	4.	Do you sometimes forget what happened while you were drinking?
___	___	5.	When drinking with other people, do you try to have a few extra drinks when others will not know it?
___	___	6.	Are there times when you feel uncomfortable if alcohol is not available?
___	___	7.	Do you sometimes gulp your drinks?
___	___	8.	Do you sometimes feel a little guilty about your drinking?
___	___	9.	Are you a binger?
___	___	10.	Do you often take a drink to help you relax?
___	___	11.	Do you drink often when you are alone?
___	___	12.	Are you untruthful about how much you have had to drink when questioned on the subject?
___	___	13.	Are you secretly irritated when family or friends discuss your drinking?
___	___	14.	Do you often find that you wish to continue drinking after your friends say they have had enough?
___	___	15.	Do you usually have a reason for the occasion when you drink heavily?
___	___	16.	When you are sober, do you often regret things you have done or said while drinking?
___	___	17.	Has your drinking ever created problems between you and your friends, between you and your parents, or with the law?
___	___	18.	Have you ever injured yourself or another person after drinking?
___	___	19.	Have you tried switching brands or following different plans for controlling your drinking?
___	___	20.	Have you often failed to keep promises you have made to yourself about controlling or cutting down on your drinking?
___	___	21.	Do you try to avoid family or close friends while you are drinking?
___	___	22.	Does drinking ever cause you to take time off work, or to miss class, scheduled meetings, or appointments?
___	___	23.	Do you sometimes have the shakes (or a hangover) in the morning and find it helps to have a little drink?
___	___	24.	Do you ever become frightened after you have been drinking heavily?
___	___	25.	After periods of drinking, do you ever see or hear things that aren't there?

Scoring: You should regard a "Yes" answer to any one of the questions as a warning sign. Questions 1–12 relate to early alcoholism. Questions 13–25 relate to more advanced alcoholism. Seek professional help if you are concerned that you may have an alcohol problem.

table 13-12 — Tips for Behavior Change: Controlling Alcohol

Stages of Change = In What Stage Are You?

1. Precontemplation = "Contrary to what others say, I don't have a problem with alcohol."
2. Contemplation = "I would probably be better off if I cut back on alcohol consumption."
3. Preparation = "I am preparing to cut back on my alcohol consumption."
4. Action = "I drink very little alcohol anymore and am hosting alcohol-free parties."
5. Maintenance = "I socialize regularly without thinking of alcohol as a necessary component."

Processes of Change =

After identifying your current stage, try using some of the following selected processes and behavior strategies that are appropriate for your particular stage—to facilitate your transition into the next stage [refer to Fig. 2-2].

- Consciousness-Raising: pay attention to media accounts of violent behavior or tragic consequences of alcohol consumption. Study strategies for dealing with alcohol in this chapter.
- Social Liberation: identify nondrinking social functions on campus.
- Emotional Arousal: spend a Saturday night in the hospital emergency room observing the consequences of too much alcohol.
- Commitment: publicly announce to your social group your nonalcoholic intentions.
- Countering: develop exotic nonalcoholic drinks for your next party.
- Helping Relationships: support and encourage others to sponsor social events without alcohol.

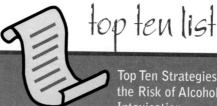

top ten list

Top Ten Strategies for Reducing the Risk of Alcoholism and Intoxication

1. Follow the Zero . . . One . . . Three Rule (Table 13.8) and remember "It's always OK not to drink."
2. Confine alcohol use to leisure activities, eating, and social functions.
3. Confine drinking to times where you are among friends or family; where social controls are more likely to function.
4. Do not drink fast! Pace your consumption by sipping and take your second drink no sooner than one hour after the first.
5. Avoid drinking on an empty stomach. Eggs, milk, cheese, ice cream, and meat are good choices to eat before consuming alcohol, and also eat while drinking.
6. Restrict your drinks, even on special occasions.
7. Drink in well-lighted, quiet places. Dark, noisy places produce tenseness, which in turn may give rise to over drinking.
8. On occasion, find some substitute for alcoholic beverages at traditional drinking times.
9. Deliberately avoid consuming alcohol when you are "stressed" or feel the need to relax.
10. Watch carefully your personal drinking pattern for early signs and symptoms of problem drinking (Table 13-11). Remember, if you need a drink to be social, that is *not* social drinking!

of over 2 million. AA is a fellowship of mutual and spiritual support that has endured in simplicity. There are no dues and no minutes; the only condition for membership is *a desire to stop drinking.*

Strategies for Dealing with Alcohol

Alcohol is an accepted drug in today's society, but you don't have to go along with the crowd. Who controls and makes decisions about your life—you or others? Take charge. One voice can make a difference; that voice is yours.

Review the top ten strategies for avoiding the chaos of intoxication and more importantly of developing alcoholism. Also, here are additional strategies for drinking less or not at all:

- Let your waistline be your incentive. Alcoholic beverages are loaded with "empty" calories (high in calories, low in nutrients). There is some evidence that alcohol not only adds calories to the diet but also keeps the body from burning dietary fat properly. Alcohol in the bloodstream slows down fat metabolism more than 30 percent while speeding up the burning of carbohydrates. This unused fat is deposited on the thighs, hips, and stomach.
- Switch to juice or soft drinks after the three-drink maximum.
- At restaurants, order food first, not an alcoholic beverage. That way you will have less time to drink.
- After exercise, or when extra thirsty, avoid carbonated alcoholic drinks. They are absorbed too fast, and you may be tempted to gulp them down. Drink a glass of cold water first.
- Don't hold the drink in your hand. Put it down somewhere—this will help slow down consumption.
- Try cocktails without the alcohol (i.e., a Bloody Mary without the vodka) or nonalcoholic beer.
- Dilute your drinks with water, ice, or extra fruit juice to slow alcohol absorption; beware of unfamiliar drinks with unknown alcohol content.
- Make sure your drinks are accurately measured.
- Volunteer to be the designated driver (you may even get free soft drinks).

If friends pass out from drinking alcohol, do the following:

1. *Put them on their side.* Stay with them.
2. *Do not give them anything to eat or drink.* They are unconscious. You could cause them to choke.
3. *Be sure they are breathing normally—not shallow, but deeply.* Shallow breathing means the brain is shutting down and involuntary bodily functions are ceasing. Call for help!
4. *Cover them with a sheet, not a blanket.* If they have overdosed on alcohol, their internal body temperature has fallen. Shivering stimulates them and helps to keep them alive. Too much external warmth will stop that vital stimulation.
5. *If they are shivering, call for medical help!*
6. Gently shake them and call them by first name. They will probably respond in some manner. *If they don't respond, call for medical help!*

Alcohol and the Law

Society has responded to the alcohol problem with legislation. All 50 states have a drinking age of 21 years. You are breaking the law if you are under the age of 21 and are using, possessing, or transporting alcohol. These laws partly discourage some students from drinking, which lowers the potential for accidents. Drinking to *any* extent reduces the ability of any driver (see Table 13-5). Fifty percent of fatal auto accidents in this country are alcohol related.

A tough new standard for drunken driving has recently become federal law. All states must comply to this new law by 2004. This new laws defines driving under the influence of alcohol as driving with a blood alcohol content (BAC) of 0.08 percent. Whether a person feels intoxicated is not the point; the point is whether he or she registers 0.08 on a breathalyzer (see Table 13-5). The rationale for the law is that it may act as a deterrent to drinking and driving. Some states have dropped the figure to 0.05 percent as presumption of intoxication. The point is, there is no safe drinking BAC. Look at Table 13-13 for some sobering statistics.

Here is the message: You could be one of the persons who dies in the next 20 minutes due to alcohol-related accidents. Or you could be crippled or permanently injured for life. Do not let it be you. Most think it won't happen to them.

Fetal Alcohol Syndrome (FAS) and Fetal Alcohol Effect (FAE)

Fetal alcohol syndrome (FAS) is a condition acquired by the unborn fetus and caused by the mother drinking alcohol during pregnancy. The alcohol passes through the placenta (within minutes) and affects the unborn child. There is no other cause for FAS. Women need to understand that the pla-

wellness flash

States that refuse to impose the new legal limit of 0.08 percent as the standard for drunken driving by 2004 will lose millions of dollars in federal funds.

table 13-13   Sobering Facts on Drinking and Driving

1. Drunk drivers are 25 times more likely than sober drivers to have accidents.
2. About 23,000 persons are killed each year in alcohol-related accidents. About 450 persons die each week, and every 20 minutes another life is lost in an alcohol-related accident.
3. More than 36 percent of the persons who die in alcohol-related accidents are passengers, drivers of the other vehicle, and pedestrians.
4. About one of every two Americans will be involved in an alcohol-related accident in their lifetime.
5. Social drinkers are a greater menace than commonly believed, as their critical judgment is impaired with a low BAC and they outnumber the obviously intoxicated drivers.
6. More people are arrested for drunken driving—1.8 million a year—than for any other crime in the United States. Yet the average drunken driver drives hundreds of times, thousands of miles, before being caught.
7. The average BAC of those arrested is 0.17 percent—equivalent to a 160-pound man drinking nearly 10 beers in 2 hours.
8. Of repeat offenders within 7 years 24 percent are convicted for a second time, 8.6 percent for a third time, and 4.3 percent for four or more times.

Source: National Highway Transportation Safety Administration.

centa does not keep unwanted chemicals away from the fetus. We know that what a mother eats, drinks, or smokes passes to her unborn child. Humans are supposed to be the wisest of creatures, yet it is not uncommon to see pregnant women drinking alcoholic beverages, smoking, and taking drugs they would never consider giving to their children. Then they expect their babies to come into the world unaffected.

Alcohol damages the vulnerable, developing brain and may impair placental function as well. This damage is irreversible. We are unsure exactly which brain cells of the fetus are destroyed; the expectant mother who drinks is denying her child development of his or her full potential. FAS is the leading known cause of mental retardation in the Western world. In addition babies born with FAS have facial deformities, smaller than normal heads, oddly shaped eyes, and flattened noses and faces. They suffer stunted growth and abnormalities of major organs such as the kid-

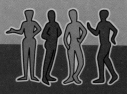

diversity issues

Racial and Ethnic Differences in College Alcohol Use

Percentages of Students Who Drank Alcohol in the Previous Year

Asian/Pacific Islanders	71%
African Americans	72%
Native Americans	83%
Hispanics	85%
Caucasians (whites)	87%

A national study found the largest number of abstainers to be among Asian/Pacific Islander and African American college students.

Percentages of Students Who Are Binge Drinkers

African Americans	21%
Asian/Pacific Islanders	22%
Hispanics	37%
Native Americans	40%
Caucasians (whites)	42%

White and Native American college students reported the highest percentage of frequent binge drinking in a national survey. African American women were the least likely to binge drink, while white males were the most likely to binge.

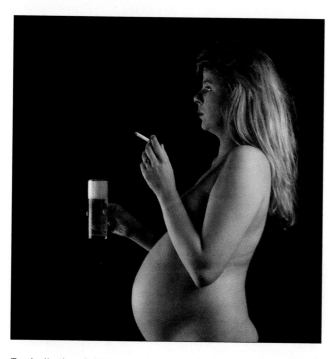

Tragically, though FAS and the related conditions are preventable and numerous warnings persist as to the hazards, at least *one in five* American women continues to drink during pregnancy.

wellness flash

A single drinking binge by a pregnant woman can be enough to permanently damage the brain of her unborn child.

neys, heart, muscles, joints, and sex organs. The effects of FAS can last a lifetime. Alcohol use during pregnancy may cause the child to have problems learning and behavioral difficulties. No one is certain how much alcohol it takes to cause damage to the fetus. Some women drink very little and their babies are still affected.

A far greater number of babies have more subtle symptoms that are sometimes—mistakenly—not attributed to their mothers' alcohol consumption. This less severe manifestation of FAS is called **fetal alcohol effect (FAE).** The mother of a child diagnosed with FAE did not necessarily drink less during pregnancy than the mother of a child with FAS, but, for some biological reason, the FAE child was not as damaged physically. The FAE child shows traits of impaired memory, poor judgment, and reduced capacity to learn from experience. Many FAE children go through life undetected and misjudged. They often drop out of school or wind up on the margins of society. Reports indicate an increasing frequency of FAS and FAE. Drinking while pregnant is like playing Russian roulette with your baby's life. Why take chances with your baby's future? The message is this: There is no known safe level of alcohol consumption during pregnancy. FAS and FAE are preventable, but abstinence is the only way to guarantee that a baby will suffer no ill effects from alcohol.

Tobacco

If you are a regular smoker, you may be losing about 6 minutes of life expectancy for every cigarette you smoke. For most smokers that means a life expectancy reduced by 5 to 8 years. The U.S. surgeon general has described cigarette smoking as "the number one preventable cause of death and health problems in our society." To put things in perspective, more people die from smoking-related diseases than from alcohol, cocaine, heroin, suicide, homicide, car accidents, and AIDS combined. Over 400,000 people die each year because they smoked cigarettes. That is more than seven times the total U.S. battle fatalities during the Vietnam War. Every day in this country, 3,000 children become regular smokers. More than one-third of these individuals will die prematurely of smoking-related diseases. For years the Federal Drug Administration and the American Medical Association have pushed for nicotine to be declared an addictive drug that should be regulated. The government has also recently banned the sale of tobacco products to anyone under the age of eighteen.

Despite the frightening statistics, the warnings, and the publicity given to the health risks of smoking, each year thousands of young people still start smoking.

Smoking Is Becoming Socially Unacceptable

Little was known about the health consequences of smoking until 1964 when the first surgeon general's report on smoking and health was published. At that time, nearly half of our population smoked. In the years since, millions of people have quit, and now smokers are less than a quarter of the population. The decline in smoking has been influenced by the proliferation of restrictive worksite and public smoking policies. Once considered sophisticated, smoking now seems to be most prevalent in the lower socioeconomic and the least-educated groups. Studies reveal that smoking is twice as high among those with less than a high school education than it is among those with a college education. However, more college students than ever are picking up the habit, despite the downward trend of cigarette smoking in this country. Overall, only 25 percent smoke in this country. That's the good news. The bad news is that nearly 30 percent of college students now smoke—that's up 25 percent in the last six years.

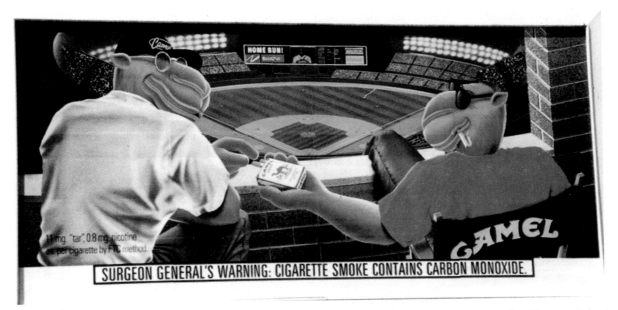

The courts have ruled that tobacco companies conspired to hide these dangers and sell a dangerous product for more than 40 years. At least one tobacco company admits that "smoking causes lung cancer, heart disease, and emphysema; is addictive; and that the industry markets to young people (ages 14–18)."

Before World War II, smoking was considered a masculine activity, and few women smoked. After World War II, with increasing emancipation, women began smoking in ever-increasing numbers. As a result, lung cancer deaths for women tripled. While proportions of adult men and women smokers have dropped since 1964, surveys indicate that men have given up smoking more often than have women.

Smoking may have been considered glamorous once, but, today, attitudes are changing. Smoking commercials have been banned from radio and television since 1971. Cigarette advertisements and packages carry health warnings. Over 70 percent of adult smokers have either tried to quit smoking or would like to try. Nonsmokers are tired of passive smoking—breathing air polluted by tobacco smoke—and are gaining the right to breathe clean air in workplaces and public areas. Nationwide, colleges are responding to nonsmokers by increasing smoke-free zones on campuses.

Why Do People Smoke?

The most important influences in starting to smoke are family and friends. In families where one or both parents smoke, children are twice as likely to be smokers than are children of parents who are nonsmokers. Many teenagers start smoking because they think everybody else does, and they want to be like their friends or appear more adult. They don't think much about the costs or health risks of smoking. Powerful advertising directed at young people (e.g., Joe Camel) deemphasizes the harmful factors. The tobacco industry spends over $4 billion on advertising to convince young people they should take up smoking. For young people, cigarettes are considered to be a gateway drug—the first drug many use as a stepping stone to illicit drugs and heavy drinking (see Table 13-1).

Nicotine, a drug in cigarette smoke, is addicting, as anyone who has tried to quit smoking has quickly discovered. Nicotine is an alkaloid drug synthesized by the tobacco plant in the same fashion that the opium poppy (the source of heroin) and the coca plant (the source of cocaine) synthesize their addictive substances. Habituation to nicotine may occur after smoking only three packs of cigarettes. Once a person is hooked on nicotine, it can be difficult for the person to quit. Indeed, experts say that addiction to nicotine can be as strong as addiction to cocaine or heroin. Without a steady supply of nicotine, withdrawal symptoms may occur. A person may become irritable, anxious, hostile, and crave tobacco. Nicotine withdrawal may also produce headaches, nausea, and inability to concentrate. Although 70 percent of smokers want to stop smoking and 34 percent attempt to quit each year, only 3 percent successfully stop smoking each year. The high rate of relapse is a consequence of the effect of nicotine dependence. Smokers' families and friends should be more aware that smoking is not only a nasty habit, but a form of drug dependence.

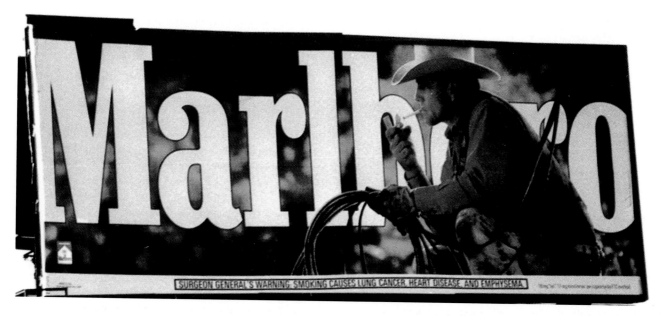

The Marlboro man rode off into the sunset on Joe Camel as billboards advertising tobacco products with these icons are history. Since 1998 tobacco companies have agreed to stop billboard advertising and to stop marketing to young people

Health Risks of Smoking

Of the 4,000 potentially toxic chemicals in cigarette smoke, the three major toxic substances are nicotine, carbon monoxide, and tar. Nicotine stimulates the cardiovascular system. Increased heart rate and blood pressure place a burden on the heart muscle, which then needs more oxygen. Carbon monoxide, a toxic gas, immediately reduces the blood's ability to carry oxygen and ultimately damages the inner surface of coronary arteries, increasing the rate of atherosclerosis. When combined with vasoconstriction, a narrowing of the arteries, this atherosclerosis can cause ischemia (lack of oxygen) and coronary tissue damage. Smoking also increases arrhythmias, increases stickiness and clotting of blood cells, and decreases levels of HDL. This is why twice as many smokers as nonsmokers die from heart attacks. Also, smoking contributes to peripheral vascular disease, which is the hardening of the arteries in the lower legs. This condition can affect the ability to walk and may eventually lead to amputation of the legs.

Tar contains potent carcinogens. It also contains chemicals that irritate lung tissue and may promote chronic bronchitis and emphysema. These substances can paralyze and destroy the cilia that line the bronchi, allowing tar and other particles to accumulate in the lungs. This causes *smoker's cough*, the body's attempt to rid itself of the buildup of particulate matter. Long-term contact between lung tissue and tar can cause cellular changes leading to the development of cancer.

The reduction in a person's life expectancy due to smoking parallels increasing cigarette use. Mortality is higher the younger a person started smoking, the longer a person has smoked, the deeper a smoker inhales, and the higher the tar and nicotine content of the tobacco used. If a smoker is overweight, has moderately elevated blood pressure, or has a high cholesterol level, the risk of having a heart attack skyrockets.

If you've smoked for many years, does it do any good to quit? Yes. Heart attack risk declines by about half in the first year after quitting. Risk continues to decrease with each year of abstinence until, after 10 to 15 years, an exsmoker has almost the same risk of dying as if he or she had never smoked (Fig. 13-2). People who quit smoking may gain weight (men gain about 10 pounds and women about 11), of course there is no comparison between the health risks of being 10 or 11 pounds overweight and the hazards of smoking. Regardless of how long or how much a person has smoked, quitting is beneficial.

Smokeless Tobacco

Cigarette smoking is not the only form of tobacco that presents health risks. Smokeless tobacco—snuff and chewing tobacco—is surging in popularity among young adult males. Often used by athletes, smokeless tobacco seems to be viewed as a safe alternative to cigarette smoking, which is forbidden by coaches on athletic teams. The tobacco industry wants you to believe that snuff and chewing tobacco provide all the pleasure of cigarettes minus the risks. But the evidence shows otherwise. Highly carcinogenic tobacco **nitrosamines** are released in concentrations 1,000 times higher in smokeless tobacco-saliva mixtures than in cigarette smoke. Snuff and chewing tobacco cause many problems ranging from bad breath to cardiovascular disease and cancer. A decrease in the ability to taste and smell, stained teeth, gum damage, tooth loss, and wear on the chewing surfaces of the teeth caused by grit in the tobacco are commonly experienced. Use of smokeless tobacco also causes leukoplakia, a precancerous condition that produces thick, rough, white patches on the gums, tongue, or inner cheek. Experts predict an oral cancer epidemic beginning in two or three decades if the trend continues.

In addition, smokeless tobacco is addictive. Nicotine from the smokeless tobacco is absorbed directly into the bloodstream from the mouth (one of the most efficient delivery systems known) and eventually produces dependency. Evidence has revealed that tobacco companies manipulated the chemical recipes of their products. These chemical changes supposedly allow more nicotine to be absorbed into the bloodstream, thus making the product gradually more addictive. Many people feel that the dependency produced by smokeless tobacco is harder to break than that produced by smoking.

Are You a Passive Smoker?

Nonsmokers, who outnumber smokers 3 to 1, are growing tired of **passive smoking**—breathing air polluted by tobacco smoke, especially when they read reports from the American Heart Association and the Environmental Protection Agency (EPA). Reports state that passive smoking causes more than 60,000 deaths per year. Nonsmokers regularly exposed to secondhand smoke have a 91 percent higher risk of heart disease than do those not exposed to this killer. Those occasionally exposed have an increased risk of 58 percent. As you learned in Chapter 7, "Maximizing Your Heart Health," secondhand smoke harms the cardiovascular systems of nonsmokers more than smokers. This is because the smoker's cardiovascular system has adapted to the ill effects of cigarette smoke. Nonsmokers exposed to secondhand smoke exhibit

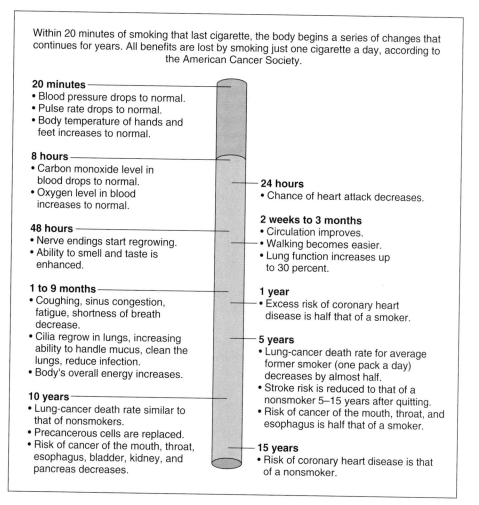

Within 20 minutes of smoking that last cigarette, the body begins a series of changes that continues for years. All benefits are lost by smoking just one cigarette a day, according to the American Cancer Society.

20 minutes
- Blood pressure drops to normal.
- Pulse rate drops to normal.
- Body temperature of hands and feet increases to normal.

8 hours
- Carbon monoxide level in blood drops to normal.
- Oxygen level in blood increases to normal.

48 hours
- Nerve endings start regrowing.
- Ability to smell and taste is enhanced.

1 to 9 months
- Coughing, sinus congestion, fatigue, shortness of breath decrease.
- Cilia regrow in lungs, increasing ability to handle mucus, clean the lungs, reduce infection.
- Body's overall energy increases.

10 years
- Lung-cancer death rate similar to that of nonsmokers.
- Precancerous cells are replaced.
- Risk of cancer of the mouth, throat, esophagus, bladder, kidney, and pancreas decreases.

24 hours
- Chance of heart attack decreases.

2 weeks to 3 months
- Circulation improves.
- Walking becomes easier.
- Lung function increases up to 30 percent.

1 year
- Excess risk of coronary heart disease is half that of a smoker.

5 years
- Lung-cancer death rate for average former smoker (one pack a day) decreases by almost half.
- Stroke risk is reduced to that of a nonsmoker 5–15 years after quitting.
- Risk of cancer of the mouth, throat, and esophagus is half that of a smoker.

15 years
- Risk of coronary heart disease is that of a nonsmoker.

figure 13-2   When smokers quit.

an increased rise of fatal and nonfatal cardiac events. This is due to the extreme sensitivity of the cardiovascular system to the many chemicals in secondhand smoke. This sensitivity accelerates atherosclerotic heart lesions and increased tissue damage following a heart attack. In 1993, the EPA officially declared secondhand smoke to be a human carcinogen that causes about 3,000 nonsmokers a year to die from lung cancer and about 12,000 a year to die from other cancers.

Nearly all employers in the United States have restricted smoking in the workplace because of the effects of smoke-filled air on the nonsmoker. The problem is that passive smokers involuntarily inhale toxic fumes produced by the cigarette of the mainstream smoker. What nonsmokers may not realize is that these highly toxic substances are found in higher concentrations in sidestream than in mainstream smoke. Even though smoke is mixed with environmental air, it still causes eye and nasal irritations, sore throats, coughing, and headaches in nonsmokers. Families of smokers have more respiratory problems and more days of absence from work or school due to illness than do families of nonsmokers. In fetuses it increases the risk of low birth

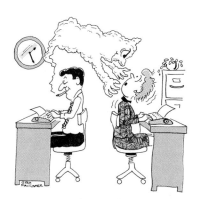

Smoking is everybody's business.

weight and is blamed for up to 300,000 cases of childhood bronchitis and pneumonia. It is also linked to childhood asthma and sudden infant death syndrome. Studies have indicated that nonsmoking spouses of heavy smokers have double the risk of lung cancer of nonsmokers. The same may be true for their risk of emphysema, bronchitis, and other respiratory diseases.

The decision to smoke can no longer be considered a private matter. Past solutions, such as separating smokers and nonsmokers within the same room, are inadequate. The surgeon general states that this helps but does not eliminate exposure. The AHA concludes, "the only sure way to protect nonsmokers from environmental tobacco smoke is to eliminate smoking from areas that smokers share with nonsmokers." This once radical step is rapidly gaining acceptance—indoor smoking may soon be a thing of the past.

It does not make sense to strengthen your heart and lungs with regular exercise only to be at the mercy of smokers when you venture into public. Get involved and start campaigning for eliminating exposure to secondhand smoke.

Here are some tips to keep others from smoking around you:

- Speak up. Make others aware of the dangers of secondhand smoke and let them know *you don't like it.*
- Suggest alternative places for others to smoke—outside.
- Display reminders. Hang "Thank you for not smoking!" signs in your home, car, office, and so on.
- Get rid of ashtrays.
- Discuss smoking cessation strategies. Many new products and strategies are available to help smokers quit. Bringing these up in conversation makes your antismoking concerns clear. It may save your life and that of someone close to you.

Why Should You Quit?

The act of quitting smoking can add years to a person's life (see Fig. 13-2). Even more important, it increases the chance that those years will be healthy and active, drastically decreasing the chances of suffering painful, incapacitating, and costly illnesses. Overall quality of life will improve. You will save money, because cigarettes are expensive. A pack-a-day habit sends over $700 a year up in smoke. You can say goodbye to tobacco stains on your teeth and fingers. Your breath, hair, clothes, and surroundings will smell fresher. Your smoke will no longer annoy or harm other people, and this will particularly benefit your family. No longer will cigarette burns or messy ashes ruin furniture, carpet, and countertops. Your risk of setting an accidental fire will be reduced. Your ability to taste and smell will return. As the effects of smoking are reversed, you will eliminate smoker's cough and increase your endurance so that you will have more energy all day. Besides reducing your health risks, you will overcome a potential drug addiction that may have taken control of your life.

How to Quit Smoking

Millions of Americans have quit smoking. Of smokers who quit, most have done it on their own. There are many ways to quit. Some people try to gradually reduce the number of cigarettes they smoke. Others quit "cold turkey." The "patch" helps many quit. A small patch worn on the skin helps minimize the usual withdrawal symptoms. It is available by prescription only. It works by painlessly releasing decreasing doses of nicotine through tiny blood vessels near the surface of the skin. Stop smoking pills (Zyban) have helped many smokers quit. An even more successful cessation program is an approach combining nicotine chewing gum, nicotine patches, and behavior modification counseling. The number one determinant of success, however, is the smoker's desire to quit, based on some strong motivational goal, like saving money or improving health. If you are a nonsmoker wishing to help a smoker trying to quit, you should know that the support of family and friends is the second most important factor in successfully breaking the grip of the nicotine habit.

Giving up smoking can be a long-term process, and some people must try several times before they quit for good. It is not easy. Smokers have about the same success rate as those trying to break alcohol or heroin addiction. This doesn't mean that a person can't quit, because every year thousands of people do. But it takes effort, desire, support, and a firm commitment. If a person quits smoking and then starts again, he or she should not be considered weak. Some former smokers say they still crave cigarettes long after they quit smoking. The smoker who does not succeed in quitting on the first try should try and try again. Mark Twain said it best: "It's easy to *quit* smoking, I should know—I've done it dozens of times."

If you're ready to toss those cigarettes, *Clearing the Air: A Guide to Quitting Smoking*, available from the American Cancer Society, gives these recommendations:

- *Identify your reasons* for quitting.
- *Set a target date for quitting.* Then list the reasons you want to quit. Review these whenever you crave tobacco.
- *Identify your barriers to quitting* (such as your spouse smokes or you have relapsed before due to stress or weight gain).
- *Make specific plans ahead of time for dealing with temptations.* Identify two or three coping strategies that work for you (such as taking a walk or calling a friend.
- Before you quit, *change to a brand you find distasteful,* and then taper off a little more each day. Smoke only half of each cigarette. Smoke only during even hours of the day.
- *Involve friends and family.* Tell them when and why you are going to quit and ask for their support.
- *On the day you quit,* toss out all cigarettes and matches. Go to the dentist to have your teeth cleaned. Keep busy and concentrate on getting through that one day without tobacco.
- After quitting, *change your normal routine.* Spend as much time as possible away from places and situations that you associate with smoking. Go jogging, drink more fluids, get plenty of rest.

- When you get the "crazies," *chew on carrots, pickles, sunflower seeds, sugarless gum.* Take a shower. Never allow yourself to think, "One won't hurt." It will.
- *Mark progress.* Each month, celebrate the anniversary of your quit date. Put aside the money you've saved by not smoking and treat yourself to something special. You deserve it.

The Clock Strategy

Another strategy for quitting smoking is to let the clock tell you when to smoke. The clock strategy was reported to be twice as successful in the long term as quitting cold turkey. This is how it works:

Step 1:   Assign yourself specific times of the day to light up.

Step 2:   Gradually lengthen the intervals between cigarettes.

Step 3:   Cut back progressively on the number of cigarettes per week (decreasing cigarettes by one-third each week).

The key to why the clock strategy seems to work so well lies in breaking the link between everyday smoking cues and the habit of lighting up. That is, smokers don't smoke when they want to. They smoke on cue. By repeatedly putting nicotine urges on hold for manageable periods, smokers gain practice and self-confidence for when they finally stop. If you wish to quit smoking, try this new strategy. We wish you success!

Psychoactive Drugs

Psychoactive drugs are mind-affecting or mind-altering drugs. They are chemical substances that change one's thinking, feelings, perceptions, and behaviors. These changes are the result of the drug's action on the brain. Psychoactive drugs are classified in this text by their effect on the CNS. The classification includes: (1) depressants, (2) marijuana, (3) narcotics or opiates, (4) stimulants, (5) psychedelics, and (6) inhalants.

Depressants

Depressants are drugs known as sedatives. They slow down the CNS, relax or tranquilize, and produce sleep. This category includes the "date rape drugs:" gamma-hydroxybutyric acid (GHB) and Rohypnol ("roofies"). Alcohol is a CNS depressant but it was discussed earlier in the chapter.

The Date Rape Drugs (GHB and Rohypnol)

GHB and **Rohypnol** (flunitrazepam) are two drugs sometimes used to cause women to become overly relaxed or pass

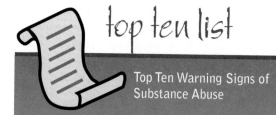

top ten list

Top Ten Warning Signs of Substance Abuse

1. Change in attendance patterns at school/work.
2. Change in behavior—previously happy individual becomes withdrawn, rebellious, depressed, tired, or aggressive.
3. Forms different friendships and association with known drug users.
4. Loss of interest in hobbies, sports, and school.
5. Eating and sleeping habits are altered.
6. Weight loss and other physical complaints.
7. Poor physical appearance (e.g., clothes, personal hygiene).
8. Increased borrowing of money from friends or family members; stealing from home, school, or employer.
9. Heightened secrecy about actions and possessions.
10. Change from typical capabilities, such as work habits, efficiency, self-discipline, mood, or attitude expression.

out and yield unknowingly in a sexual way. Both drugs are often knowingly used to intensify the effects of alcohol.

GHB is known by street names such as "liquid ecstasy," "liquid X," "gamma 10," "Georgia home boy," "G-riffick," "easy lay," "salty water," "grievous bodily harm," and "scoop." The drug is most often seen as a colorless, odorless, and tasteless liquid, but occasionally can be found as a white powder. Because GHB is odorless and tasteless it can be slipped into someone's drink without detection. GHB induces a state of dazed relaxation not unlike that caused by alcohol.

GHB first showed up in health food stores in the late 1980s as a potential aid for sleep, weight loss, and body building. After reports of adverse effects, the Food and Drug Administration took GHB off the market in 1990. It is a Schedule 1 (no approved medical use) controlled substance and illegal to manufacture, sell, or purchase. However, instructions to make GHB can be found on the Internet, and the ingredients can be purchased over the counter.

Rohypnol can be called "roofies," "roach," "rope," "la rocha," "the forget pill," and simply the "date rape drug." Rohypnol is legally prescribed outside the United States for short-term treatment of sleep disorders, but is used illegally to sedate a victim. It is a powerful sedative 10 times more potent than valium and is illegal in the United States.

Rohypnol, a small white tablet, dissolves easily in liquid and is colorless, tasteless, and odorless. The drug takes effect 10 to 30 minutes after ingestion and creates a sleepy, relaxed, and drunk feeling that lasts 2 to 8 hours. The victim may experience difficulty speaking and moving, and then may pass out. While under the drugs influence, a victim will have no memories of what happened (blackouts and amnesia). The drug, usually dissolved in a drink, can be swallowed as a pill or snorted. "Roofies" are sometimes taken to enhance a heroin high or to mellow or ease the experience of coming down after a cocaine or crack high.

Both drugs are powerful sedatives and become extremely dangerous when mixed with other CNS depressants, such as alcohol or narcotic drugs. This combination is potentially life-threatening and can be fatal. To reduce the risk of substance-related rape, practice the following suggestions:

1. Do not leave beverages unattended.
2. Do not take any beverages, including alcohol, from someone you do not know well or trust.
3. At a bar or club, accept drinks only from the bartender, waiter, or waitress.
4. At parties, do not accept open container drinks from anyone.
5. Be alert to the behavior of friends. Anyone appearing disproportionately inebriated in relation to the amount of alcohol they have consumed, may be in danger.
6. Anyone who believes they have consumed a sedativelike substance should be driven to a hospital emergency room or someone should call 9-1-1 for an ambulance. Try to keep a sample of the beverage for analysis.

Marijuana (Cannabis)

Marijuana is an intoxicating psychoactive drug that may produce both depressant and psychedelic effects.

Marijuana is the United States' most widely used illegal drug and trails only alcohol and tobacco in popularity as a social or recreational drug. At lower doses marijuana produces a variety of effects including sedation, mild euphoria, and mild analgesic. At higher doses it produces hallucinations. Marijuana is made from the leaves and flowers of the cannabis sativa plant. The leaves and flowers are dried and crushed, causing the marijuana to have a tobaccolike appearance. It is usually smoked as a cigarette (called a *joint* or a *nail*) or in a pipe or bong. In recent years marijuana has appeared in *blunts*, cigars that have been emptied of tobacco and refilled with marijuana, often in combination with another drug, such as crack. Some users also mix marijuana into foods or use it to brew tea. There are over 200 slang terms for marijuana including "pot," "grass," "herb," "weed," "boom," "Mary Jane," "gangster," and "chronic."

Although there are at least 421 ingredients in marijuana, **delta-9-tetrahydrocannabinol (THC)** is the principal psychoactive ingredient. When in smoke, THC is rapidly absorbed by blood in the lungs and transported to the brain in less than 30 seconds. Because the strength of marijuana has increased 15 percent over its strength in the 1980s, the effects of smoking a joint may last several hours

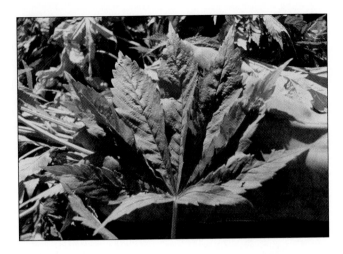

If you think "everybody's doing it," you're wrong.

with the peak occurring 20 to 30 minutes after inhalation. THC is fat soluble and is stored in fatty tissues of the body, brain, and reproductive organs. Due to this, complete elimination of a single dose is slow and may require 1 month or more before the body is drug free. During this time, marijuana residuals can be detected in the urine.

The short- and long-term negative effects of marijuana are numerous:

- Induces a false sense of well-being or euphoria and produces feelings of relaxation ("mellowing out").
- Produces sleepiness.
- Lowers resistance to both bacterial and viral infections.
- Impairs or reduces short-term memory.
- Decreases the concentration needed to master important academic skills.
- Creates difficulty keeping track of time.
- Causes brain cell damage and lowered sperm count. THC changes the cell membranes, causing it to be less efficient with less energy, particularly in the brain and testicles.
- Results in a **motivational syndrome** due to changes in the brain cell membranes. A person with this experiences low energy, apathy, and little drive to do anything. Students exhibit this syndrome by not going to class, not completing assignments, "vegetating" on a chair, or appearing not to care about anything.
- Decreases testestrone levels for men, lowers sperm counts, and increases difficulty having children.
- Increases testestrone levels in women and increases risk of infertility.
- Increases forgetfulness.
- Diminishes sexual pleasure.
- Slows physical reflexes.
- Decreases social inhibition.

table 13-14   Do You Have a Marijuana Problem?

Yes	No	
____	____	1. Are you using marijuana more often?
____	____	2. Do you think marijuana is safe and not addictive?
____	____	3. Do you use marijuana to escape from problems or to relax?
____	____	4. Do you seek out people so you can smoke marijuana with them?
____	____	5. Do you do things under the influence of marijuana that you wouldn't normally do?
____	____	6. Do you worry that you will run out of marijuana?
____	____	7. Do you think marijuana makes you more social and creative?
____	____	8. Does your throat ever feel raspy?
____	____	9. Are you finding it more difficult to remember things that recently happened?
____	____	10. Do you feel tired more often?
____	____	11. Have you noticed you react more slowly to situations, even if they are serious?
____	____	12. Do you find you are getting more colds, flus or other infections?

Scoring: Did you answer "Yes" to three or more questions? If so, you may have a problem with marijuana.

- Distorts space and distance judgment, increases fearlessness, and increases risk of injury.
- Increases heart rate. The risk of heart attack is five times higher than the usual in the hour after smoking a joint. It is particularly dangerous if user has preexisting heart disease.
- Causes bloodshot eyes and dry mouth and throat.
- Causes panic attacks; increases anxiety, paranoia, and hallucination.
- More lung and throat damage results because marijuana burns hotter than tobacco. The damage is greater even though tobacco smokers smoke 20 or more cigarettes per day, far more than marijuana smokers do. Joints don't have filters and are usually smoked to the last bit, so they deliver more irritating particles to the lungs. Damage is further magnified when users inhale the smoke deeply and hold it as long as possible.
- Increases risk of cancer. Research reveals marijuana to have 50 to 70 percent more known carcinogens than tobacco smoke.
- Increases psychological dependence and tolerance requiring more of the drug to get the same effect.

Drinking alcohol while smoking marijuana is dangerous. Marijuana inhibits vomiting, causing the alcohol to remain in your system. This increases the chance of alcohol poisoning. Use of marijuana severely reduces the ability to drive a car. It impairs motor coordination, impairs judgment and perception, and decreases awareness of external stimuli (such as flashing lights). Take the self-assessment in Table 13-14. Also, see Table 13-15.

Even though illegal, marijuana has been used in medicine for over 2,000 years. In 1965, THC was commercially synthesized. However, it was not until 1985 that the U.S. Food and Drug Administration (FDA) approved it for medical purposes. Marijuana and synthesized THC are desig-

table 13-15   Marijuana Use

One of four college students reported using marijuana within the past year

Characteristics Predicting Marijuana Use:

- Higher among students at noncommuter colleges and at colleges with pubs on campus

Student Characteristics Associated with Marijuana Use:

- Being single
- Caucasian (white)
- Spending more time at parties and socializing with friends and less time studying. Participating in other high risk behaviors such as binge drinking; cigarette smoking; having multiple sexual partners; and perceiving parties as important and religion and community service as not important.

nated as controlled substances under federal law (Controlled Substance Act of 1970). This law includes all drugs with no medical use and/or high potential for abuse. Marijuana is available only with a physician's prescription in capsule, liquid, or naturally cultivated cigarette form. It is administered orally, intravenously, as drops, or as a cigarette to be smoked. It is sometimes prescribed for relieving the nausea accompanying cancer chemotherapy. More recently, it has been used to stimulate the appetite in AIDS patients to help overcome the debilitating weight loss associated with this disease. Most medical professionals insist that there are synthetic drugs that achieve the same results as smoking marijuana for medical purposes, without the side effects.

When conventional therapies have failed, marijuana has been somewhat effective when used alone or in combination with other drugs to treat the following conditions:

- *Asthma:* It sometimes produces a bronchodilation effect.
- *Epilepsy:* It sometimes protects against minimal and maximal seizures.
- *Glaucoma:* It sometimes helps reduce the vision-threatening intraocular pressure.
- *Multiple sclerosis:* It sometimes reduces muscle spasticity.

Marijuana has not been found superior to ordinary medications in the treatment of anxiety, depression, pain relief, or drug/alcohol abuse. In some cases, it hasn't even been helpful. However, the therapeutic potential for medical marijuana merits continued study.

Marijuana is considered a gateway drug leading to possible cocaine and heroin use. Experiments with legalization of marijuana in Europe have proved unsuccessful, leading to higher crime rates, higher addiction rates, and higher health costs.

Narcotics or Opiates

Narcotics are powerful painkillers. The narcotic analgesics, often referred to as opioids, also produce pleasurable feelings (euphoria) induce sleep, and depress breathing.

Heroin

Heroin (sometimes called *smack, junk, H,* and *hard stuff*) is a psychoactive drug that depresses the CNS. It is most abused and the most rapidly acting of the opiates. Pure heroin is a white powder with a bitter taste. It may vary in color from white to dark brown due to impurities remaining in the manufacturing process or the presence of additives. Heroin is a semisynthetic drug made by treating morphine with acetic anhydride to yield diacetylmorphine. It was first introduced into medical practice in 1898 as a cough suppressant because it had fewer undesirable side effects than morphine. The drug quickly lost favor in the United States due to its great drug-dependency potential. Heroin, a controlled substance, is no longer used medically.

Users are seldom aware of precisely what they are buying on the street from pushers. It may be mixed or cut with substances such as powdered milk, sugar, starch, quinine, and even strychnine and arsenic. A cheaper and more potent form of heroin, originating in Mexico and known as *black tar* or *tootsie roll,* is being widely used in the United States.

Heroin is illegal and a highly addictive narcotic. It exerts its primary addictive effect by activating the region of the brain that is responsible for producing the pleasurable sensations of reward and the region that produces the classic physical dependence syndrome. Together, these actions account for the user's loss of control and the drug's habit-forming action.

Heroin is usually mixed into a liquid solution and injected into a vein (*mainlining*). It can also be injected under the skin, sniffed, and taken by mouth. Increases in sniffing heroin indicate that purer and cheaper forms are available on the street. Many crack users are switching to snorting heroin because it is cheaper, more plentiful, and carries less stigma than crack. Another sign of increased purity is the increasing rate of fatal overdoses. Heroin today is often 65 percent pure, 15 years ago, it was only 6 percent pure. Some pushers, to be more competitive, are offering super-pure heroin (90 percent pure) to users. This too potent heroin is known as *Poison, People's Choice, China Cat,* and *Red Sun* and has been linked to a string of overdose deaths.

Intravenous injection provides the greatest intensity and most rapid onset of euphoria (7 to 8 seconds), while intramuscular injection produces a relatively slow onset of euphoria (5 to 8 minutes). When heroin is sniffed or smoked, peak effects are usually felt within 10 to 15 minutes. All three forms of administration are addictive.

Tolerance to heroin develops quickly. After several weeks of continued use, the user needs to increase the dose to achieve the desired rush. Eight to 12 hours after the last dose is taken, withdrawal symptoms appear if another fix is not taken. The symptoms of the body's need for another fix include: watery eyes, runny nose, yawning, loss of appetite, muscle cramps, and insomnia. Elevations in blood pressure, pulse, respiration rate, and temperature occur as withdrawal progresses. Acute physical withdrawal from heroin addiction is grueling and peaks between 48 and 72 hours after the last dose. During this time symptoms include vomiting, nausea, diarrhea, cramping, muscle and bone pain, cold flashes with goose bumps, kicking movements, and severe shaking. Withdrawal takes approximately 1 week.

Many health problems related to heroin use are caused by uncertain dosage levels (due to fluctuations in purity), use of unsterile equipment, contamination by cutting agents, or use of heroin in combination with other drugs such as alcohol or cocaine. The short-term effects of heroin use include:

- "Rush" (Euphoria)
- Drowsiness
- Depressed respiration
- Constricted pupils
- Clouded mental functioning
- Nausea and vomiting
- Suppression of pain
- Spontaneous abortion
- Warm flushing of the skin
- Dry mouth
- Heavy feeling of the extremities
- Slowed, slurred speech
- Droopy eyelids
- Constipation

Any drug-abusing lifestyle may depress the strength of the immune system and the body's ability to withstand infection. The long-term effects of heroin use include:

- Addiction
- Infections and diseases (e.g., HIV/AIDS and hepatitis B and C, from sharing or using unsterile equipment)

- Collapsed veins
- Abscesses
- Infection of the heart lining and valves
- Arthritis and other rheumatologic problems
- Liver disease
- Pulmonary complications including various types of pneumonia
- Clogging of blood vessels that leads to the lungs, liver, kidneys, or brain

Symptoms of heroin overdose include shallow breathing, clammy skin, convulsions, and coma. Death may result. Heroin use during pregnancy is associated with stillbirths, sudden infant death, and below-normal birth weight. The newborn infant is likely to demonstrate the heroin withdrawal process.

Stimulants

Stimulants are chemical substances that speed up the central nervous system, resulting in alertness and excitability. This category includes: Cocaine and Crack, and Methamphetamine (a.k.a. Crank and Ice). Caffeine is a CNS stimulant but is discussed later in the chapter in "Drugs Affecting Physical Performance."

Cocaine and Crack

Cocaine and crack (a cocaine derivative) are controlled substances. They are potent, rapid-acting drugs. Cocaine comes from the coca plant, mainly harvested in Central and South America. Cocaine is extracted from the coca leaf during a two-step chemical process involving sulfuric and hydrochloric acid. This process separates cocaine from the other chemicals in the coca leaf and results in cocaine hydrochloride (or *street cocaine*). Cocaine hydrochloride is the fine, opalescent, white, fluffy, odorless, and bitter-tasting drug sold for illegal, recreational use. It is the second most widely used illegal drug in the United States. Until the early 1980s, cocaine was used mainly by the wealthy. Today, it is an equal opportunity drug used by members of all socioeconomic groups.

Cocaine (a.k.a. "blow") is a euphoriant and a central nervous system stimulant whose effects last from 20 minutes to several hours, depending on the drug's purity. There are several ways to take cocaine, and the speed with which the cocaine user achieves a high varies with each method. It may take 10 to 30 minutes to feel cocaine's effects when the drug is swallowed, 3 minutes when it is snorted, 30 seconds when it is injected, and just a few seconds when it is smoked. While it may be swallowed, this is not as effective as other methods because of poor absorption in the gastrointestinal tract. The most common method is to snort the drug (sniff it through the nose). The powder is first chopped fine with a razor blade and arranged into lines on a piece of glass. The user may then inhale the cocaine through a rolled-up dollar bill, straw, or "coke spoon." Injecting cocaine produces an intense and exhilarating rush, but one that is short-lived because of the drug's rapid metabolization by the liver. Cocaine may also be smoked in the form of either freebase cocaine or crack.

Freebase cocaine is separated from ordinary street cocaine (cocaine hydrochloride) in a process that results in a purer and more intense form that can be smoked. (Cocaine hydrochloride—the street, powder form—cannot be smoked.) In this process, the drug is freed from the parent compound by mixing it with water and ammonium hydroxide. The cocaine base is then separated from the water using a fast-drying solvent such as ether, leaving unadulterated cocaine freebase. Small amounts of the base are then placed in the neck of a specially designed water pipe and smoked at high temperature over a torch. All of the freebase components are readily available in the retail marketplace. Smoking freebase cocaine creates a rush that is rapid, powerful, and short-lived, much like the high from injected cocaine. While the euphoria and feelings of energy last only a few minutes, the other effects (such as pupil dilation, increased blood pressure and heart rate) are prolonged and can be dangerous. Also, the ether used in the process is extremely volatile and may explode.

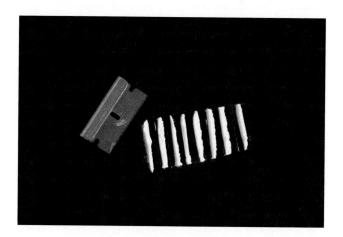

Crack is crystallized freebase cocaine sold in the form of ready-to-smoke "rocks." The rocks of processed cocaine are smoked in a pipe, or placed in cigarettes or joints of marijuana. As a ready-to-smoke drug, crack spares the user the delay and bother of having to extract the potent freebase form of cocaine from cocaine hydrochloride. The rocks are nicknamed *crack* because of the crackling sound they make as they are smoked. Before crack came on the market, cocaine smokers had to make the freebase themselves, using dangerous, highly flammable chemicals such as ether. The extraction process was complicated and costly as well. Because crack is such a pure drug (about 90 percent pure cocaine) and approximately five times more potent than using cocaine, smoking crack gives the user a far more intense and rapid euphoria than does snorting cocaine. One puff of a pebble-sized rock produces an intense high that lasts about 20 minutes. The user can generally get three or four hits off one rock. The high is always followed immediately by an equally unpleasant crash, characterized by irritability, agitation, and intense cravings for more of the drug.

Crack is usually purchased in small plastic vials containing two or three rocks, and is more affordable per dose than cocaine. However, most people cannot stop after one vial and may use five or more vials to keep the high. Although crack is sold in inexpensive units, this has nothing to do with the actual price of the drug. Crack's price per gram is almost double that of cocaine powder. Crack only appears cheaper—much as buying a single cup of coffee for 50 cents seems cheaper but is actually much more expensive than buying a whole pound of coffee for $5.99. The deceptively low initial price of crack makes it possible for just about anyone to start using the drug. Some users go on a 3-day crack binge, depleting their body and bank accounts. They quit only because they are out of money or out of crack or because their bodies cannot take it anymore.

Addiction to crack takes less time to develop than addiction to snorting cocaine. Some users can become psychologically addicted after smoking it only a few times. Crack addiction is accelerated by the speed with which it is absorbed through the lungs (it hits the brain within 4 to 6 seconds) and by the intensity of the high.

Some people may start using cocaine to lose weight (it depresses the appetite) or to enhance alertness and relieve fatigue (it stimulates the central nervous system). As a stimulant, this drug also causes blood pressure, heart rate, and body temperature to rise. Because the heart and breathing are accelerated and because cocaine acts as a vasoconstrictor (narrows blood vessels), cocaine can be dangerous to anyone with heart or respiratory problems. The increase in the number of strokes in the early 1990s has been linked to cocaine use.

Cocaine users develop tolerance and eventually need more and purer forms of the drug to achieve the same effect. If addiction occurs, withdrawal symptoms will develop.

Eventually, the addict uses cocaine to avoid the unpleasant depression or crash that always follows the rush. How do you know if you are addicted to cocaine? Put simply, and as stated earlier in this chapter, continuing to use a drug (any drug) despite negative consequences constitutes addiction.

Consequences of using any form of cocaine may be severe. Cocaine is an illegal drug, so users risk arrests, fines, and jail terms. Some states are considering prosecuting women who take drugs during pregnancy and give birth to addicted babies.

Eventually, continued smoking of crack and freebase cocaine may cause paranoia, other psychoses, lung and liver damage, depression, insomnia, impotence, nausea, vomiting, anxiety, and isolation. People who smoke crack (whether for the first or the 50th time) are risking their lives. The intense high can be too much for the body, causing respiratory arrest, heart attack, convulsions, and death. Snorting cocaine can lead to chronic rhinitis (runny nose), nasal congestion, perforation of the nasal septum, and greater vulnerability to upper respiratory infections. Injecting cocaine increases the risk of contracting AIDS, hepatitis, and other infectious diseases if needles are shared.

Methamphetamine (a.k.a. Crank and Ice)

The drug is also called speed, meth, crystal, crank, and ice. **Crank,** a term once used as a street name for cocaine, has emerged on the drug scene as an alias for **methamphetamine** (a synthetic form of amphetamine). Crank is a powerful CNS stimulant; odorless; yellow or off-white in color; and sold in capsules, chunks, or crystals. *Eightballs*, approximately one-eighth of an ounce, are considered to be a day's supply. Meth is often sniffed, inhaled, swallowed, or injected to produce a greater high. The rush, an effect greatly desired by the abuser, is a highly pleasurable sensation experienced almost immediately after intravenous injection. **Ice,** the street name for crystallized crank, sometimes called *Crystal Meth*, is smoked, like crack cocaine. It is quickly overtaking crack cocaine as the drug of choice for many addicts. Experts claim that methamphetamine is more dangerous than cocaine because it is more addictive. The high caused by using cocaine lasts about 20 to 30 minutes, but meth users can feel a high lasting from 24 to 48 hours, The effects of methamphetamine use include:

- increased heart rate and blood pressure
- increased wakefulness; insomnia
- increased physical activity (often used at raves . . . all-night dance parties)
- decreased appetite
- respiratory problems
- hyperthermia, convulsions, and cardiovascular problems, which can lead to death.
- euphoria
- irritability, confusion, tremors

- anxiety, paranoia, or violent behavior
- irreversible damage to blood vessels in the brain, producing strokes.

Methamphetamine is a cheap high. While it costs about the same as cocaine, it is cheaper to use because each dose is smaller and the effects last much longer. Also the drug is much easier to obtain.

Ice, used in Asia for years, was imported to Hawaii in the early 1980s and has since spread to the West Coast. This drug is not new. It has been around since the nineteenth century (one past user was Hitler). What is new is the source: The drug, once manufactured and aggressively marketed by youth and motorcycle gangs on the West Coast, is now controlled by Mexican crime families who are quickly spreading it eastward across the United States. The main ingredient for the manufacture of the drug, ephedrine, originates in Asia and Europe. It is then shipped to Mexico. Next, it is smuggled across the U.S. border and resold to the operators of stove-top labs located in places as varied as rural shacks and motel bathrooms. Additionally, methamphetamine can be easily manufactured in the home laboratory by a "cook" with a few hundred dollars worth of equipment by extracting ephedrine, the main ingredient from easy to obtain over-the-counter allergy, cold, and diet pills or from pseudophedrin another decongestant easy to obtain. The recipe is on the Internet, available to those who know where to look. Some law enforcement officials fear methamphetamine will be the basis for a national drug crisis in the future. The aftereffects of this drug are similar to those of crack and cocaine: lethargy, severe depression, paranoia, and cardiopulmonary damage. Many users develop a tolerance for these drugs quickly and need larger and larger doses to gain the effect they seek.

Psychedelics

Psychedelic drugs are known as mind-expanders or hallucinogens. These drugs affect an individual's perception, awareness, and emotions and can also cause *hallucinations*, completely groundless, false perceptions. They can also cause *illusions*, misinterpretations of reality or something imagined. This category includes: LSD and MDMA (*Ecstacy*).

LSD

LSD (Lysergic acid diethylamide), a controlled substance, is a dangerous and unpredictable hallucinogenic drug. LSD was discovered in 1938 by Dr. Albert Hofmann, a Swiss chemist, seeking to develop a drug to improve blood circulation. This illegal drug is manufactured from lysergic acid, found in ergot, a fungus that grows on rye or other grains.

LSD, commonly referred to as *acid*, is sold on the street in many forms, including tablets or pellets called *microdots*, gelatin chips known as *windowpanes*, and thin squares of absorbent paper soaked in liquid LSD called *blotter acid*. Sev-

eral factors account for the resurgence in popularity of this drug. First, the potency of today's LSD is less than it was at the height of its popularity in the 1960s and 1970s. Currently, the strength of LSD ranges from 20 to 80 micrograms per dose. During the 1960s and early 1970s, the dosage ranged from 100 to 200 micrograms or higher per unit. This weaker LSD tends to produce more manageable reactions. Second, the packaging of the product is more appealing to young users. Blotter acid is enticing and seems almost harmless when packaged on absorbent paper featuring cartoon characters, stars, moons, and dragons. Blotter acid is difficult to detect because it is so small and light; it can be carried in textbooks or pockets and sent in greeting cards through the mail. Third, LSD is affordable; a hit runs about $3 to $5 in most areas of the country.

The effects of LSD are unpredictable. They depend on the amount taken; the user's personality, mood, and expectations; and the surroundings in which the drug is used. Usually, the user feels the first effects in 30 to 90 minutes after taking the drug. The physical effects include dilated pupils, increased body temperature, increased heart rate and blood pressure, sweating, loss of appetite, sleeplessness, dry mouth, and tremors. Sensations and feelings change much more dramatically than do the physical signs. The user may feel several different emotions at once or swing rapidly from one emotion to another. If taken in a large enough dose, the drug produces delusions and visual hallucinations. The user's sense of self and time changes. Sensations may seem to cross over, giving the user the feeling of hearing colors and seeing sounds. These changes can be frightening and can cause panic attacks.

Users refer to their experience with LSD as a *trip* and to acute adverse reactions as a *bad trip*. Bad trips are long lasting, taking about 12 hours to end. Some LSD users experience severe, terrifying thoughts and feelings, fear of losing control, and fear of insanity. Some fatal accidents and suicides have occurred during states of LSD intoxication because of the user's highly suggestive state and feelings of invulnerability. Examples of this include users walking out in front of fast-moving automobiles and jumping out of high windows.

Many LSD users experience **flashbacks,** a recurrence of certain aspects of a person's drug experience without the user having repeated its use. A flashback occurs suddenly, often without warning, and may occur within a few days or well over a year after LSD use. Flashbacks usually occur in people who have used hallucinogens chronically or who have underlying personality problems. However, people who are apparently normal also have flashbacks.

Bad trips and flashbacks are only part of the risks of LSD use. Relatively long-lasting psychoses, such as schizophrenia, severe depression, mania, and paranoia, may afflict users. Most users of LSD voluntarily decrease or stop its use over time. LSD is not considered to be an addicting drug because it does not produce compulsive drug-seeking behavior as does use of cocaine, amphetamines, heroin, alcohol, and nicotine. LSD does produce tolerance, however, the one characteristic it has in common with many of the other addictive drugs. Thus, the user is required to take progressively higher doses to achieve the state of intoxication previously achieved. This is an extremely dangerous practice given the unpredictability of the drug.

MDMA (Ecstacy)

Known as **"Ecstacy,"** "Adam," "The Big E," "X," and "X-TC," **MDMA** (3-4 methylenedioxymethamphetamine) has enjoyed popularity because it combines the "rush," or stimulating effects of cocaine, with the hallucinogenic qualities of psychedelics. It is an illegal, synthetic "designer drug" produced mainly by underground chemists. MDA the parent drug of MDMA and of similar chemical structure, destroys the serotonin-producing neurons of the brain, as does MDMA.

Originally synthesized in 1914, as an appetite suppressant, MDMA is classified federally as a Schedule 1 drug, as is heroin, LSD, and MDA. The drug did not become a significant drug of abuse until the 1980s, when it became popular among American college students. MDMA use was common at all-night dance parties called "raves." In 1985 the federal government outlawed the drug. Ecstacy's popularity has intensified and as has marketing taken over by established drug dealers and organized crime mobsters. It can be found at raves, rock concerts, night clubs, and schools. MDMA can be used as a white powder or in tablet or capsule form. The pill form of Ecstacy often is decorated with logos such as cartoon characters or familiar brand names (e.g., Mitsubishi, Nike swoosh). Taking the drug by mouth is preferred; it is inhaled on occasion, but rarely injected. Basically, Ecstacy, increases the users sense of euphoria and energy.

Many problems users encounter with MDMA are similar to those found with the use of amphetamines and cocaine. They are:

- *Psychological difficulties* including confusion, depression, sleep problems, drug craving, severe anxiety, and paranoia—during and sometimes weeks after taking MDMA.
- *Physical symptoms* such as muscle tension, involuntary teeth clenching, nausea, blurred vision, dilated pupils, rapid eye movements, faintness, chills and sweating, and dry mouth and throat. Most problems are attributed to dehydration among novice users who don't drink enough water. In fact, some ravers have danced themselves into severe dehydration, as well as heat exhaustion, and overexertion, which can lead to heart failure, convulsions, and death.
- *Decrease in resistance to disease*
- *Increases in heart rate and blood pressure*, a special risk for people with circulatory or heart disease.

On the other hand, many users report:

- Mild visual hallucinations and distortion of the senses
- An "at peace" or happy feeling
- Decreased use of psychological defense mechanism (friendlier, more outgoing)
- Increased empathy for others
- Promotion of intimate communications
- Enhance sensual experience, especially pleasures of touching

The greatest fear is Ecstacy's potential for acting as a toxic substance within the brain causing impaired learning and brain damage.

Inhalants

Inhalants are volatile nondrug substances (often ordinary household products) that have druglike effects when inhaled. A few of these substances do have some medical uses, specifically, amyl nitrite and nitrous oxide. Inhalants are a diverse group of breathable chemicals that produce mind-altering vapors.

Inhalants are classified into three major groups, all potentially hazardous to users.

- *Commercial solvents* such as toluene, xylene, benzene, naphtha, acetone, and carbon tetrachloride are components of common commercial products that can cause a "high" when abused. They are found in airplane glue, plastic cement, paint thinner, gasoline, cleaning fluids, nail polish remover, marking pens, and typewriter correction fluid.
- *Aerosols* are suspended particles in a gas used as a propellant in many household and commercial sprays. The abused products include: cooking sprays, glass chillers, spray paints, computer sprays, fire extinguishers, deodorizers, and hair sprays. Also, in this category are Freon gas, used in refrigerators and air conditioners, and propane gas, a widely used fuel. Two additional inhalants in this category include:
  - *Amyl nitrite*, an inhalant prepared in cloth-covered glass capsules (ampules), has a legitimate medical use in treating heart patients. Upon breaking, the amyl nitrite capsules make a popping sound that has given rise to their common street names of "snappers" and "poppers."
  - *Butyl nitrite*, a substance legally produced and formerly sold as a room odorizer or liquid incense, is a clear yellow liquid and is sometimes packaged in ampules. It's known as "Rush," "Locker Room," and "Super Bullet." Although not aphrodisiacs, amyl nitrite and butyl nitrite seem to intensify sexual orgasm when inhaled close to the peak of passion.

- *Anesthetics* such as chloroform, ether, and halothane are volatile gases sometimes abused as inhalants. This category also includes nitrous oxide (laughing gas) and cyclopropane gases. When tanks of nitrous oxide cannot be obtained from legal medical sources, the intoxicating gas can be obtained from whipped cream propellants, pressurized pellets, and trace gas used to detect pipe leaks. Recently, "whippets," (canisters used to make whipped cream), have become faddish. For the past several years, nitrogen oxide has become a popular intoxicant among high school and college-age persons, as well as young urban professionals, or "yuppies." Nitrous oxide can produce permanent damage to the nervous system—this means the ability to see, hear, walk, and talk may be seriously jeopardized.

Some inhalants produce a temporary mild euphoria, because they slow down CNS function and produce a dreamlike "high" resembling drunkenness. Beware, however, that they can damage the nerves that control breathing, leading to coma or death, especially if taken with sedatives or alcohol. Bone marrow, liver, and kidney damage have also been noted. Some fumes (e.g., Freon, butane, propane) also can cause "sudden sniffing death," probably from cardiac arrest, even in first-time users.

These products are sniffed, snorted, bagged (fumes inhaled from a plastic bag), or "huffed" (inhalant-soaked rag, sock, or roll of toilet paper in the mouth) to achieve a high. Inhalants are also sniffed directly from the container. Be alert to obvious signs of inhalant abuse:

- Slow, thick, slurred speech; disorientation; general drunken appearance
- Complaints of headaches
- Signs of paint or other products where they would not normally be (face, fingers)
- Chemical odors on breath, clothing, or rags
- Rapid disappearance of household aerosol or cleaning products
- Red or runny eyes or nose (can have nosebleeds)
- Spots and/or sores around the mouth
- Nausea and/or loss of appetite

Drugs Affecting Physical Performance

In the world of competitive athletics, where the margin between winning and losing may be only a fraction of a second, athletes looking for an edge are tempted by illegal drugs. Anabolic steroids are taken to build muscle. Amphetamines may be taken to mask fatigue, caffeine to enhance performance. Diuretics may be used to cause rapid weight loss or to

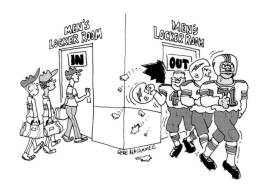

Overly aggressive behavior is a symptom of steroid use in males.

mask anabolic steroid use. These drugs can adversely affect your health.

Anabolic Steroids

Anabolic steroids are an artificial form of the male hormone **testosterone.** This hormone, secreted by male testes stimulates the bone, muscle, skin, and hair growth characteristically found in the adult male. Steroids were first developed in the 1930s to build body tissues and to prevent the breakdown of tissue that occurs in some diseases. In the 1950s, a few foreign countries experimented with giving testosterone to their male and female athletes. Because these athletes dominated many international competitions, a U.S. doctor developed a form of anabolic steroid that could help build muscle yet minimize masculinizing side effects. Initially steroids were used only by weightlifters in small doses, but athletes assumed that larger doses would build even more muscle. Today, anabolic steroids are widely used and abused by both male and female athletes, from young teens to professionals, at all levels of competition. Many athletes "stack" them—that is, take a combination of brands in quantities of 100 mg or more daily.

While these drugs increase muscle mass and have some legitimate uses (e.g., treatment of hormone disorders, treatment of multiple sclerosis and anemia), they have numerous adverse side effects (Table 13-16). Anabolic steroids can alter mood and behavior. Significant increases in depression, violence, sexual arousal, and distractibility were seen in young male athletes in one study. When taken by men, steroids shut down the body's production of testosterone, causing breast growth, testicular atrophy, prostate enlargement, and premature cessation of bone growth. Large doses of anabolic steroids trigger masculine changes in women. Deepened voice, male pattern baldness, and increased facial and body hair are irreversible. Females experience loss of body fat, enlarged clitoris, decreased breast size, and changes in or absence of menstruation. The athlete who uses steroids faces a variety of other steroid side effects: acne; mood swings; changes in sex drive; and uncontrollable, aggressive behavior, or **'roid rage.**

table 13-16 The Bad News About Steroids

Established side effects and adverse reactions from steroids follow:

- Acne
- Aggressive, combative behavior (" 'roid rage")
- Anaphylactic shock (from injections)
- Breast development (soreness or swelling in men)
- Cancer
- Cholesterol increase
- Clitoris enlargement
- Death
- Depression
- Diarrhea
- Edema (water retention in tissue)
- Fatigue
- Feeling of abdominal or stomach fullness
- Fetal damage
- Frequent or continuing erections (mature males)
- Frequent urge to urinate (in mature males)
- Gallstones
- HDL (which helps reduce cholesterol) decrease
- Heart disease
- High blood pressure
- Hirsutism (hairiness—irreversible)

- Impotence
- Increased chance of injury to muscles, tendons, and ligaments, and longer recovery period from injuries
- Increased risk of coronary artery disease (heart attack, stroke)
- Insomnia
- Kidney disease
- Liver disease
- Liver tumors
- Male pattern baldness (irreversible)
- Menstrual irregularities
- Priapism (painful, prolonged erections)
- Prostate enlargement (which can result in blockage of the urinary tract)
- Rash
- Sterility (reversible)
- Stunted growth
- Testicular atrophy
- Unnatural hair growth
- Unpleasant breath odor
- Unusual bleeding
- Yellowing of the eyes or skin

Source: Department of Health and Human Services.

The popularity of anabolic steroids is attested to by the growth of a large black market and quack steroid products. Many of the black-market brands come from underground labs and foreign countries and are of questionable quality and purity.

Steroids can be deadly. Unfortunately, to the high school junior trying to make first-string linebacker, the long-term effects of steroids may not seem important. However, steroid use can lead to sterility, kidney disease, liver tumors, bleeding ulcers, cancer, cardiovascular problems (high blood pressure, stroke, lowered high-density lipoprotein), and death. One surprising risk to the user who injects anabolic steroids is the exposure to HIV.

Even though steroids may be easily accessible through health clubs and spas, they are illegal if purchased without a physician's prescription. Some physicians have readily written prescriptions for athletes, but this practice is decreasing as doctors become more aware of the drug's dangerous side effects.

Amphetamines

Amphetamines (*speed, uppers, crank, bennies, meth,* or *crystal*) are powerful central nervous system stimulants. They are controlled drugs, meaning legislation has severely restricted even medical use. Their use without a prescription is illegal. Currently, amphetamines are legitimately used for short-term diet control in obesity and **narcolepsy** (uncontrollable attacks of deep sleep). They increase blood pressure, heart rate, respiratory rate, and metabolic rate; suppress the appetite; and place the body in a state of stress. The ability of amphetamines to relieve sleepiness and fatigue; to decrease appetite; and to increase alertness, confidence, and short-term performance has led to extensive nonmedical use, particularly by people involved in activities that demand stamina and long periods of wakefulness: long-distance truck drivers, pilots, flight attendants, and entertainers. They have also been used by students cramming for exams and by athletes trying to enhance their performance. These drugs do not increase maximal oxygen uptake. While they do enhance endurance by masking fatigue, under the influence of amphetamines, an athlete may go out in a race too hard and burn out midway. Also, a person using amphetamines in competition may be seriously injured and not be aware of it.

Common side effects include headaches, mood swings, rapid heartbeat, restlessness, insomnia, and anxiety. Use of amphetamines over a prolonged period increases tolerance of the drug and results in a need for larger doses. Large doses can lead to high blood pressure, anorexia, convulsions, and psychosis. Use of amphetamines during exercise in a hot environment may result in an elevated body temperature and death. Amphetamine injections, when needles are shared, may expose the user to needle diseases such as hepatitis and AIDS.

Diuretics

Diuretics cause the body to pass water by increasing urine output. They are useful in treating edema and mild hypertension. Diuretics are useless in producing true weight loss, because they result in loss of water, not fat. Any water lost is quickly regained over the next 24 hours. When used by wrestlers to temporarily decrease weight in order to compete, the resulting dehydration produces weakness and fatigue, along with increased susceptibility to heat illness. Diuretics have also been used, ineffectively, by some athletes attempting to mask anabolic steroid use. Urine tests for steroids are sufficiently sensitive to detect amounts as minute as a drop in a swimming pool of water.

Caffeine

Caffeine is probably the most common drug used by adults and children in our society. It occurs naturally in coffee, tea, colas, cocoa, and chocolate and is added to some prescription and nonprescription drugs. Table 13-17 lists average amounts of

table 13-17   Common Sources of Caffeine

	Milligrams		Milligrams
Coffee (6-oz. cup)		Tea (6-oz. cup)	
Brewed, drip method	80–175	Brewed	53
Decaffeinated, brewed	3	Instant	30
Instant	60–100	Oolong	36
Decaffeinated, instant	2	Green	32
Espresso (2 oz.)	90–120	Analgesics	
Cocoa beverage (5 oz.)	4	Actamin Super, Aspirin-free	
Chocolate milk (8 oz.)	5	Excedrin, Excedrin Extra	
Chocolate		Strength	65
Dark chocolate (1 oz.)	5–35	Goody's Headache Powders,	
Chocolate cake (1 slice)	20–30	Supac, Vanquish	33
Milk chocolate (1 oz.)	1–10	Anacin, Anacin Maximum	
Chocolate-flavored syrup (1 oz.)	4	Strength, Buffets II, Cope, Gelpirin,	
Soft drinks (12 oz.)		Gensan, P-A-C Revised formula,	
Jolt Cola	72	Rid-A-Pain Compound, Midol	32
Sundrop	63	Cold-allergy remedies	
Kick	58	Kolephrin, Kolephrin/DM	65
Mountain Dew	55	Fendol	32
Mellow Yellow	52	Triaminicin, Histosal	30
Coca-Cola	47	Dristan AF Decongestant	16
Diet Coke	47	Stimulants	
Mr. Pibb	41	Caffedrine, Keep Alert, NoDoz Maximum	
Dr. Pepper	41	Strength, Ultra Pep-Back, Vivarin	200
Sunkist Orange	40	Quick Pep	150
Pepsi-Cola	38	NoDoz, Pep-Back	100
Diet Pepsi	36	Enerjets	75
A&W Cream Soda	28	Weight Control	
Barq's	23	Dexatrim Extra Strength	200
Slice Cola	11	Diuretics	
Water, caffeine enhanced (12 oz.)		Permathene H_2 Off	200
Java Water	71	Aqua-Ban	100
Krank $_2$0	70		
Water Joe	46		
Aqua Java	43		
Juice drinks, caffeine enhanced (12 oz.)			
Java Juice	90		
XTC	70		

caffeine found in commonly used drinks, food, and drugs. Caffeine is a powerful central nervous system stimulant. In healthy, rested people, a dose of 100 milligrams (about 1 cup of coffee) increases alertness, banishes drowsiness, quickens reaction time, enhances intellectual and muscular effort, increases heart and respiratory rates, and stimulates urinary output.

Ingestion of 1 to 2 cups of coffee an hour before prolonged exhaustive exercise produces a glycogen-sparing effect by promoting fat use, which may enhance performance in endurance activities. It also tends to mask fatigue. This effect decreases as fitness increases, however, resulting in little or no benefit for highly trained athletes. If a competitive edge is desired, an athlete is wiser to drink a sports drink or plain water. Caffeine produces dehydration and, in some individuals, abnormalities in heart electrical function, both of which hinder performance.

While moderate use of caffeine is generally harmless, overconsumption can produce a toxic reaction known as *caffeinism*. A 300-milligram dose for many people produces sleep disruption, nervousness, irritability, restlessness, muscle twitches, headaches, heart palpitations, and gastric disturbances. In addition, some women report increased incidence of premenstrual syndrome (PMS) or fibrocystic breast disease (noncancerous breast lumps) related to caffeine consumption. How much caffeine is too much? Although tolerance varies from one person to another, intake of less than 200 milligrams per day is a wise limit.

Caffeine use is habit forming, and those who try to abruptly stop a long-term pattern of heavy consumption often experience withdrawal symptoms. Headaches, lethargy, irritability, and difficulty concentrating are common symptoms that will gradually diminish over a few days to 2 weeks.

Over-the-Counter and Prescription Drugs

Legal drugs are often subdivided into over-the-counter drugs (OTCs) and prescription drugs. There are over 300,000 OTCs available in the United States. Aspirin is the most common form, but most cold medicines, cough syrups, and laxatives also fall into this category. OTCs are not addictive if used correctly, and they must have clear warnings and instructions printed on labels for consumer use and protection. Still, there is a difference between *safe* and *harmless*. OTCs can do damage if used incorrectly, and some can lead to physical dependence if overused.

Five common kinds of nonprescription drugs are especially likely to produce adverse side effects or dependence:

1. *Nasal sprays.* After several days' use, these can produce a "rebound" effect, making your nose more congested than ever. The rebound effect is the result of increased swelling of the nasal tissues. If you use a spray, limit use to 1 or 2 days.

2. *Laxatives.* The most habit-forming laxatives are the so-called stimulants, which work by stimulating the walls of the intestines. A diet high in fruits, vegetables, and grains, plus 2 quarts of fluids a day will almost always eliminate constipation. Laxatives should not be used to induce weight loss.

3. *Eyedrops.* These blood vessel constrictors will whiten bloodshot eyes, but like nasal sprays, they can produce a rebound effect.

4. *Alcohol/codeine cough syrups.* Codeine, a narcotic, works directly on the part of the brain that controls coughing. In many drugstores, you can obtain codeine-containing cough suppressants by signing at the cash register. Some of these medications contain substantial amounts of alcohol, dangerous for anyone with an alcohol problem.

5. *Stimulants such as herbal energizers, food supplements, fatigue reducers, antihistamines, cold medications, asthma relievers, diet and exercise aids.* Caffeine, ephedrine, pseudoephedrine, and phenylpropanolamine (PPA) are the most common types of stimulants used in these drugs (Table 13-18). All of these drugs can cause an increase in physical tolerance with repeated use. Physical tolerance and prolonged use will be followed by withdrawal symptoms upon cessation of use. Withdrawal can include depression, fatigue, irritability, nausea, and headache. Adverse side effects of these stimulants can range from anxiety to agitation; alertness to disorientation; mildly elevated heart rate to dangerously elevated heart rate levels; as well as increased muscle tension and shakes, temperature elevation (from mild to severe), increased urine

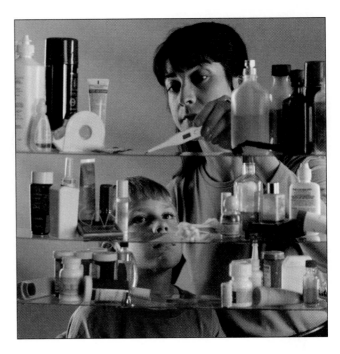

Over-the-counter drugs should be used with caution.

production, appetite suppression. Additionally, ephedrine can cause heart palpitations, hypertension, nerve damage, muscle injury, psychosis, stroke, and death.

Phenylpropanolamine (PPA) has been found to increase the risk of hemorrhagic stroke. The Food and Drug Administration (FDA) is taking steps to remove PPA from all drug products and recommends that consumers not use any products that contain PPA (Table 13-18).

OTC stimulants, frequently sold at convenience stores and truck stops or even out-of-the-home businesses, are advertised using terms such as "herbal," "natural," "performance enhancing," and "nutritional supplement." This gives the impression that they are healthful and harmless substances. However, most of these products contain powerful stimulants such as ephedrine and caffeine and carry dangerous side effects if used excessively or improperly. Some popular products in this category are: "Herbal Fen-Phen" (introduced by Nutri/System Weight Loss Centers); "kickers" (aimed for athletes, body builders, weight lifters); "Mini-Thin," "Permathin," "Dexatrim," "Diet Now," (aimed at dieters); and "Super Ener-Max," "Super Pep Extra Strength," "Mega-Blast," "Ultra Energy Now" (aimed at students studying late or drowsy drivers).

Most prescription drugs are put to good use (for example, antibiotics used for treating infection), but many are abused. Prescription drugs that are sometimes abused include amphetamines, barbiturates, narcotics, and tranquilizers. These drugs are used for a wide range of purposes such as to stimulate and/or depress the CNS, overcome fatigue, sup-

table 13-18 — Over-the-Counter Stimulants

Drug	Cold Medications/Antihistamines/ Asthma Medications	Exercise and Diet Aids
*Ephedrine (includes herbal energizer Ma Huang)	Bronkaid, Primatene, Vitronol Nose Drops	High Energy, Herbal Energy Formula, High Energy Max Strength, Diet Now, E'ola Drops
Phenylephrine Pseudoephedrine	Codimal, Coricidin, Dristan, Neo-Synephrine, Robitussin Actifed, Afrinol, Sudafed, Drixol, Chlortrimeton	
*Phenylpropanolamine (PPA)	Allerest, ARM, Contac, Dimetapp, 4 Way Formula, Nyquil, Sine-Off, Nightime Cold Medicine, Alka-Seltzer Plus Cold Medicine, Triaminic, Robitussin CF	Acutrim, Dexatrim, Metabolift, Thermo-genic Formula, Permathin-16 Maximum Strength
*Caffeine	Anacin, Excedrin, No-Doz	Caffedrine

*Most common OTC stimulants. The sale of the combination has been banned by the FDA.

press hunger, induce sleep, deaden the senses, relieve pain, and control anxieties.

There seems to be a pill for every need. Unfortunately, once prescribed, drugs are often taken in amounts and combinations not anticipated by the prescribing physician. Some physicians prescribe drugs more readily than do others, and some fail to stress the importance of reading labels carefully and taking drugs only as directed. Drugs prescribed to diminish physical or mental anguish are sometimes used for social purposes, leading to drug abuse.

Synergistic reaction, a major problem with drug use, is a phenomenon that occurs when various drugs are taken in combination, where the cumulative effect is greater than the effects of the drugs when taken separately. This results in an exaggerated drug effect or a prolonged drug reaction. Used alone, alcohol and tobacco are linked to oral cancer. Used together, the risk escalates. The same is true for alcohol and oral contraceptives in connection to increased risk of stroke and coronary heart disease. The combined effects of OTC stimulants and caffeine can be fatal. The sale of the combination of these three—ephedrine, caffeine, and phenylpropanolamine—has been banned by the FDA. This combination might be found in asthma and cold medications along with a cup of coffee (see Table 13-18).

Two of the world's most widely prescribed drugs, Zantac and Tagamet (used by millions of people with persistent heartburn and ulcers), act synergistically with alcohol. One study reported that in individuals who drank one and one-half glasses of wine with a meal and were taking Zantac, BAC increased 34 percent. For those taking Tagamet, BAC increased 92 percent. Especially hazardous is the combination of alcohol and barbiturates. This combination can kill a person or leave him or her in a persistent vegetative state.

frequently asked questions

Q. What is the definition of "Risk Reduction" or "Harm Reduction"? What does it involve?

A. The simplest definition is: A lower risk drinker does not harm anyone including himself or herself. Also, a lower risk drinker limits the amount of alcohol consumed in order to maintain sound judgment. It involves six steps:

1. Deciding why you want to reduce your risk. Some possible motivations are:
   - To avoid acting stupid
   - Family history of alcohol problems (your chances of having problems are three to four times greater than those without a family history)
   - Commitment to a healthy lifestyle
   - Cost—alcohol is expensive
   - Excessive drinking can be a roadblock to achieving life goals

2. Deciding what your limits are: The more you consume, the more your judgment is impaired. Remember, your body can only process one drink per hour!

3. Determining what places you at risk for exceeding your limits:
   - Emotions—if you are angry/anxious you may drink too much
   - Environments—certain places or people may lead you to drink too much
   - Events—recent problems/losses/stressors contribute to over drinking
   - Activities—drinking games/chugging/keg parties are associated with overdrinking

4. Developing strategies for every risk situation in Step 3:
   - Drink only if YOU want to
   - Drink only as much as YOU want to
   - Drink only the type of drink YOU want to
   - Do not drink if YOU feel negative emotions or the urge to "get drunk"
   - Be assertive—YOU can say no and not be rejected

5. Evaluation and improving upon your strategies: If you make a mistake and act irresponsibly consider it a learning experience. Explore why it happened and change your strategies accordingly.

6. Rewarding yourself for making responsible choices: Buy fun stuff with some of the money you save.

Q. Are the nicotine replacement products as bad as smoking cigarettes?

A. No, they do not have all the tars and poisonous gases found in cigarettes. Furthermore, they provide less nicotine than a smoker gets from cigarettes. These products should not be used by pregnant or nursing women. People with other medical conditions should check with their doctor before using any nicotine replacement product. Most important is that smokers quit completely before starting to use these products.

Q. Can nicotine chewing gum help me stop smoking? How much nicotine gum do quitters chew?

A. Nicotine chewing gum releases small amounts of nicotine into the body. This cuts down on withdrawal symptoms and makes it easier to break the smoking addiction. Nicotine gum is available over the counter and the recommended treatment period is 12 weeks. Usually 10 to 15 pieces of gum a day is used. Package instructions explain how the gum is to be chewed. Drinks such as coffee or soda should be avoided before, during, and after use of the gum.

Q. Cigars are so popular now. Are they safe?

A. No! Cigars, and pipes too, for that matter, may be more glamorous and acceptable than cigarettes, but they still kill. Research reveals that cigar smokers are twice as likely as nonsmokers to get cancer of the mouth, throat, and lung. They also run about 1½ times the risk of all smoking-related cancers and are more likely to develop heart disease or chronic obstructive pulmonary disease. By comparison, cigarette smokers have about three times as high a risk of coronary heart disease as nonsmokers and 20 times the risk of lung cancer. The rates for cigar and pipe smokers are lower than among people who smoke cigarettes only because those smokers consume less tobacco on average, not because cigar and pipe tobacco is less harmful.

Q. What causes hangovers, and can anything help ease or prevent them?

A. A hangover is a combination of physiological occurrences making you feel sick and hungover.
   - *Dehydration*—alcohol has caused evaporation of a vital portion of the body's water.
   - *Nervous shock*—the body is experiencing the effects of a mild overdose of a depressant drug (alcohol), so the nerves are in a hypersensitive state.
   - *Malnutrition*—the alcohol has caused a flushing away of a significant supply of the body's vitamins and nutrients. The body cannot activate its defense systems now that the essential nutrients are depleted.

   The amount needed to trigger a hangover depends partly on how much you're used to drinking. As little as one or two drinks, for example, can leave some people feeling wiped out if they seldom drink. The best way to avoid a hangover is not to drink heavily or more than usual. But several steps may reduce the likelihood and severity of a hangover. Try not to drink on an empty stomach or when you're worn out from exercise or lack of sleep. After you've indulged, the following may help:
   - Drinking lots of nonalcoholic liquids to replace lost fluids.
   - Taking a nonsteroid anti-inflammatory drug such as aspirin or ibuprofen (Advil, Motrin) may be helpful.
   - Resting. Expose the nervous system to as little stimulation as possible.
   - Eat something to help replace the vitamins and nutrients that were lost. Fruits and vegetables are best.

Summary

The wellness journey does not include substance abuse. Before drinking alcohol, smoking, or using other drugs, consider what these substances do to you. Your mind and body are capable of handling stress and emotional and physical pain without the help of drugs. You can feel happy, sexy, sad, angry, and joyous and experience love without artificial chemicals to enhance your feelings or to help you cope with life's challenges. The fact is, these substances magnify your problems. The single biggest killer of young adults is not heart disease, stroke, or cancer. It is accidents. Over half of all fatal accidents are alcohol- or drug-related. Use of many substances leads to tolerance or addiction as well as health problems. No other drug, not even alcohol, even comes close to nicotine in terms of deaths, illness, and other economic costs such as fires. Drugs do not make you a better athlete, either. On the contrary, inappropriate substance use can ruin your health, relationships, and future.

Before using any substance, whether over-the-counter, illegal, or prescribed, remember that you have choices. What you do now will affect your future. Be responsible and choose wisely.

additional information resources

Al-Anon Family Group Headquarters, 1600 Corporate Landing Parkway, Virginia Beach, VA 23454-5617, http://www.al-anon.alateen.org

Alcoholics Anonymous, P.O. Box 9999, Van Nuys, CA 91409, (818) 780-3951, http://www.alcoholics-anonymous.org.

Alcoholics Anonymous World Services, 475 Riverside Dr., 11th Floor, New York, NY, (212) 870-3400, 10115 http://www.alcoholics-anonymous.org

American Liver Association, 1425 Pompton Avenue, Cedar Grove, NJ 07009, (201) 256-2550; (800) 223-0179.

American Lung Association, (800) LUNG-USA, http://www.lungusa.org/asthma

Americans for Nonsmokers Rights 2530 San Pablo Avenue Suite J, Berkeley, CA 94702, (510) 841-3032.

Boost Alcohol Consciousness Concerning the Health of University Students (BACCHUS of the United States, Inc.), c/o Campus Alcohol Information Center, University of Florida, Gainesville, FL 32611, (800) COCAINE.

Food Addiction Hotline (1-800-872-0088).

Gamblers Anonymous, International Service Office, P.O. Box 1713, Los Angeles, CA 90017, (213)386-8789.

Marijuana Anonymous, World Services, P.O. Box 2912, Van Nuys, CA 91404, 1-800-766-6779.

Mothers Against Drunk Driving (MADD), 511 E. John Carpenter Freeway, Suite 700, Irving, TX 75062, 214-744-6233, http://www.madd.org

Narcotics Anonymous, World Service Office, P.O. Box 9999, Van Nuys, CA 91409, (818) 773-9999, http://www.na.org

National Association for Native American Children of Alcoholics, P.O. Box 18736, Seattle, WA 98118; (206) 322-5601.

National Black Alcoholism Council, Inc. 1629 K Street N.W., Suite 802, Washington, DC 20006; (202) 296-2696.

National Association for Children of Alcoholics, 11426 Rockville Pike, Suite 301, Rockville, MD 20852, 301-468-0985.

National Clearinghouse for Alcohol and Drug Information, P.O. Box 2345, Rockville, MD 20852, 800-729-6686, http://www.health.org

National Coalition for Hispanic Health and Human Services Organizations (COSSMHO), 1030 15th Street, N.W., Suite 1035, Washington, DC 20005; (202) 371-2100.

National Council on Alcoholism, and Drug Dependence (NCADD) Inc., 12 West 21st Street, New York, NY 10010, 1-800-NCA-CALL.

National Council on Compulsive Gambling, 444 West 56th Street, Room 3207S, New York, NY 10019, (212) 765-3833.

National Helpline, run by National Council on Problem Gambling, (800) 522-4700.

National Inhalant Prevention Coalition, (800) 269-4237, http://www.inhalants.org

National Institute on Alcohol Abuse and Alcoholism, Scientific Communications Branch, 6000 Executive Blvd., Suite 409, Rockville, MD 20892-7003, (301) 443-3860, http://www.niaaa.nih.gor

PRIDE (Parents' Resource Institute for Drug Education), Signal Press, 1730 Chicago Avenue, Evanston, IL. 60201.

National Institute on Drug Abuse (NIDA), U.S. Department of Health and Human Services, 5600 Fishers Lane, Rockville, MD 20857; (301) 443-6245.

Shoplifters Anonymous, P.O. Box 24515, Minneapolis, MN 55424.

Students Against Driving Drunk (SADD) P.O. Box 800, Marlboro, MA 01752; (508) 481-3568.

U.S. Department of Human Services, Public Health Service, Alcohol, Drug Abuse, and Mental Health Administration, Rockville, MD.

U.S. Environment Protective Agency (EPA) Indoor Air Quality Information Clearinghouse, Washington, D.C. 20013–7133,

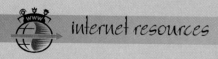

internet resources

American Lung Association Fact Sheet
http://www.Lungusa.org/
noframes/global/news/report/
smking/smkcessafac.html

Medicine Online/environmental tobacco smoke
http://www.meds.com/lung/smoking/environmental.html

Web of Addictions
http://www.well.com/user/woa

Cocaine Anonymous, World Service Office, 3740 Oveland Ave., Ste. C., Los Angeles, CA, 90034.
http://www.ca.org

Action on Smoking and Health (ASH)
http://www.ash.org

Higher Education Center for Alcohol and Other Drug Prevention
http://www.edu.org.hec

Substance Abuse
Values Clarification

1. Complete each of the following value clarification statements according to your feelings. Discuss each response in a few sentences:

   a. I view substance abuse as . . .

   b. The thought that alcohol, tobacco, and caffeine are drugs . . .

   c. If my sister continued to smoke while pregnant I would . . .

   d. If my 16-year-old brother asked me to get him some beer, I would . . .

   e. If the police picked me up for driving while intoxicated, I would . . .

   f. The next time my roommate comes in drunk and disturbs my study time (or sleep), I'm going to . . .

   g. How serious is substance abuse (on a scale of 1 to 5, 5 being most serious)?
   - in the United States: _____
   - at this university: _____
   - in my residence hall (fraternity/sorority house, apartment):_____
   - in my home: _____
   - Defend your ratings. What substances are being abused; what can/should be done to curb the abuse?

2. Discuss the pros and cons of each of the following statements:
   a. A mother should be charged with murder if she takes illegal drugs during pregnancy and her baby dies of addiction at birth.

   b. A nursing mother should be charged with child abuse if she uses illegal drugs.

   c. Any pregnant woman has a right to drink alcohol.

3. a. Do the following songs reflect society's values? Do they reflect your values? Explain your responses to both questions.

   - "I Drink Alone" by George Thoroughgood

   - "I Wanna New Drug" by Huey Lewis & The News

   - "Fight for the Right to Party" by Beastie Boys

   - "Margaritaville" by Jimmy Buffett

   b. What current music depicts substance use? List three examples and tell how.

   -

   -

   -

   c. How do music/videos/TV influence the use of drugs in our society?

Substance Abuse
Harm Reduction

Use the text (Chapter 13) to respond to the following 11 items:

1. Complete the "Do You Have a Drinking Problem?" self-assessment (Table 13-11). Are you concerned or surprised at your score?

   Yes _____ No _____ Discuss:

2. Leaving a party, you see a girl passed out on the lawn. What should you do? List six actions you should take.

3. Use five factors that affect alcohol absorption to give a profile of a person who will get drunk fastest.

4. How does alcohol change people's behavior? Give five examples from your observations.

5. You want to plan a safe party. List five ways you can help those attempting to reduce their use of or abstain from using alcohol (or drugs).

6. How can you reduce your risk of intoxication and/or alcoholism? List seven strategies.

7. What is "risk reduction" or "harm reduction"? Describe the six steps involved.

8. George can drink two six-packs before he feels drunk. Susan feels tipsy after two drinks. Should both be considered legally drunk at the same BAC? Discuss the reasons for your response.

9. Describe moderate use of alcohol.

10. What is considered abuse of alcohol?

11. Define binge drinking.

Tobacco Use Values Clarification

1. Tobacco companies spend $700,000 (or more) *an hour* to convince people that smoking is fun and exciting. List five ways they do so:

   a.

   b.

   c.

   d.

   e.

   How can you resist these tactics? How can you help others resist these tactics?

   a.

   b.

2. Young people should be angered by the overt efforts of the tobacco industry advertising campaigns to entice them to use tobacco. Yes _____ No _____. Defend your response.

3. Discuss the pros and cons of each of the following statements. Label your *pro* and *con* remarks:

   a. The tobacco *industry* should be made to compensate the cost of physical damage of the smoker (i.e., pay for the health care/medical costs due to tobacco use).

   b. The tobacco *consumer* should be made to compensate the cost of physical damage of other smokers (i.e., pay for the health care/medical costs due to using tobacco).

   c. Nonsmokers should help pay health care costs (i.e., lung cancer treatments, bypass surgeries, etc.) of coworkers who smoke when both groups share group health insurance plans.

   d. Insurance companies should drop policies of people who smoke.

   e. The age of 18 is the ideal age to be legally allowed to purchase tobacco products.

   f. Tobacco farmers should continue to be subsidized by the federal government.

   g. Congress should legislate tobacco to be an illegal drug and its manufacture and use should be controlled by the FDA.

   h. Secondhand smoke should be outlawed—no smoking inside any building.

   i. No smoking inside any home.

   j. Cigarette packages should require labeling such as "cigarettes kill"; "cigarettes cause cancer"; "this product is addictive."

4. How much should a pack of cigarettes cost? _____ Why?

5. Complete the following statement
   I won't smoke today because . . .

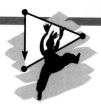

lab activity
13-4

Using HealthQuest

Directions: Insert HealthQuest CD. Click on "Alcohol" on the "Table of Contents" screen. Read "Alcohol Introduction." Click on "Specifics On." Read all eight sections of "Specifics On." Respond to the following questions.

1. What is the most abused drug in the United States? _____

2. (T or F) Ethyl alcohol needs to be digested before it is absorbed into the bloodstream. _____

3. Where in the body is the largest percentage of alcohol absorbed? _____

4. List four of seven factors that influence rate of alcohol absorption.

   _____   _____   _____   _____

5. Where is alcohol metabolized? _____

6. (T or F) It is permissible to drink small amounts of alcohol while pregnant. _____

7. What is the impact of heavy drinking on your cancer risk?

   What sites are most often affected? (List 10)

   _____   _____

   _____   _____

   _____   _____

   _____   _____

   _____   _____

8. What is the impact of drinking and breast cancer incidence?

   _____

9. What health condition is connected to long-term alcohol abuse?

   _____

10. Discuss responsible drinking behavior.

    _____

    _____

    _____

11. a. Which special U.S. population is most likely to drink and drive?

      _____

    b. Name the special U.S. population that has the lowest level of alcohol-related problems?

      _____

12. Can consumption of alcohol and wellness coexist? Explain your response.

    _____

    _____

    _____

Name

Class/Activity Section

Date

lab activity
13-5

Using HealthQuest

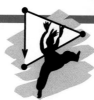

Direction: Insert CD. Click on "Alcohol" on the "Table of Contents" screen. Click on "Introduction" then "Wellness Activities." Click on "Alcohol Decision Maze." Read "Introduction." Go back and click on "Exploration" to begin. Explore and have fun.

1. Discuss the outcome of your drinking.

_____

_____

2. What feedback did you receive?

_____

_____

3. If you consumed alcohol what was your highest BAC?

What was your friends' highest BAC? _____

4. What is BAC?

5. What is the legal definition of intoxication?

_____

_____

6. What is the meaning of a BAC of 0.40?

_____

_____

7. How many beers does it take for your BAC to reach 0.10 percent? _____

lab activity @ chapter thirteen

Changing Behavior
Using the Transtheoretical Model

Using a highlighter, trace a path on the algorithm as you answer each question. Highlight your stage of change.

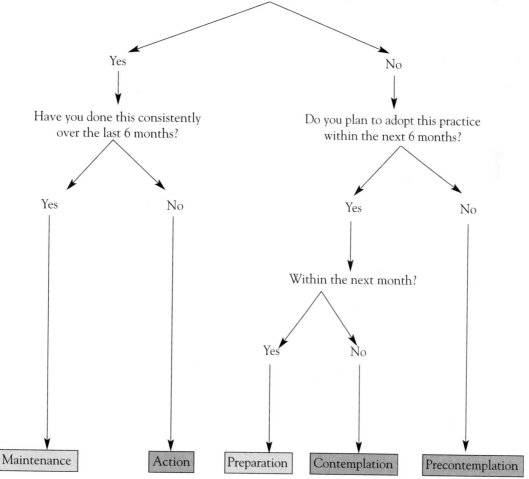

Do you refrain from driving every time you drink alcohol?

Once you've identified which stage of change you are in, it is important to use the processes most useful in progressing to the next stage—*or* remaining in maintenance.

In the box, write your stage of change. Then, list the processes that are most useful in that stage (see Fig. 2-2 in Chapter 2). Use only the number of processes that apply to your stage of behavior change. You may not need to use all six. Under each process that you use, give two specific behavior strategies (see Table 2-1 in Chapter 2) that could help you progress to the next stage—*or* maintain, if you're in the maintenance stage.

The stage I am in = _____ .

Process 1.   _____

      Behavior strategy – a.

      Behavior strategy – b.

Process 2.   _____

      Behavior strategy – a.

      Behavior strategy – b.

Process 3.   _____

      Behavior strategy – a.

      Behavior strategy – b.

Process 4.   _____

      Behavior strategy – a.

      Behavior strategy – b.

Process 5.   _____

      Behavior strategy – a.

      Behavior strategy – b.

Process 6.   _____

      Behavior strategy – a.

      Behavior strategy – b.

lab activity
13-7

Creating Balance
in Your Life

I. Calculate the amount of caffeine you consume daily. If you are using too much caffeine, develop a plan to reduce your consumption.

1. How many milligrams are you consuming per day? _____

2. List the main sources of your caffeine intake. How much caffeine is in each?

_____   _____   _____

_____   _____   _____

_____   _____   _____

3. Describe your plan for reducing your consumption. List at least four strategies.

a._____

b. _____

c._____

d. _____

II. Assess your lifestyle for addictive behaviors that do not involve drugs (e.g., gambling, Table 13-3; shopping or spending, Table 13-4; overexercising, Chapter 6, Table 6-3; or watching too much TV). Develop a plan to reduce these activities and create more balance in your life.

1. Which self-assessments did you use?

_____

_____

2. What was/were your score(s)? _____   _____   _____

3. What strategies can you initiate to reduce your involvement in these activities and how can you create more balance in your life? List at least six.

a._____

b. _____

c._____

d. _____

e._____

f. _____

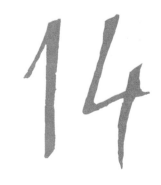

Preventing Sexually Transmitted Disease

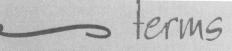

objectives

After reading this chapter, you will be able to:
1. Describe symptoms of AIDS and the most common sexually transmitted diseases.
2. Differentiate between curable and incurable sexually transmitted diseases.
3. Describe at least four ways HIV is transmitted.
4. Recognize the latency period for AIDS.

5. Differentiate between high-risk and low-risk sexual activities.
6. Describe precursors to unwanted sexual pressure and ways to deter it.
7. List actions you can take to decrease the risk of acquiring a sexually transmitted disease.

terms

- Acquired Immune Deficiency Syndrome (AIDS)
- Chancre
- Chlamydia
- Genital herpes
- Genital warts
- Gonorrhea

- Hepatitis B
- Herpes simplex virus
- Human immunodeficiency virus (HIV)
- Human papilloma virus (HPV)
- Lymphocytes
- Opportunistic diseases

- Pelvic inflammatory disease (PID)
- Sexual abstinence
- Sexually transmitted disease (STD)
- Syphilis
- T-cells
- Urethritis

Diseases spread through sexual contact were once called *venereal diseases (VD),* named for Venus, the Greek goddess of love, mother of Cupid. The term **sexually transmitted disease (STD)** refers to diseases spread primarily through sexual intercourse but also through other intimate behavior; sex play; and, occasionally, non-sexually. Understanding their symptoms and how they are spread and treated are important steps in risk reduction.

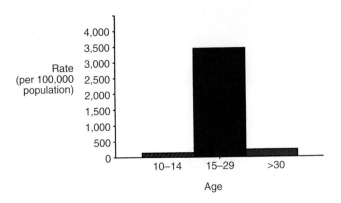

figure 14-1   STD rates by age.

Sexually Transmitted Disease

While **Acquired Immune Deficiency Syndrome (AIDS)** claims the spotlight as the most deadly and feared STD, we are experiencing a silent epidemic of other STDs in the United States. As a group, STDs are the number one communicable disease problem, but many people are unaware of this because of our cultural reluctance to discuss STDs and fear of public embarrassment. Only colds and flu, not officially reported, occur more frequently. It is estimated that one in four Americans will acquire at least one STD in their lifetime.

Changing mores appear to be a major factor in the increasing rate of STDs. Young people are becoming sexually active earlier, yet marrying later and divorce is more common. As a result, people often have more sexual partners. Increasing rates of premarital sexual intercourse among young people offer more opportunity for the spread of disease. Involvement with alcohol, a concern on many college campuses, is tied to increased sexual activity and lack of commitment to one's sex partner, which increase STD risk. Another factor may be the development of the birth control pill, which resulted in decreasing use of the condom. With concern over AIDS, however, this is changing. Both male and female condoms not only prevent conception but serve as barriers to transmission of STDs.

STDs affect people of all backgrounds and economic levels but are most common in people in their late teens to their 20s: 90 percent of reported STDs occur among persons ages 15 to 29 (Fig. 14-1). Nevertheless, your risk of acquiring an STD is determined by your behavior, not by your age or sexual orientation. Risk can be reduced or increased by personal choices that you control. If you choose to be sexually active, you are at risk. Your chances of exposure to an STD increase with multiple sexual partners and with increased frequency of sexual activity. Risk of infection is low to zero in a mutually monogamous relationship or if you abstain from sex.

Unfortunately, many people, especially young people, feel that STDs aren't serious or that "STDs only happen to others," and they fail to take precautions. A person may think, "If I get one, I'll just go get it taken care of." Many college students misjudge the risks of their sexual behavior. They feel that they are at "extremely low risk" for STDs even though they were previously diagnosed with an STD, have

had numerous sexual partners, and inconsistently use condoms. While some STDs are curable, some are not. Even some of the traditionally curable STDs are becoming antibiotic resistant making treatment more difficult. STDs may not seem to be a serious problem because you can't tell by looking at your friends who is infected and who is not. Also, your friends probably are not going to discuss STDs with you as they would discuss their last cold. But silence can be deadly. If you can't see it and don't hear about it, some think the problem isn't real. They are wrong.

STDs are spread from an infected person to a partner during sexual intercourse, oral sex, or anal sex. Nonsexual infection is possible with some STDs but uncommon. STDs are not spread on toilet seats, in hot tubs, or in swimming pools. The bacteria and viruses that cause STDs need the warmth and moisture of mucous membranes to live. That is why they infect the reproductive organs, rectum, and mouth. After transmission to a new host, the bacteria or virus quickly multiplies and may produce noticeable symptoms in 2 days to 4 weeks. Sometimes, an infected person notices no symptoms, however.

Women are particularly vulnerable to STDs, including AIDS, because they have more mucous membranes in their genital tissue than men do. Vaginal and cervical tissue can sustain microscopic tears through which viruses and bacteria, often transmitted by semen, can enter. In addition, women experience early warning signs of STDs much less frequently than men do, resulting in more advanced disease before treatment is sought. STDs are serious and, if left untreated, can cause permanent damage.

Early diagnosis and treatment is important to prevent serious physical harm and to prevent spread of the disease to other sexual partners. Symptoms of STDs vary with the type of infection and may differ between males and females. Be aware of the warning signs that may indicate the presence of an STD (Table 14-1).

Diagnosis and treatment of STDs is confidential. Contact the STD clinic of your local county health department or see a doctor immediately if you suspect that you may have an STD. Your local family planning clinic can also give in-

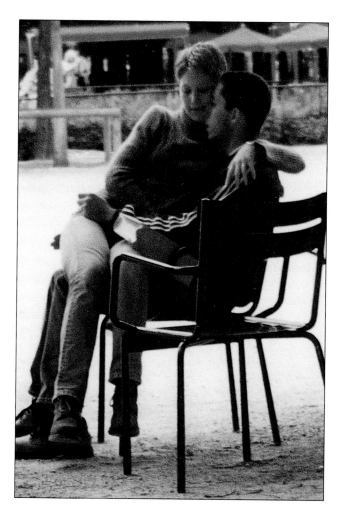

Serious relationships require serious decisions. If this couple is sexually active, using condoms will protect both from STDs.

table 14-1 — Symptoms of Sexually Transmitted Disease

Women	Women and Men
• Pelvic pain • Bleeding from the vagina between periods • Burning or itching around the vagina • Pain deep inside the vagina during sexual intercourse	• Abnormal discharge from the penis or vagina • A burning sensation during urination or bowel movements • Sores, bumps, or blisters near the mouth, rectum or genitals • Flulike feelings with fever, chills, or aches • Redness and swelling in the throat • Swelling in the groin

formation on where to go for help, or you can call one of the hotlines at the end of this chapter. Wherever you are treated, your case will be kept private.

table 14-2 — Curable and Incurable STDs

Bacterial (Curable)	Viral (Incurable)
• Chlamydia • Gonorrhea • Syphilis	• Genital herpes • Genital warts • Hepatitis B • AIDS

There are over 25 known STDs, some of which are incurable. Most STDs are either bacterial or viral. The most common bacterial STDs, which are treatable, are chlamydia, gonorrhea, and syphilis. Viral STDs, which are incurable, include genital herpes, genital warts, hepatitis B, and AIDS (Table 14-2). A person can have more than one STD at a time. Although less prevalent, AIDS is causing much concern because it is not only incurable but fatal. We will look first at the bacterial, then the viral STDs listed in Table 14-2.

Chlamydia

Chlamydia is caused by the bacterium *Chlamydia trachomatis.* It is one of the most widespread and damaging of all STDs. According to the Centers for Disease Control and Prevention, from 1984 through 1997, the last year for which reports are available, the rate of chlamydia rose from 3 to 207 per 100,000 people. This was primarily due to better screening, however, and recognition of asymptomatic infection rather than a true increase in the rate of disease. Rate of infection in women was reported as 336 per 100,000 people and in men 70 per 100,000. The lower rate reported among men probably indicates that the partners of many women with chlamydia remain untreated. Young women have the highest rate of infection, with 46 percent of infections reported in 15- to 19-year-olds and another 33 percent in 20- to 24-year old women. An estimated 1 in 10 college-age women are infected. Chlamydia is spread mainly through sexual intercourse but can be spread by the fingers from one body area to another, such as from the genitals to the eyes. It affects twice as many people as gonorrhea, although it mimics its symptoms, and both diseases often occur together. For this reason, physicians usually treat both infections if one is diagnosed. Early symptoms are usually mild, and if they occur, they appear within 1 to 3 weeks of exposure. Chlamydia causes an abnormal genital discharge and **urethritis,** an inflammation of the urethra, which produces a burning sensation during urination. In women, it can also cause lower abdominal pain. In men, chlamydia can infect the epididymis, causing painful scrotal swelling. About 80 percent of women and 10 percent of men have no noticeable symptoms and may not know they are infected. This makes the disease more difficult to diagnose and cure. As a result, the disease is often not diagnosed until it has done permanent damage.

Untreated chlamydia in women can produce a serious inflammation of the sexual organs called **pelvic inflammatory disease (PID).** PID is extremely damaging and can infect the lining of the uterus, fallopian tubes, and ovaries. This may cause fever and pain in the lower abdomen and scarring and blockage of the fallopian tubes and leave a woman unable to bear children. Of those with PID, 9 percent will have a life-threatening tubal pregnancy, 18 percent will experience chronic pelvic pain, and 20 percent will become infertile. A new urine screening test for chlamydia makes detection easier. The preferred treatment for chlamydia is tetracycline.

While anyone who is sexually active can get a chlamydial infection, highest rates occur among those who have had more than one sexual partner, have taken a new sexual partner in the past 2 months, are African American, are between 15 and 24 years of age, are of lower socioeconomic status, or are living in an inner city neighborhood.

Gonorrhea

Gonorrhea, the second most common bacterial STD, was named by Galen in 150 B.C. from Greek meaning "flow of seed." At that time, the penile discharge of men infected with gonorrhea was thought to be semen. Actually, the discharge was pus produced from inflammation of the urethra. The gonorrhea bacteria grows and multiplies quickly in mucous membranes such as in the cervix, mouth, rectum, or urinary tract. In women, the most common site of infection is the cervix, but it can spread to the ovaries and fallopian tubes, causing PID. It can be spread directly through sexual intercourse or from the genitals to the mouth with the fingers.

As with chlamydia, gonorrhea often has no symptoms, or the symptoms go undetected as the infected individual continues to spread the disease. Men are much more likely to notice the symptoms than are women. Up to 80 percent of women infected have no symptoms, compared to 20 percent of men. If they occur, symptoms usually appear within 2 to 14 days of infection. Gonorrhea often strikes the urethra, causing a burning sensation during urination. Males may notice an unusual penile discharge, as well as swollen lymph glands in the groin. Women may experience an abnormal vaginal discharge, abdominal pain, or vaginal bleeding. A rectal infection may produce anal itching or discharge. Oral infections usually produce no symptoms, though a few victims may get a sore throat. Early symptoms may clear up on their own, but a person can still be infected and spread the disease to others.

If not treated, gonorrhea may cause permanent damage to the reproductive organs and cause sterility. In men, it may damage the penis, making urination difficult and erection impossible. It can also infect the epididymis, leaving scar tissue that can block the flow of semen from the infected testicle. In women, it can scar the fallopian tubes, making it impossible to bear children. In both sexes, the bacteria can spread to the bloodstream, producing a generalized bacterial infection. It can infect joints with gonococcal arthritis and irreversibly damage heart valves, spinal cord, or the brain. It can be spread from an infected mother via the birth canal to her baby, causing eye infection and blindness if not treated immediately.

Gonorrhea is usually treated with penicillin and antibiotics, although penicillin-resistant strains have developed. Fifteen to 75 percent of cases in some regions are penicillin-resistant, making treatment more difficult. This increasing occurrence of penicillin-resistant gonorrhea underscores the need for taking protective measures during sexual activity and for being tested once or twice a year even if there are no symptoms.

While overall rates of infection have declined, infection rates for minority adolescents and young adults remain high, especially in high-density urban areas among those who have unprotected sex or multiple sexual partners.

Syphilis

For when it has once been received into the body, it does not immediately declare itself; rather it lies dormant for a certain time and gradually gains strength as it feeds.

—Fracastoro (1483–1553), *Syphilis, the "French Disease"*

Syphilis was rampant in Europe in the late 1400s, spread during times of war by soldiers who frequented prostitutes and then returned home to their wives and mistresses. It was also reported spread by soldiers who sailed with Columbus to the New World and by many Renaissance explorers who took it beyond the boundaries of Europe. It was first known as the "great pox," in contrast to which "smallpox" was later named, and was at first thought to be a special divine punishment for sexual transgressions. In the eighteenth century, syphilitics wore wigs and high collars to hide hair loss and throat lesions. Many early treatments used mercury or arsenic but produced side effects that were as bad as the disease. Although syphilis has been a serious health problem during all major wars, it was not until after World War II began that the U.S. Public Health Service started using penicillin to combat it.

Some social problems such as poverty, lack of access to health care, and lack of education are associated with high levels of syphilis in some populations. The infection rate among African Americans, particularly those living in inner cities, is nearly 24 times higher than the rate for whites, according to the Centers for Disease Control and Prevention.

Nevertheless, risk of acquiring any STD is determined by behavior, not by racial or ethnic factors. Avoiding risky behavior and making responsible choices are keys to reducing STD rates even in high-risk groups. Like other bacterial STDs, syphilis is easily spread because its symptoms are often unnoticed or confused with other diseases. Syphilis is known as "the great imitator" because it mimics so many other diseases.

Syphilis occurs in four stages—primary, secondary, latent, and tertiary—depending on how long a person has had it and how far it has progressed. We turn now to a brief discussion of each stage.

Primary Syphilis

The first sign of syphilis is a **chancre,** or small painless sore, which appears within 1 to 12 weeks of sexual contact. It may appear on the penis, in the vagina, in the mouth, or in any other area that contacted the bacteria, and it lasts 1 to 5 weeks. It is often accompanied by painless swelling of the lymph nodes in the groin. The initial sore may go unnoticed and will disappear if left untreated. The disease then enters a secondary stage 2 weeks to 6 months later.

Secondary Syphilis

In the secondary stage, skin rash, fever, headache, sore throat, swollen lymph glands, flulike symptoms, and patchy hair loss may occur. The symptoms are so general that the disease can be misdiagnosed even if medical help is sought. The rash may appear as pink spots or small raised bumps on the palms, soles of the feet, back, chest, arms, legs, face, or abdomen. Small, moist sores may appear in the mouth, and lesions may appear on the genital area. Secondary symptoms, if they occur, may clear up in 2 to 6 weeks without treatment but may recur for up to 2 years. During this time, an infected individual can still spread the disease. If untreated, although the initial symptoms may subside and a person can feel normal, the disease progresses.

Latent Syphilis

In latent syphilis, the third stage, a person is generally no longer infectious to others unless there is a relapse of moist lesions or unless the disease is passed to a baby during pregnancy. This stage can last for several years with no symptoms, but the infecting bacteria can continue to multiply.

Tertiary Syphilis

While two-thirds of untreated people will have no more symptoms, the one-third who are affected may suffer permanent damage to the cardiovascular or nervous systems. Tertiary syphilis can occur anywhere from 3 to 40 years after initial infection. Complications include heart disease, blindness, brain damage, paralysis, insanity, and death.

Penicillin was discovered to be effective against syphilis in the 1940s. It is still considered the treatment of choice.

Genital Herpes

Genital herpes, a viral infection, is another major contributor to human misery. It has no cure, thus, often brings feelings of shame, depression, regret, anxiety, and personal anguish, as well as physical pain. Once you have it, you have it for life. Symptoms usually occur within 2 to 30 days of having sex. Early signs include itching, tingling, or burning on the legs, buttocks or genitals. This is followed by small, painful genital sores or blisters that break open and crust over, causing intense itching and extreme pain. In addition, active herpes may be accompanied by fever, swollen glands, and general flulike feelings. Herpes virus is shed from the sores, which are highly contagious. After the blisters appear, they last from 1 to 3 weeks and then heal and disappear. The first episode is usually the most painful, and most people can expect to have four or five recurrences a year. Once established, the herpes virus migrates into nerve cells, where it may lie dormant or reactivate to cause recurring outbreaks of sores from time to time. New attacks of the disease appear at intervals, triggered by lowered resistance, fever, sunburn, or stress.

Genital herpes is caused by the **herpes simplex virus.** A virus invades body cells to live and reproduce. Nearly all herpes infections are caused by Herpes Simplex Type II, transmitted from one infected individual to another by direct contact including kissing, sexual contact (vaginal, oral, or anal sex), or skin-to-skin contact. This is different from the common Herpes Simplex Type I, which causes cold sores to appear on or around the mouth. However, it is possible to spread Type I to the genitals or Type II to the mouth by touching the sores and scratching or rubbing somewhere else. You can also become infected by both types of herpes at the same time. Consistent use of latex condoms is the best protection against infection. However, they *do not* provide complete protection because herpes is spread by skin-to-skin contact rather than blood or body fluids. A herpes lesion may not be covered by a condom. It is important to avoid letting the lesions contact someone else's body through touching, kissing, or sexual contact. Touching an eye after touching a sore can cause a severe eye infection called *ocular herpes*. Washing the hands thoroughly after touching a sore can prevent transmission of the virus.

At least two-thirds of the infected individuals are unaware that they have genital herpes—their symptoms are so mild that they go unnoticed. Because many unreported cases exist, experts estimate that the nationwide infected population may be as large as 30 million Americans. Infections are most common between the ages of 18 and 25 years. Risk factors for genital herpes include having more than one sexual partner, being sexually active for a number of years, exposure

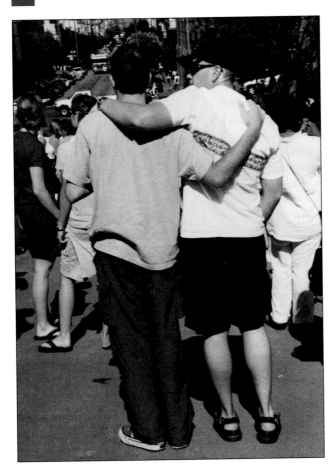

STD infection is related to behavior, not ethnic group or sexual orientation.

highest risk time is ages 16 to 28. The problem doesn't seem real on most college campuses because people silently infected with HIV are not likely to appear ill." Many students who carry HIV look fine and have no symptoms. They may not even know they are infected. However, during intercourse, they can spread the disease to others.

Among gay men, the group with the highest HIV infection rate, significant behavioral change is already dropping the rate of infection and diagnosis. There has been no behavioral change among the next two highest infected groups: IV drug users and their partners and young heterosexuals with multiple partners. Surveys of young people show that while most know how to prevent spread of HIV, over 50 percent report having sexual intercourse with more than one partner and sporadic or no use of condoms. HIV infections among young heterosexuals have increased dramatically in the past 5 years.[24] Most students know the facts about AIDS, but many do not use condoms or know their sexual partners. Why? Keeling states that there are six reasons:

1. *They feel invincible.* They think, "Things like that don't happen to people like me."

wellness flash

Women now account for over 40 percent of HIV-infected people over age 15. The highest rate of new infections is among young women.

2. *They lack social skills and have low self-esteem.* Many people don't feel comfortable with sexual feelings or behavior and don't feel comfortable talking about these matters or negotiating with a sexual partner to take precautions.
3. *They engage in unwanted sexual behavior.* They become involved in sex without really wanting to—due to peer pressure, role expectations, or alcohol. Alcohol is involved in a tremendous amount of risky sexual behavior on campus. Alcohol increases risk taking and decreases ambivalence and judgment. It is impossible for sex under the influence of alcohol to be safe in terms of prevention of STDs.
4. *They are victims of sexual assault.* Date rape is a common unreported campus problem. If there is no consent, no precautions can be taken.
5. *Society sends mixed messages.* Our society may say, "Just say no," but in advertising and media, it screams, "Just say yes. It will be OK. Just try it."
6. *They share needles.* On campus, this is less a problem of recreational drugs than of anabolic steroids. If needles are shared, it doesn't matter what's in them; they can still spread HIV.

It doesn't matter who you are. It is not who you are that causes AIDS, but what you do. If you do things that can spread HIV, consider the risks. The problem with HIV is that if you make a mistake in judgment, it's irreversible. When you risk AIDS and lose, you lose it all.

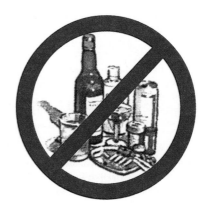

Is sex under the influence worth it?

How Can I Protect Myself from STDs?

While the facts about AIDS and other STDs are sobering, the good news is that you can reduce your risk of exposure to zero by personal choices. The best prevention for any STD is sexual abstinence or a mutually monogamous sexual relationship with an uninfected partner. There is no safe sex, only less risky sex. No orgasm is worth dying for. Unless you are willing to throw away your future, you must weigh the choices and consequences. If you are sexually active with more than one partner, there are steps that you can take to avoid becoming a victim of AIDS and other sexually transmitted diseases.

Abstinence

Sexual abstinence is a choice to refrain from sexual activity. The choice of abstinence is a personal decision based on what you feel is right for you. People do this for different reasons: religious, social, moral, health, or other reasons. Some of those reasons may be they:

- Do not feel ready for a sexual relationship
- Want time to develop friendship and trust in a relationship before having sex
- Feel that sex belongs only in marriage or a close, committed relationship
- Do not have the time or energy to put into a sexual relationship
- Do not have to deal with feelings of guilt, hurt, or confusion if the relationship ends
- Want to avoid the risk of pregnancy
- Want to avoid the risk of contracting a sexually transmitted disease
- Have a sexual health concern or infection that needs to be addressed

Abstinence can mean different things to different people. To some it means "Just say no" or "Wait until marriage" and these choices should be respected. To others it means waiting for the right person, place, and time to have sex. Discuss sexual values and beliefs with your partner before you find yourself in a sexual situation, especially in a new relation-

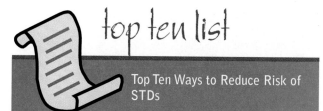

top ten list

Top Ten Ways to Reduce Risk of STDs

1. Abstain from sexual contact with others or have a mutually monogamous relationship with an uninfected sexual partner.
2. Communicate assertively about sexual feelings, activities, partners, and STDs.
3. Choose lower-risk sexual activities that have less likelihood of transmitting STDs.
4. Separate alcohol and drugs from sexual activity. Drunk sex can't be safe sex.
5. Protect yourself. Use latex condoms or dental dams and a spermicide.
6. Be selective. Limit the number of partners you have sex with. The fewer partners you have, the lower your risk.
7. Do not have sex with someone who has several sex partners or with prostitutes. Prostitutes may also use IV drugs, increasing their chances of exposure to HIV.
8. Do not use intravenous drugs. If you do, do not share drug needles and syringes. Don't have sex with people who shoot drugs.
9. Observe a partner discreetly for discharge, sores, or rash. While it may not seem romantic, if you see anything that concerns you, don't have sex!
10. If you are sexually active, have an STD checkup every time you have a health exam. This is especially important for women, who often have no signs of an STD. Have an STD checkup every 6 months if you have more than one partner.

In addition: Know the symptoms of STDs, and if you notice a symptom that concerns you, abstain from sex and see a physician. If you do acquire an infection, make sure that all partners are notified and treated. To prevent infecting others, don't have sex until you have completed treatment and your doctor says you are cured.

ship. Some questions that you might ask yourself to clarify your feelings and values include:

- Why am I choosing to be abstinent?
- What does abstinence mean to me? What are my "do's and don'ts"?
- Am I comfortable with my current level of involvement and intimacy with my partner?
- Do I feel pressured into a sexual relationship?

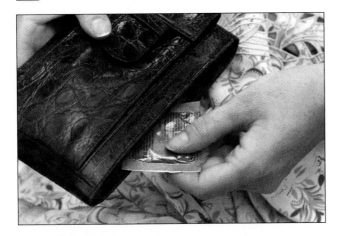

If you are sexually active, carry your own condoms, even if you don't plan to have sex."

table 14-6	Levels of Risk in Sexual Activities

No Risk
- Kissing with the mouth closed
- Hugging
- Touching
- Holding hands
- Massage
- Fantasy
- Masturbation

Low Risk
- Vaginal or oral sex using a condom and spermicide
- Masturbating a partner partner using a latex barrier

Risky
- Wet kissing with your mouth open
- Anal sex with or without a condom
- Vaginal or oral sex without a condom

- Do I feel physically and emotionally ready for a sexual relationship?
- Am I comfortable talking with my partner about sex? If not, am I ready to have sex?
- What do I want from this relationship? How will I feel if I have sex and the relationship ends?
- Are my partner and I ready and willing to use protective measures against STDs and unexpected pregnancy?

You can choose to be abstinent at any time, even if you have had sex in the past. The choice of abstinence may be for a short time or for years, but being abstinent doesn't mean that you give up being loving or sensual. There are many ways to physically express affection besides sexual intercourse (see "No Risk" activities in Table 14-6). Many people enjoy dating even more when they have agreed sexual intercourse is off limits. It gives partners a chance to develop creative ways to show love for each other; to focus more on feelings, shared interests, values, and goals and less on sex. Sex isn't an emergency. Abstinence is an important and personal choice and an excellent way to avoid exposure to sexually transmitted diseases.

Choosing Lower-Risk Sexual Activities

There are many ways to show someone you care besides having sex: respect, sharing, trust, commitment. Lasting relationships are built on alternative ways of expressing love and affection. Even if you have decided to have sex, there are lower-risk sex techniques you can use to protect yourself from STDs. Keep in mind that your skin is your largest sexual organ, and your imagination is your most important sexual asset. Consider these options in Table 14-6.

Planning Ahead for Safer Sex

When you are in the midst of a passionate embrace, it may not seem convenient to discuss safer sex or how to use a condom, and using condoms takes practice. Before beginning a sexual relationship, plan ahead. Think about what you'll say to your partner about using condoms. It may help to use a news story about AIDS to bring up the subject of safer sex. Make your feelings about condom use clear. Tell your partner you want to take precautions because you care about both of you. If your partner won't agree to use condoms, don't have sex. Preventing STDs impacts dimensions of wellness in many ways (Table 14-5).

How to Use Condoms

If abstinence or a mutually faithful, single-partner relationship is not your choice, the next best way to protect yourself from sexually transmitted diseases including AIDS is to use a latex condom during sex. While condoms are not 100 percent effective in preventing STDs, if used correctly, it is estimated that they can reduce risk by up to 98 percent. Condom breakage rates are low, around 2 in 100. Most condom failures are due to incorrect or inconsistent use. Unfortunately, few people know how to use condoms correctly, resulting in a failure rate of 40 percent or more. If you are a woman, carry condoms, even if you don't plan to have sex (few young adults who have sex plan it). Do not store condoms in a hot place such as a glove compartment or carry them in a wallet for more than 1 week (they need to be fresh). Use a condom every time, including for oral or anal sex. Avoid skin con-

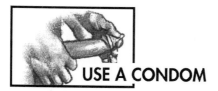

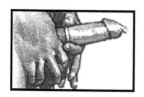

USE A CONDOM

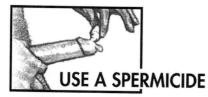

USE A SPERMICIDE

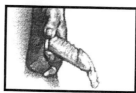

figure 14-3 How to use a condom.

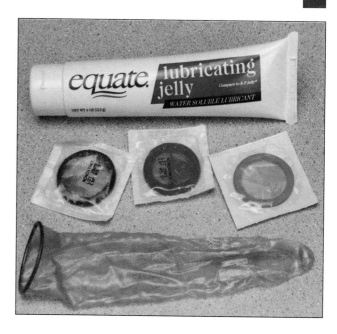

Condoms protect against pregnancy and STDs.

doms (lambskin)—they do not provide protection from all STDs, though they do prevent pregnancy.

To maximize condom effectiveness, follow these steps (Fig. 14-3):

1. Be careful when opening the package. Be especially careful not to tear the condom with a fingernail or teeth.
2. Put the condom on before penetration, even if ejaculation is not planned. Withdrawal is not effective in preventing STDs. Unroll the condom on the erect penis. Squeeze the air from the top of the condom, leaving about 1/2-inch space for semen at the tip. Hold the tip as you unroll the condom, making sure there is no air inside. If there is no space at the tip, the force of semen coming out of the penis can break the condom.
3. Apply a water-based lubricant or spermicide onto the tip of the condom. Do not use an oil-based lubricant. Vaseline or baby oil quickly deteriorate latex. A few people have allergic reactions to certain spermicides. Do not use a spermicide that causes a rash or irritation, as this could increase chance of infection.
4. Withdraw while the penis is still erect. Hold the rim of the condom to avoid spilling semen. Throw the used condom away. Do not reuse it.

If you or your partner don't like male condoms, you can try a female condom, which works like an extra-large male condom inserted into a woman's vagina. It consists of a 6 1/2-inch long plastic tube with a large ring on each end. One ring holds it in the vagina, and the other ring fits outside the vaginal lips. It is as effective in preventing conception and STDs as the male condom, and it gives a woman the ability to protect herself and her partner, however it is more expensive, is somewhat unwieldy, and has not proved popular.

Coping with Unwanted Sexual Pressure and Avoiding Sexual Assault

Carlos is invited to a party at an off-campus apartment by Maria, whom he met at a football game. He doesn't know anyone at the party but doesn't want to miss the fun. The music is lively and the drinks are free so he has a few drinks

wellness flash

Alcohol has been used by either the rapist or the victim in 90 percent of campus rapes.

and starts feeling relaxed. Maria shows up and invites him to go to her room so they can talk. He agrees. They take their drinks and head toward the bedroom.

Is a woman "asking for it" if she has been drinking? Is consent implied if Maria invites Carlos into her room? If she closes the bedroom door and sits on the bed? Unfortunately, the double standard is alive and well in the United States. Many people come to campus with little experience in sexual matters. What can a person do to prevent unwanted sexual behavior? Dr. Richard Keeling states, "We need to build skills in assertiveness, self-esteem, decision making, running a relationship, and dealing with intimacy. We need a personal commitment that says my life, my future, my potential are more valuable than what's going to happen in this relationship or on this date or in the next 10 minutes." What do you do when he or she wants to have sex and you don't?

An estimated 80 percent of rape victims are attacked by someone they know, either a date, a former partner, or a casual acquaintance. Many people with active social lives involve themselves in parties and activities with the expectation of meeting new friends and dating partners. There is a tendency to assume this is a safe way to meet people, but placing trust in someone you know only casually can put you in an unsafe situation, particularly if alcohol is involved. Some people have trouble understanding how a person can be raped by someone known. Date rape has been characterized as a four-stage process, and while these stages do not always occur, they show how sexual assault can happen even to someone who exercises caution:

1. *Intrusion.* The offender begins by violating the victim's space in one way or another. He (men can also be raped, but most rapes involve men assaulting women, so we'll use that scenario for our discussion) may start by interrupting while she is talking, talking about personal topics she feels uncomfortable with, or touching her unnecessarily or inappropriately.

2. *Desensitization.* The victim lets down her guard. While the intrusion makes her uncomfortable, she ignores the feelings and thinks, "That's just the way he is" or "He doesn't mean anything by it."

3. *Isolation.* The offender tries to get the victim alone, such as in a car or her home, where she might think she is safe, and uses tactics that put her at greater risk, such as encouraging her to drink alcohol.

4. *Offender denial.* The offender justifies his actions to himself and others by insisting that the victim gave consent and encouraged his behavior. This also increases the victim's feelings of confusion and guilt.

Here is how it might happen: Marcus and Kari were introduced by mutual friends. Marcus has invited Kari to go out to a movie with him. He seems to be a nice guy, so she accepts. They go to the movie and have a couple of beers afterward. Then Marcus takes Kari home. Parked by her home, Marcus engages Kari in a conversation that grows increas-

wellness flash

About 90 percent of campus rape victims know their attackers and 57 percent of them are attacked by dates.

ingly personal, and he begins making advances that make Kari uncomfortable (intrusion). Assuming that this is typical behavior for him (desensitization), she puts up with it for a while and gently tries to discourage him. She had intended to go to her apartment alone, but Marcus has a long drive home and he asks for a cup of coffee. This seems reasonable, so Kari accepts and Marcus accompanies her to her apartment (isolation). Her belief that she can control the situation and her desire to spare his feelings put her at risk. As soon as they are inside the door, Marcus pins her to the wall with a kiss and becomes increasingly aggressive. When she finally tells him to stop, he becomes verbally abusive, calling her a "tease" and a "bitch." Then he forces himself on her. Afterward, he asks her why she invited him to her apartment if she didn't want sex and he insists that it was consensual sex (offender denial).

Unfortunately, these scenes too common, and the victim is left feeling somehow responsible for the rape and wondering what she did to cause it or why she didn't head it off. Men can be raped too—about 10 percent of reported rapes are of men. Many go unreported because of homophobia (in men-on-men rape) and the myth that rape is a crime of desire rather than of violence.

If you are sexually assaulted, follow these steps:

- Once out of immediate danger, call the police.
- Do not change clothes, shower, urinate, defecate, gargle, take medication, drink alcohol, or do anything else that might destroy evidence.
- Go with a trusted friend to a hospital emergency room, where a doctor will ask for information about the assault, conduct a rape exam, and collect physical evidence to be used in court.

If a friend of yours is a victim of date rape, remember the following:

- Rape is not a result of uncontrolled passion. It is a violent assault using sex as a weapon.
- No one wants to be forced to have sex. No matter what happened, no one wants to be a victim of a crime. A person has handled the situation right if he or she is alive.
- You can't control what others think or say about it. Do not isolate yourself or the victim from friends who know about the rape. Neither you nor the victim have any reason to feel shame,

embarrassment, or guilt. Your understanding and support are important.

- If the assault is reported to the police, the victim is not responsible for what happens to the rapist, regardless of what pressure is brought by family or friends of the assailant. The courts are responsible for the outcome and the rapist is responsible for the rape.

To avoid coercive sexual pressure or sexual assault, you must break the chain of circumstances that lead to these outcomes. Here are some tips from the Santa Monica Rape Treatment Center.

Women and Men

- *Attend parties with friends you can trust.* Look out for each other. Leave together, rather than alone or with a new acquaintance. If you are attracted to someone you'd like to get to know better, agree to meet for lunch the next day.
- *Be selective.* Even if a person you just met seems nice, find out about him or her from friends and family.
- *Avoid isolation.* Don't go to a secluded place or to a wild party with a new acquaintance. Go to concerts, movies, lectures, or restaurants; double date; and stay around people. When you get to know the person well, then you can relax the rules.
- *Communicate.* Don't lead someone on. Don't expect a person to know how you feel unless you speak up. Make your feelings, limits, and intentions clear. You have a right to say no to any unwanted sexual contact. If you are being pressured and feel uncertain, ask the person to respect your feelings.
- *Listen closely to what a person is saying.* If you think she or he is giving you a mixed message, ask for clarification. On a date when neither person stops to check out what the other person is feeling, the situation can get out of hand.
- *Make sure how you say something agrees with what you say.* Your body language may come across louder than your words. If you say no with downcast eyes and a smile to soften the refusal, you may end up giving the other person a mixed message. You are more likely to

get your message across if you look a person directly in the eyes and say no assertively.
- *Be aware.* Pay attention to what is happening. Rely on your gut instinct. If a situation doesn't feel right, exit as quickly as you can and go to a safe place.
- *Speak up if you believe someone is at risk.* If you see a friend in trouble at a party or if someone is using force and pressuring a friend, don't be afraid to intervene. You may save your friend from the trauma of sexual assault and that person from criminal prosecution.
- *Stay sober.* You'll be more likely to make wise decisions if you are sober.

Men

- *Don't fall for the stereotype* that when a woman says no she means yes. If she says no to sexual contact, believe her and stop.
- *Don't make assumptions about a person's behavior.* Just because a person drinks heavily, dresses provocatively, or goes with you to your room, don't assume she wants sex. Just because she had sex with you once, don't assume she is willing now. Also, don't assume that because she willingly engages in kissing or other intimate behavior that she wants sexual intercourse.
- *Don't assume that silence is consent.* Having sex with someone who is intoxicated, passed out, drugged, or otherwise incapable of giving consent is rape.

Both men and women must be especially careful in situations involving drinking or drugs. These decrease reasoning ability and your ability to make a decision and to communicate effectively. They increase willingness to take risks you wouldn't normally take. Alcohol, a social lubricant par excellence, sets you up for unwanted sexual behavior and STDs. It is involved in approximately half of the incidents of coercive sexual behavior. It decreases the ability to recognize an unsafe situation and to react appropriately. It also decreases the likelihood that you will use a condom. Even if you have one, you may be too drunk to put it on.

 frequently asked questions

Q. Can I get genital herpes from a person who had it once but who hasn't had an outbreak in over a year?

A. Yes. Between outbreaks, the herpes virus is still in the body. Active virus can be shed at any time, even if there are no symptoms, so it is important to use latex condoms to reduce risk of spreading the virus. Because herpes is a lifelong infection, it can still be transmitted even after years of monogamy.

Q. My partner had genital warts but they were removed. Is he cured? Can he still infect me?

A. Genital warts are caused by a human papilloma virus. While the external warts can be treated and removed, the virus can still be present and cause recurrence. There is no cure for HPV infection, so it is important to use condoms during any sexual activity to prevent becoming infected.

Q. I once had pelvic inflammatory disease. I was treated for chlamydia and cured. How does PID affect a person's chances to have children?

A. The risks of pelvic inflammatory disease include scarring, constriction, and blockage of the fallopian tubes. Complete blockage results in sterility. Partial blockage increases risk of an ectopic (tubal) pregnancy. This occurs when a fertilized egg implants in an area other than the uterus, such as a fallopian tube. This is a serious complication that can rupture a fallopian tube, causing internal bleeding, even death. However, PID affects people differently, so it is important to consult your physician.

Q. Where can a person go to be tested for HIV?

A. Confidential testing is available at several places. Check with your family doctor, the university health center, your local public health agency, or call the AIDS hotline listed at the end of this chapter under "additional information resources."

summary

Sexually transmitted diseases reached epidemic levels in the 1990s. Young adults are at greatest risk. Chlamydia, gonorrhea, syphilis, genital herpes, and human papilloma virus are the most common STDs. AIDS, a deadly STD, makes preventative measures more important than ever for those who are sexually active. To reduce risk of STDs, people must take responsibility for their sexual behavior and take protective measures, for themselves and their partners. It is also important to learn skills in communication, assertiveness, negotiation, and relating to others. Awareness of the risk of sexual assault and guidelines for recognizing and preventing it can make dating relationships safer for all.

additional information resources

AIDS Task Force for the American College Health Association, c/o Dr. Richard P. Keeling, Dept. of Student Health, Box 378, University of Virginia, Charlottesville, VA 22908, (804) 924-2670.

CDC AIDS Hotline (U.S. Public Health Service), English, 24 hours daily, (800) 342-AIDS; Spanish, 8 A.M. to 2 A.M. daily, (800) 344-SIDA; deaf and hearing impaired, Mon.-Fri., 10 A.M. to 10 P.M., (800) AIDS-TTY.

CDC National AIDS Information Clearinghouse, (800) 458-5231.

CDC National STD Hotline, (800) 227-8922.

ETR Associates, pamphlets on STDs, (800) 321-4407.

National Gay Task Force AIDS Crisis Line, (800) 227-8922.

National Herpes Hotline, (919) 361-8488.

National Herpes Resource Center, Mon.-Fri., 9 A.M. to 7 P.M., (800) 230-6309.

Teens Teaching AIDS Prevention, (800) 234-TEEN.

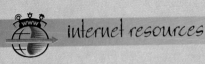

internet resources

onhealth.com
goaskalice.com
cdc.gov
go.drkoop.com

lab activity
14–1

Values Clarification Statements

Complete or respond to the following statements. They may be used for class discussion.

1. AIDS is _____

2. STDs are _____

3. If I found out I had an STD, I would _____

4. If I found out my partner had an STD, I would _____

5. Five ways to show someone you care about them without having sex are

_____

_____

_____

_____

_____

6. Money for AIDS research should be cut because people get AIDS due to immoral lifestyles. Agree or disagree? Explain. _____

_____

_____

_____

_____

7. HIV infection is not a significant risk for college students. Agree or disagree? Explain. _____

_____

_____

_____

_____

8. My peers are changing their sexual behavior because of AIDS. Agree or disagree? Explain. _____

_____

_____

_____

_____

9. Condoms are not used much to prevent STDs on this campus. Agree or disagree? Explain. _____

_____

_____

_____

10. Because of the AIDs crisis, it is easier to talk to my peers about sex. Agree or disagree? Explain. _____

_____

_____

_____

11. Both men and women should share responsibility for safer sex. Agree or disagree? Explain. _____

_____

_____

_____

12. "Just Say No" is the right message to give young people about how to prevent STDs. Agree or disagree? Explain.

_____

_____

_____

_____

13. Schools should distribute condoms to students. Agree or disagree? Explain. _____

_____

_____

_____

14. Sexual intercourse improves a relationship. Agree or disagree? Explain. _____

_____

_____

_____

15. Condom ads should be allowed on television. Agree or disagree? Explain. _____

_____

_____

_____

16. The media responsibly portray sex. Agree or disagree? Explain. _____

_____

_____

Self-Test on STD Prevention

Answer true or false to the following questions. Correct answers follow and are explained in the chapter.

1. STDs are most common in people over 30   T   F
2. Some STDs are antibiotic resistant, making cure difficult   T   F
3. Both lambskin and latex condoms are effective against HIV   T   F
4. Sexual abstinence is the most effective prevention for STDs   T   F
5. Oral sex cannot transmit STDs   T   F
6. Herpes is spread by skin-to-skin contact   T   F
7. Genital herpes and genital warts are curable   T   F
8. Vaseline or oil are good lubricants with latex condoms   T   F
9. Giving blood puts you at risk for AIDS   T   F
10. Burning during urination is a symptom of gonorrhea   T   F
11. Chlamydia causes small painful genital blisters   T   F
12. Having other STDs increases the risk of acquiring HIV   T   F
13. A person may have HIV 10 years before it progresses to AIDS   T   F
14. HIV is more infectious than other STDs such as hepatitis B   T   F
15. Open-mouth, French kissing cannot spread STDs   T   F
16. A person may be infected with HIV and not appear ill   T   F
17. STDs in women may be associated with cervical cancer   T   F
18. Often, STDs cause no symptoms, particularly in women   T   F
19. Untreated STDs may cause infertility   T   F
20. Syphilis and chlamydia are curable STDs   T   F

Answers: 1—F, 2—T, 3—F, 4—T, 5—F, 6—T, 7—F, 8—F, 9—F, 10—T, 11—F, 12—T, 13—T, 14—T, 15—F, 16—T, 17—T, 18—T, 19—T, 20—T

Scoring:

18 - 20 Excellent

16 - 17 Good

14 - 15 Average

< 13 Reread the chapter

Results:

1. My score was _____, which is _____.

2. Were you surprised? Why or why not?

Using HealthQuest

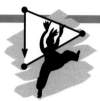

1. Insert the HealthQuest CD into your computer

2. Click on "Communicable Diseases" from the menu. Click on "Introduction" and read.

3. Click on "Introduction" again and go to "Wellness Activities." Click on the "STDs: Are You at Risk?" activity. Read the introduction, then click on "Assess Yourself." This activity enables you to assess your STD risk related to your sexual behaviors. After you complete the series of questions, HealthQuest will give feedback on your risk level and how you can reduce your risk in the future.

4. What is your risk of acquiring an STD?

5. What are three specific actions that you can take to decrease your STD risk in the future?
   a.

   b.

   c.

6. What are three specific STD protective behaviors that you currently practice?
   a.

   b.

   c.

lab activity @ chapter fourteen

7. Close this out (bottom left corner) and click on "Wellness Activities" again, then on "Topics."

8. Click on either: "Specifics On," "Our Changing World," or "Key Articles." Peruse the topics under these three categories. Select three topics and read the information. Summarize what you learned.

a. Topic = _____

b. Topic = _____

c. Topic = _____

15

Planning Wellness for a Lifetime

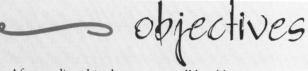 objectives

After reading this chapter, you will be able to:

1. Define *quackery* and list six of its nine common characteristics.
2. Identify the four premises on which corporate wellness programs are based, and give examples of wellness programs that corporations might offer their employees.
3. Describe three ways parents can foster wellness habits in their children, and give two examples of behaviors within each dimension of wellness that parents can develop in a young child.
4. List five guidelines for wearing a seat belt properly.
5. List two responsible precautions that you can take to minimize your risk of injury/trouble in each of the following situations:
   a. Walking alone on campus at night
   b. Apartment or home fire
   c. In the home
   d. In a hotel
   e. On an airplane
6. Describe seven responsible precautions you can take to minimize your risk of being attacked, assaulted, or robbed.
7. Identify three trends and describe how they will affect wellness in the future.
8. Identify and describe three future challenges we face about wellness.
9. List six environmental concerns that may affect our wellness.

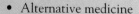 terms

- Alternative medicine
- Altruism
- Complementary medicine
- Psychoneuroimmunology (PNI)
- Quackery

The purpose of this book is to present wellness as a lifestyle where positive choices result in optimal functioning and enhanced living. You have gained knowledge that will help you make informed decisions and you have learned skills for making behavioral change. You are now "wellness educated." With knowledge comes responsibility, so you no longer have the luxury of saying, "I didn't know!" You know what choices contribute to wellness and which ones do not. You can choose to eat right, exercise, and manage stress or you can choose not to. You know the possible consequences of such choices. The challenge of wellness is ongoing, whereas college coursework eventually comes to an end. A new career, different living environments, and family responsibilities will bring many changes to your life. During these changes, the wellness lifestyle can prevail. We hope it will grow for you. Wellness is a process, not a solution. It is a journey, not a destination. A major part of wellness is adapting to change and maximizing your potential amidst change.

Remember that wellness involves a balance among and integration of all seven dimensions of wellness. Too often, *physical fitness* is thought of synonymously with *wellness*. Admittedly, being physically fit has a positive effect on the other dimensions. However, your job satisfaction, family relationships, social ties, emotional health, and spiritual health are equally linked to wellness. This final chapter focuses on some important issues for you to consider as you plan for the future.

Taking Charge

Following a great musician's performance, an admirer said to him, "I'd give my life to play like that." The brilliant performer hesitated for a moment and then replied, "I did." We often view a performance of an athlete or artist with envy. Accomplishment is often deceptive, because we don't see the perseverance that produces it. Pursuing wellness also involves a certain amount of perseverance and discipline. Many desire the benefits of wellness living but fail to commit to its precepts. As you take charge of your lifestyle, focus on the positive outcomes of changing a health-robbing behavior, rather than the effort involved. Remember, you do not pay the price for having wellness; you pay the price for *not* having it.

Knowledge and good intentions are a good start. Then focus on self-management techniques and behavior-changing skills (Chapter 2) that put your knowledge into practice through maintainable habits. Many people muddle through life making compromises or excuses, and passing up opportunities for self-improvement. Be aware of the power of cultural norms, the media, advertising, and sources of social support. Become a leader and example of wellness to those around you.

Partners in Prevention

The *Healthy People 2010* document sets high goals for the health and well-being of the American people. It emphasizes personal responsibility and self-empowerment as the means for increasing the quality and quantity of life. Some people need to know the facts to make informed decisions. Others need positive influences to motivate them toward appropriate choices. For the wellness lifestyle to permeate our culture, support systems within communities must be available. While emphasizing personal responsibility, we cannot overlook the importance of the collective burden of responsibility of governmental policies, wellness curriculum in the schools, corporate action, and the American family. Although personal behaviors contribute to the leading causes of death, behaviors occur in and are influenced by the environment. Advertisements, television programs, and popular songs that glamorize drinking, violence, sex, and immoral behavior undermine our nation's health and well-being. For example, cigarette ads show likable young people in upscale settings enjoying smoking. The subliminal message is that cigarettes must not be so bad if such bright, attractive people are not afraid to smoke. In these ads, though, there are never dirty ashtrays, nicotine-stained teeth, or anyone coughing or getting chemotherapy. There is no dangerously underweight baby lying in intensive care. There is no one dying. An important part of wellness education is deciphering these messages and knowing what promotes well-being.

Individuals, families, communities, corporations, and the government share the task of enhancing the well-being of Americans. You are wellness educated, so part of this challenge of culture change rests with you. How will you affect this change?

Understanding Quackery

The concept of wellness has widespread appeal. Most everyone is attracted to the thought of enhancing the quality of their lives. The expanse of the wellness concept invites a considerable amount of quackery and shortcut schemes. **Quackery** is the promotion of a misleading and fraudulent health claim that is unproven. Most quackery products are foods, drugs, gadgets, or cosmetics that promote physical change—baldness cures, bust enhancers, wrinkle removers, miracle cancer treatments, instant weight loss schemes, bogus AIDS cures, youth elixirs, arthritis cures. These products and schemes are usually developed for the purpose of financial gain. Health fraud is big business in the United States. It is estimated that Americans spend $27 billion per year on quack products or treatments.

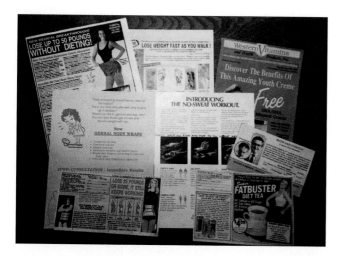

Are you able to recognize quackery?

table 15-1   How to Recognize Quackery

Some products use scientific jargon and carry professional-looking logos and endorsements (many are bogus).

Watch for the following characteristics common in quackery:

1. It sounds too good to be true.
2. It is quick and painless.
3. It has a "secret," "special," "foreign," "magical," "exclusive," or "ancient" formula.
4. It is available only through the mail (most often through a P.O. box number) or telephone and only from one supplier.
5. It is a scientific "breakthrough" or "miracle cure" that has been overlooked by the medical community.
6. It uses testimonials or case histories from "satisfied customers" as the only proof of its effectiveness.
7. It is a single product effective for a wide variety of ailments.
8. It uses pseudoscientific languages: "detoxifies," "revitalizes immunities," "offers enzymatic protection," and so on.
9. It displays degrees, credentials, or titles from unaccredited or unknown schools.

Many people erroneously believe that product advertisements are screened by government agencies and that claims on television or in print must be true. This is not so. It is hard to resist the "promise" of effortless, quick shortcuts to health and wellness. Many promoters are wealthy as a result of our willingness to spend money for miracle solutions. Unfortunately, the results are often shattered hopes and wasted money and sometimes endangered health. Misconceptions and half-truths fuel these promotional fires. As an educated wellness consumer, you should be able to evaluate products and plans with intelligence and realism. See Table 15-1 for common characteristics of quackery.

Remember, if it sounds too good to be true, it probably is. Sometimes, television personalities or well-known celebrities write books, represent products in advertisements, or are portrayed as experts in the field of health and fitness. Be wary of the credibility of this type of product/information marketing.

Many hospitals, schools, corporations, community wellness centers, and health organizations offer legitimate programs that can assist you in pursuing a wellness lifestyle. Investigate references and sources before falling for any fly-by-night scheme. Your physician, the Better Business Bureau, local consumer office, or nearest office of the Food and Drug Administration (FDA) can offer professional advice if you suspect a product makes untrue claims.

psychological well-being, career planning, spiritual discovery, health-risk assessment, and lifetime fitness. It is not uncommon for colleges to offer programs for stress management, alcohol education, weight management, smoking cessation, eating disorders, and investment counseling. Some universities have wellness residence halls, nutrition-controlled food services, academic wellness courses, and fitness standards for students. Day-care services, family counseling, and flexible class scheduling are common on campuses because many students have child-care responsibilities and other jobs. Attending college is a part-time pursuit for many full-time parents and workers. The college campus is no longer viewed as an isolated haven for learning, void of the challenges and realities of life. In response to the diverse needs of students, faculty, and staff, the college environment can enhance your pursuit of wellness with wellness services, information, and programs. Investigate your campus for wellness resources. The variety of expertise and resources found at most universities can prepare you not only for a lifetime career but also for lifetime wellness. Attending a wellness-oriented university is an example of how choosing a supportive environment can enhance your quest for wellness.

Campus Wellness

Many colleges and universities have voiced a commitment to wellness and, as a result, offer a variety of wellness programs to students. Many programs are also available to faculty and staff. Realizing that the collegiate experience involves more than intellectual growth, universities are providing services and activities to promote self-discovery,

Career Wellness

Your job will be a prominent facet of your adult life. You will spend at least 50 percent of your waking hours at work, if you maintain a full-time job or career. Cellular/digital phones, computers, e-mail, and fax machines have altered the complexion of American work. Twenty-four hour manufacturing and retail shopping, the Internet, home-based businesses, voice mail, and telemarketing have revolutionized the business place. Even with enhanced technology and conveniences, the working hours of most Americans are longer than they were 50 years ago. These realities make the workplace a likely place to receive information and support regarding personal health improvement and wellness living. Leaders in business and industry are beginning to see employee wellness as an asset to be maintained and enhanced. When employees are happy and healthy, productivity increases. The promotion of wellness programs in business and industry is based on four related premises:

1. Prevention is preferable to curing.
2. Teaching people to stay healthy is generally less expensive than treating them when they are ill.
3. Healthful lifestyles offer a better quality of life, higher morale, increased productivity, and possibly increased longevity.
4. Health promotion programs promote a favorable corporate image and help attract healthy, capable employees who see these programs as a valuable employee benefit.

Rising medical insurance costs, employee absenteeism, and sick leaves cut deeply into profits and lead to increases in the costs of doing business. On average, U.S. Fortune 500 corporations spend 61.2 percent of after-tax profits on medical care for employees, dependents, and retirees. As a result, corporate officials are experimenting with ways of incorporating wellness into the workplace. This exciting avenue for health promotion can bring about changes in behavior for an improved lifestyle and enhance personal relationships. Wellness in the workplace can be promoted in a variety of ways. Programs can involve:

- Diagnosis (assessment of current health and habits)
- Education (give information about health enhancement)
- Behavior Modification (give help and support in making a specific behavior change)

Regardless of how they are organized, most corporate health promotion programs aim to facilitate behavior change. These programs include, among others, smoking cessation, health risk appraisals, back care, stress management, fitness classes, nutrition education, weight management, and cholesterol screening.

Employers realize that the work and nonwork parts of our lives are interactive. That is, job satisfaction is also dependent on family happiness, leisure pursuits, and feelings of worth. Knowing this, employers are actively pursuing a multidimensional approach to supporting employee wellness. Examples are flexible work hours, child care, on-the-job retraining, sports team participation, job sharing, smoke-free work sites, parental leaves, family hikes and picnics, and children's fitness classes. Several forward-thinking companies are responding to the needs of employees with elderly

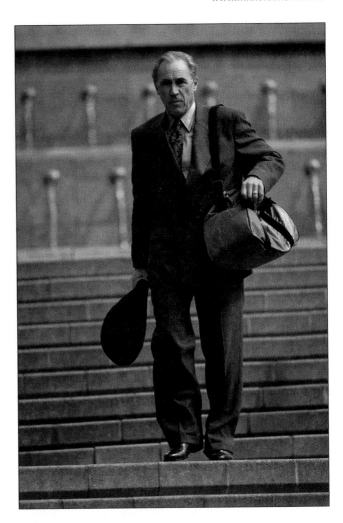

Many companies support employee wellness.

parents by providing elder care, as well as providing substance abuse and marital counseling. Spouses and children of employees account for 40 to 60 percent of a company's health-care expenditures, so such multidimensional programs can be cost-effective.

Due to the growing interest in and emphasis on wellness in business and industry, many employers prefer hiring personnel who have already adopted a wellness lifestyle—not smoking, being physically fit, maintaining a reasonable weight. This knowledge is added incentive for you to continue a wellness lifestyle. As a potential employee, your confirmed dedication to wellness may also influence your final selection of a job and your chances of getting hired. You may favor a company that is highly supportive of wellness and provides wellness programs for employees and that company may favor you. Remember how important a supportive environment is in the maintenance of positive lifestyle choices.

Many college students, pressured by school demands, feel they will have more time to exercise and eat right once they graduate. Your life will most likely be as busy, if not more so, once you begin your career. Time restraints and demands will always be with you. Making wellness living an important part of your current lifestyle will help you to maintain it after graduation, as a habit.

Family Wellness

In all cultures, the family unit is the primary transmitter of values and attitudes in the society. Each partner in a relationship comes with values, norms, and expectations derived from his or her family. Couples continue to grow, interact, and develop a value framework. If and when children come along, the parental role of maintaining the culture from generation to generation is created. The interacting dynamics of a family unit promote the spiritual, physical, psychological, and social growth of each member.

The family units in today's society are not identical. Single parents, divorce, combined families, and joint custodies are realities that have changed the American family structure. Dual careers have altered the role of women within the family. Such changes affect the balance between work life and family life, often creating role conflicts, stress, and changing values. Regardless of the makeup of the family unit, nurturance remains essential for all members to strive toward full potential.

The Well Relationship

Many romantic fairy tales conclude with "... and they lived happily ever after." Whereas these words *end* the story, marriage is most often the *beginning* of the story of a relationship in real life. Whom you marry or choose to spend your life with is one of your most important life decisions. Much of your happiness and life satisfaction will be based on the success of this relationship. Like the wellness lifestyle, a relationship demands conscious effort, commitment, and sacrifice. It is a partnership that involves change and growth. Many factors influence the success of a marriage relationship. Look at the top ten list of key elements that help build a strong and lasting relationship.

As in wellness growth, partner growth is a process. It doesn't happen all at once. Enjoy each step along the path.

The Well Child

It will be your challenge as a parent to initiate wellness living within your child. All dimensions (emotional, social, physical, intellectual, spiritual, environmental, and occupational) demand your attention. If you favor behaviors that promote wellness, your children will follow your example. Family wellness patterns can set the stage for a lifelong pattern of self-responsibility. Self-responsibility relies on learning and practicing skills, therefore you can be the master

top ten list

Top Ten Elements for Building a Strong and Lasting Relationship

1. *Communication:* Partners must be able to share their true feelings.
2. *Compromise:* Each partner must be willing to give a little. Sometimes it's 50:50, sometimes 100:0.
3. *Common values:* Common values and shared goals help maintain focus during tension-filled times.
4. *Likability and respect:* Enjoying each other's company and respecting each other's needs is essential.
5. *Shared responsibilities:* In a world where the two-parent career is the norm, each partner must be willing to share in the responsibilities of home and child care.
6. *Finances:* Having a common financial philosophy or strategy in handling money can prevent many emotional confrontations.
7. *Trust:* Partners need to feel secure in their commitment and devotion to one another—without deception, secrets, or lies.
8. *Space:* Each partner needs to have his or her identity and be allowed to grow individually.
9. *Sense of humor:* Laughing and having fun are ways to keep daily problems in proper perspective.
10. *Love:* Unselfish love and devotion to each other will stand the test of time!

teacher of wellness and help your child grow as a decision maker. Children do not learn just in school. They learn by watching you, too. If you exercise, eat nutritiously, read instead of watch television, handle stress, communicate your feelings, and display attitudes of cooperation and respect, your child will, too. Studies show that the strongest predictors of lifetime exercise activity in children are enjoyment of physical activity, family support of physical activity, and direct parental modeling of physical activity.

Nearly half of youths ages 10 to 18 do not engage in enough physical activity to derive any aerobic or endurance benefit. Forty percent of children ages 5 to 8 have at least one major heart disease risk factor. Obesity in children and teens is rising rapidly. Children with unhealthy habits have a greater likelihood of growing up to be unhealthy adults, so part of every parent's responsibility should be to create an environment for children that is conducive to optimum health and wellness. This includes being a positive role model. Aristotle expressed it best when he wrote, "good habits formed at youth make all the difference."

The self-concept of most children is formed by the time they start kindergarten, therefore you as parents will be

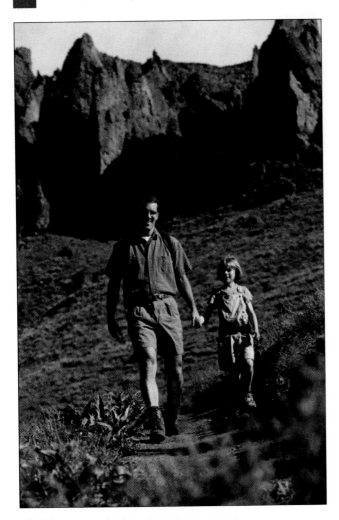

Parents are important role models for wellness.

table 15-2 — Wellness Behaviors That Can Be Developed by the Young Child

Physical Dimension
- Forms habits of regular, vigorous exercise
- Establishes healthy eating habits and preferences
- Forms self-care habits (seat belts, fire, bike riding, etc.)
- Establishes attitudes about smoking, drug use, alcohol

Social Dimension
- Seeks companionship with others
- Senses responsibility for behavior
- Shows concern and respect for others
- Displays willingness to share work responsibilities with others

Emotional Dimension
- Forms feelings of self-worth and self-confidence
- Talks freely about feelings
- Develops appropriate coping behaviors for a variety of situations
- Displays the capacity to give and receive love

Spiritual Dimension
- Develops an awareness of life vs. death
- Develops a sense of the importance and expanse of life
- Begins establishing a value system; can distinguish right from wrong
- Begins showing compassion and forgiveness

Intellectual Dimension
- Develops creativity and curiosity
- Establishes listening skills
- Learns cause-and-effect concepts
- Recognizes the expanse of the world through a variety of experiences

Occupational Dimension
- Identifies a variety of jobs/careers
- Understands the importance of work and effort
- Begins developing work habits
- Begins understanding the importance of money

Environmental Dimension
- Develops habits of recycling bottles, papers, cans, and so on
- Displays habits of energy conservation (water, electricity, etc.)
- Develops an appreciation for nature (plants, wildlife, etc.)
- Learns to maintain a clean environment by not littering

prime molders of this self-concept. A positive self-esteem is an important foundation as the child moves into larger social spheres beyond the family. The child with a high degree of self-worth is able to confront life's situations with confidence and optimism. Optimism and self-confidence are the building blocks for wellness living.

Although it is popularly believed that risk-taking behavior among teenagers and preteens is most strongly influenced by peer pressure, research by adolescent medicine specialists concludes that family closeness plays a key role. Young people who have a balance of strong attachment to family and parental encouragement to be independent are least likely to take part in high-risk activities (alcohol and drug use, sexual activities, cigarette experimentation) that could seriously affect their well-being.

Although the broad concept of wellness is difficult for young children to understand, they can become aware and learn the value of specific wellness choices. Their capacity to understand the cause and effect of certain choices depends on their age and maturity level. Can children learn to habitually fasten their seat belts? Select fruits for snacks? Show respect for others? Appreciate nature? Enjoy vigorous exercise? Of course, they can. Look at Table 15-2 for examples of wellness behaviors that parents are instrumental in developing in their children.

Personal Safety Issues

Throughout this book we have tried to increase your awareness of risks and personal choices that affect your wellness. Injuries and illnesses stemming from accidents and environ-

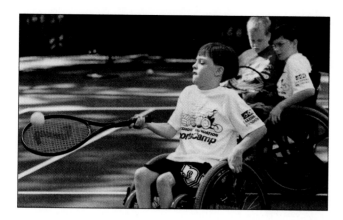

Every child deserves an opportunity to grow in all dimensions of wellness. (Photo courtesy of The Lakeshore Foundation, Birmingham, AL.)

table 15-3	Why I Don't Buckle Up

1. *"Seat belts are uncomfortable."* Unlike the original floor-anchored belts, new belts are designed to let you move freely until a collision occurs. And, they are a lot more comfortable than a body cast or traction!
2. *"I'm only going to the store down the street."* Seventy percent of crashes occur within 25 miles of home, and 80 percent occur at speeds less than 40 mph. People not wearing seat belts have been killed at speeds less than 12 mph!
3. *"The belt will prevent me from being thrown clear of the accident."* Exactly! Your chances of being killed are 25 times greater if you're thrown out of the car.
4. *"The seat belt will trap me in a burning or submerged car."* Only one-half of 1 percent of crashes result in fire or submergence. Unfortunately, television action shows capitalize on such scenes. If you find yourself in this terrifying predicament, wouldn't it be better to have been restrained and thus be conscious enough to get out of the vehicle, rather than to have had your head smashed into the windshield, leaving you unconscious and incapable of escaping?

mental hazards sometimes seem to be beyond the average person's control. Especially accidents—which are the fifth overall cause of death in the United States (and the number one cause of death among teens and young adults)—often appear to be a matter of chance. You can substantially reduce the risks you are exposed to while driving, traveling, getting around campus, and working around your apartment or house by heeding basic safety precautions. Some of these precautions seem like common sense. Yet, for whatever reason, many people fail to follow even common sense precautions. Federal, state, and local regulations have been established to help protect us from a variety of traffic, fire, water, and air travel tragedies. But laws and regulations cannot *make* people act. When you strive for high-level wellness, you must take seriously *all* lifestyle choices. The wellness concept is centered on an ongoing personal commitment to positive choices, so safety awareness and responsibility cannot be excluded.

We tend to focus solely on the impact an accident has on our physical dimension of wellness. The truth is, such a trauma can equally affect our emotional, social, occupational, and even spiritual dimensions. The following personal safety issues will focus on choices that can help you control risks in your immediate environment.

Automobile Seat Belts

Motor vehicle crashes are the leading cause of death among people age 40 and younger. In talking about motor vehicle collisions, we deliberately chose not to use the word *accident*, which would imply a luck/fate approach to the topic. Instead, we use *crash* because it is well understood what specific actions you can take to reduce risks. Drunk-driving laws, child car-restraint regulations, seat belt laws, availability of air bags, and designated driver programs have done much to curtail traffic fatalities. Still, approximately 48,000 Americans die annually in car crashes, costing the nation $40 bil-

lion per year. Of these casualties, half of the people could have been saved if they had used their seat belts *and* half of the serious injuries incurred in collisions could have been prevented by the use of seat belts. Although drivers initially resisted seat belt use, compliance is growing. The National Transportation Department in Washington, D.C., reports that 67 percent of Americans buckle up (the highest rate ever), and that this growing habit has saved 55,600 lives over the last ten years. The importance of using seat belts cannot be overstated. Even if you practice all the other advice in this book (exercise regularly, eat a nutritious diet, don't smoke, etc.), *one* accident without a seat belt could immediately and irrevocably end your wellness program. It does not make sense, if we care about health and wellness, to not buckle up. Table 15-3 lists the most common excuses people give for choosing not to use their seat belts. We hope you do not use the same flimsy excuses.

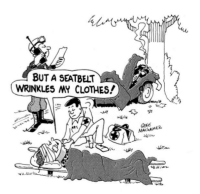

What is your excuse for not wearing a seat belt?

To prevent injury, seat belts must not only be worn but must be worn properly every time. You are most likely to survive an automobile crash without injury if you follow these recommendations:

1. *Wear the seat belt low across the pelvis*, not the abdomen. In a crash, a force of 20 to 50 times your body weight is exerted against the belt. The bony pelvis can withstand this load, whereas internal organs would be injured if the belt were higher, across the abdomen.
2. *Keep the belt snug.* A loose belt offers little protection and may compound injuries if you are thrown against it. You can also slide forward under a loose belt and suffer head or neck injuries from the shoulder strap.
3. *Never wear the shoulder strap under your arm or behind your back.* When properly worn, this strap rests on the middle of the collarbone and the upper chest.
4. *Never share a belt.* In a crash, a parent sharing a belt with a child can crush the child. Each passenger must have his or her own belt. Also, it is impossible to hold a child in your arms in the event of a collision. In a crash, a 20-pound baby is propelled forward with the force of 400 pounds.
5. *If you are pregnant, wear the seat belt under the abdomen*—across the upper thighs and as low on the hips as possible. The shoulder strap should go across your shoulder and chest. The fetus is at *much greater* risk when the mother does not wear a seat belt. The leading cause of fetal death in a crash is death of the mother.

Most newer automobile models include two front seat inflatable airbags as standard equipment and some have optional side airbags. These bags will be valuable in preventing thousands of deaths and injuries. Your seat belt, however, is still your first line of defense in all crashes. Air bags inflate with great speed and force. Therefore, infants and young children should ride in the *back* seat of a car—in proper safety seats or restraints. Children and even small, frail adults riding in the passenger side have suffered injuries as a result of air bag deployment. Remember, an air bag can never substitute for a seat belt or for defensive driving.

Driving Safety

Driving is, on average, approximately 10 times more dangerous than traveling by airplane or train. However, if you are a low-risk driver, you are far less likely to die in a car crash than a high-risk driver is. Statistics define a low-risk driver to be a 40-year-old who is sober when driving and who wears a seat belt; a high-risk driver is an 18-year-old, intoxicated male traveling in a lightweight car without wearing a seat belt. The best driver is also a defensive driver—one who can anticipate potential danger and respond appropriately. Attitude is a key ingredient in defensive driving. Speeding, following too closely, and improper lane changing are the

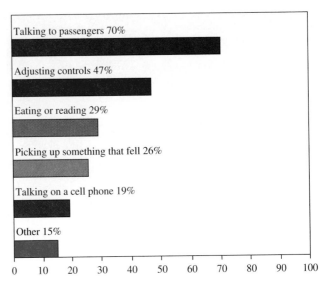

figure 15-1   Not paying attention. Distracted drivers cause an estimated 4,000 to 8,000 accidents everyday. Here are the biggest causes for distraction.
Source: Network of Employees for Traffic Safety

most common traffic infractions leading to crashes. Driver inattention has also become a major contributor to crashes.

Drivers focusing on newspapers, makeup, snacks, cellular phones, and CD players cause an estimated 50 percent of crashes (see Fig. 15-1). Cars have become mobile offices and living rooms, causing driver inattention to be the fourth most serious detriment to safe driving, behind drunken driving, aggressive driving, and speeding.

A driving risk causing new concern is *driving while drowsy (DWD)*. DWD has been an underrated risk factor in crashes. DWD accounts for as many as 100,000 car crashes and 10,000 traffic fatalities annually in the United States; surveys show that 25 percent of drivers have fallen asleep at the wheel, causing 1 in 10 of them to crash. For a variety of reasons, more Americans (even teenagers) are juggling jobs (sometimes more than one), school, and family responsibilities. Loss of sleep and driving at odd hours have become commonplace. Today's economy and high-tech boom have increased the number of people who work at night. Data indicates that one in five workers reports to work at night. A "24/7 world" demands an around-the-clock workforce. As a result, many Americans do not get enough sleep. Sleep deprivation affects many aspects of personal well-being, including driving safety. Getting 6 to 8 hours less sleep than usual over a week not only impairs mental efficiency and reaction time, but also decreases the immune system, and causes depression, anxiety, and irritability. Combining drowsiness with the comforts in modern day vehicles (cruise control, cellular phones, compact disc players, contoured reclining seats), it is easy to lose sight that driving a powerful automobile carries tremendous responsibility and demands constant attention.

wellness flash

A 1997 study found that talking on a phone while driving quadrupled the risk of an accident and was almost as dangerous as being drunk behind the wheel.

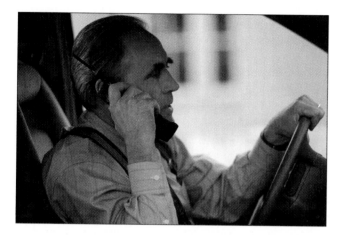

In some parts of the country it is illegal to talk on a car phone while driving.

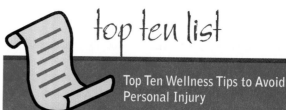

top ten list

Top Ten Wellness Tips to Avoid Personal Injury

1. *Fall-proof your home/apartment.* Falls are the second leading cause of accidental death in the United States. Stairs, loose carpeting, icy sidewalks, improper lighting, and wet tile help contribute to these statistics. Take charge of your environment to make it safe.
2. *Install smoke detectors throughout your home/apartment.* Test them periodically and replace batteries at least once a year. Plan and rehearse evacuation procedures in preparation for a fire. The heat and toxic gas buildup from a fire can be even more threatening than the flames. In most cases, you only have a few minutes after the smoke detector goes off to safely escape a building.
3. *When checking into a hotel, locate the nearest fire exits to your room.* Count and memorize the number of doorways between your room and these fire exits.
4. *Always wear a helmet when riding a motorcycle or bicycle.*
5. *Learn to swim.* Never swim alone or dive into shallow water (or water of unknown depth).
6. *Always wear a life preserver when boating.*
7. *Find shelter immediately during a lightning storm.* Once inside, stay away from telephones, metal objects, and open doors and windows.
8. *Never use electrical appliances near a sink or tub filled with water.*
9. *When walking, jogging, or cycling at night, always wear light clothing or reflective apparel.*
10. *Fasten your seatbelt whenever you get into a car.*

Finally, keeping your automobile in good running order with routine maintenance, as well as carrying emergency supplies (tools, flashlight, blankets, a first-aid kit, flares, "send help" signs, jumper cables), shows a preventive and preparedness mindset.

Personal Safety Awareness

Falls, drownings, fires, tornadoes, floods, rape, lightning, thefts, chokings, bicycle accidents, assaults, vandalism—these predicaments don't just happen to *other* people. You may find yourself facing any of these situations at some time. Though chance is one factor, you do have some control over your fate. You have the capacity to handle a variety of emergencies, possibly minimizing any ill effects. Advanced planning and preparation is the key. Look carefully at the top ten list of ways to avoid personal injury and think seriously about each item as it relates to you. Do you adhere to these common-sense safety precautions?

Crime Prevention

As much as we hate to admit it, crime and violence are a real part of contemporary U.S. life. Whether you are at school, traveling, at work, or going about daily living routines, you can become a victim. Even in the idyllic setting of a college campus, assaults, sexual attacks, and thefts occur. You can help protect yourself from being a victim with some basic precautions. A constant awareness of your environment is the best weapon for guarding your personal safety. Always be alert to your surroundings whether in your car, on the street, or at home. There is nothing extraordinary about the following personal safety tips. They are simple examples of assuming self-responsibility for your wellness.

1. *Always lock your house, apartment, residence hall room, and car—even when you are there.*
2. *At night, park in well-lit spots and walk in brightly lit areas.*
3. *Never walk alone at night or in unpopulated areas.* Nearly one in five rapes occur on unfamiliar, darkened, isolated streets. Use a campus escort service if available. Even during daylight hours,

always enlist the company of at least one other person when jogging or exercising outside.

4. *Beware of suspicious persons in buildings, hallways, parking areas, elevators, stairwells, and restrooms.* Note their description and contact the police or security.

5. *Don't let strangers know when you are home alone.*

6. *Glance into your car, checking the seats and floor, before getting in.*

7. *Never hitchhike or pick up hitchhikers.*

8. *If you are being harassed, turn and proceed toward lights and people.* If someone accosts you, yell "fire" instead of "help," because more people are likely to respond.

9. *Watch your alcohol consumption.* Drinking puts you at risk and makes you vulnerable to assault, robbery, and rape.

10. *Secure all valuables and don't flaunt expensive possessions.*

11. *When you are walking alone, walk with your shoulders back and your head held high.* Keep a strong and steady pace. Remain alert and be aware of your surroundings. Muggers and rapists rarely attack those who appear assured and confident. Also, walk facing traffic, even if you're on the sidewalk. This prevents an assailant in a car from sneaking up on you from the rear.

12. *Don't wear headphones or other devices that would make it difficult for you to predict and avoid a confrontation.*

13. *Let a roommate or a friend know where you are going and how long you might be gone when you leave campus.*

Not all accidents and injuries are preventable. Some just happen. However, many accidents and personal traumas *are* preventable with some basic precautions. Too often after an accident or tragic event someone says, "I wish I would have . . . ." Always have a plan of action. Play a mental game of "what if . . ."—where you would go and what you would do should a dangerous situation occur. Trust your instincts. Research shows that a large percentage of people who have been assaulted had a feeling something was wrong just before being attacked. Being careful may seem boring to some, but it *is* the wellness way.

Wellness Trends and Challenges for the Future

Some regard wellness as a passing fad, but we disagree. In his highly acclaimed book, *Megatrends*, John Naisbitt predicted, "The focus of health care is shifting from the short-term treatment of illness to the long-term attainment of wellness. Regarded by some as fad, wellness is a trend that is here to stay." We have already seen the wellness trend give impetus to societal changes. Designated smoking areas, seat belt laws, shopping mall wellness screenings, community walk-

ing clubs, and low-fat food choices in groceries and restaurants are examples of positive wellness changes. What else is down the road for wellness? What other changes and trends will you see in your lifetime? Also, what are the challenges that will continue to demand attention? The remainder of this chapter addresses these questions.

Trend 1: Changes in Health Care

One of the biggest trends is the changing focus in hospitals and the health-care profession. Medical care is shifting from the sickness business to the wellness business. Many community hospitals offer a variety of wellness programs with the intention of preventing individuals from becoming ill and needing hospitalization. Cholesterol testing, nutrition workshops, family counseling, drug rehabilitation, weight-management classes, and exercise prescription are examples of such programs. Some hospitals offer support services for a variety of specific groups (e.g., cancer survivors, families with Alzheimer members, diabetes education, etc.).

Some health facility administrators have found that a simple name change attracts clients to some of their programs. For example, a *mental health center* renamed a *stress center* has an easier time drawing individuals searching for help in dealing with personal problems. The counseling services of such a center may not be altered, but the connotation of learning ways to handle personal stress rather than trying to maintain mental health (often erroneously linked to mental illness) better attracts individuals needing such services.

Another change in medical care deals with the medical education of physicians. Some medical schools are expanding their physician training to include studying lifestyle and preventive influences on health and disease, rather than solely learning to identify and cure illness. There is compelling evidence showing that physicians exert a strong influence on their patients' behavior patterns. By incorporating preventive services and counseling into their patient encounters, physicians can dramatically affect the well-being of the nation. In this way, the physician can become a prime force in advocating a wellness lifestyle.

One of the most interesting evolutions occurring in health care is the emergence and acceptance of more natural medical therapies. Called "alternative," "complementary," "holistic," "integrative," or "naturopathic" medicine, treatments involving acupuncture, nutritional and herbal supplementation, massage, homeopathy, hypnosis, therapeutic touch, and biofeedback are being introduced into hospitals and medical research centers across the country. Many of these therapies are ancient medicine traditions from Oriental, Native American, Asian, and European cultures. With or without their doctor's blessings, Americans are flocking to these therapies. A national survey revealed that 42 percent of Americans used at least one alternative therapy in 1997. These 629 million visits to alternative med-

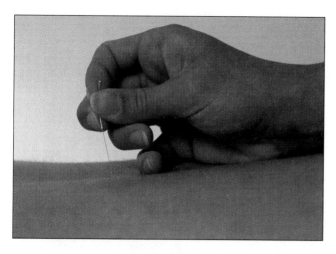

Some alternative therapies such as acupuncture are gaining respectability as emerging research supports their effectiveness.

icine practitioners exceeded the total visits to all primary care physicians. In addition, Americans spent more than $27 billion on these therapies in 1997, exceeding out-of-pocket spending for U.S. hospitalizations. Forty-seven percent of physicians report using alternative therapies themselves.

As evidence that the medical and scientific community are recognizing these previously unorthodox methods, the National Institutes of Health (NIH) established the National Center for Complementary and Alternative Medicine (NCCAM). NCCAM has defined **complementary** and **alternative medicine** (CAM) as "healing philosophies, approaches, and therapies that mainstream Western (conventional) medicine does not commonly use, accept, study, understand, or make available." The overriding mission of the NCCAM is to support rigorous research and objective inquiry into which complementary and alternative practices work, which do not, and why they work or don't work. This will give Americans reliable information about the safety and effectiveness of these practices. As a result of the emerging research, many of these therapies are gaining a more mainstream image among a multitude of skeptical medical doctors. Seventy-five out of 117 U.S. medical schools now offer courses in various alternative therapies.

Why are people attracted to alternative therapies? A survey out of Stanford University reported that people use such therapies not only because they are dissatisfied with conventional medicine, but because these health care alternatives mirror their values, beliefs, and philosophical orientations toward health and life. People use CAM therapies alone (as an *alternative* to conventional treatments), or in addition to conventional, mainstream therapies (referred to as *complementary* or an *integrative* approach).

Results from many studies are validating these natural therapies. Because most of these alternative treatments are far less expensive and less physically invasive than standard med-

ical procedures, their use and popularity will continue to grow dramatically. With new scientific journals such as *Complementary Medical Research* and *Alternative Therapies in Health and Medicine* appearing, it is evident that science is beginning to direct medicine back toward the principles of enabling the body to heal itself with more natural and preventive practices—*including* personal lifestyle changes. The visionary words spoken by Thomas Alva Edison represent this wellness trend: "The doctor of the future will give no medicine, but will interest his patients in the care of the human frame, in diet and in the cause and prevention of disease."

The high cost of medical care and the rising cost of health insurance have initiated another related trend. Insurance companies are beginning to provide incentives for staying well. Insurance benefits are being expanded and costs are being lowered for those who actively strive for optimal well-being by refraining from smoking, participating in periodic health screenings, maintaining a healthy weight, and exercising regularly. Some health insurance companies are even covering the costs of the new, emerging complementary therapies such as acupuncture and massage therapy. Group health benefits at reduced rate will be sought by companies that promote wellness in their workplaces and have predominantly healthy employees.

The underlying theme is that *preventing* ill health is more efficient and effective than *treating* illness. Prevention saves money, lives, and suffering, and, most important, it enhances human vitality and potential.

Trend 2: Aging America

All demographic studies document that the population of the United States is getting older. In January 2011, the first baby boomer will turn 65. Baby boomers (those born after World War II between 1946 and 1964) make up the largest segment of our population—approximately 76 million Americans. In 2000, 13 percent of the U.S. population was 65 years of age or over. Among these 35 million persons, nearly 4 million were 85 years of age and over. It is estimated that by 2030, seventy million persons will be 65 years of age or older, representing 20 percent of the population (see Fig. 15-2). It is estimated that the population of 85 years of age and older will more than double to approximately 8.5 million persons! This oldest of the old is the fastest growing segment of our population. These figures verify that the older population is growing at a faster rate than the population as a whole. And, women constitute the majority of this older group.

People are living longer because of healthier habits, the use of antibiotics and vaccinations, and modern medical treatments for heart disease and cancer. Death rates from heart disease among persons ages 65 to 84 have been reduced by half. This is all good news as far as your life expectancy is concerned, but could lead to huge shortfalls in available health care, pensions, and social services.

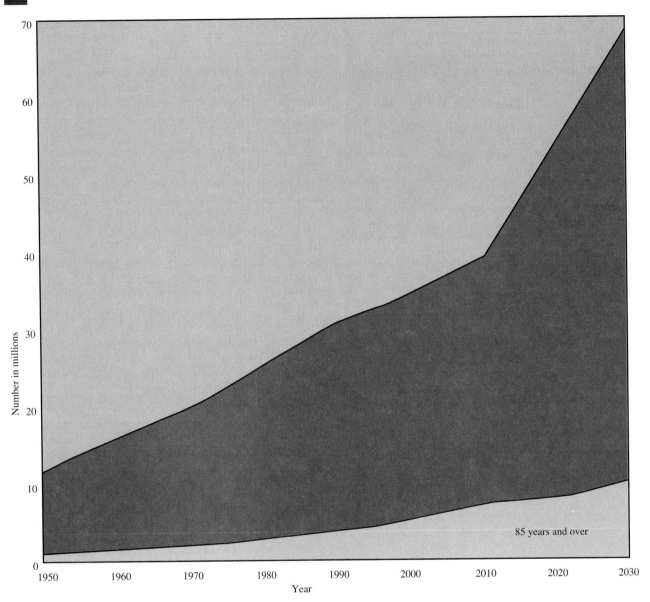

figure 15-2   Population 65 years of age and over: United States, 1950–2030

Notes: Figures for 1950–1990 are based on decennial censuses. Figures for 2000–2030 are middle series population projections of the U.S. Bureau of the Census.
Sources: See *Health, United States, 1999*, table 1 for data years 1950–90. For data years 2000–30, see U.S. Bureau of the Census. Day JC. Population projections of the United States by age, sex, race, and Hispanic origin: 1995 to 2050. Current population reports; P25-1130. Washington: U.S. Department of Commerce. 1996.

Describing the 60-plus age group is not an easy task. This diverse group can be described as "rich and poor, college-educated and illiterate. Some are vibrant and young; others are sick and elderly. They are not one unified consumer group with similar needs and attitudes." Most of this population is not, as many would think, senile or confined to nursing homes. Many older Americans are healthy, self-sufficient, and physically capable. A study released by the National Academy of Sciences found a 14.5 percent decline in the proportion of older people who cannot take care of themselves. Many senior citizens have money to spend and desire to continue as active contributors to society. Some have retired, remarried, and begun second careers. Consider

the impact this will have in the working world! They want and need programs for nutrition education, exercise, personal enrichment, and financial management. They want

wellness flash

People who survive to age 65 today can expect to live on average nearly 17.6 more years (19.0 years for females; 15.8 years for males).

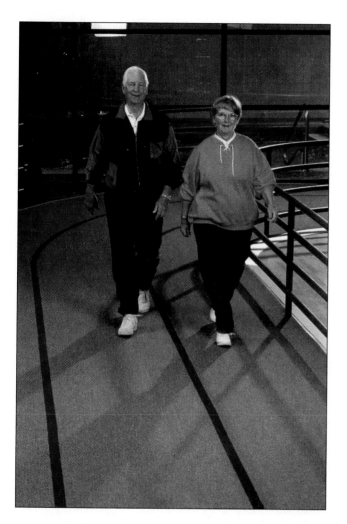

Americans are living longer.

housing alternatives. Experts say we should plan for a time when it's fairly common to see people who are 100 years old. The older population is one of the top markets perceived by health promotion analysts to be important during the next 20 years. As wellness becomes a way of life, you, too, will want programs as you reach older adulthood, whether they be special exercise classes, social activities, or special living environments.

Trend 3: The Mind-Body Connection

There has been an explosion of research in **psychoneuroimmunology (PNI),** the study of how emotions, behavior, and mental attitudes affect the immune system and the onset and course of illness. At one time, physiologists thought the immune system functioned independently from the central nervous and endocrine systems. Now it is clear that emotional states affect us right down to our cells. Researchers have shown that nerve cells connect directly to organs of the immune system, that hormones responsive to stressful expe-

riences affect the immune response, and that psychological and social factors can affect the immune system's responsiveness. Additional research into the chemicals produced by the brain has shown that the immune system and brain communicate chemically. Mental states such as loneliness, depression, fear, and pessimism alter the responses in the immune system. Stress is considered to be one of the top contributors to a lowered immune system. In contrast, experiencing close relationships, hope, compassion, humor, and social support enhance the body's ability to fight diseases. Owning a pet has even been found to have a positive effect on health. The immune system is most active during sleep. During your deepest states of sleep, your body releases compounds that greatly benefit immune function. Therefore, sleep deprivation is harmful to your immune system. The most important and rigorous study in support of psychoneuroimmunology was conducted by Dr. David Spiegel, a psychiatrist at the Stanford University School of Medicine. He and his colleagues found that weekly group therapy sessions dramatically increased the life expectancy of women with advanced breast cancer.

This area of research brings a fascinating approach to health care. Mind-body interventions, including relaxation techniques, meditation, biofeedback, autogenic training, and visualization, are being given credibility thanks to sophisticated research. Clinical applications of these techniques have shown promise in arresting the development of heart disease, cancer, AIDS, gastrointestinal problems, asthma, and chronic pain. Pioneers in this emerging area—Dr. Dean Ornish, Dr. Herbert Benson, and Dr. Andrew Weil—view mind-body therapies as mainstream medicine (rather than "alternative") that provides as much symptom relief as drugs or any other modern medical treatment has to offer. This exciting news clearly solidifies the strong connection between spirituality and physical well-being. Look at the top ten list of strategies that can boost the immune system. How many of these traits do you possess?

Challenge 1: Diversity

One of the biggest challenges we face is making wellness information and services available to *everyone*—and making wellness a priority in *all* people's lives, despite our many differences. The racial and ethnic composition of the United States is changing dramatically. The United States is perhaps one of the most multiracial countries in the world. In the year 2000, whites (not including Hispanic Americans) declined from 76 to 72 percent of the population. African Americans, presently comprising the largest minority, increased from 12.4 to 13.1 percent of the population. Hispanics, one of the fastest-growing population groups, rose from 8.0 to 11.3 percent.

Our diversity should be celebrated and recognized as a basis for national strength; it also presents challenges in meeting the health and wellness needs of everyone. Ideally,

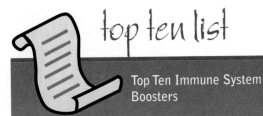

Top Ten Immune System Boosters

1. *Optimism.* Health can be a self-fulfilling prophecy. Good things happen to people who expect them. Pessimism, fatalism, and resignation are linked to poorer health.
2. An *unsinkable spirit.* Belief in the ability to make it through any crisis is essential.
3. *Taking charge.* Whereas a fighting spirit provides motivation, a take-charge attitude (also termed *active coping*) puts that spirit into action.
4. *Stress reduction.* By using exercise, relaxation, meditation, or other personal coping strategies, you give your immune system a big boost.
5. *Altruism.* Giving to others and making the world a better place have physical and mental benefits.
6. A *sense of humor.* Being able to laugh at yourself—as opposed to ridiculing others—is health enhancing.
7. *Absence of malice.* Those who have a lot of hostility are especially susceptible to disease.
8. *Social connectedness.* How would you answer the question, "Can you count on anyone to provide you with emotional support?" A yes means your relationships with people make a real difference in your health.
9. *Sleep.* Getting 7 to 9 hours of sleep every night allows your immune system to function optimally.
10. *Nutritional Support.* Just as a Ferrari can't run on kerosene, your system needs good fuel to function adequately.

other groups. Nearly one out of every eight Americans lives in a family with an income below the federal poverty level; and for virtually all of the chronic diseases that lead the nation's list of killers, low income is a special risk factor.

Everyone deserves a high level of functioning and well-being. Showing how small lifestyle changes can enhance well-being, providing wellness information, and changing attitudes toward self-responsibility in our diverse population is difficult. But making wellness available to all Americans is a wellness issue. In today's world, television is a common learning environment, especially for the uneducated. While there is a considerable amount of health-related information in television programming and commercials, many times, for our vastly diverse population, the suggestions seem impersonal, impractical, and unrealistic. This presents a considerable challenge to those in health promotion. Perhaps the biggest payoff would be to integrate wellness information, behaviors, and attitudes into all segments of primary and secondary school curricula, reaching all youth before unhealthy life habits develop. Wellness information should also be integrated into America's workplaces and community centers.

In *Healthy People 2010*, the U.S. government prioritized "eliminating health disparities" as one of its foremost goals. However, it is not enough to ask or expect every individual to accept responsibility for health and well-being without communities, businesses, health organizations, families, and civic organizations joining with the *government* to bring about national wellness. Dr. Kenneth Pelletier states that "The critical challenges remain to implement established knowledge, to increase awareness and motivation for healthy living, and to provide resources for equitable access to appropriate care. By supporting and reinforcing individual choices with innovations in policy and programs, we *can* achieve health."

Challenge 2: The Environment

Environmental policy has long been an important part of public health. Throughout history, regulations regarding safe food, water, and sewage management have substantially improved our well-being. However, rapid technological changes have resulted in new environmental hazards, many whose effects on the body may remain unrecognized for years. Worldwide consumption has had a tremendous effect on the world's resources and energy supplies. Cartoon character Pogo's insightful quip, "We have met the enemy and he is us," is particularly appropriate in addressing the challenge we face in saving and protecting the environment. This opens new opportunities for you to make an impact on your wellness—and that of others.

Being apathetic or becoming accustomed to environmental pollution is a serious matter. That you cannot do everything is no excuse for doing nothing. There is a lot you can do to limit, or at least minimize, the pollution and over-

wellness has no race, class, or income. However, the gulf is widening between the haves and have-nots, the insured and the uninsured, and whites and minorities. For example, the death rate for chronic diseases is more than twice as high among adults with fewer than 12 years of education than among those with more than 12 years of education. And, blue-collar workers, low socioeconomic and low education groups, and persons with the most risk for coronary heart disease (particularly smokers) are the individuals most resistive to public health promotion. These people cannot afford health club memberships and specialized medical screenings. Many of these people are more concerned about maintaining decent housing and feeding their families than about their cholesterol levels.

Generalizations about various subgroups from local studies can be misleading because of the disparities among subgroups living in different geographic locations. Nevertheless, the most striking aspect of health comparison rates is the tremendous gap between low-income people and all

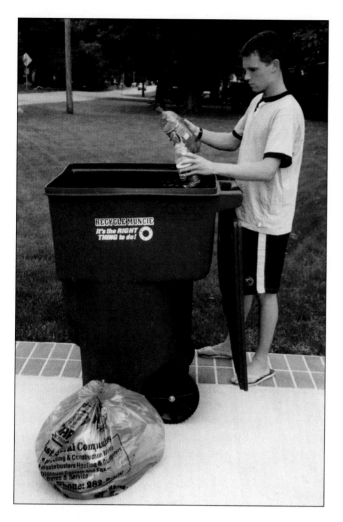

When it comes to caring for the environment, you make a difference each time you recycle.

consumption in your "little world." As in all areas of wellness improvement, form a personal plan to combat environmental hazards. Look at the following list of environmental concerns, and consider ways you could make changes in your daily living to make the world a better place in which to live.

1. The earth's protective ozone layer—our shield against the sun's hazardous ultraviolet rays—is being eaten away by human-made chemicals. The result is damaged food crops and ocean plants, increased skin cancer and cataracts, and decreases in human immunities. Aerosol sprays, refrigerants, plastic foam, and cleaning fluids contain chlorofluorocarbons (CFCs)—the chief agents of ozone destruction.

2. Our excessive use of paper, plastic, glass, and aluminum continues to add to our landfills. Consider that 10 years ago there were only about 500,000 fax machines in the United States. Now there are over 13 million business fax machines sending and receiving 35 billion sheets of office paper every year.

Recycling can decrease the need for more landfills and cut down on the pollution from the manufacture of new products.

3. Residues of harmful pesticides can be found in the air, on crops, in the ground, and in water supplies. Lawn and garden chemicals are significant contributors to this.

4. Water and air, essentials for life, face increasing contamination. Fish caught in polluted waters may be contaminated.

5. Loud rock music is associated with hearing loss.

6. Traffic sounds, aircraft noise, and noisy industrial areas are associated with stress and stress-related physical symptoms.

7. Radon gas and asbestos have been linked to cancer. Radon is a naturally occurring radioactive gas emitted by soil and rocks. Radon is diluted to safe levels outdoors but can be dangerously concentrated if trapped in poorly ventilated basements, houses, and buildings. Asbestos, a commonly used insulating material, has been linked to a variety of lung diseases. By order of the U.S. government, no asbestos has been manufactured since 1997.

8. Exposure to high levels of lead is toxic to the central nervous system and can be fatal. House paints used before 1980 often contained lead. Also, people who live near airports, battery factories, and landfills are at risk.

We often take too many things for granted. Part of your challenge in wellness living will be to assume some responsibility for preserving the environment. This personal challenge must then progress to the next level: more social and political action nationwide. Remember the 3 R's . . . Reduce, Reuse, and Recycle.

Challenge 3: Cultivating a Wellness Mindset in Everyone

Throughout this book we have addressed many effective strategies that nearly all individuals can use to pursue optimal well-being. However, the challenge of wellness extends beyond these commendable personal habits. Wellness goes beyond human physiology; it is also humility, compassion, and true happiness. Complete wellness includes possessing a deep altruistic commitment to the betterment of humankind. **Altruism** means having a regard for the interest of others without concern for oneself. Unfortunately, in this world the residues of self-gratification are visible—cheating; violence; family breakdown; loss of personal character, integrity, and values; drug use; and vanity. Is this the road to happiness? Is this a mindset for personal excellence?

In his book *The Pursuit of Happiness*, social psychologist Dr. David Myers uncovers the underlying recipe for personal happiness and well-being. His recipe includes three ingredients:

"Well-being is found in the renewal of *disciplined lifestyles, committed relationships*, and *receiving and giving of acceptance*." Myers' three ingredients intertwine with wellness-living: giving to others, achieving personal excellence, going beyond mediocrity, shaping your environment, seizing life. Wellness is not something to have. Rather it is something to be. The challenge we face is to achieve a wellness mindset, as well as creating a wellness mindset in everyone—where just getting by is intolerable. Rather than muddling through life making compromises and excuses, or passing up opportunities, take charge of your life! Be the best you can be! Instill this attitude in those around you. Perhaps Hugh Downs said it best: "A happy person is not a person in a certain set of circumstances, but rather a person with a certain set of attitudes."

A Parting Thought

Suppose you are the owner of a fine show dog. To make this dog a champion, you handle her in special ways: you make sure she gets proper exercise every day, her coat is brushed and groomed, and her diet is carefully monitored (at the grocery store you walk past the doggie treats and junk food to Be Lean and Win Dog Food). Her living environment is regulated to make her the best show dog possible. Do you treat yourself as you would a champion show dog? Do you walk past the treats and junk food to the "be lean and win" food? Are you managing your environment in such a way that it makes you the best you can be? You have 24 hours a day 365 days a year to make choices. Our society provides you the opportunity to make many positive choices. Our society also allows for choices that are not in your best interest. You now have the knowledge and skills to make choices that enhance your well-being.

Remember, wellness is a journey in which the benefits are gained along the trip. It is not a life of self-sacrifice and delayed gratification. It is being the most you can be every day of your life. It is reveling that you have considerable control over your well-being and happiness. Go to it! We wish you well.

frequently asked questions

Q. I feel confident that I can distinguish quackery or bogus health products from those that are legitimate. What confuses me are the health reports that emerge almost daily that often contradict a previous report. One day coffee is good for you; the next day it is linked to heart attacks. Beta-carotene supplements prevent cancer in one report. Another report shows it increases cancer risk in smokers. How do I know what to believe?

A. Part of well-informed wellness is distinguishing good quality health research from flimsy or biased data. However, it can be confusing because the modern media often sensationalizes, misinterprets, overgeneralizes, or gives only partial results from research studies. The more you know about the economics, politics, and methodology of research, the better able you are to form a sound opinion. Ask yourself the following questions as you weigh the evidence:

- Where is the work published? In a supermarket tabloid? In a homemaker's magazine? In a scientific journal that uses a board of experts to review the article?
- Who paid for the research? (Some companies and foundations might profit from certain outcomes, e.g., a ginseng manufacturer touting their researched benefits of ginseng.)
- Do my biases lead me to want to believe this information?
- Are advertisers using this information to sell a product?
- Is this only a preliminary finding that has not been fully tested?
- Are the researchers from respectable institutions?

- Was good scientific methodology used? What was the number of subjects involved in the study? Was there a control group?

Remember, it takes more than headlines to draw a sound conclusion. Many repeated studies are often necessary. Only after weighing *all* of the scientific evidence can sound public health policy be recommended. Unfortunately, you cannot believe everything you read and hear.

Q. It seems like the incidence of commercial airplane crashes is rising. Is there any way to minimize my risk when traveling by plane?

A. Unfortunately, many people take a fatalistic attitude toward airplane crashes. Despite sensational headlines, deaths due to airplane crashes are low when compared to those occurring with other modes of transportation. According to the National Transportation Safety Board, passengers who think systematically in advance about their safety are more likely to survive an airplane accident. Many airplane travelers settle into their seats, bury their heads in a newspaper, and ignore the safety instructions given by the flight attendants. Taking the first few minutes on a plane to review all safety instructions, observe safety features on the plane, and make an escape plan are responsible wellness behaviors. The following steps will help prepare you for an emergency:

- Locate the nearest exit and count the number of rows to the exit, so you can find it if the lights are out.
- Keep your seat belt fastened throughout the flight.
- Study the seat-pocket safety card.
- If possible, wear comfortable clothes and shoes.

Contrary to popular belief, where you sit in the plane has not been found to be a significant survival factor; however, sitting in an aisle seat may quicken an escape.

Q. I am interested in trying complementary and alternative therapies, especially acupuncture. How can I find more information about such practices or find a practitioner in my area?

A. Increasingly, traditional healthcare providers are becoming familiar with alternative treatments or are able to refer you to someone. If your healthcare provider cannot provide information, medical libraries, public libraries, and popular bookstores are good places to find information about

particular CAM practices. The NCCAM's online database (*www.nccam.nih.gov*) includes research and information on various disease conditions and links directly to MEDLINE's alternative medicine information. As far as finding a qualified practitioner, you may want to contact medical regulatory and licensing agencies in your state. Many states license acupuncture, naturopathy, herbal medicine, homeopathy, and massage therapy. Many CAM specialties have professional associations with websites that provide information about the specialty and listings for licensed practitioners close to your locale.

summary

Everyone is born with a genetic blueprint. However, personal lifestyle choices have a great impact on whether you maximize your potential. You, as an educated citizen, know the choices that enhance wellness. You, as an informed consumer, must be able to evaluate wellness products and programs. No doubt your campus offers activities and facilities that can support your quest for wellness. The business world has also discovered the value of wellness in the workplace, in terms of increased productivity, lessened health insurance costs, and enhanced employee morale. Knowing how important a supportive environment is in pursuing wellness, you may want to consider working for a company that supports and values employee wellness. After all, you will spend at least one-third of your life at work.

Wellness is an integral part of a productive family life. Family wellness involves meeting the various physical, psychological, and social needs of all members, regardless of ages, as they strive toward full potential. You, as a parent, will be the master teacher of lifestyle habits to your children. Your example will have a strong influence on your children's ability to make responsible wellness choices.

Accidents are the fifth most common cause of death in the United States. However, accidents (especially automobile crashes) are the number one cause of death among young people. All accidents and crime are not only a matter of chance. You can substantially reduce your risks of being a victim by heeding basic precautions. Acting to control risks in your immediate environment is a powerful way to enhance your total wellness.

Wellness is not a passing craze. The wellness trend is revolutionizing the medical care system. The broad scope of wellness creates opportunities for life enhancement for everyone: young, old, poor, rich, black, and white. New research in the mind-body relationship, including how attitudes, beliefs, and emotional states can affect the immune system, is creating increased interest in the *total* wellness concept of health. Wellness becomes a global issue as we work together to protect the environment. The ultimate challenge is to get the word to everyone (especially to those who need wellness the most) and get it to them while they are young. Empowering people to have a mind-set of self-responsibility along with an attitude of altruism is the only guaranteed way to perpetuate wellness as the undisputed way of life for everyone.

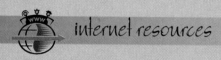 internet resources

Organizations

CNN's Health Report
www.cnn.com/HEALTH

National Center for Complementary and Alternative Medicine
www.nccam.nih.gov

National Health Information Center
www.healthfinder.gov

National Institute on Aging Information Center
www.aoa.gov

National Safety Council
www.nsc.org

U.S. Consumer Products Safety Commission
www.cpsc.gov/

U.S. Environmental Protection Agency
www.epa.gov/

Websites

www.alternativemedicine.com
www.altmedicine.com
www.discoveryhealth.com
www.drkoop.com
www.healthy.net
www.kidshealth.org
www.virtualrecycling.com
www.wellnessjunction.com
www.wholehealthmd.com

Quackery Detection

Doctors Accidentally Discover "Lazy Way" to Remove Cellulite

Discovery Astounds Scientific Community

Swedish researchers at the University of Pelento have discovered (accidentally) a secret formula that ACTUALLY SHRINKS CELLULITE! This astounding discovery has virtually *eliminated the need for dieting or torturous exercise!* This miracle formula is being marketed exclusively under the trade name SHRINK-It 5000.

Clinically Tested

Exhaustive medical tests at a world famous medical center in Burgess, Australia, have proven that **SHRINK-IT 5000** has no harmful side effects and is the most effective cellulite-reducing formula of all time. Like a magnet, the chemical molecules in **SHRINK-IT 5000** tie up and trap undigested fat particles many times their size. And it begins happening almost instantly! In fact, it is so effective that some people tend to overdo it and become too thin—within days!!

6 Week Supply
(Was $79.90)
NOW ONLY

$59.90
SAVE $20!!

Eat All You Want and Keep Losing Cellulite

This amazing formula was discovered by scientists searching for a compound to shrink varicose veins. Researchers were amazed to find the test group actually lost a considerable amount of cellulite fat—all while eating anything they wanted. Dr. Garth Robbins stated in the *Universal Journal of Clinical Science:* "This formula will virtually revolutionize the way people typically try to lose fat (with deprivating diets and exhaustive exercise)."

Act Now

This is a limited time offer. Since news of this product is sweeping the country, send in your order today. Don't let this golden opportunity get away. Imagine being the thin, attractive person you've dreamed about! **SHRINK-IT 5000** is only available from Powers Pharmaceuticals, which holds exclusive North American rights. Call now. Orders accepted by phone only.

1-800-987-6543
ALL CREDIT CARDS ACCEPTED

Answer the following questions:

1. List signs of quackery in the advertisement for SHRINK-IT 5000.

2. What makes this advertisement attractive or seem legitimate to the uninformed consumer?

3. If your sister were ready to send away for this product with the hope of reducing fat thighs, what would you tell her? How would you advise anyone wanting to reduce the fat on his or her thighs?

Look to the Future

Imagine that you are 10 years older, married with two children, and working in your chosen field.

1. Describe four wellness programs that you want your employer/company to offer. (If you plan to be self-employed or involved in a small business, describe the wellness programs you would want your hospital or community to offer.)
    a.

    b.

    c.

    d.

2. List five family activities that are important to you to promote family wellness.
    a.

    b.

    c.

    d.

    e.

3. Describe how you manage a regular fitness program. (Where?, When?, What type of activity?, etc.)

4. Not including fitness, what other lifestyle and wellness habits are you committed to for your lifetime? (Your answer may involve the entire wellness spectrum.)

lab activity
15-3

The Environment

Steve and Jane Brown have a 3-month-old baby and a 9-year-old Oldsmobile with a leaky air conditioner. They live in a 50-year-old house (with a basement) near a large shopping mall. The battery factory where they work is about 1 mile from their home.

Steve has not had a lawn grub or mole problem since he hired a company to take care of his lawn. He is considering buying a lawn tractor.

For recreation, the Browns like to fish in the nearby White River. They also enjoy working in their large garden and taking long drives in the country.

1. Using the information in Chapter 15 of your text, list six or more environmental concerns that affect the Browns' wellness.

   a.   d.

   b.   e.

   c.   f.

2. For each concern, list at least two steps they can take to protect the environment and, in turn, enhance their wellness.

   a.   d.

   b.   e.

   c.   f.

3. List three ways you consciously protect the environment. Explain why you choose to do so.

    a.

    b.

    c.

4. Name three actions you are *not* taking now but could begin to take to contribute to a better environment.

    a.

    b.

    c.

A Pop Quiz on Life

To discover an important lesson on life, take this quiz:

1. Name the four wealthiest people in the world.

2. Name the last four Heisman Trophy winners.

3. Name the last four winners of the Miss America contest.

4. Name four people who have won the Nobel Prize or Pulitzer Prize.

5. Name the last four Academy Award winners for best actor and actress.

How Did You Do?

The Point: No one remembers the headlines of yesterday, even though they are the best in their fields. Applause dies; awards tarnish; achievements are forgotten.

Now . . . . turn the page and take a second, more important quiz.

1. Name four teachers who aided your journey through school.

2. Name four people who taught you something worthwhile.

3. Name four people who have made you feel appreciated and special.

4. Name four people with whom you enjoy spending time.

5. Name four heroes whose stories have inspired you.

MUCH EASIER, HUH?

The Lesson: The people who make a difference in most lives are not always the ones with the most awards, money, or credentials.

appendix 1

Nutritive Values of Popular Fast Foods

Arby's

	Calories	%Calories From Fat	Total Fat (g)	Saturated Fat (g)	Cholesterol (mg)	Protein (g)	Total Carbohydrate (g)	Fiber (g)	Sugars (g)	Sodium (mg)	Calcium (mg)
Regular Roast Beef	400	45%	20	7	40	23	36	3	N/A	1030	50
Super Roast Beef	530	46%	27	9	40	24	50	5	N/A	1190	80
Beef 'N Cheddar	510	49%	28	9	50	26	45	3	N/A	1250	150
Grilled Chicken Deluxe	420	34%	16	4	60	30	42	3	N/A	930	80
Big Montana	720	50%	40	17	110	50	44	7	N/A	2270	80
French Dip Sub	490	40%	22	8	56	30	43	3	N/A	1440	120
Philly Beef 'N Swiss Sub	780	55%	48	16	90	39	52	4	N/A	2140	350
Turkey Sub	670	52%	39	10	60	29	49	2	N/A	2130	350
Light Roast Chicken Deluxe	260	17%	5	1.5	40	23	32	4	N/A	950	60
Light Grilled Chicken Salad	190	19%	4	.5	40	25	16	1	N/A	530	200
Broccoli 'N Cheddar Baked Potato	550	41%	25	13	50	14	71	7	N/A	730	250
Chicken Broccoli Baked Potato	830	51%	47	8	60	35	68	7	N/A	970	500
Med. Homestyle Fries	420	41%	19	3	0	5	57	4	N/A	830	*
Med. Curly Fries	380	45%	19	4.5	0	5	49	0	N/A	1100	*
Cheddar Curly Fries	450	50%	25	6	5	7.5	52	0	N/A	1420	80
Potato Cakes (2)	220	57%	14	3	0	2	21	3	N/A	460	*
Mozzarella Sticks	470	56%	29	14	60	18	34	2	N/A	1330	400
Tangy Southwest Sauce	250	90%	25	4	30	0	3	0	N/A	280	0
French Toastix (6)	370	41%	17	4	0	7	48	4	N/A	440	70
Jamocha Shake	380	21%	9	6	10	8	66	0	N/A	300	250

N/A = Not Available

* Contains Less Than 2% of the Daily Value

Burger King
Additional food items listed at: www.burgerking.com/nutrition (click on "Nutritional Tables")

	Calories	% Calories from Fat	Total Fat (g)	Saturated Fat (g)	Cholesterol (mg)	Protein (g)	Total Carbohydrate (g)	Fiber (g)	Sugars (g)	Sodium (mg)	Calcium (mg)
Whopper	640	55%	39	11	90	27	45	3	8	870	100
Whopper with Cheese	780	54%	47	17	105	34	55	4	9	1390	250
Double Whopper with Cheese	960	59%	63	24	195	52	46	3	8	1420	150
BK Big Fish Sandwich	710	48%	38	14	50	24	67	4	4	1200	80
BK Broiled Chicken Sandwich	550	41%	25	5	105	30	52	3	5	1100	60
Whopper Jr.	420	51%	24	8	55	20	32	2	6	520	80
Chicken Tenders (8 pieces)	340	50%	19	5	50	22	20	<1	0	840	0
Jalapeno Poppers (4)	230	51%	13	5	20	7	22	2	1	790	150
Ranch Dipping Sauce	120	98%	13	2	5	1	1	N/A	N/A	85	150
Barbeque Dipping Sauce	35	0	0	0	0	0	9	N/A	N/A	400	N/A
Broiler Chicken Salad (No Dressing)	190	38%	8	4	75	20	9	3	5	500	N/A
Garden Salad (No Dressing)	100	45%	5	3	15	6	8	4	4	115	N/A
Blue Cheese Salad Dressing	160	90%	16	4	30	2	1	<1	0	260	N/A
Med. French Fries (Salted)	370	41%	17	5	0	4	49	4	0	760	0
Med. Onion Rings	330	44%	16	4	0	5	41	3	5	470	100
Chocolate Shake (Medium)	440	20%	10	6	30	12	75	4	67	330	300
French Toast Sticks (5)	390	46%	20	4.5	0	6	46	2	11	440	60
Cini-Minis (4) Without Icing	440	47%	23	6	25	6	51	1	20	710	60
Croissan'wich w/Sausage, Egg & Cheese	500	65%	36	13	190	19	26	1	5	1020	150
Dutch Apple Pie	340	48%	18	13	0	2	52	1	23	470	0

N/A = Not Available

Domino's Pizza
1 serving = 2 of 8 slices or 1/4 of 14" (large)

	Calories	% Calories from Fat	Total Fat (g)	Saturated Fat (g)	Cholesterol (mg)	Protein (g)	Total Carbohydrate (g)	Fiber (g)	Sugars (g)	Sodium (mg)	Calcium (mg)
6-inch Deep Dish, Cheese	597	41%	27	10	36	23	68	4	6	1341	334
Classic Hand-Tossed, Cheese	516	26%	15	7	31	21	75	4	6	1080	261
Thin Crust, Cheese	382	38%	16	6	31	16	43	2	5	1171	315
Deep Dish, Cheese	676	39%	29	10	40	26	80	4	8	1575	334
Classic Hand-Tossed, Extra Cheese	583	31%	20	9	47	26	76	4	6	1308	378
Thin Crust, Extra Cheese	450	44%	22	9	47	21	44	2	5	1399	432

	Calories	% Calories from Fat	Total Fat (g)	Saturated Fat (g)	Cholesterol (mg)	Protein (g)	Total Carbohydrate (g)	Fiber (g)	Sugars (g)	Sodium (mg)	Calcium (mg)
Deep Dish, Extra Cheese	744	42%	35	13	56	31	81	5	9	1803	451
Classic Hand-Tossed, Mushroom	524	26%	15	6	31	22	76	4	7	1081	263
Thin Crust, Mushroom	390	37%	16	6	31	17	45	3	6	1172	316
Deep Dish, Mushroom	685	39%	30	11	40	27	82	5	9	1576	336
Topping Per Serving:											
Pepperoni	66	82%	6	2	14	3	<1	<1	<1	212	*
Ham	17	53%	1	<1	7	2	<1	0	<1	156	*
Italian Sausage	44	61%	3	1	9	2	1	<1	<1	137	*
Bacon	75	72%	6	2	11	4	<1	0	<1	207	*
Beef	44	82%	4	2	8	2	<1	<1	<1	123	*
Barbeque Wings (1)	50	36%	2	.6	26	6	2	<1	1	175	5
Hot Wings (1)	45	40%	2	.6	26	6	<1	<1	<1	354	5
Breadsticks (1)	116	31%	4	.8	0	3	18	<1	<1	152	6
Double Cheese Bread (1)	141	38%	6	2	6	4	17	<1	<1	183	47

*Contains Less Than 2% of The Daily Value

Added to a cheese pizza, each of the following toppings supply only about 10 additional calories per serving: green peppers, onions, olives, and pineapple.

Jack in the Box

	Calories	% Calories from Fat	Total Fat (g)	Saturated Fat (g)	Cholesterol (mg)	Protein (g)	Total Carbohydrate (g)	Fiber (g)	Sugars (g)	Sodium (mg)	Calcium (mg)
Breakfast Jack	280	39%	12	5	195	17	30	1	3	920	150
Supreme Croissant	520	55%	32	13	245	21	39	2	6	1240	100
Hamburger	280	35%	11	4	45	13	31	1	5	560	100
Jumbo Jack	590	55%	36	11	80	25	42	4	6	720	150
Sourdough Jack	690	60%	46	15	110	31	38	3	3	1180	300
Chicken Fajita Pita	280	29%	9	4	75	24	25	3	5	840	150
Grilled Chicken Fillet	520	45%	26	6	140	27	42	4	9	1240	200
Chicken Supreme	680	60%	45	11	85	23	46	4	8	1500	200
Chicken Caesar Sandwich	490	48%	26	6	55	24	41	3	6	1050	200
Garden Chicken Salad	200	41%	9	4	65	23	8	3	4	420	200
Blue Cheese Dressing	210	64%	15	2.5	25	1	11	0	4	750	20
Chicken Teriyaki Bowl	670	5%	4	1	15	26	128	3	27	1730	100
Monster Taco	270	57%	17	6	30	12	19	4	2	678	200
Egg Rolls (3 pieces)	440	49%	24	6	35	15	40	4	5	1020	80
Chicken Breast Pieces (5)	360	43%	17	3	80	27	24	1	0	970	20
Stuffed Jalapenos (10)	750	53%	44	17	80	20	65	5	7	2470	450
Barbeque Dipping Sauce	45	0	0	0	0	1	11	0	7	310	0
Seasoned Curly Fries	410	50%	23	5	0	6	45	4	0	1010	40
Onion Rings	460	49%	25	5	0	7	50	3	3	780	40
Cappuccino Shake	630	41%	29	17	90	11	80	0	58	320	350

KFC

Additional food items listed at:
www.kfc.com/food/nutrition.asp

	Calories	% Calories from Fat	Total Fat (g)	Saturated Fat (g)	Cholesterol (mg)	Protein (g)	Total Carbohydrate (g)	Fiber (g)	Sugars (g)	Sodium (mg)	Calcium (mg)
Original Recipe: Breast	400	54%	24	6	135	29	16	1	0	1116	40
Thigh	250	65%	18	4.5	95	16	6	1	0	747	20
Extra Tasty Crispy: Breast	470	54%	28	7	80	31	25	1	0	930	40
Thigh:	370	61%	25	6	70	19	18	2	0	540	20
Hot and Spicy: Breast	530	59%	35	8	110	32	23	2	0	1110	40
Thigh	370	66%	27	7	90	18	13	1	0	570	*
Tender Roast: Breast (as served)	251	39%	11	3	151	37	1	0	<1	830	*
Breast (skin removed)	169	21%	4	1	112	31	1	0	0	797	*
Thigh (as served)	207	52%	12	4	120	18	<2	0	<1	504	*
Thigh (skin removed)	106	51%	6	2	2	84	13	<1	0	<1	312*
Hot Wings Pieces	471	63%	33	8	150	27	18	2	0	1230	40
Colonel's Crispy Strips (3)	261	55%	16	4	40	20	10	3	0	658	*
Chunky Chicken Pot Pie	770	49%	42	13	70	29	69	5	8	2160	100
Corn on the Cob	150	12%	2	0	0	5	35	2	8	20	*
Mashed Potatoes with Gravy	120	45%	6	1	<1	1	17	2	0	440	*
Mean Greens	70	39%	3	1	10	4	11	5	1	650	200
BBQ Baked Beans	190	14%	3	1	5	6	33	6	13	760	80
Potato Salad	230	55%	14	2	15	4	23	23	9	540	20
Cole Slaw	180	45%	9	1.5	5	2	21	3	20	280	40
Biscuit (1)	180	50%	10	2.5	0	4	20	<1	2	560	20

*Contains Less Than 2% of the Daily Value

McDonald's

Additional food items listed at:
www.mcdonalds.com/countries/
/usa/food/nutrition_facts

	Calories	% Calories from Fat	Total Fat (g)	Saturated Fat (g)	Cholesterol (mg)	Protein (g)	Total Carbohydrate (g)	Fiber (g)	Sugars (g)	Sodium (mg)	Calcium (mg)
Hamburger	260	31%	9	3.5	30	13	34	2	7	580	150
Cheeseburger	320	37%	13	6	40	15	35	2	7	820	200
Quarter Pounder	420	45%	21	8	70	23	37	2	8	820	300
Quarter Pounder with Cheese	530	51%	30	13	95	28	38	2	9	1290	150
Big Mac	560	50%	31	10	85	26	45	3	8	1070	250
Fish Filet Deluxe	560	45%	28	6	60	23	54	4	5	1060	80
Grilled Chicken Deluxe	440	41%	20	3	60	27	38	4	6	1040	60
Chicken McNuggets (6 pieces)	290	53%	17	3.5	60	18	15	0	0	510	20
French Fries (large)	450	44%	22	4	0	6	57	5	0	290	20

Garden Salad (no dressing)	35	0	0	0	0	2	7	3	3	20	40
Grilled Chicken Salad (no dressing)	120	11%	1.5	0	45	21	7	3	3	240	40
Ranch Dressing (1 pkg.)	230	82%	21	3	20	1	10	0	6	550	40
Fat-Free Herb Vinaigrette (1 pkg)	50	0	0	0	0	0	11	0	9	330	*
Chocolate Shake (small)	360	23%	9	6	40	11	60	1	54	250	350
Egg McMuffin	290	37%	12	4.5	235	17	27	1	3	790	200
Bacon, Egg, & Cheese Biscuit	540	57%	34	10	250	21	36	N/A	N/A	1550	N/A
Ham, Egg, & Cheese Bagel	550	38%	23	8	255	26	58	N/A	N/A	1490	N/A
Hot Cakes with Marg. & Syrup	570	25%	16	3	15	9	100	2	42	750	100
Hash Brown	130	55%	8	1.5	0	1	14	1	0	330	*
Low-Fat Apple Bran Muffin	300	9%	3	.5	0	6	61	N/A	N/A	380	N/A

N/A = Not Available

* Contains Less than 2% of the Daily Value

Papa John's Pizza

1 serving = 1 of 8 slices or 1/8 of 14" (large)

	Calories	% Calories from Fat	Total Fat (g)	Saturated Fat (g)	Cholesterol (mg)	Protein (g)	Total Carbohydrate (g.)	Fiber (g.)	Sugars (g.)	Sodium (mg.)	Calcium (mg.)
Original Crust:											
Cheese	270	30%	9	3	17	12	37	2	N/A	660	163
Pepperoni	305	35%	12	5	24	13	37	2	N/A	800	165
Sausage	335	38%	14	5	28	15	37	2	N/A	900	171
All the Meats	390	44%	19	7	21	19	37	2	N/A	1110	170
Garden Special	290	31%	10	4	17	12	39	3	N/A	720	170
The Works	345	37%	14	5	31	16	38	2	N/A	920	185
Thin Crust:											
Cheese	225	48%	12	4	17	9	22	1	N/A	440	180
Pepperoni	260	52%	15	5	24	11	22	1	N/A	580	180
Sausage	285	54%	17	6	28	12	22	1	N/A	680	185
All the Meats	345	57%	22	8	41	16	22	1	N/A	890	185
Garden Special	240	45%	12	4	17	10	24	2	N/A	500	185
The Works	295	52%	17	6	31	13	23	1	N/A	700	200
Sides:											
Cheesesticks-2 (1/7 of an order)	180	40%	8	3	13	8	20	1	N/A	380	120
Breadsticks-1 (1/8 of an order)	140	13%	2	0	0	4	26	1	N/A	260	8
Nacho Cheese Dip (1 T.)	30	60%	2	1.5	7.5	1.5	0	*	N/A	115	*
Garlic Sauce (1 T.)	75	96%	8	1	0	0	0	*	N/A	115	*
Pizza Sauce (1 T.)	10	45%	.5	0	0	0	1	*	N/A	50	*

N/A = Not Available

* Contains Less Than 2% of the Daily Value

Added to a cheese pizza, each of the following toppings supply only about 10 additional calories per serving: green peppers, onions, olives, mushrooms, pineapple, tomatoes.

Subway

Additional food items listed at: www.subway.com

(click on "nutrition information," "U.S. Nutrition Guide")

	Calories	% Calories from Fat	Total Fat (g)	Saturated Fat (g)	Cholesterol (mg)	Protein (g)	Total Carbohydrate (g)	Fiber (g)	Sugars (g)	Sodium (mg)	Calcium (mg)
*6" Cold Subs: Tuna	378	33%	14	3	32	18	45	3	4	942	N/A
Seafood & Crab	338	24%	9	2	14	14	51	4	5	1034	N/A
Classic Italian BMT	450	42%	21	8	52	21	45	3	5	1579	N/A
Cold Cut Trio	374	34%	14	5	47	19	45	3	5	1435	N/A
Veggie Delite	232	12%	3	1	0	9	43	3	4	582	N/A
Turkey Breast	282	13%	4	1	20	17	45	3	5	1170	N/A
Turkey & Ham	288	13%	4	2	23	18	45	3	5	1256	N/A
Subway Club	304	15%	5	2	26	21	46	3	5	1239	N/A
6" Hot Subs: Subway Melt	370	27%	11	5	41	23	46	3	6	1619	N/A
*Meatball	413	33%	15	6	35	19	50	5	7	1025	N/A
Chicken Parmesan Ranch Wrap	333	14%	5	2	45	17	56	2	N/A	1393	N/A
Steak & Cheese Wrap	353	23%	9	4	37	16	53	2	N/A	1450	N/A
Turkey Breast Salad (no dressing)	101	18%	2	0	20	11	12	1	1	896	N/A
Roasted Chicken Breast Salad (no dressing)	162	22%	4	1	48	20	13	1	2	693	N/A
2 Triangles of Cheese	41	66%	3	2	10	2	0	0	0	204	N/A
Chocolate Chip or Chunk Cookie	215	42%	10	3	13	3	29	1	17	144	9
Peanut Butter Cookie	223	48%	12	2	0	3	27	1	15	214	7
Regular Mayonnaise (1 T)	111	97%	12	3	9	0	0	0	0	81	N/A
Light Mayonnaise (1 T)	54	83%	5	0	6	0	0	0	0	99	N/A
Mustard (2 tsp.)	7	0%	0	0	0	0	1	0	0	115	N/A

N/A = Not Available

*Values Do Not Include Cheese or Condiments

Taco Bell

Additional food items listed at: www.tacobell.com

	Calories	% Calories from Fat	Total Fat (g)	Saturated Fat (g)	Cholesterol (mg)	Protein (g)	Total Carbohydrate (g)	Fiber (g)	Sugars (g)	Sodium (mg)	Calcium (mg)
Taco	180	50%	10	4	25	9	12	3	1	330	80
Taco Supreme	220	57%	14	6	35	10	14	3	2	350	100
Double Decker Taco Supreme	390	44%	19	8	35	15	40	9	3	760	150
BLT Soft Taco	340	61%	23	8	40	11	22	2	3	610	100
Burrito Supreme	440	39%	19	8	35	17	51	10	4	1230	150
Big Beef Burrito Supreme	520	40%	23	10	55	17	54	11	4	1520	150
Chili Cheese Burrito	330	35%	13	6	35	10	37	5	2	870	200
Beef Gorditas Supreme	300	39%	13	6	35	21	31	3	3	390	80

	Calories	% Calories from Fat	Total Fat (g)	Saturated Fat (g)	Cholesterol (mg)	Protein (g)	Total Carbohydrate (g.)	Fiber (g.)	Sugars (g.)	Sodium (mg.)	Calcium (mg.)
Chicken Gorditas Supreme	290	37%	12	5	55	14	30	2	4	420	80
Big Beef Meximelt	290	47%	15	7	45	21	23	4	0	850	200
Taco Salad with Shell	850	55%	52	15	60	9	65	16	1	1790	300
Taco Salad without Shell	420	45%	21	11	60	5	32	15	1	1520	250
Chicken Fajita Wrap	470	40%	21	6	60	9	51	4	N/A	1290	150
Veggie Fajita Wrap	420	41%	19	5	20	N/A	53	3	N/A	980	150
Steak Fajita Wrap Supreme	510	44%	25	8	50	N/A	52	3	N/A	1200	150
Big Beef Nachos Supreme	450	48%	24	8	30	N/A	45	9	N/A	810	150
Nachos Bell Grande	720	49%	39	11	35	N/A	84	17	N/A	1310	200
Pintos 'N Cheese	190	43%	9	4	15	N/A	18	10	N/A	650	150
Chalupa Supreme (chicken)	360	50%	20	7	45	17	28	2	3	500	N/A
Chalupa Sante Fe (beef)	440	55%	27	6	35	18	29	2	2	580	N/A

N/A = Not Available

Wendy's

Additional food items listed at: www.wendys.com (click on "nutritional information")

	Calories	% Calories from Fat	Total Fat (g)	Saturated Fat (g)	Cholesterol (mg)	Protein (g)	Total Carbohydrate (g.)	Fiber (g.)	Sugars (g.)	Sodium (mg.)	Calcium (mg.)
Single with Everything	420	43%	20	7	70	25	37	3	9	920	130
Big Bacon Classic	580	47%	30	12	100	34	46	3	11	1460	250
Jr. Hamburger	270	33%	10	3.5	30	15	34	2	7	610	110
Jr. Bacon Cheeseburger	380	45%	19	7	60	20	34	2	7	850	170
Grilled Chicken Sandwich	310	23%	8	1.5	65	27	35	2	8	790	100
Caesar Side Salad (no dressing)	110	41%	5	2.5	15	10	7	1	1	650	150
Grilled Chicken Salad (no dressing)	200	36%	8	1.5	50	25	9	3	6	720	190
Taco Salad (no dressing)	380	45%	19	10	65	26	28	7	9	1040	370
Ranch Dressing, reduced fat (2T)	60	75%	5	1	10	1	2	0	1	240	10
Soft Breadstick	130	21%	3	.5	5	4	23	1	N/A	250	40
Med. French Fries	390	44%	19	3	0	5	50	5	0	120	20
Baked Potato w/Broccoli & Cheese	470	27%	14	2.5	5	9	80	9	6	470	210
Baked Potato w/Chili & Cheese	630	34%	24	9	40	20	83	9	7	770	350
Small Chili, plain	210	30%	7	2.5	30	15	21	5	5	800	80
Large Chili w/Cheese & Crackers	405	37%	16.5	7	60	28	37	7	8	1380	250
Chicken Nuggets (5)	230	63%	16	3	30	11	11	0	0	470	20
Barbeque Sauce	45	0	0	0	0	1	10	0	7	160	10
Chicken Club Sandwich	470	38%	20	4	70	31	44	2	6	970	110
Garden Veggie Pita	400	38%	17	3.5	20	11	52	5	8	760	170
Medium Frosty	440	22%	11	7	50	11	73	0	56	260	410

N/A = Not Available

appendix 2

Outside Reading Assignment

Note—You may want to make extra copies of this form for future outside reading assignments.

Name _____

Class/Activity Section _____

Select a research article on fitness, health, or wellness. This article should be from a professional/scientific journal (not a popular, newstand magazine). A copy of the article should be attached to this form. Use a current journal, that is, dated 1999 to present. Complete the following:

I. Bibliographic information:
example: Powers, Debbie, Gwen Robbins, and Sharon Burgess. "Living the Wellness Way of Life." *Journal of Health Behavior* 25 (June 2000): 25–31.

II. Summarize the research/study and its most important findings (in your words):

III. Explain how you can apply this information to your life:

appendix 2

Outside Reading Assignment

Note—You may want to make extra copies of this form for future outside reading assignments.

Name _____

Class/Activity Section _____

Select a research article on fitness, health, or wellness. This article should be from a professional/scientific journal (not a popular, newstand magazine). A copy of the article should be attached to this form. Use a current journal, that is, dated 1999 to present. Complete the following:

I. Bibliographic information:
    example: Powers, Debbie, Gwen Robbins, and Sharon Burgess. "Living the Wellness Way of Life." *Journal of Health Behavior* 25 (June 2000): 25–31.

II. Summarize the research/study and its most important findings (in your words):

III. Explain how you can apply this information to your life:

appendix 3

Reaction Paper to Guest Speaker

Note—You may want to make extra copies of this form for future guest speakers.

Name _____

Class/Activity Section _____

Answer the following questions concerning the presentation by _____
                                                                                    (name of speaker)

entitled _____on _____.
            (name of presentation)   (date)

  I. List and discuss three important points the speaker made.

    a.

    b.

    c.

  II. What was the *most* important information you heard at this presentation?

 III. Was there anything that the speaker said that you disagreed with? (Explain)

 IV. How can you incorporate what you learned into your lifestyle?

appendix 3

Reaction Paper to Guest Speaker

Note—You may want to make extra copies of this form for future guest speakers.

Name _____

Class/Activity Section _____

Answer the following questions concerning the presentation by _____
(name of speaker)

entitled _____on _____.
(name of presentation)   (date)

 I. List and discuss three important points the speaker made.

  a.

  b.

  c.

 II. What was the *most* important information you heard at this presentation?

III. Was there anything that the speaker said that you disagreed with? (Explain)

IV. How can you incorporate what you learned into your lifestyle?

glossary

a

Acquired Immune Deficiency Syndrome (AIDS) is the final stage in a human immunodeficiency virus (HIV) infection and a group of symptoms resulting from infections due to a weakened immune system. These may include pneumocystis carinii pneumonia, Kaposi's sarcoma, persistent infections, and damage to the brain and spinal cord. AIDS is spread through sexual intercourse; sharing infected needles; and, rarely, through tainted blood products. It can be spread from a pregnant woman to her fetus.

action stage is the fourth stage in the transtheoretical model of behavior change. In this stage, individuals are overtly changing their behaviors; taking conscious action; and using strategies to resist temptations, remain motivated, and cope with everyday challenges.

addiction is a pathological or abnormal relationship with an object or event. It is an illness that progresses from a definite, though often unclear, beginning toward an end. Beginning as a voluntary, pleasurable act, it then becomes a reflective and compulsive behavior.

aerobic literally means "with oxygen." Aerobic activities are those that demand large amounts of oxygen, follow the FITT prescription, and improve cardiorespiratory endurance.

agonist is a muscle primarily responsible for producing a movement. For example, in a biceps curl, the biceps muscle is the agonist.

alcohol (ethyl alcohol/ethanol) is a beverage and a CNS depressant. Alcohol slows reaction time, dulls alertness, and impairs body coordination. It intensifies emotions, lowers inhibitions, and increases risk-taking behaviors. Alcohol is the most abused legal drug in our society.

alcoholism is a chemical dependence on (an addiction to) alcohol that causes physical, mental, emotional, social, and economic damage to the alcoholic's life and to the lives of those close to him or her.

alternative medicine is a healing philosophy, approach, or therapy that conventional medicine does not commonly use, accept, study, understand, or make available. (Sometimes referred to as complementary or integrative medicine.)

altruism is having an unselfish interest in the welfare of others.

amenorrhea is a menstrual abnormality that results in absent menses.

amotivational syndrome is characterized by low energy, apathy, and little drive to do anything. It is linked to marijuana use which, after time, results in changes in brain cell membranes.

amphetamines (speed, uppers, crank, bennies, meth, or crystal) are powerful CNS stimulants. They are controlled substances legitimately used for short-term diet control in obesity and for narcolepsy. They have the ability to relieve sleepiness and fatigue and to increase alertness, confidence, and short-term performance. Truck drivers, pilots, entertainers, and athletes may use amphetamines nonmedically to enhance their performance.

anabolic steroids are artificial forms of the male hormone testosterone. They are used legitimately in the treatment of anemia, hormone disorders, and multiple sclerosis. They are also used to increase muscle mass by both male and female athletes at all levels of competition, and they have numerous adverse side effects.

anaerobic means "without oxygen." This type of activity demands more oxygen than the body can supply while exercising, causing an oxygen debt. Start and stop activities, such as sprinting, are examples of anaerobic exercise.

angina pectoris is chest pain and is primarily caused by atherosclerosis.

anorexia nervosa is an eating disorder characterized by self-inflicted starvation and dramatic weight loss. The anorexic is obsessed with achieving thinness.

antagonist is a muscle opposing a movement. For example, in a biceps curl, the triceps muscle is the antagonist.

antioxidants are compounds that help protect the body's cells from the damaging effects of the normal oxygenation process. Vitamin C, vitamin E, beta-carotene, and selenium are antioxidants.

arteriosclerosis is thickening and hardening of the arteries.

atherosclerosis is a type of arteriosclerosis and is a progressive condition that results in a buildup of plaque in the blood vessels.

atrophy is the condition of diminished muscle size and strength due to lack of use.

autogenic training and imagery is a self-generating or self-induced relaxation technique. This method uses mental concentration exercises to bring about sensations of warmth and heaviness in the limbs and torso and then uses relaxing images (e.g., clouds drifting by) to expand the relaxed state.

b

ballistic stretching involves jerking and bouncing movements and is not the recommended type of stretching.

basal metabolic rate (BMR) is the amount of energy (calories) expended by the body at rest to sustain vital functions.

behavior modification is the use of techniques to enhance awareness or consciousness about a behavior and to subsequently alter the behavior. For example, a behavior modification technique for weight management would be refraining from grocery shopping while hungry.

benign tumors are lumps of cells that are usually nonthreatening and seldom cause death. They usually resemble surrounding tissue; remain localized; and spread by expansion, like a wart or mole. They do not spread to other parts of the body.

beta-carotene is a plant substance that the body uses to make vitamin A, an antioxidant that helps prevent cellular damage from free radicals.

binge drinking is alcohol abuse. It is consuming *five* or more drinks at one setting for males or *four* or more at one setting for females.

binge eating disorder is recurrent episodes of eating characterized by eating, in a discrete period, an amount of food much larger than most people would eat in a similar period—and accompanied by a sense of lack of control or a feeling that one cannot stop.

biofeedback training is a technique in which machines measure certain physiological processes of the body. The machines convert this information to an understandable form and feed it back to the individual. This process allows a person access to biological information not usually available through consciousness alone.

blackout an inability to remember a period of time, may result after a night of abusive alcohol consumption.

blisters are inflamed burns caused by the friction of skin against a fabric or surface (like a shoe).

blood alcohol concentration (BAC) or blood alcohol level (BAL), is the amount of alcohol in the blood and is expressed as a percentage. A recently passed federal law has defined drunk driving as driving with a BAC of 0.08

percent or greater. All states must comply to this new standard by 2004.

body composition refers to the amount of body fat in proportion to fat-free weight.

body fat is tissue made up of billions of cells filled with varying amounts of triglyceride. If triglyceride is added to or removed from a fat cell, the cell will increase or shrink in size accordingly.

body mass index (BMI) is a ratio between weight and height. It is calculated as weight (in kg) divided by the square of height (in m). The BMI is used by many health professionals as a measure of overweight and obesity.

bulimia nervosa is an eating disorder characterized by alternating bouts of eating large quantities of food (binging), followed by purging through vomiting, use of laxatives, or fasting.

bursitis is inflammation of a bursa, a fluid-filled sac that lies between tissues and allows tendons, ligaments, muscles, and skin to glide smoothly over one another during activity.

c

caffeine is a powerful CNS stimulant. In healthy, rested people, a dose of 100 milligrams (about one cup of coffee) increases alertness, banishes drowsiness, quickens reaction time, enhances intellectual and muscular effort, increases heart and respiratory rates, and stimulates urinary output. It occurs naturally in coffee, tea, colas, cocoa, and chocolate and is added to some drugs. It is probably the most common drug used by adults and children in our society.

calorie (kcal) is a measure of food energy. One pound of body fat equals 3,500 calories.

cancer is a group of over 100 different diseases, all characterized by abnormal cell growth and replication. It has a lethal tendency to invade and destroy normal tissues and spread to other parts of the body. While cancer is the second leading cause of death in the United States, about half of cancers can be cured.

carbohydrates are the major source of energy for the body. Starches (such as potatoes, rice, and grains) and sugars are the main sources of carbohydrates in our diet.

carcinogens are substances that cause cancer, such as tobacco, UV radiation from sunlight, and certain chemicals.

cardiorespiratory endurance (CRE) is the ability to deliver essential nutrients, especially oxygen, to the working muscles of the body and to remove waste products during prolonged physical exertion. It involves efficient functioning of the heart, blood vessels, and lungs.

cardiovascular disease is a condition in which blood flow through the heart is impeded.

catecholamines are powerful, adrenalinelike chemicals pumped into the bloodstream during stressful situations. These stress chemicals are damaging to the cardiovascular system.

CD4+ or **T-cells** are lymphocytes (white blood cells) important in immune system response. They are destroyed by the AIDS virus, weakening a person's immunity to disease.

cellulite is a slang term used to describe dimpled fat found primarily on the buttocks and thighs of women. It is no different from any other body fat.

chancre is a small painless sore that appears at the site of infection within 1 to 12 weeks of infection with syphilis.

chlamydia is the most common bacterial STD, causing inflammation of the urethra. Symptoms include burning during urination, painful scrotal swelling, and pelvic inflammatory disease.

cholesterol is a fatlike waxy substance found in animal tissue. Although it plays a vital role as a structural component of cell membranes, too much cholesterol has been linked to coronary artery disease.

cocaine is a euphoriant and a CNS stimulant whose effects last from 20 minutes to several hours, depending on the drug's purity. It is a fine, opalescent, white, fluffy, odorless, and bitter-tasting drug sold for illegal, recreational use. It is the second most widely used illegal drug in the United States. Cocaine may be snorted, injected, swallowed, or smoked.

collateral circulation is a process in which new blood vessels develop to nourish the areas of the heart muscle that are starved of oxygen and other nutrients.

complementary medicine is a healing philosophy, approach, or therapy that conventional medicine does not commonly use, accept, study, understand, or make available. Complementary therapies are often used in conjunction with mainstream therapies.

complex carbohydrates are nutritionally dense foods (grains, rice, pasta, potatoes, fruits, and vegetables) that are a rich source of vitamins and minerals and provide a steady amount of energy for many hours. Complex carbohydrates are an important source of fiber.

concentric contraction occurs when a muscle shortens as it overcomes resistance. For example, the biceps muscle contracts concentrically during arm flexion in a biceps curl.

conditioning bout is the middle part of a three-segment workout. It contains vigorous aerobic exercise that stimulates the cardiorespiratory system and should follow the FITT formula.

contemplation stage is the second stage in the transtheoretical model of behavior change. In this stage, individuals have an awareness about their problem behavior and are thinking about changing it—but are not ready to do it.

contraindicated exercises are exercises indicated to be injurious to some people.

cool-down is the final segment of the three-segment workout. The purpose of the cool-down is to safely ease your body back to its resting state.

crack is crystallized, freebase cocaine sold in the form of ready-to-smoke "rocks." The rocks are nicknamed *crack* because of the crackling sound they make as they are smoked. The drug is an illegal CNS stimulant. Because crack is such a pure drug (about 90 percent pure cocaine) and approximately five times more potent than cocaine, smoking crack gives the user a far more intense and rapid euphoria than does snorting cocaine.

cramp is a sharp, painful, involuntary muscle contraction.

crank is a powerful CNS stimulant. The drug, also known as methamphetamine (a synthetic form of amphetamine), is often sniffed, inhaled, or injected. It is odorless; yellow or off-white in color; and sold in capsules, chunks, or crystals.

cross training involves developing all five health-related components of fitness.

crucifera vegetables are members of the mustard family, such as broccoli and cabbage, and contain powerful phytochemicals that help prevent certain cancers.

d

daily hassles are the events or interactions in daily life that are bothersome, annoying, or negative in some way. Examples are losing things, having too many things to do, and filling out paperwork.

daily uplifts are the counterpart to daily hassles. These are the positive events that make us feel good. Examples are payday; being visited, phoned, or sent a letter; being complimented; having fun with a friend.

delta-9-tetrahydrocannabinol (THC) is the principal psychoactive ingredient in marijuana.

depressants are drugs known as sedatives. They slow down the CNS, relax or tranquilize, and produce sleep.

diabetes mellitus is a condition characterized by the body's inability to produce insulin or to use the hormone properly.

diastolic blood pressure is the resting blood pressure and is the force of blood against the artery wall when the heart relaxes between beats. It is recorded as the lower number.

distress refers to unpleasant or harmful stress under which health and performance begin to decline.

diuretics cause the body to pass water by increasing urine output. They are used in treating edema and mild hypertension.

drug is a chemical that alters a person's physical or mental condition.

dynamic flexibility is the range of motion achieved by quickly moving a limb to its limits as in a bouncing hamstring stretch.

dysmenorrhea is painful menstruation.

e

eating disorder is a disturbance in eating behavior that jeopardizes a person's physical or psychosocial health.

eccentric contraction occurs when a muscle lengthens and contracts at the same time, gradually allowing a force to overcome muscular resistance. For example, the biceps contracts eccentrically during the lowering phase of a biceps curl.

electrolytes are chemicals, such as calcium, potassium, or sodium, dissolved in blood or cellular fluids that act as a vital messenger for many bodily processes. Electrolytes are essential for example, in maintaining heart rhythm and kidney function, dehydration and certain drugs can disrupt electrolyte balance.

emotional dimension is the dimension of wellness that deals with the ability to control or cope with the vast array of human feelings/emotions. Adjusting to life's ongoing changes is one sign of emotional wellness.

endorphins are pain-relieving chemicals produced by the brain. Some individuals report experiencing their effects during aerobic exercise.

environmental dimension is the dimension of wellness that deals with the preservation of natural resources and the protection of plant and animal wildlife, as well as the defining of your relationship with the environment. Practicing recycling shows evidence of environmental wellness.

essential fat is the body fat required for normal functioning. This fat is stored in major body organs and tissues such as the heart, muscles, intestines, the nervous system, and breasts.

estrogen is a female sex hormone.

ethyl alcohol (or ethanol) is the technical term for alcohol.

eustress refers to happy or pleasant events under which health and performance improve even as stress increases.

exercise addiction is a chronic loss of perspective of the role of exercise in a full life.

exercise tolerance test is a test of aerobic capacity in which a person exercises while heart rate and oxygen consumption are measured. A maximal effort on a treadmill or bicycle ergometer is an example. This test gives an excellent measure of overall physiological functioning.

extrinsic motivation refers to external rewards such as trophies, certificates, and recognition that often stimulate one to action toward a goal.

f

fast-twitch (FT) muscle fiber contracts quickly and strongly. It is recruited and developed mainly in short-burst anaerobic activities such as sprinting and weight training.

fat cells (adipose cells) are storage sites for energy. This type of cell shrinks and enlarges depending on the amount of excess calories (energy) in storage.

fat is the most concentrated form of food energy, providing 9 calories per gram— more than twice the energy provided by carbohydrates and proteins. Diets high in fat have been linked to coronary heart disease, some cancers, and obesity.

fat-free mass is all body tissue except fat (muscle, bones, etc.).

fat soluble vitamins are vitamins that are stored in the fatty tissues of the body. Vitamins A, D, E, and K are fat soluble.

female athlete triad is a life-threatening syndrome marked by three disorders: eating habits disordered (inadequate food energy intake to meet metabolic demands), amenorrhea, and osteoporosis. This condition may be found in extremely physically active women.

fetal alcohol effect (FAE) is a less severe manifestation of fetal alcohol syndrome and is a condition acquired by the fetus. It is caused by the mother drinking alcohol during pregnancy.

fetal alcohol syndrome (FAS) is a condition acquired by the fetus and is caused by the mother drinking alcohol during pregnancy. Alcohol irreversibly damages the developing brain. The damage can range from severe physical deformity, clumsiness, behavioral problems, and stunted growth to mental retardation.

fiber is the part of plant food that is not digested in the small intestine. It helps the movement of solid waste through the digestive tract.

fight-or-flight response (Alarm Reaction Stage) is the first stage in the Stress Response, in which the body prepares to cope with a stressor. Physiological and psychological responses appear. It is a basic survival mechanism.

FITT prescription factors should be followed to develop cardiorespiratory endurance. The factors include recommendations about frequency, intensity, time, and type of exercise.

flashbacks are recurrences of certain aspects of a person's drug use without the user having repeated the use of the drug. They are experienced by many LSD users.

flexibility refers to the movement of a joint through a full range of motion.

free radicals are singlet oxygen molecules that can produce tissue and cellular damage.

g

gamma-hydroxy butyrate (GHB) is a drug most often seen as a colorless, odorless, and tasteless liquid. GHB produces a state of dazed relaxation similar to that of alcohol. It is also known as a "date rape drug," "liquid ecstasy," "liquid X," and "gamma 10."

General Adaptation Syndrome (GAS) was described by Hans Selye and is today known as the Stress Response. It is the body's reaction or adaptation to stress and includes three stages: the fight-or-flight response, the stage of resistance, and the stage of exhaustion.

genital herpes is an STD that produces small painful genital sores or blisters that break open and crust over, causing intense itching and pain. Active herpes may also be accompanied by fever, swollen glands, and flulike feelings. Symptoms usually occur within 2 to 30 days of having sex with an infected person, last from 1 to 3 weeks, and then subside, only to recur later.

genital warts are flat or rounded bumps with a cauliflowerlike appearance resulting from a human papilloma virus infection. They are highly contagious and take 1 to 8 months to appear after exposure. They may appear on the genitals, mouth, throat, or anus.

glycogen is the storage form of carbohydrates, found in the muscles and liver.

gonorrhea is a bacterial STD that can cause inflammation in the cervix, mouth, rectum, or urinary tract. Symptoms include burning during urination, penile discharge, swollen lymph glands in the groin, abnormal vaginal discharge, and abdominal pain.

h

Hatha yoga, or physical yoga, is the most familiar form of yoga. It is a discipline that involves the use of various exercises or postures (called *asanas*) in combination with proper breathing rhythm to remove tension and inflexibility in the body.

health, in a simplistic view, is a state of not being ill. If you show no signs or symptoms of illness, you are considered healthy.

health promotion involves the systematic efforts made by organizations to help people change their lifestyles toward a state of optimal well-being. Smoking cessation workshops, stress management classes, low-fat cooking demonstrations, and bulletin boards with cholesterol information are examples of health promotion activities.

heart rate reserve is the difference between your maximal and resting heart rates.

heel spur is a bony growth found on the underside of the heel.

hemoglobin is the oxygen-carrying component of red blood cells.

hepatitis B formerly called *serum hepatitis*, is an inflammatory disease that can be spread through sexual contact and that destroys liver tissue.

heroin (sometimes called *smack, junk, H, and hard stuff*) is a psychoactive drug and an opiate. Pure heroin is a white powder with a bitter taste. It is a semisynthetic drug made by treating morphine with acetic anhydride to yield diacetylmorphine. Heroin is an illegal and highly addictive narcotic.

herpes simplex virus type I is the virus that produces cold sores. Type II produces genital herpes. Both may be spread through sexual contact.

high-density lipoprotein (HDL) is considered to be the good form of cholesterol because of its dense structure. It cleans out plaque and debris (e.g., atherosclerotic buildup) from the blood vessel walls.

homocysteine is an amino acid in the blood and a natural by-product of protein metabolism. Too much homocysteine in the blood is related to a higher risk of CHD, stroke, and peripheral vascular disease. Homocysteine levels in the blood are strongly influenced by diet and genetic factors.

hot reactors are apparently healthy individuals who are prime candidates for stress-related heart attack or stroke because of the extreme reactions they demonstrate in response to daily stress.

human immunodeficiency virus (HIV) attacks white blood cells (T-cells), weakening the immune system. It has an incubation period of up to 12 years during which a person feels fine and may have no symptoms. When enough of the immune system is destroyed, symptoms may include chronic fatigue, swollen lymph glands, weight loss, fevers or night sweats, poor appetite, and diarrhea.

human papilloma virus (HPV) is a group of viruses that may produce genital warts and genital tract cancers.

hydrogenation is a manufacturing process in which hydrogen atoms are added to unsaturated fats, making them more saturated. Manufacturers use hydrogenated oils to extend the shelf life of products. Consumption of hydrogenated oils has been shown to increase blood cholesterol levels.

hypercholesterolemia is the term for high cholesterol levels in the blood.

hypertension is high blood pressure that is acknowledged to be equal to or greater than 140/90.

hyperthermia is a life-threatening condition in which the body temperature rises to a dangerously high level.

hypertrophy is an increase in muscle size due to enlargement of existing muscle fibers. Muscles hypertrophy when exercised.

hypokinetic diseases are lifestyle diseases resulting from inadequate physical fitness. Examples are heart disease, diabetes, osteoporosis, stroke, back pain, and cancer.

hypothermia is a life-threatening condition in which the body temperature drops to a dangerously low level.

i

ice is the street name for the crystallized (and smokable) form of crank (also known as methamphetamine). It is sometimes called *crystal meth*. The drug is more addictive than crack cocaine.

iliotibial band syndrome causes tightness, burning, and pain on the side of the knee or hip. It is caused by inflammation of a long tendon that begins in the buttocks, runs down the outside of the thigh, and attaches just below the knee.

inhalants are volatile nondrug substances (often ordinary household products) that have drug-like effects when inhaled.

insoluble fiber absorbs water as it passes through the digestive tract, increasing fecal bulk. By quickening the passage of food through the system, insoluble fiber is a good deterrent to digestive disorders, including cancer.

intellectual dimension is the dimension of wellness that involves ongoing curiosity and the pursuance of knowledge. Attending lectures, reading newspapers, discussing new ideas with people, and visiting museums are a few practices that reflect intellectual wellness.

intervertebral disc is a fluid-filled cushion that separates each bony vertebra in the back.

intrinsic motivation refers to internal feelings of accomplishment that help one persist or sustain action toward a goal.

ischemia means "insufficient oxygen." It is used in reference to conditions in which cells are deprived of oxygen, resulting in pain or discomfort (heart angina, side stitch, etc.).

isokinetic muscle contraction occurs when speed of movement is controlled as force is applied through a range of motion. Cybex or Orthotron equipment employs isokinetic contraction to strengthen muscles.

isometric muscle contractions are those in which the muscle does not change length and no movement occurs. If you pushed your palms together hard, your pectoral muscles would contract and try to shorten, but your arms would not move.

isotonic muscle contractions are those in which the muscle tension or force of contraction is controlled throughout the motion, as in a bench press.

k

Karvonen equation is used to determine the target heart rate (THR) for exercise. It takes into account the current fitness level of the exerciser by using his or her resting heart rate. (Karvonen was a Finnish researcher.) The formula is THR = MAX HR − RHR × IF + RHR.

Kegel exercises strengthen the pelvic floor muscles and may prevent or cure stress incontinence. They are done by contracting the perineal muscles, which surround the bladder and vagina. The exercises are named after the physician who invented them.

ketone bodies is a toxic waste product that builds up in the body if fats are burned for energy in the absence of carbohydrates. This buildup, or *ketosis*, can result in fatigue, nausea, and nerve and brain damage.

l

LDL cholesterol receptors, primarily in the liver cells, bind and remove cholesterol from the blood.

lean-body mass (muscle mass) is specifically the *muscle* part of the fat-free body mass.

ligament is the fibrous connective tissue that binds bones together to form a joint.

liposuction is a surgical procedure in which fat is removed/suctioned from selected parts of the body.

low-density lipoprotein (LDL) is considered to be the bad form of cholesterol because it more easily

attaches to the blood vessel wall, thereby increasing the atherosclerotic process.

LSD (lysergic acid diethylamide) is a controlled substance and a dangerous and unpredictable hallucinogenic drug. This illegal drug is manufactured from lysergic acid found in ergot, a fungus that grows on rye or other grains. It is commonly referred to as *acid* on the street and is sold in many forms, including tablets, gelatin chips, and thin squares of absorbent paper soaked in liquid LSD.

lymphocytes are white blood cells that are an important part of the body's immune system.

m

macrominerals are minerals needed in large doses (more than 100 mg daily). Examples are calcium, magnesium, and potassium.

maintenance stage is the fifth and final stage in the transtheoretical model of behavior change. In this stage, individuals have been able to sustain their new behavior for over 6 months. Their habits are becoming automatic.

malignant (cancerous) cells tend to spread from their origin to other sites in the body where they continue to grow, invade, and destroy normal tissue.

marijuana is (sometimes called *pot* or *grass*) a psychoactive drug (i.e., mind-affecting) made from the leaves and flowers of the cannabis sativa plant. The principal psychoactive ingredient is delta-9-tetrahydrocannabinol (THC).

maximal heart rate (Max.HR) is the highest possible heart rate. Maximal heart rate can be estimated by subtracting age from 220 bpm.

maximal oxygen uptake (max VO$_2$) is the greatest amount of oxygen that can be used by the body during intense exercise.

MDMA, also Ecstasy, is an illegal, synthetic "designer drug" that combines the "rush" or stimulating effects of cocaine with the hallucinogenic qualities of psychedelics. It destroys the serotonin-producing neurons of the brain.

meditation is a mental exercise that elicits the body's relaxation response. The purpose of meditation is to gain control over one's attention—to internally quiet down, allowing the individual to choose what to focus upon and to block out distracting thoughts.

melanoma is a type of skin cancer that usually starts out as a dark wart or mole, has a tendency to metastasize, and may be fatal.

menarche is the start of a young female's menstrual cycle. Menarche is usually experienced between 11 and 12 years of age.

metastasis is a process by which cancer cells break away from the primary tumor and migrate to other tissues through the lymph or blood systems where they continue to grow.

methamphetamine (a.k.a. crank, ice, meth, speed) is a powerful CNS stimulant and a synthetic form of amphetamine. It is odorless; yellow or off-white in color; and sold in capsules, chunks, or crystals. It can be manufactured in the home laboratory by a "cook" with a few hundred dollars worth of equipment by extracting ephedrine, the main ingredient, from easy to obtain over-the-counter allergy, cold, and diet pills.

mindfulness meditation involves focusing on whatever a person happens to be experiencing at the time and learning to experience anything calmly, whether it is pleasant or unpleasant. This type of meditation was popularized by Dr. Jon Kabat-Zinn. Traditional meditation involves training the mind on a single point of focus, such as a word or phrase.

minerals are inorganic substances critical to many enzyme functions in the body.

moderate physical activity is activity that uses approximately 150 calories of energy per day, equivalent to walking 2 miles in 30 minutes. This produces significant health benefits, but not physical fitness.

monounsaturated fats are fatty acids that have one double bond between carbon atoms, thus reducing the number of hydrogen atoms attached. Monounsaturated fats are better for the heart than are saturated fats. Olive oil and peanut oil are monounsaturated.

muscular endurance is the ability of the muscle to exert a submaximal force repeatedly against resistance or to sustain muscular contraction.

muscular power, a function of strength and speed, is the ability to apply force rapidly. Jumping requires muscular power.

muscular strength is the ability of the muscle to exert one maximal force against resistance.

myocardial infarction is a heart attack.

n

narcolepsy is a condition involving uncontrollable attacks of deep sleep.

narcotics are powerful painkillers. The narcotic analgesics, often referred to as opioids, also produce pleasurable feelings (euphoria), induce sleep, and depress breathing. Heroin is the most rapidly acting opiate.

nitrosamines are highly carcinogenic ingredients found in tobacco products.

o

obesity is an excessive accumulation of body fat. A woman over 30 percent body fat or a man over 25 percent body fat is considered obese. Having a body mass index (BMI) of 30 or over is generally classified as obesity.

occupational dimension is the dimension of wellness that entails the ability to integrate skills, interests, and values that will heighten job satisfaction. Being able to identify a "well" work environment and balancing work time and personal leisure time are important skills in the occupational dimension.

oligomenorrhea is a menstrual abnormality that results in infrequent or irregular menses.

omega-3 is a polyunsaturated fat that is prevalent in fish. Omega-3 fatty acids inhibit atherosclerosis and can reduce blood cholesterol levels.

opportunistic diseases are produced by common bacteria, viruses, parasites, and fungi that surround but do not usually have the opportunity to infect people with healthy immune systems. If a person is infected with HIV and enough of the immune system is destroyed, he or she will be more susceptible to unusual infections such as pneumocystis carinii pneumonia, an uncommon parasitic lung infection.

optimal stress is the point at which stress is intense enough to motivate and physically prepare us to perform optimally yet not intense enough to cause the body to overreact or to sustain harmful effects.

orthotics are shoe inserts specially molded to the foot to correct foot, arch, or leg abnormalities.

osteoporosis is an age-related condition in which the formation of bone fails to keep pace with lost bone tissue. The result is brittle, porous bone susceptible to fracture.

overpronation is a condition in which the foot rolls inward excessively upon contact with the ground during walking, jogging, or running.

overuse is a condition of excessive overloading of fitness activities, resulting in nagging injuries. It often means doing too much, too soon—before the body is ready. The body and muscles must be given time to gradually adapt to new demands with *gradual* overloading.

overweight is a term that refers to an excess of body weight compared to a set standard. A body mass index (BMI) of 25–29.9 is considered overweight.

ovo-lactovegetarian is the type of vegetarian who will consume plant foods, dairy products, and eggs.

p

passive smoking occurs when nonsmokers breathe air polluted by tobacco smoke.

patellofemoral syndrome causes pain and stiffness around and under the kneecap.

pelvic inflammatory disease (PID) is an inflammation of the sexual organs that may cause fever and pain in the lower abdomen and scarring and blockage of the fallopian tubes and leave a woman unable to bear children. PID is sometimes a result of an untreated infection of chlamydia or gonorrhea.

physical dimension is the dimension of wellness that deals with the functional operation of the body. Committing to a regular exercise program, not smoking, and low-fat eating are signs of physical wellness.

physical fitness is the capacity of the heart, lungs, blood vessels, and muscles to function at optimal efficiency.

phytochemicals are "plant chemicals" that we consume when we eat vegetables, fruits, grains, legumes, garlic, soy, and green tea. Regular consumption of these natural pigments and enzymes help protect against cardiovascular disease, diabetes, and some cancers.

phytoestrogens are plant estrogens that have a similar structure to the body's hormones. Found particularly in soy products, they may help reduce the risk for some cancers.

plantar fasciitis is an inflammation of the plantar fascia—the long thick band of connective tissue on the undersurface of the foot.

plaque is an accumulation of cholesterol on the inner walls of coronary arteries.

polyunsaturated fats are fatty acids that have two double bonds between carbon atoms, thus reducing the number of hydrogen atoms attached. Corn oil, soybean oil, and safflower oil are examples.

precancerous cells exhibit potentially cancerous changes such as abnormal growth.

precontemplation stage is the first stage in the transtheoretical model of behavior change. In this stage, individuals deny any need to change or they resist change.

preparation stage is the third stage in the transtheoretical model of behavior change. In this stage individuals are intending to take action in the immediate future and are putting together a plan of action.

P.R.I.C.E. an acronym for Protect, Rest, Ice, Compress, and Elevate, is the recommended treatment for many injuries.

primary risk factors are linked directly to the development of CHD; they increase the possibility of having a heart attack more so than do the secondary risk factors. All primary risk factors are controllable.

progressive overload is the gradual increase in physical activity to stress a muscle group or body system beyond accustomed levels. Gradual adaptation occurs, resulting in improved physiological functioning. The FTI order of overload and 10 percent increase per week rules should be followed to overload correctly.

principle of specificity means that only the muscles or body systems being exercised will show beneficial change.

processes of change are the covert and overt activities and experiences that individuals engage in when they attempt to modify problem behaviors.

progressive relaxation is a series of exercises designed by physician Edmund Jacobson for his tense patients. The method emphasizes the relaxation of the voluntary skeletal muscles by contracting a muscle group and then relaxing it, progressing from one muscle group to another until the total body is relaxed. Individuals eventually learn to recognize tenseness and to consciously relax whenever needed.

pronation is the slight inward roll of the foot as it contacts the ground. It is natural for the foot to pronate slightly.

proprioceptive neuromuscular facilitation (PNF) is a type of flexibility exercise in which you perform a static stretch, contract the muscle to produce fatigue, and then relax while a partner stretches your limb.

protein builds and repairs tissue; maintains chemical balance; and regulates the formation of hormones, antibodies, and enzymes. Good sources of protein are found in both animal sources (meat, dairy) and plant sources (beans, nuts, grains).

psychedelic drugs have mind-expanding or mind-affecting capabilities and include hallucinogens such as LSD.

psychoactive drugs are mind-affecting or mind-altering chemical substances that change one's thinking, feelings, perceptions, and behaviors. Depressants, marijuana, narcotics, stimulants, psychedelics, and inhalants are classifications of psychoactive drugs.

psychoneuroimmunology is the study of the effects of emotions, behavior, and mental attitudes on the immune system and the onset/course of illness.

psychosomatic disease is a physical ailment that is mentally induced. *Psycho* refers to the mind and *somatic* refers to the body. This type of disease is frequently called a *stress disease.*

q

quackery is the promotion of a misleading and fraudulent health claim that is unproven. Most quackery products are foods, drugs, gadgets, or cosmetics that promote physical change.

r

rate of perceived exertion (RPE) is a method of measuring exercise intensity developed by Gunnar Borg. Using this method, exercisers are able to accurately sense (or perceive) their exercise intensity levels.

reframing is a way of looking at life in a positive manner. For example, seeing the glass half full is a reframing of seeing it as half empty.

relaxation response is the body's built-in defense mechanism against the harmful effects of the inappropriate elicitation of

the fight-or-flight response caused by everyday living. Dr. Herbert Benson of Harvard University discovered that, with training, the healing mechanism can be summoned at will.

repetition (rep) is the performing of an exercise one time, such as lifting a weight once.

repetition maximum (1 RM) is the heaviest weight you can lift once with correct form.

risk factors are the conditions, situations, and behaviors that increase the likelihood that an undesirable outcome (injury, illness, or death) will occur.

Rohypnol ("roofies") is a powerful sedative and is also known as the "date rape drug." It is illegal, usually seen in the form of a small white tablet that dissolves easily in liquid, becoming colorless, tasteless, and odorless.

roid rage is uncontrollable, aggressive behavior and can be a side effect of anabolic steroid use.

s

saturated fats are fatty acids that have hydrogen atoms attached to every carbon atom. Consumption of saturated fats has been shown to increase blood cholesterol levels. Coconut oil, butter, cheese, bacon, and meats are high in saturated fat.

secondary hypertension is high blood pressure caused by a specific condition, such as kidney disease, tumor of the adrenal gland, or a defect of the aorta.

secondary prevention refers to early detection of cancer, such as by knowing cancer's warning signals and performing a monthly self-exam.

secondary risk factors contribute to the development of CHD but not as directly as primary risk factors.

semivegetarian is the type of vegetarian who only excludes red meat from his or her diet.

set is a group of several repetitions of an exercise. For example, lifting a weight eight times might be one set.

set point is a fat amount or weight level that the body physiologically works to maintain. It is thought that the brain regulates a "weight thermostat" for the body's metabolism. The set point can be altered, especially by engaging in regular exercise.

sexual abstinence is a choice not to have sex.

sexually transmitted disease (STDs) is a disease spread primarily through sexual intercourse but also through other intimate behavior and sex play and, occasionally, nonsexually.

shin splint is a condition of pain along the front of the lower leg (shin). Involving the anterior tibialis muscle, the pain may range from mild discomfort to acute burning.

side stitch is pain that sometimes occurs on the side of the body just below the ribs during vigorous exercise. A variety of conditions may contribute to this spasm of the diaphragm—poor conditioning, shallow breathing, inadequate warm-up, exercising too soon after eating.

simple carbohydrates are sugars that provide energy but lack much nutritional value. Honey, corn syrup, sucrose, fructose, dextrose, and brown sugar are examples.

skinfold calipers are devices that measure skinfold thickness to determine body fat percentage.

slow-twitch (BT) muscle fibers have good endurance but low power. They are recruited mainly in endurance-type activities.

social dimension is the dimension of wellness that deals with the ability to get along with other people—regardless of race, ethnic background, or beliefs. It involves appreciating the uniqueness of others, as well as demonstrating a sensitivity to the needs of others. Regular community volunteerism demonstrates social wellness.

societal norms are those behaviors or practices expected in a culture and accepted and supported by its members. The practice of giving candy in heart-shaped boxes on Valentine's Day is an example of an American cultural norm.

soluble fiber travels through the digestive tract in a gel-like form, pacing the absorption of carbohydrates. This prevents dramatic shifts in blood sugar levels.

spiritual dimension is the dimension of wellness that involves looking within and exploring one's values and beliefs to discover a source of inner strength and serenity. It includes the ongoing search for personal meaning and purpose in life. Exhibiting honesty and having a clear sense of right and wrong are signs of spiritual wellness.

sprain is a partial or complete tear of a ligament. Both ankles and knees are vulnerable to sprains because of the sudden force or twisting motion that these joints often endure.

stage of exhaustion is the third stage of the General Adaptation Syndrome (GAS), now known as the Stress Response. During this stage, adaptation energy is exhausted and the organ system involved in the repeated stress response breaks down. Disease or malfunction of the organ system or death may occur.

stage of resistance is the second stage of the General Adaptation Syndrome (GAS), now known as the Stress Response. During this stage, the body actively resists and attempts to cope with the stressor.

static flexibility refers to the range of motion you can achieve through a slow controlled stretch, as in a sitting hamstring stretch that you hold for 15 to 30 seconds.

static stretching is the recommended method of stretching for flexibility. Each stretch is held for 15 to 30 seconds with no bouncing or jerking movements.

stimulants are chemical substances that speed up the central nervous system, resulting in increased alertness and excitability.

storage fat is the extra fat that accumulates in fat (adipose) cells around internal organs and beneath the skin surface to insulate, pad, and protect the body from trauma and extreme cold.

strain is a partial or complete tear of muscle fibers and/or a tendon. Sometimes referred to as a *pull*, a strain is often a result of a violent contraction of a muscle.

stress is the response of the body to any type of change and to any new, threatening, or exciting situation. Dr. Hans Selye, one of the foremost authorities on stress, defined stress as the "nonspecific response of the human organism to any demand made upon it." *Nonspecific* means that the body reacts the same regardless of the cause.

stress fracture is a microscopic break in a bone caused by overuse. Rather than a result of a distinct traumatic event, a stress fracture results from cumulative overload on a bone (typically the lower leg and foot) that has not been able to adjust to the repeated force.

stress incontinence is an involuntary leakage of urine when laughing, coughing, sneezing, or exercising. It is a common problem particularly in women over 30 who have given birth.

Stress Response, once known as the General Adaptation Syndrome (GAS), is the body's adaptation (reaction) to stress. Regardless of the cause, the reaction to stress is psychological and physiological.

stressors are factors causing stress. They may be pleasant or unpleasant; real or imagined; and physical, psychological, or emotional in nature.

stretch reflex is a reflex tightening of a muscle (to protect it from injury) when it is quickly stretched. For example, when you do a bouncy stretch, the muscle reflexively tightens as you reach the limits of your range of motion to prevent muscle strain.

strict vegetarian (vegan) is the type of vegetarian who consumes only plant foods.

stroke occurs when blood flow to the brain is blocked. It is primarily caused by atherosclerosis.

subcutaneous fat is fat that underlies the skin.

supination is the rolling outward of the foot upon contact with the ground.

synergistic reaction is a phenomenon that occurs when various drugs are taken in combination, so the cumulative effect is greater than the effects of the drugs when taken separately.

syphilis is a bacterial STD that has four stages. The primary stage is a chancre, the secondary may produce skin rash, fever, headache, sore throat, swollen lymph glands, flulike symptoms, and patchy hair loss.

systolic blood pressure is the pumping pressure of the heart as it pushes the blood out of the heart. It is recorded as the upper number.

t

target heart rate (THR) is the recommended heart rate range (or intensity level) for exercise. It is the range of intensity that assures adequate stimulation of the cardiorespiratory system yet is not so strenuous that symptoms of overtraining develop.

task specific activity is an exercise (or activity) using the same muscles that will be used in the conditioning bout. Warm-up and cool-down should be task specific. For example, if you jog during the conditioning bout, a period of jogging at a lower intensity should precede (warm-up) and follow (cool-down).

T-cells are a type of lymphocyte (white blood cell) destroyed by HIV.

tendinitis is the inflammation of a tendon from repeated stress.

tendons are the fibrous cords that connect muscle to bone. The most familiar tendon in the body is the Achilles tendon, which connects the calf muscle to the heel.

testosterone is a male hormone secreted by the testes.

three-segment workout is the recommended pattern for exercise workouts. It should include a warm-up, conditioning bout, and cool-down.

tolerance is the body's physical adjustment to the habitual use of a chemical.

trace minerals are minerals needed in small amounts. Examples are iron, zinc, copper, iodine, and fluoride.

training effect is the total beneficial change or physiological adaptation that results from regular aerobic exercise.

transcendental meditation (TM) is a form of meditation that originated in the eastern cultures of India and Tibet. It was exported to the western world by the Maharishi Mahesh Yogi. It involves training the mind on a single point of focus, such as a word or phrase.

trans-fatty acids (transfats) are a type of fat found in many processed foods. During the manufacturing process of hydrogenation, some fatty acid molecules become rearranged into transfats. Foods typically high in transfats include margarine, crackers, cookies, doughnuts, french fries, chips, and candy.

transtheoretical model of behavior change is a five-stage progression that one passes through on the way to making a permanent lifestyle change. The five stages are precontemplation, contemplation, preparation, action, and maintenance.

triglycerides are known as *free fatty acids* and contribute to the atherosclerotic process. They are manufactured in the body and stored as excess fats.

tumor is a lump of cells. It can be either benign or malignant.

Type A emotional behavior is described as competitive, ambitious, driven, impatient, and workaholic and demonstrates a high degree of time urgency. Type As put big demands on themselves to accomplish more and more in less and less time. These demands may lead to angry, cynical, and hostile behavior, which is a risk factor of CHD.

Type B emotional behavior is relaxed, noncompetitive, patient, and slow to anger, the opposite of Type A emotional behavior.

Type C emotional behavior is Type A emotional behavior in individuals who demonstrate stress-resistant, "hardiness" traits and who are thus not prone to the deleterious effects of stress, even though they live highly stressed lives. These traits are called the *Five Cs* (control, commitment, challenge, choices in lifestyle, and connectedness).

Type A personality is described as competitive, ambitious, driven, impatient, workaholic, and always rushed. Type As put big demands on themselves to accomplish more and more in less and less time. They have little time for or interest in hobbies or leisure pursuits and have few intimate friends. The key problem with Type A behavior is stress. Type As put themselves under constant pressure and their bodies react by producing extra amounts of stress hormones, which can be harmful.

Type B personality is the opposite of Type A personality. Type Bs are relaxed, casual, unaggressive, and patient. Most Type Bs build time in the day for absorbing activities such as exercise, hobbies, and friendship. They speak more softly, are less obsessed with success, and tend to deal more effectively with stressful situations.

Type C personality is a Type A personality who has stress-resistant, "hardiness" traits and who thus is not prone to the deleterious effects of stress, even though he or she lives a highly stressed life. Type Cs have five common traits called the *Five Cs* (control, commitment, challenge, choices in lifestyle, and connectedness).

U–Z

urethritis is an inflammation of the urethra that causes a burning sensation during urination. May be symptomatic of chlamydia or gonorrhea.

Valsalva maneuver involves holding your breath while you strain against a closed epiglottis, as in holding your breath while lifting a weight. You should avoid doing this because it can cause a dangerous elevation of blood pressure. When you lift weights, exhale on the exertion.

vigorous physical activity is exercise that follows the FITT formula and provides not only health benefits, but also increases cardiorespiratory fitness.

vitamins are the organic catalysts necessary to initiate the body's complex metabolic functions.

warm-up is the first part of the three-segment workout. It prepares the body physically and mentally for the conditioning bout.

water soluble vitamins are vitamins that remain in the body tissues for a short time. Excesses are excreted out of the body.

weight cycling (yo-yo syndrome) is the repetitive cycle of weight loss and weight gain. Off and on fad dieters typically experience weight cycling.

wellness is an integrated and dynamic level of functioning oriented toward maximizing potential, dependent on self-responsibility. It is a mindset of self-empowerment and lifelong growth in the emotional, spiritual, physical, occupational, intellectual, environmental, and social dimensions.

bibliography

1. Adams, Troy, Janet Bezner, Mary Drabbs, Robert Zambarano, and Mary Steinhardt. "Conceptualization and Measurement of the Spiritual and Psychological Dimensions of Wellness in a College Population." *Journal of American College Health* 48 (January 2000): 165–173.

2. Allison, David, et al. "Annual Deaths Attributable to Obesity in the United States." *Journal of the American Medical Association* 282 (October 27, 1999): 1530–1538.

3. American Cancer Society. *Cancer Facts and Figures—1995.* New York: American Cancer Society, 1992.

4. American Cancer Society. *Cancer Facts and Figures—2001* (American Cancer Society, 1599 Clifton Road, N.E., Atlanta, GA, 30329-4251).

5. American Cancer Society. "The Importance of Nutrition in Cancer Prevention." www.cancer.org. (May 1999).

6. American Heart Association, American Cancer Society, and American Lung Association. "Smoke-Free Class of 2000 FACTS." Dallas: 2000.

7. American Heart Association. *An Eating Plan for Healthy Americans: The New 2000 Food Guidelines.* Dallas, 2000.

8. American Heart Association. *Heart and Stroke Facts: 1995 Statistical Supplement.* Dallas, Tex.: American Heart Association National Center, 1995 (7272 Greenville Avenue, Dallas, TX 75231-4596).

9. American Institute for Cancer Research. *A Healthy Weight for Life.* Washington, D.C., 1998.

10. American Institute for Cancer Research. "AICR Introduces The New American Plate." www.aicr.org. (September 2000).

11. American Institute for Cancer Research. "A Weighty Problem." *AICR Science News* 11 (March 1999).

12. American Institute for Cancer Research. "Cancer Researchers Agree: New Colon Cancer Studies Send Wrong Message." www.aicr.org. (April 2000).

13. American Institute for Cancer Research. "Food, Nutrition and the Prevention of Cancer: A Global Perspective." www.aicr.org/report2.htm. (Sept. 1997).

14. American Institute for Cancer Research. "Growing Evidence Clarifies Numerous Cancer-Fighting Benefits of Exercise, Say Experts." www.aicr.org. (December 1999).

15. American Institute for Cancer Research. "New Survey Shows Americans Ignore Importance of Portion Size in Managing Weight." www.alcr.org Washington, D.C., March 24, 2000.

16. American Social Health Association. www.ashastd.org. (January 2000).

17. Andersen, R. E. "Exercise, an Active Lifestyle, and Obesity: Making the Exercise Prescription Work." *The Physician and Sportsmedicine* 27 (October 1999): 41–48.

18. "A New Spin on Yo-Yo Diets." *University of California, Berkeley Wellness Letter* 11 (January 1995): 1–2.

19. Ardell, Donald B. "Definition of Wellness." *Ardell Wellness Report* 37 (Winter 1995): 1.

20. Artal, Raul, M. D., and Carl Sherman. "Exercise During Pregnancy." *The Physician and Sportsmedicine* 27, no. 8 (August 1999): 51–60.

21. "Are Sports Drinks Better Than Water?" *The Physician and Sportsmedicine* 20, no. 2 (February 1991): 415.

22. Arthritis Foundation. *Osteoporosis.* Atlanta, 1997.

23. Astin, John A. "Why Patients Use Alternative Medicine: Results of a National Study." *The Journal of the American Medical Association* 279 (May 20, 1998): 1548–1553.

24. Babyak, M., et al. "Exercise Treatment for Major Depression: Maintenance of Therapeutic Benefit at 10 Months." *Psychosomatic Medicine* 62 (Sept–Oct 2000): 633–638.

25. Bairati, Isabelle. "Lifetime Occupational Physical Activity and Incidental Prostate Cancer (Canada)." *Cancer Causes and Control* 11 (September 2000): 765–771.

26. Balady, Gary J., et al. ACSM's *Guidelines for Exercise Testing and Prescription,* 6th ed. Barry A. Franklin, ed. Philadelphia, PA: Lippincott Williams & Williams, 2000.

27. Ball State University Health Education "Sexual Responsibility." www.bsu.edu/students/health_education/sexual.htm. 2000.

28. Bassett, David R., and Edward T. Howley. "Limiting Factors for Maximum Oxygen Uptake and Determinants of Endurance Performance." *Medicine & Science in Sports & Exercise* 32 (January 2000): 70.

29. Becton, Wendell W. "Daily Accumulated Exercise Improves Adult Fitness." *The Physician and Sportsmedicine* 27, no. 5 (May 1999): 27.

30. Bennett, William Ira. "Beyond Overeating." *The New England Journal of Medicine* 332 (March 9, 1995): 673–674.

31. Benson, Herbert. *The Relaxation Response.* New York: Avon Books, 1976.

32. Benson, Herbert, M.D., et al. *The Wellness Book.* Boston: Mind and Body Medical Institute, Carol Publishing Group, A Birch Land Press Book, 1992.

33. Berg, Frances M. *Afraid to Eat.* Hettinger, N.D.: Healthy Weight Journal, 1997.

34. "Bioelectrical Impedance Analysis in Body Composition Measurement: National Institutes of Health Technology Assessment Conference Statement." *American Journal of Clinical Nutrition* 64, no. 3S (September 1996): 524S–532S.

35. Bishop, George D. *Health Psychology: Integrating Mind and Body.* Boston: Allyn and Bacon, 1994.

36. Blair, S., et al. "Physical Fitness and All-Cause Mortality: A Prospective Study of Healthy Men and Women." JAMA 66, no. 17 (November 3, 1989): 2395–2401.

37. Blair, Steven N., et al. "Influences of Cardiorespiratory Fitness and Other Precursors on Cardiovascular Disease and All Cause Mortality in Men and Women." *Journal of American Medical Association* 276, no. 3 (July 17, 1996): 205–210.

38. Blanke, Daniel. "Flexibility." *Sports Medicine Secrets.* Morris B. Mellion, ed. Philadelphia: Hanley & Belfus, Inc., 1995.

39. Block, Abby, and Cynthia A. Thomson. "Position of the American Dietetic Association: Phytochemicals and Functional Foods." *Journal of the American Dietetic Association* 95 (April 1995): 493–496.

40. Blumenthal, James, et al. "Effects of Exercise Training on Older Patients with Major Depression." *Archives of Internal Medicine* 159 (October 1999): 2349–2356.

41. Borg, G. "Psychophysical Bases of Physical Exertion." *Medicine and Science in Sports and Exercise* 14 (1982): 707.

42. Bowden, Rodney, Dawn Ella Rust. "A Review of Fetal Alcohol Syndrome for Health Educators." *Journal of Health Education* 31, no. 4 (July/August 2000): 231–237.

43. Brand-Miller, Jennie, et al. *The Glucose Revolution.* New York: Marlow & Co., 1999.

44. Breast Cancer.com. "Coping: Friends & Family." breast.cancer.com (2000).

45. Breast Cancer.com. "Coping: Help Yourself Cope." breast.cancer.com (2000).

46. Breast Cancer.com. "Coping: Support Groups." breast.cancer.com (2000).

47. Brill, P. A., et al. "Muscular Strength and Physical Function." *Medicine & Science in Sports & Exercise* 32 (February 2000): 412.

48. Burgess, Donna. "Fetal Alcohol Syndrome and Fetal Alcohol Effect: Principles for Educators." *Phi Delta Kappan* 74, no. 1 (September 1993): 49–51.

49. Buschbacker, Ralph M., M.D., and R. L. Braddom, M.D., eds. *Sports Medicine and Rehabilitation: A Sports Specific Approach.* Philadelphia: Hanley and Belfus, Inc. Publishers, 1994.

50. "Businesses Promote Family Health." *The Futurist* 24 (November/December 1990): 48.

51. Butler, Lesley M., et al. "Menstrual Risk Factors and Early-Onset Breast Cancer." *Cancer Causes and Control* 11 (July 2000): 451–458.

52. Campbell, Sharon. "Six Reasons Why People Don't Buckle Up." *Safety and Health* 143 (February 1991): 78–80.

53. Canavan, L. C. *Rehab in Sports Medicine.* Upper Saddle River, N.J.: Prentice Hall, 1997.

54. *Cancer Facts and Figures—2000.* Atlanta, Ga.: American Cancer Society, 2000.

55. Carroll, Charles R. *Drugs in Modern Society,* 3d ed. Dubuque, IA: Brown & Benchmark Publishers, 1993.

56. Carstensen, Earl J. "VO2 Max Tops Total Exercise as Risk Reducer" *The Physician and Sportsmedicine* 27, no. 2 (February 1999): 16–17.

57. Caspersen, Carl J., et al. "Changes in Physical Activity Patterns in the United States, by Sex and Cross-Sectional Age." *Medicine and Science in Sports and Exercise* 32 (September 2000): 1601–1609.

58. Cecil, Heather, and Steven D. Pinkerton. "Reliability and Validity of a Self-Efficacy Instrument for Protective Sexual Behaviors." *Journal of American College Health* 47 (November 1998): 113–121.

59. Centers for Disease Control and Prevention. "AIDS Among Racial/Ethnic Minority Men Who Have Sex with Men—United States, 1989–1998." *Morbidity and Mortality Weekly Report* 49, no. 2 (January 14, 2000): 5–11.

60. Centers for Disease Control and Prevention. "Breast and Cervical Cancer." www.cdc.gov. (July 1999).

61. Centers for Disease Control and Prevention. "Combating Complacency in HIV Prevention." www.cdc.gov/nchstp/hiv_aids/pubs/facts. (June 1998).

62. Centers for Disease Control and Prevention. "Comprehensive HIV Prevention Messages for Young People." www.cdc.gov/nchstp/hiv_aids/pubs/facts/compyout.htm. (April 2000).

63. Centers for Disease Control and Prevention. "Condoms and Their Use in Preventing HIV Infection and Other STDs." www.cdc.gov/nchstp/hiv_aids/pubs/facts/condoms.htm. (September 1999).

64. Centers for Disease Control and Prevention. "Dating Violence." www.cdc.gov/ncicp/factsheets/datviol.htm. (April 2000).

65. Centers for Disease Control and Prevention. "Genital Herpes." www.cdc.gov/nchstp/dstd/Genktal_Herpes_facts.htm. (October 1997).

66. Centers for Disease Control and Prevention. "HIV and Its Transmission." www.cdc.gov/nchstp/hiv_aids/pubs/facts/transmission.htm. (July 1999).

67. Centers for Disease Control and Prevention, National Center for Health Statistics, "Health and Aging." Atlanta, GA, November 1999.

68. Centers for Disease Control and Prevention, National Center for Health Statistics, "Health Status." Atlanta, GA, September 1999.

69. Centers for Disease Control and Prevention, National Center for Health Statistics. "Nutrition Monitoring in the United States." www.cdc.gov/nchs March 2000.

70. Centers for Disease Control and Prevention, National Center for Health Statistics. "Prevalence of Overweight and Obesity Among Adults: United States, 1999." www.cdc.gov/nchs Hyattsville, MD. (December 2000).

71. Centers for Disease Control and Prevention. "Neisseria gonorrhoeae Gonorrhea." www.cdc.gov/ncidod/dastlr/gcdir/gono.html. (April, 2000).

72. Centers for Disease Control and Prevention. "Physical Activity and Health Fact Sheets: Adolescents and Young Adults." www.cdc.gov/nccdphp/sgr/adolesc.htm (November 17, 1999).

73. Centers for Disease Control and Prevention. "Prevention and Treatment of Sexually Transmitted Diseases as an HIV Prevention Strategy." www.cdc.gov/nchstp/hiv_aids/pubs/facts/hivstd.htm. (July 24, 1998).

74. Centers for Disease Control and Prevention. "Primary and Secondary Syphilis—United States, 1998." Morbidity and Mortality Weekly Report 48, no. 39 (October 8, 1999): 872–879.

75. Centers for Disease Control and Prevention. "Sexually Transmitted Diseases." www.cdc.gov/od/owh/whstd.htm. (November 1997).

76. Centers for Disease Control and Prevention. "Some Facts About Chlamydia." www.cdc.gov/nchstp/dstd/chlamydia_facts. (October 1999).

77. Centers for Disease Control and Prevention. "Some Facts About Syphilis." www.cdc.gov/nchstp/dstd/Fact_Sheets/Syphilis_Facts.htm. (October 1999).

78. Centers for Disease Control and Prevention. "STD Prevention—Syphilis Facts." www.cdc.gov/nchstp/dstd/Syphilis_Facts.htm. (January 2000).

79. Centers for Disease Control and Prevention. "Summary of Notifiable Diseases, United States 1998." Morbidity and Mortality Weekly Report 47 (December 1999): vi–xv, 20–21, 36–37, 62–65, 78–79.

80. Centers for Disease Control and Prevention. "The Burden of Chronic Diseases as Causes of Death." Atlanta, GA, 1996.

81. Centers for Disease Control and Prevention. "The Deadly Intersection Between TB and HIV." www.cdc.gov/nchstp/hiv_aids/pubs/facts/hivtb.htm. (April 2000).

82. Centers for Disease Control and Prevention. "Viral Hepatitis B—Fact Sheet." www.cdc.gov/ncidod/diseases/hepatitis/b/fact.htm. (January 2000).

83. Centers for Disease Control and Prevention. "Young People at Risk: HIV/AIDS Among America's Youth." www.dcd.gov/nchstp/hiv_aids/pubs/facts/youth.htm. (August 1999).

84. "Chewing the Fats: AHA Conference Prompts New Look at Monos, Polys, Trans." Environmental Nutrition 23 (July 2000): 1, 6.

85. "Cigarette Smoking Among Adults." Journal of American Medical Association 273, no. 5 (February 1, 1995).

86. Cinciripini, Paul, et al. "The Effects of Smoking Schedules on Cessation Outcome: Can We Improve on Common Methods of Gradual and Abrupt Nicotine Withdrawal?" Journal of Consulting and Clinical Psychology 63, no. 3 (June 1995): 388–392.

87. Colditz, G. A., et al. "Harvard Report on Cancer Prevention Volume 4: Harvard Cancer Risk Index." Cancer Causes and Control 11 (July 2000): 477–488.

88. Colditz, Graham. "Illnesses Caused by Smoking Cigarettes." Cancer Causes and Control 11 (January 2000): 93–97.

89. Collacott, Edward A., et al. "Bipolar Permanent Magnets for the Treatment of Chronic Low Back Pain." JAMA 283 (March 8, 2000): 1322–1323.

90. Costill, David L. Inside Running: Basics of Sports Physiology. Indianapolis, IN: Benchmark Press, Inc., 1986.

91. Courneya, K. S., J. R. Mackey, and L. W. Jones. "Coping with Cancer: Can Exercise Help?" The Physician and Sportsmedicine 28 no. 5 (May 2000): 49–73.

92. Critelli, Joseph W., and David M. Suire. "Obstacles to Condom Use." Journal of American College Health 46 (March 1998): 215–219.

93. Davis, J. L. "Sun and Active Patients." The Physician and Sportsmedicine 28 no. 7 (July 2000): 79–85.

94. Davis, Judi, and Kim Sherer. Applied Nutrition and Diet Therapy for Nurses, 2nd ed. Philadelphia: W. B. Saunders Co., 1994.

95. Delongis, A., et al. "Relationship of Daily Hassles, Uplifts and Major Life Events to Health Status." *Health Psychology* 1 (January 1982): 210–214.

96. Dembo, Laura, and Kathleen McCormick. "Exercise Prescription to Prevent Osteoporosis." *ACSM's Health and Fitness Journal* 4, no. 1 (January/February 2000): 32–38.

96a. DeRoin, Dee Ann. "Sexual Abstinence." www.lib.utexas.edu/uhs/AHA/sex absti.crs.html. University of Texas Health Services, 2000.

97. *Diagnostic and Statistical Manual of Mental Disorders*. 4th ed, (revised). Washington, D.C.: American Psychiatric Association, 1994.

98. Dienstfrey, Harris. "The Mind Body Connection." *Healing and the Mind with Bill Moyers*. Kalamazoo, MI: The Fetzer Institute, 1993.

99. DiFiori, John P., M.D. "Overuse Injuries in Children and Adolescents." *The Physician and Sportsmedicine* 27 (January 1999): 75–84.

100. DiNubile, N. A. "Exercise and the Bottom Line: Promoting Physical and Fiscal Fitness in the Workplace: A Commentary." *The Physician and Sportsmedicine* 27 (February 1999): 37–43.

101. Dionne, Isabelle, et al. "The Association Between Vigorous Physical Activities and Fat Deposition in Male Adolescents." *Medicine & Science in Sports & Exercise* 32 (February 2000): 392–395.

102. Dipietro, Loreta, and James Dziura. "Exercise: A Prescription to Delay the Effects of Aging." *The Physician and Sportsmedicine* 28 (October 2000): 77–78.

103. Dolezal, Brett A. "Muscle Damage and Resting Metabolic Rate After Acute Resistance Exercise With an Eccentric Overload." *Medicine & Science in Sports & Exercise* 32 (July 2000): 1202–1207.

104. DrKoop.com. "AIDS Tips for Teens."

Go.dRKoop.com/conditions/ AIDS. (November 1998.)

105. Dunn, Halbert L. "High-Level Wellness for Man and Society." *American Journal of Public Health* 49 (June 1959): 786–92.

106. Dunn, Patricia C., et al. "What Date/Acquaintance Rape Victims Tell Others: A Study of College Student Recipients of Disclosure." *Journal of American College Health* 47 (March 1999): 213–219.

107. "DWD: Driving While Drowsy." *University of California, Berkeley Wellness Letter* 11 (May 1995): 5.

108. "Education for Health: A Role for Physicians and the Efficacy of Health Education Efforts." *The Journal of the American Medical Association* 263 (April 4, 1990): 1816–1819.

109. Eisenberg, David, et al. "Trends in Alternative Medicine Use in the United States, 1990–1997." *The Journal of the American Medical Association* 280 (November 11, 1998): 1569–1575.

110. "Elderly Living Longer, Better." *Fitness Management* 13 (May 1997): 8.

111. Eliot, Robert S., M.D. *From Stress to Strength*. New York: Bantam Books, 1994.

112. *Facts About Crank. Prevention Information Series*. Bloomington, Ind.: Indiana Prevention Resource Center for Substance Abuse, Indiana University, 1990.

113. "FAX Facts." *One Man's Trash* . . . . Indiana Department of Environmental Management (Winter 1997): 3.

114. Federal Interagency Forum on Aging-Related Statistics. "Older Americans 2000: Key Indicators of Well-Being." (August 2000).

115. Fletcher, Anne M. *Eating Thin for Life*. Shelburne, VT: Chapters Publishing Ltd., 1997.

116. Flood, Danna M., et al. "Colorectal Cancer Incidence in Asian Migrants to the United States and Their Descendants." *Cancer Causes and Control* 11 (July 2000): 403–411.

117. Fontaine, Kevin R. "Physical Activity Improves Mental

Health." *The Physician and Sportsmedicine* 28 (October 2000): 83–84.

118. Fontanarosa, Phil. "Patients, Physicians, and Weight Control." *Journal of the American Medical Association* 282 (October 27, 1999): 1581–1582.

119. Foubert, John D. "The Longitudinal Effects of a Rape-Prevention Program on Fraternity Men's Attitudes, Behavioral Intent, and Behavior." *Journal of American College Health* 48 (January 2000): 158–162.

120. Fredericson, M., Marc Guillet, and Len DeBenedictis. "Quick Solutions for Iliotibial Band Syndrome." *The Physician and Sportsmedicine* 28 (February 2000): 53–68.

121. Frezza, Mario, M.D., et al. "High Blood Alcohol Levels in Women: The Role of Decreased Alcohol Dehydrogenase Activity and First-Pass Metabolism." *The New England Journal of Medicine* 322 (April 11, 1990): 95–99.

122. Friedman, M., and R. H. Rosenman. *Type A Behavior and Your Heart*. New York: Knopf, 1994.

123. Fuchs, C. S. "Alcohol Consumption and Mortality Among Women." *The New England Journal of Medicine* 332, no. 19 (May 11, 1995): 671–680.

124. Gardner, John N., et al. "Binge Drinking: From Understanding to Action." Teleconference Resource Packet. (March 16, 2000).

125. Gibbons, Boyd. "Alcohol the Legal Drug." *National Geographic* 181, no. 2 (February 1992): 291–295.

126. Gibbons, Boyd. "The Preventable Tragedy—Fetal Alcohol Syndrome." *National Geographic* 181, no. 2 (February 1992).

127. Gilkeson, Robert, M.D. "Effects of Drugs on Learning." Sixth Annual Conference of the Indiana Federation of Communities for Drug-Free Youth, Inc. Indianapolis, Ind. (October 30, 1987).

128. Glantz, S. A., et al. "Passive Smoking and Heart Disease:

Mechanisms at Risk." *Journal of American Medical Association* 273, no. 13 (April 13, 1995).

129. Go Ask Alice. "Herpes Transmission." www.goaskalice. (May 2000).

130. Golub, Catherine. "Sleep-Starved Americans: How to Keep Your Body Clock on Schedule." *Environmental Nutrition* 23 (October 2000): 1, 6.

131. Greene, Geoffrey, et al. "Stages of Change for Reducing Dietary Fat to 30% of Energy or Less." *Journal of the American Dietetic Association* 94 (October 1994): 1105–1110.

132. Gutin, B., et al. "Body Composition Measurement in 9- to 11-Year Old Children by Dual-Energy X-ray Absorptiometry, Skinfold Thickness Measurements, and Bioimpedance Analysis." *American Journal of Clinical Nutrition* 63, no. 3 (March 1996): 287–292.

133. Haberman, Shirley, et al. "Weighing in College Students' Diet and Exercise Behaviors" *Journal of American College Health* 46 (January 1998): 189–191.

134. Hass, C. J., et al. "Single Versus Multiple Sets in Long-Term Recreational Weightlifters." *Medicine & Science in Sports & Exercise* 32 (January 2000): 235.

135. Hawks, Steven. "Spiritual Health: Definition and Theory." *Wellness Perspectives: Research, Theory, and Practice* 10 (Summer 1994): 3–13.

136. *Healthy People 2010, National Health Promotion and Disease Prevention Objectives.* Washington, D.C.: U.S. Department of Health and Human Services, Public Health Service, 2000.

137. *Heart and Stroke Facts 2000.* American Heart Association. National Center (7272 Greenville Avenue, Dallas, Texas 75231-4596).

138. Hennessy, Michael, et al. "Identifying the Social Contexts of Effective Sex Refusal." *Journal*

of *American College Health* 46 (July 1997): 27–29.

139. Hendriksen, Ingrid, et al. "Effect of Commuter Cycling on Physical Performance of Male and Female Employees." *Medicine & Science in Sports & Exercise* 32 (February 2000): 5.

140. Hicks, N., J. Martin, and C. E. Webber. "Resistance Training in Older Persons." *Journal of Gerontology* 51A (1996): B425–B433.

141. Holmes, T. H., and R. H. Rahe. "The Social Readjustment Rating Scale." *Journal of Psychosomatic Research* 11 (November 1967): 213–218.

142. Hreljac, Alan, et al. "Evaluation of Lower Extremity Overuse Injury Potential in Runners." *Medicine & Science in Sports & Exercise* 32 (September 2000): 1655–1661.

143. "Improving America's Diet and Health: From Recommendation to Action." *Nutrition Today* 27 (January/February 1992): 23–36.

144. "Issues in Weight Control." *Journal of the American Dietetic Association* (supplement) 92 (January 1992): 17–22.

145. Jakicic, John, et al. "Effects of Intermittent Exercise and Use of Home Exercise Equipment on Adherence, Weight Loss, and Fitness in Overweight Women." *Journal of the American Medical Association* 282 (October 27, 1999): 1554–1560.

146. Jenkins, Andrew P. "Herbal Energizers: Speed By Any Name." *The Journal of Physical Education, Recreation and Dance* 68, no. 2 (February 1997): 39–45.

147. Jones, C. S., Carin Christensen, and Michael Young. "Weight Training Injury Trends." *The Physician and Sportsmedicine* 28 (July 2000): 61–72.

148. Juhn, Mark S. "Oral Creatine Supplementation: Separating Fact from Hype." *The Physician and Sportsmedicine* 27 (May 1999): 47–56.

149. Kabat-Zinn, Jon. *Full Catastrophe Living: Using the Wisdom of Your Body and Mind to Face Stress, Pain*

and Illness. New York: Dell Publishers, 1991.

150. Kabat-Zinn, Jon. *Wherever You Go You Are There.* New York: Hyperion Publishers, 1994.

151. Kampman, Ellen, et al. "Calcium, Vitamin D, Sunshine Exposure, Dairy Products and Colon Cancer Risk." *Cancer Causes and Control* 11 (July 2000): 459–466.

152. Kannus, Pekka. "Immobilization or Early Mobilization After an Acute Soft-Tissue Injury?" *The Physician and Sportsmedicine* 28 (March 2000): 55–62.

153. Kantor, Mark A. "Nutrition, Cholesterol, and Heart Disease, Part III: How Diet Affects Blood Cholesterol Levels." *Nutrition Forum* 6 (May/June 1989): 17–20.

154. Karvonen, M., K. Kentala, and O. Mustala. "The Effects of Training on Heart Rate: A Longitudinal Study." *Annals of Medicine and Experimental Biology* 35 (1957): 307–315.

155. Keeling, Richard P. "Medical Issues." *AIDS in the College Community: From Crisis to Management.* Teleconference. Columbus: Ohio State University (November 16, 1989).

156. Keener, E., et al. Undergraduate Student Physical Fitness Assessment, Ball State University, Muncie, Ind. (Spring 1989).

157. Kim, Daniel J., et al. "Premorbid Diet in Relation to Survival from Prostate Cancer." *Cancer Causes and Control* 11 (January 2000): 65–77.

158. Kime, Robert E. *The Informed Wellness Consumer.* Guilford, CT: The Dushkin Publishing Group, 1992.

159. King, Abby, and Diane Tribble. "The Role of Exercise in Weight Regulation in Nonathletes." *Sports Medicine* 11 (May 1991): 331–349.

160. Kligman, Evan W., et al. "Recommending Exercise to Healthy Older Adults: The Preparticipation Evaluation and Exercise Prescription" *The Physician and Sportsmedicine* 27, no. 11 (October 15, 1999): 42–61.

161. Kobasa, S. C. "The Hardy Personality: Toward a Social Psychology of Stress and Health." *Social Psychology of Health and Illness*. R. S. Sanders, and J. Suls, eds. Hillsdale, N.J.: Erlbaum, 1982.

162. Kohl, H. W., III, et al. "Changes in Physical Fitness and All-Cause Mortality; A Prospective Study of Healthy and Unhealthy Men." *Journal of American Medical Association* 273, no. 14 (April 12, 1995): 1093–1098.

163. Kriketos, Adamandia D., et al. "Effects of Aerobic Fitness on Fat Oxidation and Body Fatness." *Medicine & Science in Sports & Exercise* 32 (April 2000): 805–811.

164. Lamb, Anna. Alcohol Education, Coordinator, Ball State Health Center, Ball State University, Muncie, Ind.

165. Lanier, Cynthia, et al. "Evaluation of an Intervention to Change Attitudes Toward Date Rape." *Journal of American College Health* 46 (January 1998): 177–198.

166. Lazarus, R. *Psychological Stress and the Coping Process*. New York: McGraw-Hill, 1966.

167. Lee, I. M., C. Hsieh, and R. S. Paffenbarger. "Exercise Intensity and Longevity in Men: The Harvard Alumni Health Study." *Journal of American Medical Association* 273, no. 15 (April 19, 1995): 1179–1184.

168. Leibel, Rudolph, Michael Rosenbaum, and Jules Hirsch. "Changes in Energy Expenditure Resulting from Altered Body Weight." *The New England Journal of Medicine* 332 (March 9, 1995): 621–628.

169. Leslie, Maryann, and Richard W. St. Pierre. "Osteoporosis: Implications for Risk Reduction in the College Setting." *Journal of American College Health* 48 (September 1999): 67–71.

170. Marcus, Bess H., Bernardine Pinto, Matthew Clark, Judith DePue, Michael Goldstein, and Laurey Silverman. "Physician-Delivered Physical Activity and Nutrition Interventions." *Medicine, Exercise, Nutrition, and Health* 4 (July 1995): 325–34.

171. Marcus, Bess H., and Laurey R. Simkin. "The Transtheoretical Model: Applications to Exercise Behavior." *Medicine and Science in Sports and Exercise* 26 (1994):1400–1404.

172. Margen, Sheldon, Joyce Lashof, and Patricia Buffler, eds. *Nutrition For Optimal Health and Weight Control*. Berkeley, CA: The University of California at Berkeley, 1995.

173. Margolis, Simeon, and Lawrence Cheskin. *Weight Control*. Baltimore: The Johns Hopkins Medical Institutions, 1997.

174. McFarland, M., et al. "Olecranon and Prepatallar Bursitis." *The Physician and Sportsmedicine* 28 (March 2000): 40–52.

175. McTiernan, Anne. "Associations between Energy Balance and Body Mass Index and Risk of Breast Carcinoma in Women from Diverse Racial and Ethnic Backgrounds in the US." *Cancer* 88 (March 1, 2000): 1248–1255.

176. Miller, Mark, and Richard Rahe. "Life Changes Scaling for the 1990s." *Journal of Psychosomatic Research*. 43, no. 3 (1997): 279–392.

177. Miller, Roger W. "Athletes and Steroids: Playing a Deadly Game." *FDA Consumer*. Washington, D.C.: Department of Health and Human Services, 1986.

178. Miserandino, Marianne. "Turning Work Into Play." *Healthline* 16 (June 1997): 6–7.

179. Moradi, Tahereh, et al. "Breast Cancer Risk and Lifetime Leisure-Time and Occupational Physical Activity (Sweden)." *Cancer Causes and Control* 11 (July 2000): 523–531.

180. Moradi, Tahereh, et al. "Physical Activity and Postmenopausal Endometrial Cancer Risk (Sweden)." *Cancer Causes and Control* 11 (November 2000): 829–837.

181. Mokdad, Ali, et al. "The Continuing Epidemic of Obesity in the United States." *Journal of the American Medical Association* 284 (October 4, 2000): 1650–1651.

182. Mokdad, Ali, et al. "The Spread of the Obesity Epidemic in the United States, 1991–1998." *Journal of the American Medical Association* 282 (October 27, 1999): 1519–1522.

183. Morris, Jeremy N. "Exercise in Prevention of Coronary Heart Disease: Today's Best Buy in Public Health." *Medicine and Science in Sports and Exercise* 26, no. 7 (1994): 807.

184. Moyers, Bill D. *Healing and the Mind*. New York: Doubleday, 1993.

185. Murray, Michael T. *Encyclopedia of Nutritional Supplements*. Rocklin, CA: Prima Publishing, 1996.

186. Murray, Robert. "Drink More! Advice from a World Class Expert." *ASCM's Health and Fitness Journal* 1, no. 1 (January/February 1997): 19–23.

187. Must, Aviva, et al. "The Disease Burden Associated With Overweight and Obesity." *Journal of the American Medical Association* 282 (October 27, 1999): 1523–1529.

188. Myers, David. *The Pursuit of Happiness: Who Is Happy and Why*. New York: Morrow, 1993.

189. Myers, Jane, J. Melvin Witmer, and Thomas Sweeney. "Spirituality: The Core of Wellness." *Wellness Connections* 4 (October 1993): 1, 6–8.

190. Naisbitt, John. *Megatrends*. New York: Warner Books, 1982.

191. Nakken, Craig. *The Addictive Personality: Understanding Compulsion in Our Lives*. Center City, Minn.: Hazelton Foundation. New York: Harper and Row Publishers Inc., 1988.

192. Napolitano, Melissa, and Bess Marcus. "Breaking Barriers to Increased Physical Activity." *The Physician and Sportsmedicine* 28 (October 2000): 88, 93.

193. Nash, Joyce D. "Binge Eating: The Newest Eating Disorder." *Healthline* 16 (September 1997): 6–7.

194. National Academy of Sciences. "Summary: Weighing the Options—Criteria for Evaluating

Weight-Management Programs." *Journal of the American Dietetic Association* 96 (January 1995): 96–105.

195. National Association for Sport and Physical Education. "Shape Up America." *NASPE News* 42 (Spring/Summer 1995): 4.

196. National Institutes of Health. "Clinical Guidelines on the Identification, Evaluation, and Treatment of Overweight and Obesity." NIH Publication No. 98-4083, Washington, D.C., (September 1998).

197. National Task Force on the Prevention and Treatment of Obesity. "Weight Cycling." *Journal of the American Medical Association* 272 (October 19, 1994): 1196–1202.

198. Nesbitt, L. "Correcting Overpronation: Help for Faulty Foot Mechanics." *The Physician and Sportsmedicine* 27 (May 1999): 95–96.

199. Nesbitt, L. "How to Buy Athletic Shoes." *The Physician and Sportsmedicine* 27 (November 1999): 133–134.

200. Nichols, Jeanne, Christopher L. Sherman, and Ellen Abbott. "Treading." *ACSM's Health and Fitness Journal,* 4, no. 2 (March/April, 2000): 13–17.

201. Nicklas, Theresa, et al. "Dietary Fiber Intake of Children and Young Adults: The Bogalusa Heart Study." *Journal of the American Dietetic Association* 95 (February 1995): 209–214.

202. Nordenberg, Tamar. "Chlamydia's Quick Cure." *FDA Consumer Magazine* www.fda.gov. (July–August 1999).

203. Nottingham, Suzanne. "Working with Pain and Injury." *Fitness Management* 13 (February 1997): 26–28.

204. Nutrition Action Healthletter. "Diet & Cancer." (December 1998): 4–5.

205. O'Donnell, Michael P. "Definition of Health Promotion: Part III: Expanding the Definition." *American Journal of Health Promotion* 3 (Winter 1989): 5.

206. Olivera, S. A., et al. "The Association Between Cardiorespiratory Fitness and Prostate Cancer." *Medicine and Science in Sports and Exercise* 28 (January 1996): 97–104.

207. Ornish, Dean, M.D., "Can Lifestyle Changes Reverse Coronary Heart Disease?" *Lancet* 336 (July 1990): 129–133.

208. Ornish, Dean, M.D., *Dr. Dean Ornish's Program for Reversing Heart Disease.* New York: Random House, 1990.

209. Ornish, Dean, M.D., et al. "Lifestyle Changes Reverse Coronary Heart Disease." *Lancet* 336 (1990): 61.

210. Ottis, Carol, M.D., FACSM. "Too Slim, Amenorrheic, Fracture-Prone: The Female Athlete Triad." *ACSM's Health and Fitness Journal* 2, no. 1 (January/February 1998): 20–25.

211. Pace, Brian. "Managing Pain." *JAMA* 283 (April 5, 2000): 1778.

212. Pacy, P. J., et al. "Body Composition Measurement in Elite Heavyweight Oarswomen: A Comparison of Five Methods." *Journal of Sports Medicine and Physical Fitness* 35, no. 1 (March 1995): 67–74.

213. Pate, Russell, et al. "Physical Activity and Public Health. A Recommendation from The Centers for Disease Control and Prevention and The American College of Sports Medicine." *Journal of American Medical Association* 273, no. 5 (February 1, 1995): 402–407.

214. Pelletier, Kenneth R. *Sound Mind, Sound Body: A New Model for Lifelong Health.* New York: Simon and Schuster, 1994.

215. Petrella, Robert J. "Exercise for Older Patients with Chronic Disease" *The Physician and Sportsmedicine* 27, no. 11 (October 15, 1999): 79–101.

216. "Physiological and Health Effects of Oral Creatine Supplementation." *Medicine & Science in Sports & Exercise* 32 (March 2000): 706–717.

217. Platz, Elizabeth A., et al. "Proportion of Colon Cancer

Risk That Might be Preventable in a Cohort of Middle-Aged United States Men." *Cancer Causes and Control* 11 (July 2000): 579–588.

218. Pope, R. P., et al. "A Randomized Trial of Preexercise Stretching for Prevention of Lower-Limb Injury." *Medicine & Science in Sports & Exercise* 32 (February 2000): 271.

219. Porcari, John. "Pump Up Your Walk." *ACSM's Health and Fitness Journal* 3, no. 1 (January/February, 1999): 25–29.

220. Powers, Scott, and Edward Howley. *Exercise Physiology,* 4th ed. Dubuque, IA: McGraw-Hill, 2001.

221. Powers, Scott, K., and Edward T. Howley. *Exercise Physiology Theory and Application to Fitness and Performance,* 4th ed. St. Louis, Mo.: McGraw-Hill Publishers, 2001.

222. Pratt, Michael, et al. "Higher Direct Medical Costs Associated with Physical Inactivity." *The Physician and Sportsmedicine* 28 (October 2000): 63–69.

223. Pribut, Stephen M. "Dr. Stephen M. Pribut's Sports Pages." www.clark.net/pub/pribut. (August 2000).

224. Prince, Alice, and Amy L. Bernard. "Sexual Behaviors and Safer Sex Practices of College Students on a Commuter Campus." *Journal of American College Health* 47 (July 1998): 11–21.

225. Princeton University Health Services. "Abstinence: Making the Choice." www.princeton.edu/puhs/SECH/abstain.html. (1998/99).

226. Prochaska, James O., John C. Norcross, and Carlo C. DiClemente. *Changing For Good.* New York: William Morrow and Co., 1994.

227. Prochaska, James O., and Wayne F. Velicer. "The Transtheoretical Model of Health Behavior Change." *American Journal of Health Promotion* 12 (September/October 1997): 38–48.

228. Prochaska, James O., W. F. Velicer, J. S. Rossi, M. G. Goldstein, B. H. Marcus, W. Rakowski, C. Fiore, L. L. Harlow,

C. A. Redding, D. Rosenbloom, and S. R. Rossi. "The Stages of Change and Decisional Balance for Twelve Problem Behaviors." *Health Psychology* 13 (1994): 39–46.

229. "Protect Yourself Against Cancer: A Diet Guide Especially for Women." *Environmental Nutrition* 23 (May 2000): 1, 4.

230. Ramon, Joseph, et al. "Dietary Fat Intake and Prostate Cancer Risk: A Case-Control Study in Spain." *Cancer Causes and Control* 11 (September 2000): 679–685.

231. Rein, Micheal, M.D. "Stress and Genital Herpes Recurrences in Women: Journal of the American Medical Association." www.ama-assn.org/special/std. (January 17, 2000).

232. Rich, Brent S. "Exercise Lifts Depression for Women With CAD." *The Physician and Sportsmedicine* 27, no. 9 (September 1999): 12.

233. Robinson, Thomas N. "Reducing Children's Television Viewing to Prevent Obesity." *Journal of the American Medical Association* 282 (October 27, 1999): 1561–1567.

234. Robison, Jonathon, et al. "Redefining Success in Obesity Intervention: The New Paradigm." *Journal of the American Dietetic Association* 95 (April 1995): 422–423.

235. Roden, M., and G. Abarbanel. *How it Happens.* Santa Monica, California: Rape Treatment Center, Santa Monica Hospital Medical Center, 1987.

236. Rohan, Thomas E., et al. "Alcohol Consumption and Risk of Breast Cancer: A Cohort Study." *Cancer Causes and Control* 11 (May 2000): 239–247.

237. Ross, Michael. "Delayed-Onset Muscle Soreness: Work Out Now, Pay Later?" *The Physician and Sportsmedicine* 27 (January 1999): 107–108.

238. Rothenberger, James H., and Henry Buck, M.D. "College Health Needs to Participate in the National STD Debate." *Journal of American College Health* 47 (November 1998): 140–142.

239. Salazar-Martinez, Eduardo, et al. "Case-control Study of Diabetes, Obesity, Physical Activity and Risk of Endometrial Cancer in Mexican Women." *Cancer Causes and Control* 11 (September 2000): 707–711.

240. Sallis, James F. "A Review of Correlates of Physical Activity of Children and Adolescents." *Medicine and Science in Sports & Exercise* 32 (May 2000): 963–975.

241. Sallis, James F. "Overcoming Inactivity in Young People." *The Physician and Sportsmedicine* 28 (October 2000): 31–32.

242. Sanders, Mary. "On the Floor: Land Training + Water Training = Best Results." *ACSM's Health and Fitness Journal* 4, no. 2 (March/April, 2000): 34–36.

243. Sattler, Thomas P., and Julie E. Mullen. "Reducing Health Care Costs." *Fitness Management* 13 (May 1997): 20–21.

244. Schlaat, Richard, and Peter Shannon. *Drugs*, 3d ed. Englewood Cliffs, N.J.: Prentice Hall, 1990.

245. Schrier, I. "Stretching Before Exercise Does Not Reduce the Risk of Local Muscle Injury: A Critical Review of the Clinical and Basic Science Literature." *Clinical Journal of Sports Medicine* 9 (April 1999): 221–227.

246. Schubert, Steven R. "Lower Leg Pain: Shin Splints or Stress Fracture?" *Emergency Medicine* (August 1999): 47–50.

247. Schwellnus, M. P. "Skeletal Muscle Cramps During Exercise." *The Physician and Sportsmedicine* 27 (November 1999): 109–115.

248. Schwenk, Thomas L. "Hamstring Flexibility Decreases Overuse Injuries." *The Physician and Sportsmedicine.* 27 (August 1999): 26–27.

249. Selye, Hans. *Stress Without Distress.* New York: J. B. Lippincott, 1984.

250. Shephard, Roy J. "Physical Activity, Fitness, and Health: The Current Consensus" (American Academy of Kinesiology and Physical Education Papers). *Quest* 47, no. 3 (August 1995): 288–303.

251. Shrier, Ian, and Kav Gossal. "Myths and Truths of Stretching." *The Physician and Sportsmedicine* 28 (August 2000): 57–63.

252. Sillum, Julie, Matthew M. Clark, and Teresa K. King. "Predictors of Exercise Relapse in a College Population." *Journal of American College Health* 48 (January 2000): 175–80.

253. Simons, Stephen M., M.D. "Foot Injuries of the Recreational Athlete." *The Physician and Sportsmedicine* 27 (January 1999): 57–70.

254. Skender, Martha, et al. "Comparison of 2-Year Weight Loss Trends in Behavioral Treatments of Obesity: Diet, Exercise, and Combination Interventions." *Journal of the American Dietetic Association* 96 (April 1996): 342–346.

255. Slattery, Martha, et al. "Colon Cancer Screening, Lifestyle and Risk of Colon Cancer." *Cancer Causes and Control* 11 (July 2000): 555–563.

256. Sloan, A. W., and J. Weir. "Nomograms for Prediction of Body Density and Total Body Fat from Skinfold Measurements." *Journal of Applied Physiology* 28 (1970): 221–222.

257. Sobel, Jeffrey, and Donna Maurer, eds. *Interpreting Weight: The Social Management of Fatness and Thinness.* New York: Aldine de Gruyter, 1999.

258. Stall, S. H., et al. "Comparison of Five Body Composition Methods in Peritoneal Dialysis Patients." *American Journal of Clinical Nutrition* 64, no. 2 (August 1996): 125–30.

259. Stucky-Ropp, Renee, and Thomas M. DiLorenzo. "Determinants of Exercise in Children." *Preventive Medicine* 22 (November 1993): 880–889.

260. Su, T. P., et al. "Neuropsychiatric Effects of Anabolic Steroids in Male Normal Volunteers." *Journal of American Medical Association* 269 (1993).

261. Sulum, Julie, et al. "Predictors of Exercise Relapse in a College Population." *Journal of American College Health* 48 (January 2000): 175–180.

262. *Survey of American Dietetic Habits: 1993 Executive Summary.* Chicago: The American Dietetic Association, 1993.

263. Svedenhag, Jan, and Jan Seger. "Running on Land and in Water: Comparative Exercise Physiology." *Medicine and Science in Sports and Exercise* 24, no. 10 (1992): 1155–1169.

264. Synovitz, Linda B., and T. Jean Byrne. "Antecedents of Sexual Victimization: Factors Discriminating Victims from Nonvictims." *Journal of American College Health* 46 (January 1998): 151–156.

265. Talbot, Laura, et al. "Leisure-time Physical Activities and Their Relationship to Cardiorespiratory Fitness in Healthy Men and Women 18–95 Years Old." *Medicine & Science in Sports & Exercise* 32 (February 2000): 417.

266. "Teen Risk-Taking Behavior." *Healthline* 9 (August 1990): 9.

267. "The Effect of Ethanol on Fat Storage in Healthy Subjects." *The New England Journal of Medicine* 326, no. 15 (April 9, 1992): 671–675.

268. "The Fact Is . . .." Rockville, MD: National Clearinghouse for Alcohol and Drug Information, 1990.

268a. "The Growing Allure of Antioxidants." *Environmental Nutrition* 23 (January 2000): 1, 6.

269. Thigpen, L. Kay. "Building Strength." *Sports Medicine Secrets.* Morris B. Mellion, ed. Philadelphia: Hanley & Belfus, Inc., 1995.

270. Tijhuis, M. A., et al. "Prospective Investigation of Emotional Control and Cancer Risk in Men (The Zutphen Elderly Study) (The Netherlands)." *Cancer Causes and Control* 11 (July 2000): 589–595.

271. "Trends in Fetal Alcohol Syndrome." *Journal of American Medical Association* 273, no. 18 (May 10, 1995).

272. Trenthom-Dietz, Amy, et al. "Weight Change and Risk of Postmenopausal Breast Cancer (United States)." *Cancer Causes and Control* 11 (July 2000): 523–531.

272a. *2000 Heart and Stroke Statistical Update.* American Heart Association, National Center 1996: (7272 Greenville Avenue, Dallas, TX 75231-4596).

273. " 'Unhappy' Fat Cell Seeks Balance." *Obesity & Health* 6 (March/April 1992): 25.

274. University of California, Berkeley. *The Wellness Encyclopedia.* Boston: Houghton Mifflin Co., 1991.

275. U.S. Department of Agriculture, U.S. Department of Health and Human Services. "Nutrition and Your Health: Dietary Guidelines for Americans," 5th ed. *Home and Garden Bulletin* No. 232 (2000).

276. U.S. Department of Health and Human Services. *Healthy People 2010: Understanding and Improving Health.* Washington, D.C., January 2000.

277. U.S. Department of Health and Human Services Public Health Services. *Healthy People 2010: National Health Promotion and Disease Prevention Objectives.* D.H.H.S. Publication No. 19-50212 (2000).

278. U.S. Department of Health and Human Services. *If Your Kids Think Everybody Smokes, They Don't Know Everybody: A Parent's Guide to Smoking and Teenagers.* Washington, D.C.: U.S. Government Printing Office, 1995.

279. U.S. Department of Health and Human Services. *Physical Activity and Health: A Report of the Surgeon General.* Atlanta, GA: U.S. Department of Health and Human Services, Centers for Disease Control and Prevention, 2000.

279a. U.S. Department of Health and Human Services. *Physical Activity and Health: A Report of the Surgeon General.* Atlanta, GA: U.S. Department of Health and Human Services, Centers for Disease Control and Prevention, National Center for Chronic Disease Prevention and Health Promotion, 1999: 8.

280. U.S. Department of Health and Human Services. *The Health Consequences of Smoking: Cardiovascular Disease.* Washington, D.C.: U.S. Government Printing Office, 1983.

281. VanLoan, Marta Ph.D. "What Makes Good Bones? Factors Affecting Bone Health." ACSM's *Health and Fitness Journal* 2, no. 4 (July/August 1998): 27–34.

282. Voomps, Laura, et al. "Vegetable and Fruit Consumption and Lung Cancer Risk in the Netherlands Cohort Study on Diet and Cancer." *Cancer Causes and Control* 11 (February 2000): 101–115.

283. Watts, Carolyn, and Johnathan Watts. "An Argument for Abstinence." www.chebucto.ns.ca/Health/Teen Health/Hsex/abstain.html. (September 1996).

284. Wechsler, Henry, et al. "College Binge Drinking in the 1990s: A Continuing Problem. Results of the Harvard School of Public Health 1999 College Alcohol Study," 2000.

285. Weil, Andrew. *Dr. Andrew Weil's Self Healing 1999 Annual Edition.* Mt. Morris, IL: Thorne Communications Inc, 1999.

286. Weil, Andrew. *Dr. Andrew Weil's Self Healing 2000 Annual Edition.* Mt. Morris, IL: Thorne Communications Inc, 2000.

287. Wetzel, M. S., David Eisenberg, and Ted Kaptchuk. "Courses Involving Complementary and Alternative Medicine at U.S. Medical Schools." *The Journal of the American Medical Association* 280 (September 2, 1998): 784–787.

288. Willett, Walter, et al. "Weight, Weight Change, and Coronary Heart Disease in Women." *Journal of the American Medical Association* 273 (February 8, 1995): 461–465.

289. Williams, Janice, et al. "Anger Proneness Predicts Coronary Heart Risk." *Circulation 2000,* 101 (March 2000): 20–34.

290. Williams, Mark A. "Cardiovascular and Respiratory Anatomy and Physiology: Responses to Exercise." *Essentials of Strength Training and Conditioning.* T. R. Baechle, ed. Champaign, Ill.: Human Kinetics, 1994.

291. Williams, Melvin H. *Nutrition for Health, Fitness, and Sports,* 5th ed. Dubuque, IA: McGraw-Hill, 1999.

292. Williams, Redford. *Anger Kills.* New York: Times Books, 1993.

293. Williamson, David F. "The Prevalence of Obesity." *The New England Journal of Medicine* 341 (October 7, 1999): 1140.

294. Wiseman, Claire, et al. "Cultural Expectations of Thinness in Women: An Update." *International Journal of Eating Disorders* 11 (January 1992): 85–89.

295. Wood, Peter, et al. "The Effects on Plasma Lipoproteins of a Prudent Weight-Reducing Diet, With or Without Exercise, in Overweight Men and Women." *The New England Journal of Medicine* 325 (August 15, 1991): 461–466.

296. Woznicki, Katrina. "Soy May Help Prevent Breast Cancer." www.onhealth.com. (April 4, 2000).

297. Wu, Anna H. "Diet and Breast Carcinoma in Multiethnic Populations." *Cancer* 88 (March 1, 2000): 1239–1244.

298. Yeomans-Kinney, Anna, et al. "Alcohol Consumption and Breast Cancer Among Black and White Women in North Carolina (United States)." *Cancer Causes and Control* 11 (April 2000): 345–357.

299. Young, A., and D. A. Skelton. "Applied Physiology of Strength and Power in Old Age." *International Journal of Sports Medicine* 15 (April 1994): 149–151.

index

Flexibility Exercises

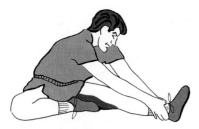

(a) Hamstring stretch

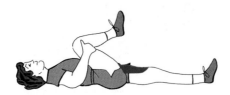

(b) Lower back/hip flexor stretch

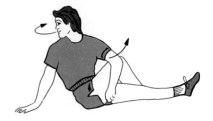

(c) Spinal twist

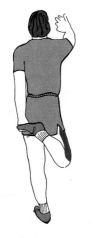

(d) Quadriceps stretch

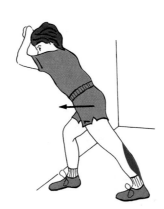

(e) Calf stretch

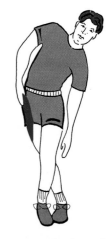

(f) Iliotibial band stretch

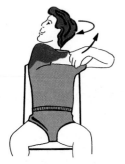

(g) Deltoid stretch

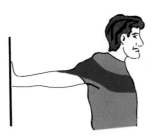

(h) Pectoral stretch

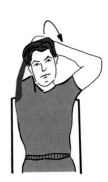

(i) Triceps stretch

Exercises for the Lower Back

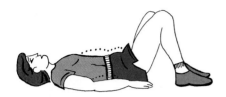

(a) Pelvic tilt
Lie on back, knees bent. Press small of back firmly down to floor by tightening the abdominal muscles. Hold for a count of 5.

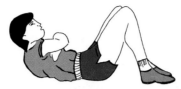

(b) Pelvic tilt with curl
Do a pelvic tilt and, while holding this position, curl head and shoulders up until shoulder blades have been lifted from the floor. Hold briefly. Lower slowly.

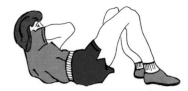

(c) Pelvic tilt with twist
Do a pelvic tilt and, while holding this position, curl head and shoulders up, twisting right shoulder toward left knee. Hold briefly. Lower slowly. Repeat other side.

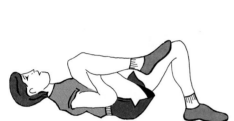

(d) Low back stretch
(a) Lie on back. Pull one knee toward chest. Hold for a count of 5. Repeat other leg.
(b) Double knee pull. Pull both knees to chest; hold for a count of 5.

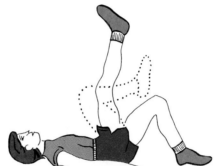

(e) Lying hamstring stretch
Lie on back. Bring knee toward chest and extend leg toward ceiling. Flex foot. (You may grasp the back of your thigh with your hands.) Hold 20 seconds. Repeat with other leg.

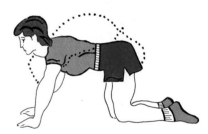

(f) Cat stretch
Start on all fours. Round the back upward like a cat. Tighten abdominals. Hold for 5 seconds. Relax and return to starting position. Do not let back sag.

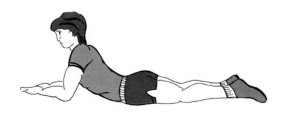

(g) Upper back lift
Lie on your stomach with forearms flat on the ground. Tighten abdominals. Lift upper body using back muscles. Do not press with arms. Hold for a count of 5.

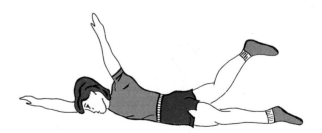

(h) Alternate arm/leg lift
Lie on your stomach with arms extended in front. Raise one arm overhead toward ceiling while simultaneously lifting the opposite leg. Hold for a count of 5. Repeat with the other arm and leg.

Free Weight Exercises

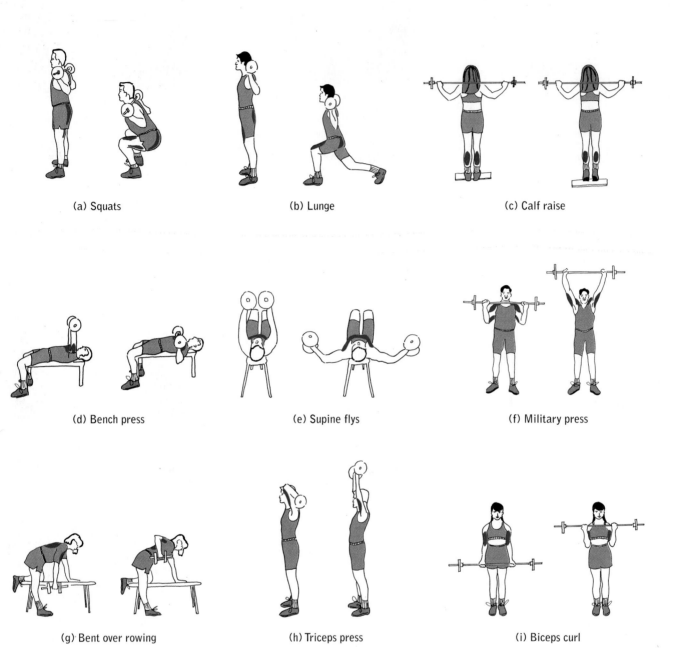

(a) Squats

(b) Lunge

(c) Calf raise

(d) Bench press

(e) Supine flys

(f) Military press

(g) Bent over rowing

(h) Triceps press

(i) Biceps curl

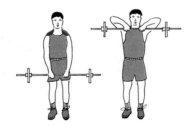

(j) Upright rowing

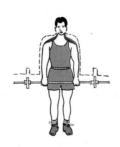

(k) Shoulder shrugs